Oxidative Stress
in Diabetic Retinopathy

Oxidative Stress in Diabetic Retinopathy

Editor

Ángel Luis Ortega

MDPI • Basel • Beijing • Wuhan • Barcelona • Belgrade • Manchester • Tokyo • Cluj • Tianjin

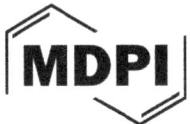

Editor
Ángel Luis Ortega
Faculty of Pharmacy,
Department of Physiology,
University of Valencia
Spain

Editorial Office
MDPI
St. Alban-Anlage 66
4052 Basel, Switzerland

This is a reprint of articles from the Special Issue published online in the open access journal *Antioxidants* (ISSN 2076-3921) (available at: https://www.mdpi.com/journal/antioxidants/special_issues/Oxidative_Diabetic_Retinopathy).

For citation purposes, cite each article independently as indicated on the article page online and as indicated below:

LastName, A.A.; LastName, B.B.; LastName, C.C. Article Title. *Journal Name* **Year**, *Volume Number*, Page Range.

ISBN 978-3-0365-0448-3 (Hbk)
ISBN 978-3-0365-0449-0 (PDF)

© 2021 by the authors. Articles in this book are Open Access and distributed under the Creative Commons Attribution (CC BY) license, which allows users to download, copy and build upon published articles, as long as the author and publisher are properly credited, which ensures maximum dissemination and a wider impact of our publications.

The book as a whole is distributed by MDPI under the terms and conditions of the Creative Commons license CC BY-NC-ND.

Contents

About the Editor vii

Ángel L. Ortega
Oxidative Stress in Diabetic Retinopathy
Reprinted from: *Antioxidants* **2021**, *10*, 50, doi:10.3390/antiox10010050 1

David J. Miller, M. Ariel Cascio and Mariana G. Rosca
Diabetic Retinopathy: The Role of Mitochondria in the Neural Retina and Microvascular Disease
Reprinted from: *Antioxidants* **2020**, *9*, 905, doi:10.3390/antiox9100905 5

Gemma Aragonès, Sheldon Rowan, Sarah G Francisco, Wenxin Yang, Jasper Weinberg, Allen Taylor and Eloy Bejarano
Glyoxalase System as a Therapeutic Target against Diabetic Retinopathy
Reprinted from: *Antioxidants* **2020**, *9*, 1062, doi:10.3390/antiox9111062 35

Mong-Heng Wang, George Hsiao and Mohamed Al-Shabrawey
Eicosanoids and Oxidative Stress in Diabetic Retinopathy
Reprinted from: *Antioxidants* **2020**, *9*, 520, doi:10.3390/antiox9060520 61

Marcella Nebbioso, Alessandro Lambiase, Marta Armentano, Giosuè Tucciarone, Vincenza Bonfiglio, Rocco Plateroti and Ludovico Alisi
The Complex Relationship between Diabetic Retinopathy and High-Mobility Group Box: A Review of Molecular Pathways and Therapeutic Strategies
Reprinted from: *Antioxidants* **2020**, *9*, 666, doi:10.3390/antiox9080666 81

Ana Karen López-Contreras, María Guadalupe Martínez-Ruiz, Cecilia Olvera-Montaño, Ricardo Raúl Robles-Rivera, Diana Esperanza Arévalo-Simental, José Alberto Castellanos-González, Abel Hernández-Chávez, Selene Guadalupe Huerta-Olvera, Ernesto German Cardona-Muñoz and Adolfo Daniel Rodríguez-Carrizalez
Importance of the Use of Oxidative Stress Biomarkers and Inflammatory Profile in Aqueous and Vitreous Humor in Diabetic Retinopathy
Reprinted from: *Antioxidants* **2020**, *9*, 891, doi:10.3390/antiox9090891 105

Beatriz Martins, Madania Amorim, Flávio Reis, António Francisco Ambrósio and Rosa Fernandes
Extracellular Vesicles and MicroRNA: Putative Role in Diagnosis and Treatment of Diabetic Retinopathy
Reprinted from: *Antioxidants* **2020**, *9*, 705, doi:10.3390/antiox9080705 141

Patricia Fernandez-Robredo, Jorge González-Zamora, Sergio Recalde, Valentina Bilbao-Malavé, Jaione Bezunartea, Maria Hernandez and Alfredo Garcia-Layana
Vitamin D Protects against Oxidative Stress and Inflammation in Human Retinal Cells
Reprinted from: *Antioxidants* **2020**, *9*, 838, doi:10.3390/antiox9090838 167

Sanghyeon Oh, Young Joo Kim, Eun Kyoung Lee, Sung Wook Park and Hyeong Gon Yu
Antioxidative Effects of Ascorbic Acid and Astaxanthin on ARPE-19 Cells in an Oxidative Stress Model
Reprinted from: *Antioxidants* **2020**, *9*, 833, doi:10.3390/antiox9090833 185

Tso-Ting Lai, Chung-May Yang and Chang-Hao Yang
Astaxanthin Protects Retinal Photoreceptor Cells against High Glucose-Induced Oxidative Stress by Induction of Antioxidant Enzymes via the PI3K/Akt/Nrf2 Pathway
Reprinted from: *Antioxidants* 2020, 9, 729, doi:10.3390/antiox9080729 201

Ying-Jung Hsu, Chao-Wen Lin, Sheng-Li Cho, Wei-Shiung Yang, Chung-May Yang and Chang-Hao Yang
Protective Effect of Fenofibrate on Oxidative Stress-Induced Apoptosis in Retinal–Choroidal Vascular Endothelial Cells: Implication for Diabetic Retinopathy Treatment
Reprinted from: *Antioxidants* 2020, 9, 712, doi:10.3390/antiox9080712 217

Manuel Saenz de Viteri, María Hernandez, Valentina Bilbao-Malavé, Patricia Fernandez-Robredo, Jorge González-Zamora, Laura Garcia-Garcia, Nahia Ispizua, Sergio Recalde and Alfredo Garcia-Layana
A Higher Proportion of Eicosapentaenoic Acid (EPA) When Combined with Docosahexaenoic Acid (DHA) in Omega-3 Dietary Supplements Provides Higher Antioxidant Effects in Human Retinal Cells
Reprinted from: *Antioxidants* 2020, 9, 828, doi:10.3390/antiox9090828 233

Young Sook Kim, Junghyun Kim, Chan-Sik Kim, Ik Soo Lee, Kyuhyung Jo, Dong Ho Jung, Yun Mi Lee and Jin Sook Kim
The Herbal Combination CPA4-1 Inhibits Changes in Retinal Capillaries and Reduction of Retinal Occludin in db/db Mice
Reprinted from: *Antioxidants* 2020, 9, 627, doi:10.3390/antiox9070627 249

Hugo Ramos, Patricia Bogdanov, Joel Sampedro, Jordi Huerta, Rafael Simó and Cristina Hernández
Beneficial Effects of Glucagon-Like Peptide-1 (GLP-1) in Diabetes-Induced Retinal Abnormalities: Involvement of Oxidative Stress
Reprinted from: *Antioxidants* 2020, 9, 846, doi:10.3390/antiox9090846 263

Sushma Vishwakarma, Rishikesh Kumar Gupta, Saumya Jakati, Mudit Tyagi, Rajeev Reddy Pappuru, Keith Reddig, Gregory Hendricks, Michael R. Volkert, Hemant Khanna, Jay Chhablani and Inderjeet Kaur
Molecular Assessment of Epiretinal Membrane: Activated Microglia, Oxidative Stress and Inflammation
Reprinted from: *Antioxidants* 2020, 9, 654, doi:10.3390/antiox9080654 275

Hossameldin Abouhish, Menaka C. Thounaojam, Ravirajsinh N. Jadeja, Diana R. Gutsaeva, Folami L. Powell, Mohamed Khriza, Pamela M. Martin and Manuela Bartoli
Inhibition of HDAC6 Attenuates Diabetes-Induced Retinal Redox Imbalance and Microangiopathy
Reprinted from: *Antioxidants* 2020, 9, 599, doi:10.3390/antiox9070599 291

About the Editor

Ángel Luis Ortega is Researcher and Associate Professor of Physiology and Pathophysiology in the Department of Physiology at the University of Valencia. He received his degrees in Biology and Biochemistry from the University of Valencia, Spain, in 1999 and 2004, respectively. Here, he also completed his Ph.D. in Biology in 2004. He has ample experience in working with animal models, microscopy, biochemistry, cell culture and cellular and molecular biology, cell isolation by flow cytometry, and the use of antisense oligonucleotides in experimental therapies. In the last few years, his research activity has focused on the effects of natural antioxidants on protection against early retinal damage caused by diabetes. He serves on the Editorial Board of *Antioxidants*.

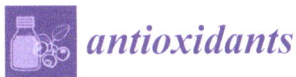

Editorial

Oxidative Stress in Diabetic Retinopathy

Ángel L. Ortega

Department of Physiology, Faculty of Pharmacy, University of Valencia, Vicente Andrés Estellés Av. s/n, 46100 Burjassot, Spain; angel.ortega@uv.es

Received: 29 December 2020; Accepted: 31 December 2020; Published: 4 January 2021

Diabetic Retinopathy (DR) is a progressive asymptomatic neuro-vascular complication of diabetes that triggers irreversible retinal damage. This common complication is the leading cause of vision loss in working-age adults (20–65 years) and, consequently, in economically active people [1–3]. Although DR is not a life-threatening illness, it leads to emotional distress and reduces daily life functionality, and thus significantly affects the individual's quality of life [1]. With the worldwide prevalence of diabetes increasing, the number of people with DR is estimated to increase from 424.9 million in 2017 to 628 million by 2045 [4]. This increase in prevalence will make DR one of the main public health burdens.

It is well known that chronic exposure to hyperglycemia induces low-grade inflammation and increases the production of reactive oxygen species with the subsequent loss of redox homeostasis. This contributes to early neuronal retinal cell death [5] and pericytes demise, followed by rupture of the blood retinal barrier, increased vascular permeability [6] and progression to advanced DR stages [6–8]. This Special Issue shows DR as a multifactorial disease with a common and complex etiology, including oxidative stress, which calls for a wide range of therapeutic approaches. Miller et al. review the current knowledge on the role of mitochondrial energetic metabolism alteration in the diabetic neural retina and its consequences on retinal function, and suggest the importance of maintaining mitochondrial integrity as a therapeutic strategy [9]. Aragonés et al. summarize the main role of advanced glycation end products (AGEs) in the progression of DR and the potential benefits of enhancing the detoxifying activity of the glyoxalase system as a therapeutic strategy against DR [10]. The harmful role and the involvement of eicosanoids derived from the oxidation of arachidonic acid by the enzymes cyclooxygenase, lipoxygenase, and cytochrome P450 in the development of DR is reviewed by Wang et al. They also propose potential targets and therapies to prevent the development of early-stage DR and progression to proliferative DR [11]. Nebbioso et al. report, as a new therapeutic target, the modulation of the high-mobility group box 1 (HMGB1), a non-histone nuclear protein involved in the inflammatory response and overexpressed under hyperglycemia, contributing to both development and progression to proliferative stages of DR [12].

Current treatments mainly target late-stage DR, when there are already serious vascular alterations and the retina shows neuronal irreparable damages [5]. An earlier diagnosis is therefore key to preventing the ongoing development of DR. López-Contreras et al. highlight the need to study classic and new biomarkers in fluid ocular matrices (tears, aqueous humor, and vitreous), and improve and optimize the sample processing and analysis methods, in order to obtain an early diagnosis and find new therapeutic targets [13]. Adding to new biomarkers and epigenetic modifications, Martins et al. review the little-known role of extracellular vesicles and miRNA in DR development and suggest the potential usefulness of miRNA in combination with anti-inflammatory and/or antioxidant drugs and nutraceutical agents in achieving a personalized therapy [14].

This Special Issue presents nine original research articles showing antioxidant strategies to protect against DR development. The first five manuscripts discuss in vitro approximations. Fernández-Robredo et al. report results showing the antioxidant and anti-inflammatory properties of vitamin D, suggesting its usefulness in moderating the chronic low-grade inflammation and oxidative stress in the development of DR [15]. Oh et al. show the antioxidant capacity of two supplements, ascorbic acid and astaxanthin, using two different oxidative models on a human retinal pigment epithelia cell line (ARPE-19) [16]. Likewise, Lai et al. study the protective pathway induced by astaxanthin against oxidative damage caused by high glucose in mouse photoreceptor cells (661W) [17]. The results show the ability of the carotenoid to activate the PI3K/AKT/Nrf2 pathway and increase the expression of the phase II enzymes NAD(P)H dehydrogenase (NQO1) and heme oxygenase-1 (HO-1), suggesting the use of astaxanthin as a nutritional supplement to prevent visual loss in DR [17]. Hsu et al. study the antioxidant and antiapoptotic properties of a peroxisome proliferator-activated receptor type α (PPAR-α) agonist, fenofibrate, on a monkey choroidal–retinal vascular endothelial cell line (RF/6A) [18]. Fenofibrate enhances thioredoxins 1 and 2 expression and suppresses apoptosis signal-regulated kinase-1 (Ask-1) activity, inhibiting subsequent apoptotic signals [18]. Saenz de Viteri et al. compare different formulations of docosahexaenoic acid and eicosapentaenoic acid supplements mixed in different proportions for the most powerful antioxidant effect on ARPE-19 [19]. Authors suggest that supplements with a higher proportion of eicosapentaenoic acid than docosahexaenoic acid may be more beneficial in preventing or delaying DR progression [19].

Another set of manuscripts presents in vitro experiments combined with in vivo. Kim et al. show the ability of CPA4-1, a herbal combination of *Cinnamomi Ramulus* and *Paeoniae Radix*, to inhibit AGE formation [20]. Moreover, CPA4-1 is able to ameliorate blood-retinal barrier leakage and retinal acellular capillary formation in a mouse model of obesity-induced type 2 diabetes (db/db mice), suggesting CPA4-1 as a potential therapeutic supplement against retinal vascular permeability observed in DR [20]. Ramos et al. examine the possibility of the use of eye drops of glucagon-like peptide-1 (GLP-1) to modulate the antioxidant response in db/db mice. This treatment increases the expression of retinal antioxidant enzymes and prevents DNA/RNA damage, showing neuroprotective activity [21]. Vishwakarma et al. explore the cellular profile and the gene expression related to oxidative stress and pro-inflammatory signaling on the fibrocellular membrane of the eye in three groups of patients: healthy, with proliferative diabetic retinopathy, and with retinal detachment. The analysis shows that oxidative stress and inflammation-associated gene expression increased in patients suffering from proliferative diabetic retinopathy and retinal detachment, providing new information for developing therapies against fibrocellular membrane formation in the late stages of DR [22]. Abouhish et al. show an increase in the expression and activity of histone deacetylase 6 (HDAC6) in human retinal endothelial cells exposed to a high concentration of glucose, in retinas of a rat model of type 1 diabetes, and in human postmortem retinal samples from diabetic patients [23]. Moreover, HDAC6 is related to retinal microvascular hyperpermeability and up-regulation of inflammatory markers, and is presented as a key mediator in hyperglycemia-induced retinal oxidative/nitrative stress in microangiopathy such as DR [23].

Funding: This research received no external funding.

Conflicts of Interest: The author declares no conflict of interest.

References

1. Simó-Servat, O.; Hernández, C.; Simó, R. Diabetic Retinopathy in the Context of Patients with Diabetes. *Ophthalmic Res.* **2019**, *62*, 211–217. [CrossRef] [PubMed]
2. Maniadakis, N.; Konstantakopoulou, E. Cost Effectiveness of Treatments for Diabetic Retinopathy: A Systematic Literature Review. *Pharmacoeconomics* **2019**, *37*, 995–1010. [CrossRef] [PubMed]
3. Ting, D.S.; Cheung, G.C.; Wong, T.Y. Diabetic retinopathy: Global prevalence, major risk factors, screening practices and public health challenges: A review. *Clin. Exp. Ophthalmol.* **2016**, *44*, 260–277. [CrossRef] [PubMed]
4. International Diabetes Federation. *IDF Diabetes Atlas*, 8th ed.; International Diabetes Federation: Brussels, Belgium, 2017.

5. Rodríguez, M.L.; Pérez, S.; Mena-Mollá, S.; Desco, M.C.; Ortega, Á.L. Oxidative Stress and Microvascular Alterations in Diabetic Retinopathy: Future Therapies. *Oxid. Med. Cell. Longev.* **2019**, *2019*. [CrossRef]
6. Semeraro, F.; Morescalchi, F.; Cancarini, A.; Russo, A.; Rezzola, S.; Costagliola, C. Diabetic retinopathy, a vascular and inflammatory disease: Therapeutic implications. *Diabetes Metab.* **2019**, *45*, 517–527. [CrossRef]
7. Ahsan, H. Diabetic retinopathy–biomolecules and multiple pathophysiology. *Diabetes Metab. Syndr.* **2015**, *9*, 51–54. [CrossRef]
8. Rangasamy, S.; McGuire, P.G.; Das, A. Diabetic retinopathy and inflammation: Novel therapeutic targets. *Middle East. Afr. J. Ophthalmol.* **2012**, *19*, 52–59. [CrossRef]
9. Miller, D.J.; Cascio, M.A.; Rosca, M.G. Diabetic Retinopathy: The Role of Mitochondria in the Neural Retina and Microvascular Disease. *Antioxidants* **2020**, *9*, 905. [CrossRef]
10. Aragonès, G.; Rowan, S.; G Francisco, S.; Yang, W.; Weinberg, J.; Taylor, A.; Bejarano, E. Glyoxalase System as a Therapeutic Target against Diabetic Retinopathy. *Antioxidants* **2020**, *9*, 1062. [CrossRef]
11. Wang, M.H.; Hsiao, G.; Al-Shabrawey, M. Eicosanoids and Oxidative Stress in Diabetic Retinopathy. *Antioxidants* **2020**, *9*, 520. [CrossRef]
12. Nebbioso, M.; Lambiase, A.; Armentano, M.; Tucciarone, G.; Bonfiglio, V.; Plateroti, R.; Alisi, L. The Complex Relationship between Diabetic Retinopathy and High-Mobility Group Box: A Review of Molecular Pathways and Therapeutic Strategies. *Antioxidants* **2020**, *9*, 666. [CrossRef] [PubMed]
13. López-Contreras, A.K.; Martínez-Ruiz, M.G.; Olvera-Montaño, C.; Robles-Rivera, R.R.; Arévalo-Simental, D.E.; Castellanos-González, J.A.; Hernández-Chávez, A.; Huerta-Olvera, S.G.; Cardona-Muñoz, E.G.; Rodríguez-Carrizalez, A.D. Importance of the Use of Oxidative Stress Biomarkers and Inflammatory Profile in Aqueous and Vitreous Humor in Diabetic Retinopathy. *Antioxidants* **2020**, *9*, 891. [CrossRef] [PubMed]
14. Martins, B.; Amorim, M.; Reis, F.; Ambrósio, A.F.; Fernandes, R. Extracellular Vesicles and MicroRNA: Putative Role in Diagnosis and Treatment of Diabetic Retinopathy. *Antioxidants* **2020**, *9*, 705. [CrossRef] [PubMed]
15. Fernandez-Robredo, P.; González-Zamora, J.; Recalde, S.; Bilbao-Malavé, V.; Bezunartea, J.; Hernandez, M.; Garcia-Layana, A. Vitamin D Protects against Oxidative Stress and Inflammation in Human Retinal Cells. *Antioxidants* **2020**, *9*, 838. [CrossRef] [PubMed]
16. Oh, S.; Kim, Y.J.; Lee, E.K.; Park, S.W.; Yu, H.G. Antioxidative Effects of Ascorbic Acid and Astaxanthin on ARPE-19 Cells in an Oxidative Stress Model. *Antioxidants* **2020**, *9*, 833. [CrossRef]
17. Lai, T.T.; Yang, C.M.; Yang, C.H. Astaxanthin Protects Retinal Photoreceptor Cells against High Glucose-Induced Oxidative Stress by Induction of Antioxidant Enzymes via the PI3K/Akt/Nrf2 Pathway. *Antioxidants* **2020**, *9*, 729. [CrossRef]
18. Hsu, Y.J.; Lin, C.W.; Cho, S.L.; Yang, W.S.; Yang, C.M.; Yang, C.H. Protective Effect of Fenofibrate on Oxidative Stress-Induced Apoptosis in Retinal-Choroidal Vascular Endothelial Cells: Implication for Diabetic Retinopathy Treatment. *Antioxidants* **2020**, *9*, 712. [CrossRef]
19. Saenz de Viteri, M.; Hernandez, M.; Bilbao-Malavé, V.; Fernandez-Robredo, P.; González-Zamora, J.; Garcia-Garcia, L.; Ispizua, N.; Recalde, S.; Garcia-Layana, A. A Higher Proportion of Eicosapentaenoic Acid (EPA) When Combined with Docosahexaenoic Acid (DHA) in Omega-3 Dietary Supplements Provides Higher Antioxidant Effects in Human Retinal Cells. *Antioxidants* **2020**, *9*, 828. [CrossRef]
20. Kim, Y.S.; Kim, J.; Kim, C.S.; Lee, I.S.; Jo, K.; Jung, D.H.; Lee, Y.M.; Kim, J.S. The Herbal Combination CPA4-1 Inhibits Changes in Retinal Capillaries and Reduction of Retinal Occludin in db/db Mice. *Antioxidants* **2020**, *9*, 627. [CrossRef]
21. Ramos, H.; Bogdanov, P.; Sampedro, J.; Huerta, J.; Simó, R.; Hernández, C. Beneficial Effects of Glucagon-Like Peptide-1 (GLP-1) in Diabetes-Induced Retinal Abnormalities: Involvement of Oxidative Stress. *Antioxidants* **2020**, *9*, 846. [CrossRef]
22. Vishwakarma, S.; Gupta, R.K.; Jakati, S.; Tyagi, M.; Pappuru, R.R.; Reddig, K.; Hendricks, G.; Volkert, M.R.; Khanna, H.; Chhablani, J.; et al. Molecular Assessment of Epiretinal Membrane: Activated Microglia, Oxidative Stress and Inflammation. *Antioxidants* **2020**, *9*, 654. [CrossRef] [PubMed]
23. Abouhish, H.; Thounaojam, M.C.; Jadeja, R.N.; Gutsaeva, D.R.; Powell, F.L.; Khriza, M.; Martin, P.M.; Bartoli, M. Inhibition of HDAC6 Attenuates Diabetes-Induced Retinal Redox Imbalance and Microangiopathy. *Antioxidants* **2020**, *9*, 599. [CrossRef] [PubMed]

Publisher's Note: MDPI stays neutral with regard to jurisdictional claims in published maps and institutional affiliations.

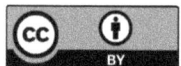

© 2021 by the author. Licensee MDPI, Basel, Switzerland. This article is an open access article distributed under the terms and conditions of the Creative Commons Attribution (CC BY) license (http://creativecommons.org/licenses/by/4.0/).

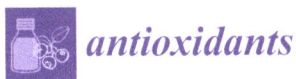

Review

Diabetic Retinopathy: The Role of Mitochondria in the Neural Retina and Microvascular Disease

David J. Miller, M. Ariel Cascio and Mariana G. Rosca *

Department of Foundational Sciences, Central Michigan University College of Medicine, Mount Pleasant, MI 48858, USA; mille15d@cmich.edu (D.J.M.); ariel.cascio@cmich.edu (M.A.C.)
* Correspondence: rosca1g@cmich.edu; Tel.: +1-989-774-6556

Received: 19 August 2020; Accepted: 18 September 2020; Published: 23 September 2020

Abstract: Diabetic retinopathy (DR), a common chronic complication of diabetes mellitus and the leading cause of vision loss in the working-age population, is clinically defined as a microvascular disease that involves damage of the retinal capillaries with secondary visual impairment. While its clinical diagnosis is based on vascular pathology, DR is associated with early abnormalities in the electroretinogram, indicating alterations of the neural retina and impaired visual signaling. The pathogenesis of DR is complex and likely involves the simultaneous dysregulation of multiple metabolic and signaling pathways through the retinal neurovascular unit. There is evidence that microvascular disease in DR is caused in part by altered energetic metabolism in the neural retina and specifically from signals originating in the photoreceptors. In this review, we discuss the main pathogenic mechanisms that link alterations in neural retina bioenergetics with vascular regression in DR. We focus specifically on the recent developments related to alterations in mitochondrial metabolism including energetic substrate selection, mitochondrial function, oxidation-reduction (redox) imbalance, and oxidative stress, and critically discuss the mechanisms of these changes and their consequences on retinal function. We also acknowledge implications for emerging therapeutic approaches and future research directions to find novel mitochondria-targeted therapeutic strategies to correct bioenergetics in diabetes. We conclude that retinal bioenergetics is affected in the early stages of diabetes with consequences beyond changes in ATP content, and that maintaining mitochondrial integrity may alleviate retinal disease.

Keywords: diabetic retinopathy; mitochondria; oxidative stress; redox; photoreceptor

1. Introduction

Diabetes mellitus is a growing public health problem, reaching pandemic proportions in the United States and worldwide [1]. Diabetic retinopathy (DR) is the leading cause of irreversible visual impairment and blindness in the working-age population [2]. The Diabetes Control and Complications Trial concluded that tight metabolic control can delay the development and slow the progression of DR. However, good metabolic control is often difficult to achieve and does not guarantee complete protection against DR, suggesting that there are additional contributing factors that remain to be discovered [3,4]. While targeted therapies are effective in mitigating the sight-threatening complications of proliferative diabetic retinopathy (PDR) [5], new therapeutic approaches are needed to manage the milder non-proliferative disease. Thus, there is an urgent need to better understand the early stages of DR in order to develop new strategies to halt its progression.

DR is clinically defined as a microvascular disease [6], and can be broadly classified into two distinct stages on the basis of the presence of neovascularization. While non-proliferative diabetic retinopathy (NPDR) is characterized by blood flow alterations, pericyte loss, downregulation of endothelial cell tight junctions [7], and thickening of the basement membrane [8], PDR presents with sight-threatening neovascularization that may precipitate retinal detachment and blindness. Recent work has shown that retinal neurodegeneration precedes clinically detectable microvascular damage [9–13]. Since Wolter's first observation of neuronal cell death in the diabetic retina [14], numerous studies have described early neuronal apoptosis and alterations in visual signaling. Retinal ganglion cells (RGCs) of the optic nerve undergo apoptosis at a rate higher than any other retinal cell [15]. These changes are associated with a subjective decline in the quality of vision including impaired contrast sensitivity and color vision [16–18], and altered visual signaling as assessed by the electroretinogram (ERG). In addition to changes in the a- and b-waves on the ERG, alterations in the amplitude of the oscillatory potential (photopic and scotopic oscillatory potentials, which are initiated in the inner retina [19]) have been suggested to predict the progression of DR [20,21].

In light of these findings, new discoveries into retinal physiology have emphasized the role of the neurovascular unit in DR [6], which refers to the physical and biochemical interaction between neurons (RGCs, amacrine cells, bipolar cells, and horizontal cells), glia (Müller cells and astrocytes), and the microvascular network (endothelial cells and pericytes) [22,23]. The key role of this interaction in neurodevelopment [24] and normal neurovascular signaling [25] has led to the hypothesis that DR may result from the uncoupling of the neurovascular unit [26,27]. Nevertheless, the effect and timing of cellular dysfunction throughout the neurovascular unit in DR has yet to be determined.

One of the classical and prevailing theories explaining the pathogenesis of DR is that diabetes enhances oxidative stress, which in turn damages the retinal microvasculature [28]. The term oxidative stress refers to an imbalance between reactive oxygen species (ROS) production and antioxidant defenses. Because of their role in oxidative metabolism, mitochondria are key sources of increased ROS in diabetes [29–31]. Oxidative stress originating in mitochondria of endothelial cells has been reported to enhance multiple seemingly independent pathways, each contributing to the development of microvascular complications [32,33]. Most current knowledge is derived from this "unifying theory" that was developed on cultured aortic endothelial cells and has since been extrapolated to the retinal microvasculature. However, recent work by Du et al. [34] determined that diabetes-induced oxidative stress originates from the photoreceptors rather than endothelial cells. In this model, photoreceptor-induced oxidative stress was associated with increased inflammation, which is widely regarded as an important pathogenic mechanism of DR, and contributes to vascular regression in the diabetic retina [35]. The critical role of the neural retina in the development of microvascular disease is further supported by studies of patients with retinitis pigmentosa who exhibit both photoreceptor degeneration and protection against DR [36,37].

While performing the core metabolic function of energy production, mitochondria are critical gears in a currently expanding number of cellular functions including redox homeostasis [38] and programmed cell death [39]. An increased mitochondrial oxidative stress reveals a change in mitochondrial function. The importance of understanding the role of bioenergetics in the diabetic neural retina is supported by the knowledge that inherited mitochondrial diseases cause retinal disease and visual impairment [40], and is further highlighted by the heterogeneity of the neural retinal cells regarding the contribution of their mitochondria to cellular ATP and oxidative stress [41,42]. This review will summarize the recent developments related to alterations in mitochondrial bioenergetics in the neural retina, as well as the consequences of these alterations on retinal function. We will conclude by acknowledging emerging therapeutic approaches to correct mitochondrial bioenergetic-related functions and maintain the mitochondrial integrity in diabetes.

2. Normal Retinal Structure

The retina is a highly organized tissue consisting of at least 10 distinct layers, which can be broadly divided into an inner and outer retina (Figure 1).

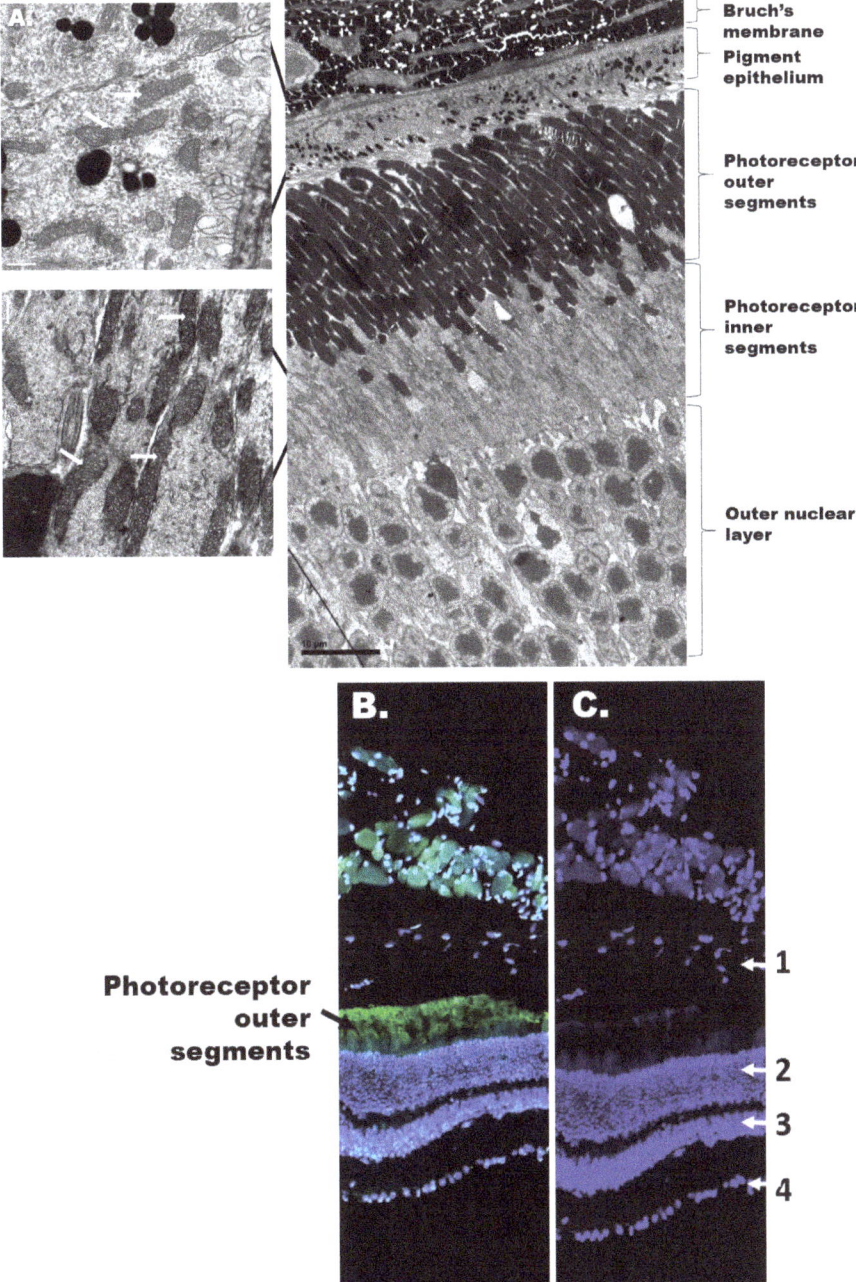

Figure 1. The structure of the retina. (**A**) Electron microscopy images of the mouse outer retina. Mitochondria are shown in the figure inset and are indicated by white arrows. (**B**) Confocal image of the mouse retina depicting rhodopsin (green) and cell nuclei (blue). (**C**) Distribution of cell nuclei (blue) in the mouse retina. The numbers represent the retinal layers: 1—retinal pigment epithelium (RPE, detached); 2—outer nuclear layer; 3—inner nuclear layer; 4—ganglion cell layer. Rhodopsin (green fluorescence) is present in stacks of membranous disks of the photoreceptor outer segments (OS). 4′,6-diamidino-2-phenylindole (DAPI, blue) stains the nuclei in all nuclear layers and the RPE.

The inner retina includes the RGCs as well as two nuclear layers with the photoreceptor soma. Photoreceptors are the light-sensitive cells responsible for phototransduction and present as either rods and cones expressing the visual pigments rhodopsin and opsin, respectively. The outer retina includes the photoreceptor outer segments (OSs) and the underlying retinal pigment epithelium (RPE). The RPE rests on Bruch's membrane, a multi-layered structure that separates the outer retina from the choroid choriocapillaris. The inner retina receives blood from three local vascular plexuses, while photoreceptors are primarily supplied by the choriocapillaris. Therefore, although the photoreceptors are physically distant from the inner retina where DR manifests as a microvascular disease, both structures contribute to the pathophysiology of DR but their cooperative signals are yet to be identified.

3. Pathophysiology of DR

The pathogenesis of the early stages of DR remains poorly understood. Pericyte death has been considered the central mechanism for the loss of retinal vascular integrity in diabetes [43]. However, the seminal work of Mizutani et al. [44] revealed early and accelerated death of both retinal pericyte and endothelial cells in diabetic rodents and humans. While endothelial cells are replaced by proliferation, migration, or neighbor cell redeployment, pericytes do not regenerate, and their absence is evidenced by the presence of "pericyte ghosts" in the capillary wall. Dynamic high resolution microscopy determined that the decrease in blood flow favors the process of vasoregression [45,46]. As an indisputable event in the diabetic retina, pericyte loss has been observed in all rodent models of both type 1 (T1D) and type 2 (T2D) diabetes [47–49]. Moreover, genetic pericyte elimination recapitulates the early features of experimental DR, including acellular capillaries, microaneurysms, and blood–retinal barrier abnormalities, all of which underline the seminal role of pericytes to maintain retinal capillary integrity [50]. While pericytes likely play a similar role in humans [51], progress in this area is limited by the scarcity of human retinal tissue and the inherent difficulties of translational research [52].

Previous studies have focused primarily on the retinal microvasculature. However, a recent growing body of literature indicates that diabetes causes cellular dysfunction and loss of virtually all retinal cell populations [13,53–58], as measured qualitatively by ERG and quantitatively by optical coherence tomography, revealing a decrease in retinal thickness [10,59]. Diabetes-induced alterations of neuronal cells and photoreceptors are particularly important as the death of these cells is not matched by similar rates of regeneration [60]. Due to the large surface area of outer segments (OS), photoreceptors are highly sensitive to incident photons and have a high capacity for ion exchange that must be supported by ATP. Abnormalities in photoreceptors have been reported in multiple models of insulin-dependent diabetes in both rodents [61,62] and rabbits [63]. Similar observations have been reported in zebrafish exposed to hyperglycemia [64]. In diabetic patients, photoreceptor integrity is altered and the OS length shortened, changes that have been associated with decreased visual acuity [65–67]. While altered photoreceptor morphology appears modest at 3–6 months of hyperglycemia [62,68], the functional abnormalities are more severe and include impaired function of the Na^+/K^+ ATPase pump [69,70]. In photoreceptors, the Na^+/K^+ ATPase pump is critical not only for normal ion homeostasis, but also for the "dark current", a physiologic event that can be assessed by the a-wave on the ERG. Subsequent studies have expanded upon this work and observed changes in the amplitude and latency of the a-wave as early events in streptozotocin (STZ)-induced diabetes [71]. Similar abnormalities in the ERG have also been noted in diabetic patients, and suggested to precede and predict the microvascular histopathology [72]. These findings are consistent with the hypothesis that early visual dysfunction precedes morphologic neurodegeneration and vascular regression in DR (Figure 2).

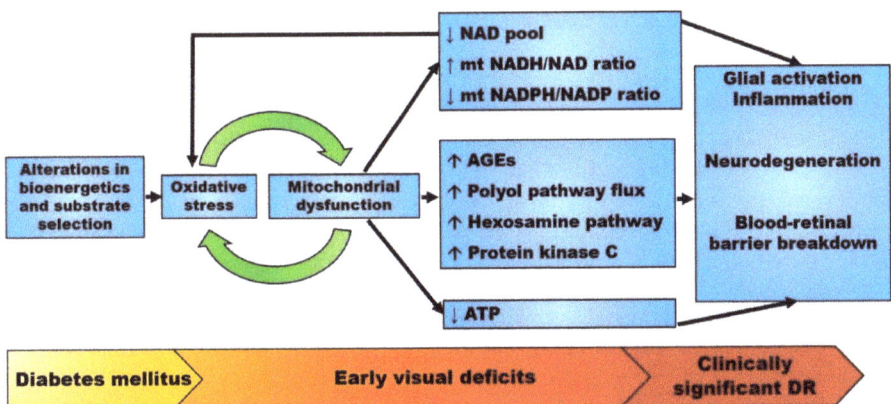

Figure 2. Proposed pathophysiology of diabetic retinopathy (DR). The early stages of diabetes mellitus are characterized by alterations in bioenergetics and substrate selection in a variety of cell types. In the retina, these changes cause oxidative stress and are associated with early visual deficits such as impaired contrast sensitivity. Mitochondrial oxidative stress alters mitochondrial metabolism and upregulates multiple seemingly independent pathways leading to retinal disease. Mitochondrial dysfunction also changes the redox state that further enhances oxidative stress. Therefore, mitochondrial-generated oxidative stress may precede overt neurodegeneration and microvascular disease. Abbreviations: AGEs, advanced glycation end products; DR, diabetic retinopathy; mt, mitochondrial. ↑: increased; ↓: decreased.

4. Retinal Bioenergetics and Mitochondrial Substrate Selection

4.1. ATP-Consuming Processes in the Retina

While all retinal cells rely on ATP as a fuel source, the photoreceptors are the largest consumers. Photoreceptors use more than 75% of oxygen of the retina and contain more than 75% of retinal mitochondria to produce large amounts of ATP by oxidative phosphorylation (Oxphos), which is necessary for phototransduction [73]. Phototransduction, the process by which photons are converted into electrical signals in photoreceptors, relies on the cycling of 11-*cis* retinal, a vitamin A derivative bound to an opsin G-protein-coupled receptor (GPCR). In the presence of light, 11-*cis* retinal is isomerized to all-*trans* retinal. This photoisomerization results in a conformational change of the opsin GPCR, leading to a signaling cascade that causes the closure of sodium ion channels, hyperpolarization of the cell, and decreased glutamate release with depolarization of bipolar cells initiating phototransduction. In the dark, 11-*cis* retinal holds the opsin GPCR in an inactive conformation allowing the entry of sodium ions with glutamate release, thus inhibiting bipolar cells. This latter process is referred to as the "dark current", a high ATP consuming process needed to maintain a steady influx of sodium ions and keep a constant membrane potential.

In order to provide a constant supply of 11-*cis* retinal, all-*trans* retinal must be converted back to 11-*cis* retinal through a series of redox reactions collectively referred to as the visual cycle [74]. The visual cycle involves proteolysis of the visual pigment (opsin or rhodopsin) and release of all-*trans* retinal into the RPE, where it is converted to 11-*cis* retinal. The rate of 11-*cis* retinal regeneration is determined by the availability of ATP and nicotinamide adenine dinucleotide phosphate (NADPH) [75], further supporting the proposition that the visual cycle is highly dependent on bioenergetic support. Photoreceptors undergo daily shedding, losing approximately 10% of their OS to phagocytosis by the RPE [76]. Continuous shedding of "used" OS discs and replacement with newly assembled discs, a critical process to maintain normal photoreceptor function, also consumes a large amount of ATP and NADPH. Photoreceptors are supported by adjacent Müller cells [77]; studies have shown that disruption of Müller cell metabolism results in impaired assembly of nascent photoreceptor OS [78].

Thus, the retina is a highly active tissue and requires a remarkable amount of oxygen and ATP to sustain its normal functions.

4.2. ATP-Generating Processes in the Retina and the Heterogeneity of Retinal Bioenergetics

The major sources of ATP in the retina are extramitochondrial glycolysis and mitochondrial Oxphos (Figure 3). In the 1920s, Warburg and Krebs reported that the mammalian retina, as a whole, has a metabolism largely based on aerobic glycolysis, converting 80–96% of glucose to lactic acid [79]. However, more recent research has demonstrated that the distribution of glycolysis and oxidative metabolism varies throughout the retina [80]. While neurotransmission in the inner retina is supported almost entirely by glycolysis, phototransduction in the outer retina is supported by mitochondrial Oxphos [80]. Mitochondrial Oxphos occurs in the inner mitochondrial membrane in which invaginations called cristae greatly increase the surface area for electron transport and ATP production. The electron transport chain (ETC) consists of four complexes (I-IV) that oxidize nicotinamide adenine dinucleotide (NADH) and flavin adenine dinucleotide ($FADH_2$) to NAD^+ and FAD^+, respectively. Through a series of redox reactions, the ETC transfers electrons towards molecular oxygen and H^+ into the intermembrane space. This process creates a transmembrane electrochemical gradient, which is used by ATP synthase (complex V) for the phosphorylation of adenosine diphosphate (ADP) to ATP. In addition to the ETC complexes, mitochondrial Oxphos also relies on ubiquinone (coenzyme Q) and cytochrome c (cyt c), two mobile electron carriers that shuttle electrons between ETC complexes [81].

A comprehensive investigation into oxidative metabolism revealed that retinal mitochondrial Oxphos operates in basal conditions at maximal capacity without a significant reserve capacity [82], suggesting that mitochondrial defects have a significant impact on retinal energy homeostasis. In most tissues, Oxphos is a tightly coupled process in which substrate oxidation is paired by ATP synthesis [81]. In the retina, mitochondria are reportedly less coupled, allowing proton leakage through the inner membrane without ATP synthesis [82]. Weak coupling between electron transport and ATP synthesis suggests that mitochondrial oxidative metabolism in the retina supports other functions in addition to ATP production, such as maintaining the $NADH/NAD^+$ and $FADH_2/FAD^+$ redox ratios. This concept is one of the core focus of our review, and will be further detailed in the following sections.

Despite the high demand for ATP and NADPH described previously, photoreceptor OSs have limited glycolytic capacity and are devoid of mitochondria (Figure 1), relying on the inner segments (IS) for their energetic needs. Accordingly, photoreceptor ISs have the highest capacity for glycolysis, tricarboxylic acid (TCA) cycle, mitochondrial Oxphos, and creatine phosphate-mediated shuttling of ATP into the cytosol [80]. Photoreceptor ISs contain high amounts of hexokinase 2 (HK2) on the mitochondrial outer membrane, which catalyzes the rate-limiting step of glycolysis, namely, the conversion of glucose into glucose-6-phosphate. From here, a portion of glucose proceeds through glycolysis and the TCA cycle, which provides the GTP needed for phototransduction. Glucose-6-phosphate is also utilized in the pentose phosphate pathway, which is the primary source of NADPH used in anabolic reactions and the regeneration of cytosolic reduced glutathione (GSH), a major antioxidant defense mechanism. Between the two photoreceptor populations, cones contain 10-fold more mitochondria and thus have a much greater ATP-generating capacity than rods. Cone ISs also contain greater amounts of creatine phosphate, suggesting that cones provide the cytosolic ATP more efficiently than rods in the setting of high energetic demand [80].

The outer retina exhibits light-induced changes in oxygen consumption and ATP production [82]. As mentioned previously, phototransduction requires a steady influx of ATP and NAPDH both for the regeneration of 11-*cis* retinal and photoreceptor OS. Light has been shown to stimulate the accumulation of ribose-5-phosphate, an intermediate in the pentose phosphate pathway, which likely reflects increased NADPH production and anabolic metabolism. Oxygen consumption also correlates with the rod dark current, which imposes a high energetic demand in mammals [83], accounting for 41% of total retinal oxygen consumption [84]. When oxygen supply is inadequate, the dark current may be partially supported by glycolysis, indicating that more ATP is needed and extracted in the dark from energetic fuel substrates through their oxidation.

In contrast to the outer retina, the inner retina does not exhibit significant light-induced changes in oxidative metabolism. Nevertheless, neurons and glia of the inner retina also require a steady state [ATP] for neurotransmission. Müller cells, the most abundant glial cell in the retina, are critical to the maintenance of the neurovascular unit and perform important functions such as synaptic transmission regulation, handling of nutrients and waste products, maintenance of the "tightness" of the blood-retinal barrier, and survival of neurons and endothelial cells. Müller cells rely primarily on glycolysis and are rich in glycogen reserves [85,86]. Although glucose is their preferred substrate, Müller cells also utilize extracellular glutamate [87], and for this reason are believed to play a role in preventing glutamate excitotoxicity. Cell culture experiments have confirmed that Müller cells exhibit aerobic glycolysis and provide lactate that can be transferred to retinal neurons for metabolic support [88]. Their Oxphos capacity, however, is limited. It is suggested that this metabolic heterogeneity of the retina likely plays an important role in the cell-specific vulnerability to diabetes.

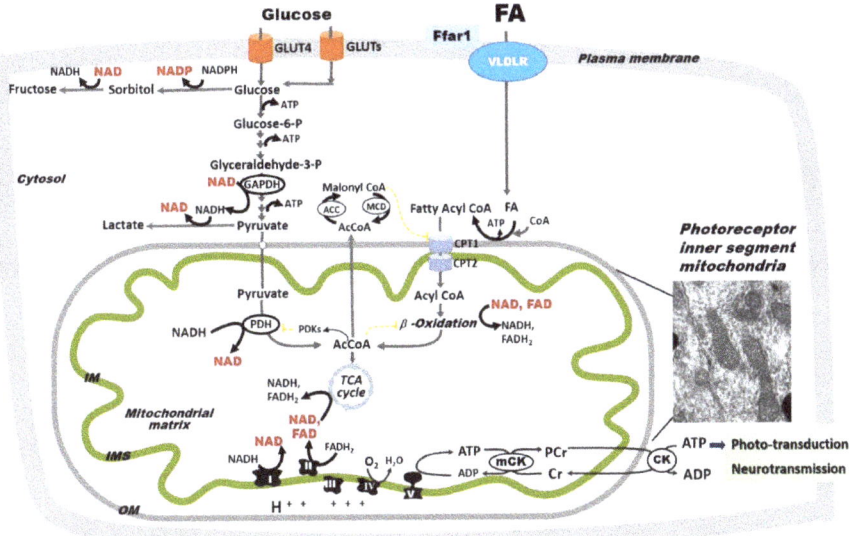

Figure 3. Glycolysis and oxidative phosphorylation in the retina. The retina relies on glycolysis and mitochondrial oxidative phosphorylation (Oxphos) as sources of ATP. Glucose uptake into retinal cells occurs via insulin-dependent glucose transporter 4 (GLUT4) and insulin-independent glucose transporter 1 (GLUT1). Fatty acid (FA) uptake is not hormonally regulated, but rather potentially driven by circulating availability (FA$_{circ}$) [89,90]. In the retina, FA uptake is regulated by a lipid sensor, the free fatty acid lipid receptor 1 (Ffar1), and mediated by the very low density lipoprotein receptor (VLDLR). In retinal cells, glucose follows multiple metabolic pathways, including glycolysis and the polyol pathway, the latter of which leads to the production of sorbitol and ultimately fructose. Pyruvate is either converted to lactate or transported into mitochondria where it is converted by pyruvate dehydrogenase (PDH) to acetyl coenzyme A (AcCoA), which enters the tricarboxylic acid (TCA) cycle. PDH is inhibited by pyruvate dehydrogenase kinases that are activated by excessive acetyl-CoA and nicotinamide adenine dinucleotide (NADH). For simplicity, other glucose metabolic pathways are not shown. FAs, which are released from triglycerides and imported into retinal cells via the VLDLR, are converted to fatty acyl-CoA, shuttled into the mitochondria via carnitine palmitoyltransferases 1 and 2 (CPT1 and 2), and oxidized via FA β-oxidation. FA β-oxidation yields NADH, flavin adenine dinucleotide (FAHD$_2$), and AcCoA, which are further oxidized by the electron transport chain (ETC) complexes in the process of Oxphos

with ATP synthesis. FA β-oxidation is inhibited by malonyl-CoA (an intermediate of FA synthesis), $FADH_2/FAD^+$ ratios, and $NADH/NAD^+$ ratios. Malonyl-CoA is degraded by malonyl-CoA decarboxylase (MCD), thus decreasing its inhibitory effect on CPT1. Although described in other organs, these regulatory steps are yet to be identified in the retina. Mitochondrial Oxphos provides the bulk of retinal ATP. As electrons transfer NADH and $FADH_2$ to molecular oxygen by ETC complexes, an electrochemical gradient is built across the mitochondrial inner membrane (IM). This gradient is used by the complex V to produce ATP. Mitochondria-generated ATP is transferred to the cytosol by the creatine kinase (CK) shuttle to sustain the normal functions of the retinal cells. The inset included here is an electron micrograph of a mouse rod photoreceptor and shows the inner segment mitochondria. For simplicity, the nicotinamide nucleotide transhydrogenase, a mitochondrial inner membrane enzyme that reduces nicotinamide adenine dinucleotide phosphate ($NADPH^+$) by oxidizing NADH and using the mitochondrial proton-motive force, is not shown in this figure. The oxidized NAD^+ and $NADP^+$ are shown in red.

4.3. Substrate Selection and Energy Production

Tissues with a high metabolic rate, such as the heart, often utilize multiple energy sources (glucose, amino acids, fatty acids), which confers some degree of metabolic flexibility during periods of scarcity and surplus [91]. The retina also uses multiple fuel sources to generate the electron carriers NADH and $FADH_2$, which donate their electrons directly to complex I and coenzyme Q-complex III, respectively, and ultimately establish the electrochemical gradient that drives ATP synthesis [81].

In addition to glucose, palmitate (C16:0), one of the most abundant fatty acids (FAs) in the human body, can also be used as a fuel substrate for retinal mitochondrial energy production [92]. In the retina, cellular FA uptake is mediated by the very low density lipoprotein receptor (VLDLR) that is expressed on both photoreceptor and RPE cells. Moreover, the expression of proteins involved in FA β-oxidation has been reported throughout the retina, including RGCs, photoreceptors, and Müller cells, albeit in varying amounts [93,94], indicating that retinal cells possess the machinery to oxidize lipids as fuel sources. FA oxidation is essential for retinal metabolism and function. In support of this concept, genetic mutations in specific enzymes involved in β-oxidation cause mitochondrial dysfunction, pigmentary retinopathy, and ultimately vision loss [95]. In mice, knockout of the peroxisome proliferative-activated receptor-α (PPARα), a nuclear receptor that modulates lipoprotein lipase expression and triglyceride metabolism, causes decreased lipid metabolism and retinal neurodegeneration [96]. Despite recognizing FA as a fuel source, the involvement of potential changes in FA β-oxidation remain largely unexplored in the retina in diabetes, a disease associated with increased FA availability. Nevertheless, two large-scale clinical trials known as the Fenofibrate Intervention and Event Lowering in Diabetes (FIELD) and Action to Control Cardiovascular Risk in Diabetes (ACCORD) studies have shown that the PPARα-agonist fenofibrate slows the progression of DR [97,98]. These findings raise the possibility that diabetes-induced alterations in mitochondrial FA β-oxidation may contribute to retinal dysfunction.

Further research has investigated the role of FA β-oxidation in the retinal microvasculature. Surprisingly, impaired FA oxidation in retinal endothelial cells neither results in energy depletion nor does it disturb redox homeostasis [99], suggesting that FA oxidation in these cells likely supports cellular functions in addition to ATP production. Using isotope labeling experiments, Schoors et al. [99] demonstrated that FA-derived carbon units are incorporated into aspartate (a nucleotide precursor) and eventually DNA. The same group also showed that blockade of carnitine palmitoyl transferase 1 (CPT1), the rate-limiting enzyme in FA β-oxidation, inhibits pathological neovascularization in mice. These data suggest a novel role of FA oxidation in endothelial cell proliferation and maintenance of the neurovascular unit. These findings raise the important question of whether, in diabetes, the retina exhibits a "metabolic switch" towards increased FA oxidation, similar to other high-energy consuming organs (e.g., heart, kidney). While such data are scarce, at least one study has indicated that the retina can increase the expression of FA oxidation enzymes in diabetic rats [100]. Subsequent studies will be needed, however, to characterize and quantify the relative contribution of individual energetic substrates to energy production in the diabetic retina.

Diabetes is characterized by decreased insulin action (a decrease in either secretion or sensitivity) and increased availability of energetic substrates (i.e., glucose and FAs). In the heart, also a highly energy consuming organ, increased availability of FAs is associated with a rapid decrease in glucose oxidation [101], thus reducing metabolic flexibility and increasing reliance on FAs for ATP production. In hepatocytes and adipocytes, increased availability of glucose leads to increased flux through the TCA cycle and increased production malonyl coenzyme A (malonyl-CoA), which inhibits CPT1 and spares lipids from β-oxidation. Similar to the heart, these changes indicate a decrease in metabolic flexibility. In the retina, glucose uptake occurs via both insulin-independent glucose transporter 1 (GLUT1) and insulin-dependent glucose transporter 4 (GLUT4) [102,103]. The retina also expresses a lipid sensor known as free fatty acid receptor 1 (Ffar1) (Figure 3) [92]. Ffar1 regulates insulin secretion in the islets of Langerhans [104] and neuronal function in the brain [105]. Interestingly, Ffar1 has been shown to downregulate GLUT1 expression in *VLDLR*-deficient photoreceptors, resulting in a dual glucose and lipid substrate uptake [92], which predictably leads to low levels of TCA cycle intermediates. Several TCA cycle intermediates including α-ketoglutarate and succinate have been shown to modulate the stabilization of hypoxia-inducible factor 1α [106]. In *VLDLR*-deficient photoreceptors, low α-ketoglutarate stabilizes hypoxia-inducible factor 1α and promotes neovascularization [92]. While similar studies have yet to be performed in the context of DR, these findings suggest multiple mechanisms by which the selection of energetic substrates, all plentiful in diabetes, may change retinal disease progression.

5. Alterations in Mitochondrial Oxidative Metabolism in the Neural Retina

5.1. Localization of Mitochondria in the Retina

An increasingly popular view is that diabetic milieu leads to the uncoupling of the retinal neurovascular unit [6], a concept that implies impaired crosstalk between neurons, glia, and the microvascular network [23]. While Müller cells rely primarily on glycolysis for ATP, those located in highly vascularized portions of the retina are rich in mitochondria [107], raising the possibility that mitochondrial dysfunction in Müller cells may have neurovascular consequences. Mitochondria also concentrate in the photoreceptor IS and the most external ends of the RPE (Figure 1), which likely reflects their migration toward the oxygen-rich choriocapillaris during neurodevelopment [108]. The specific distribution of mitochondria in the retina may explain, at least in part, the regional susceptibility to neurodegeneration and microvascular lesions in DR.

5.2. Diabetes Alters Mitochondrial Function in the Retina

The function of healthy and diseased mitochondria can be evaluated by measuring oxygen consumption rates in isolated mitochondria, retinal explants, or cultured retinal cells. However, due to limitations imposed by the small sample volume, many studies have resorted to studying mitochondrial function in retinal homogenate rather than individual cells or specific retinal layers. Retinal mitochondria exhibit a biphasic response to diabetes, characterized by an early and transient activation followed by a later decline. Masser et al. [100] showed that basal and ATP-linked oxygen consumption rates were significantly elevated in the retina of 3-month-old diabetic rats. In the same study, proteomic analysis revealed elevated levels of several FA β-oxidation enzymes and antioxidant proteins, suggesting a positive adaptive response of the retina to the diabetic milieu. This response mirrors the diabetic heart in that it indicates an energetic shift toward reliance on FA β-oxidation and metabolic inflexibility [101]. Another study reported increased mitochondrial oxygen consumption in diabetic rats at 3 weeks of hyperglycemia [109], which was associated with increased specific activities of complexes I, II, and III. Despite an increase in oxygen consumption and ETC complex activity, ATP generation was unchanged due to mitochondrial uncoupling, suggesting mitochondrial activation and inefficiency rather than mitochondrial defects. Similarly, in a model of spontaneous T2D in the cone-rich diurnal Nile rat, a short-term (2 month) hyperglycemia increased complex I-dependent mitochondrial respiration and was associated with increased cytochrome c access to cytochrome c oxidase, suggesting a change in composition or organization of the mitochondrial inner membrane [110]. Increased mitochondrial membrane permeability was confirmed in isolated mitochondria from retinas of Zucker diabetic fatty rats with 6 weeks of persistent hyperglycemia and was associated with a concomitant decrease in mitochondrial complex III-specific activity [111].

Osorio-Paz et al. [109] reported that longer (approximately 6 weeks) durations of STZ-induced diabetes in rats caused a decreased cytochrome c-reducing activity of complex III, while complexes II and IV were hyperactive when measured in isolated retinal mitochondria. These changes in ETC complex-specific activities reflect a decrease in oxygen consumption of retinal mitochondria energized with a combination of energetic substrates (glutamate and malate) that are generating NADH to be oxidized by complex I. Intriguingly, the generated ATP was unchanged. Mitochondrial respiration in the presence of substrates feeding electrons into complex I (NADH pathway) and II (succinate pathway) involves complexes III and IV, as well as mobile electron carriers such as co-enzyme Q and cytochrome c. Therefore, it is expected that a change in individual components will affect the whole Oxphos pathway. However, the effect of individual components on the whole integrative function depends upon the control of that component on the Oxphos. In comparison with heart, where the impact of individual components on the Oxphos and ATP synthesis has been determined, this control has yet to be investigated in the normal and diabetic retina. While it is unclear if complex III defect is limiting for the Oxphos in the diabetic retina, a decreased complex III activity led to increased superoxide in a mouse model of STZ-induced diabetes; both were normalized by overexpressing the mitochondrial antioxidant enzyme, manganese superoxide dismutase (MnSOD) [112].

In contrast with short-term diabetes, a long-term (18 months) sustained hyperglycemia in T2D Nil diurnal rats caused a decrease in NADH-supported mitochondrial respiration accompanied by an increase in succinate contribution to the maximal Oxphos capacity in the whole retinas, thus confirming a partial decline in mitochondrial bioenergetics [110]. As NADH-induced mitochondrial respiration is supported by complex I, co-enzyme Q, complex III, cytochrome c, and complexes IV and V, these results suggest a potential defect in any of these Oxphos subunits.

Mitochondrial DNA (mtDNA) follows a similar response in the diabetic retina. Alterations in the morphology and function in the neural retina occurring within the first 3 months of diabetes in rats are not associated with changes in mtDNA in isolated retinal synaptosomes. These findings suggest that alterations of mtDNA in synaptosomes are not causative for the early neural retina dysfunction in diabetes [100]. In addition, in a model of T1D in rats, while an elevated oxidative stress was detected as early as 15 days of diabetes, mtDNA damage was observed much later at 6 months due to inactivation of the DNA repair/replication enzymes [113]. A similar temporal relationship was observed in endothelial cells exposed to high glucose [114]. These data suggest that the oxidative damage of mtDNA is fully compensated in early stages of diabetes while the altered mtDNA in later stages leads to a decline in mitochondrial transcription and secondary ETC defects. A summary of the mitochondrial alterations in DR is presented in Tables 1 and 2.

Table 1. Summary of investigations into altered mitochondrial homeostasis in the diabetic retina by cell type *.

Cell Type	Oxidative Stress	Mitochondrial Morphology	Mitochondrial Turnover	References
RGCs	✓	✓	Unknown	[115–117]
Bipolar cells	✓	✓	Unknown	[117]
Müller cells	✓	✓	✓	[118–124]
Photoreceptors		✓	✓	[121]
Endothelial cells	✓	✓	✓	[113,114,125–131]

* Not an exhaustive list. Abbreviations: RGC, retinal ganglion cell. ✓: this feature was confirmed in the respective cells, as supported by references.

Table 2. Summary of electron transport chain protein expression and activity in the diabetic retina by cell type *.

Cell Type	Complex I	Complex II †	Complex III	Complex IV	Complex V (ATP Synthase)	References
RGCs	→	→	Unknown	→	Unknown	[132,133]
Bipolar cells	Unknown	Unknown	Unknown	Unknown	Unknown	[119]
Müller cells	Unknown	↔	Unknown	↔	Unknown	[121]
Photoreceptors	Unknown	Unknown	Unknown	Varies	Unknown	[100,109–112,121]
Retinal homogenate	Biphasic ‡	Biphasic	Biphasic	Biphasic	Varies	[134]
Pericytes	Unknown	→	Unknown	Unknown	Unknown	[135]
Endothelial cells	→	→	→	→	→	[129,136–139]

* Not an exhaustive list. † The activity of complex II was inferred in this study from the 3-(4,5-dimethylthiazol-2-yl)-2,5-diphenyltetrazolium bromide (MTT) assay, which measures the ability of succinate dehydrogenase in complex II to reduce tetrazolium salts [140]. ‡ Biphasic changes in electron transport complex activity are characterized by early activation followed by a later decline. The exact timing varies by model. Abbreviations: RGC, retinal ganglion cell. ↓: decreased; ↔: unchanged.

6. Mitochondria-Derived Oxidative Stress in the Diabetic Retina

Oxidative stress is a critical component of altered homeostasis across multiple cell types involved in DR [141]. ROS are defined by the presence of a highly reactive oxygen molecule, and are generated as normal byproducts of cellular redox reactions. Mitochondria generate superoxide during oxidation-reduction reactions as some electrons may leak to univalently reduce molecular oxygen. A number of mitochondrial antioxidant defense mechanisms are in place to prevent the increase in oxidative stress, including MnSOD, catalase, reduced glutathione, and thioredoxin. Mitochondria are both the producers and targets of oxidative stress, with the latter altering mtDNA and mitochondrial proteins leading to mitochondrial dysfunction. Defects in the ETC further amplify the risk of increased oxidative stress. In the retina, this self-perpetuating cycle has been referred to as the "metabolic memory" phenomenon, a hypothesis that is supported by the persistence of altered mtDNA, decreased activity of ETC complexes, and increased oxidative stress throughout the retina despite the reinstitution of good glycemic control [142].

The proposition that increased oxidative stress is a key pathogenic factor in the development of DR is supported by finding of insufficient antioxidant defenses in diabetic patients [143]. Antioxidant approaches alleviate diabetes-induced vascular lesions in the retina [112,144,145]. Moreover, the causal link between increased mitochondrial-generated oxidative stress and retinal microvascular disease in diabetes is supported by the effect of overexpressing the mitochondrial antioxidant enzyme, MnSOD, to decrease the number of acellular capillaries in diabetic mice [112]. Therefore, mitochondria are directly implicated in the development of diabetic microvascular lesions.

Mitochondrial dysfunction in retinal endothelial cells has been identified as the upstream contributor to diabetic vascular disease in diabetes [146,147]. Recent evidence indicates that the neurovascular unit is functionally affected before the onset of retinal microvascular disease, and that the neural retina is affected by oxidative stress originating from the photoreceptors [148]. The role of photoreceptors as oxidative stress generators is supported by the observation that human patients with photoreceptor degeneration and retinitis pigmentosa have less severe DR than diabetics with intact photoreceptors as well as diabetic mice lacking photoreceptors due to opsin deficiency [34]. The work of Du et al. [34] unequivocally identified photoreceptors as the major source of superoxide generated by retinas of diabetic mice, and showed that mitochondria contributes to at least 50% of oxidative stress, thus complementing the NADPH oxidase. Their deletion inhibited the expected increase in superoxide and inflammatory proteins in the remaining retina in diabetic mice. Of note, Müller cells cultured in high glucose also exhibit increased oxidative stress [149], but their contribution to DR in vivo is unknown.

There are two potential mechanisms explaining the increased superoxide production by the diabetic photoreceptors. The first hypothesis is that defects of the mitochondrial ETC interrupt the normal electron flow to fully reduce oxygen, thus leading to accumulation of electrons at sites within the ETC, which are accepted by oxygen to generate superoxide [150]. The ETC sites prone to leak electrons to oxygen are complexes I and III [151,152]. In support of this hypothesis, we recently reported that correcting the electron flow within the complex I-deficient ETC decreased oxidative stress and photoreceptor damage [153]. The second hypothesis is that an early increase in mitochondrial oxidative phosphorylation fed by an increased FA β-oxidation brings additional sites of electron leak to oxygen, as was shown for the heart [154,155] and kidney tubules in diabetes [156]. These possibilities are not mutually exclusive, but they are yet to be investigated in the retina.

Superoxide is dismutated to hydrogen peroxide, a highly permeable compound that may support the crosstalk between retinal cells and affect neighbor cells, thus providing a link between neural retina and microvasculature. However, this crosstalk has not yet been investigated in the retina. Oxidative stress increases the expression of pro-inflammatory proteins [157] and enhance retinal inflammation [158] that contributes to early DR [159]. In addition, in the microvasculature, increased oxidative stress is also associated with increased apoptosis [114,160,161], further compromising the integrity of the neurovascular unit.

7. NAD Pool and the NADH/NAD⁺ Redox Ratio in the Diabetic Retina

7.1. NAD Pool

Nicotinamide adenine dinucleotide (NAD) is a coenzyme for redox enzymes, shuttling electrons from glycolysis and the TCA cycle to complex I in the ETC. The oxidized form, NAD$^+$, is also a co-substrate for non-redox reactions such as those catalyzed by sirtuin (SIRT) and poly (ADP-ribose) polymerase (PARP) families of proteins [162,163]. This link represents a highly conserved mechanism by which redox status influences a wide range of cellular and metabolic functions, including cell signaling, DNA transcription, and programmed cell death. Recent work by Lin et al. [164] suggest that NAD is essential for vision. In this study, specific deficiency of NAD in rod photoreceptor for 6 weeks led to massive atrophy of the entire neurosensory retina, affecting the microvasculature, RPE, and optic nerve. The complete absence of the outer nuclear layer (photoreceptor nuclei) indicates that cone photoreceptors are also secondarily affected by rod NAD deficiency. These results strongly suggest that retinal photoreceptors are essential for the integrity of the whole retina. Although similar studies have not yet been conducted in the context of DR, these findings suggest that alterations of the photoreceptors precede the vascular regression in diabetes. During a short (3-week) period of NAD deficiency, mitochondrial morphology was maintained as normal, whereas at 4 weeks, mitochondrial cristae were lost, and photoreceptor OS were disrupted. Metabolomic analysis showed that NAD deficiency causes dysregulation of multiple metabolic pathways including the TCA cycle, mitochondrial protein biosynthesis, and propionate metabolism with accumulation of acylcarnitines, and also decreased ATP production. Both glycolysis and mitochondrial Oxphos were affected. These results highlight the critical role of metabolism and bioenergetics to maintain the photoreceptor integrity. The same research group identified the decreased retinal NAD pool as an early feature in retinal disease caused by STZ-induced diabetes at 3 weeks of sustained hyperglycemia [164]. NAD deficiency caused photoreceptor death and diminished rod ERG recordings. These data support the concept that mitochondrial dysfunction in photoreceptors in the neural retina proceed the vascular regression in the diabetic retina.

7.2. NADH/NAD⁺ Redox Ratio

The "hyperglycemic pseudohypoxia" hypothesis [165,166] suggests that diabetes is associated with an increased cellular NADH/NAD$^+$ redox ratio attributed to an increased flux through the polyol pathway and resulting in altered metabolism and neurovascular dysfunction. The polyol pathway is a two-step reaction involving the reduction of glucose to sorbitol and the subsequent oxidation of sorbitol to fructose [167]. The rate-limiting step in this pathway is catalyzed by aldose reductase, which is expressed in all cells and utilizes NADPH as an electron donor. Importantly, aldose reductase is activated by hyperglycemia. The second step in the polyol pathway is catalyzed by sorbitol dehydrogenase, which uses NAD$^+$ as an oxidizing agent to produce fructose and thus increases the NADH/NAD$^+$ redox ratio. Studies have shown that both sorbitol and fructose accumulate in diabetic tissues, including the retina [168,169], suggesting that the polyol pathway may contribute to oxidative stress in DR. This finding is supported by the observation that genetic knockout of aldose reductase protects retinal endothelial cells from oxidative stress [170].

The redox state is compartmentalized between cellular organelles. The cytosolic NADPH/NADP$^+$ is maintained in a reduced state necessary for drive biosynthetic and antioxidant processes. In energized mitochondria NADH exceeds NAD$^+$ to provide electrons for the ETC while the cytosol has a higher NAD$^+$, reflecting a relatively oxidized redox state [171]. Mitochondrial NADH/NAD$^+$ redox ratio is closely related with mitochondrial function. We recently reported that a mitochondrial complex I defect directly results in an increased NADH/NAD$^+$ ratio in cultured photoreceptor cells [153]. Diederen et al. [172] found no significant differences in NADH/NAD$^+$ redox ratios in the whole retina of 6-month-old STZ-induced diabetic mice. The redox status in specific cellular organelles including mitochondria was not assessed in this study. It may be predicted that mitochondrial redox state is unchanged in early stages of DR when considering the biphasic response of retinal mitochondria to the diabetic milieu. An early enhanced mitochondrial function would be expected to maintain a normal NADH/NAD$^+$ redox ratios until ETC defects begin to manifest. While complex I and IV defects are associated with the accumulation of NADH and an increased NADH/NAD$^+$ ratio [173,174], measures taken to correct ETC defects can be used to decrease NADH and restore redox balance [175]. These data are consistent with the hypothesis that ETC defects cause an increase in NADH and a reduced redox microenvironment in retinal mitochondria.

A potential mechanism that may increase cellular NADH/NAD$^+$ redox ratio is the activation of poly (ADP-ribose) polymerases (PARPs), a family of proteins best known for their role in DNA repair. PARPs are activated in response to DNA damage and catalyze the transfer and polymerization of ADP-ribose to DNA repair enzymes. This reaction requires NAD$^+$, leading some to hypothesize that PARP activation could lead to NAD$^+$ depletion and altered redox homeostasis. PARP-deficient mice are protected against diabetes [176], and exhibit preserved redox homeostasis and mitochondrial function [177]. The mitochondrial protective effect is mediated by activating the NAD$^+$-dependent deacetylases, sirtuins (SIRTs). Among the large family of SIRT proteins, SIRT1 is an extramitochondrial protein with a wide range of functions in both metabolism and aging. Recent work by Mishra et al. [178] have shown that the *SIRT1* promoter is hypermethylated in STZ-induced diabetic mice. *SIRT1* overexpression protected the mice against mitochondrial damage, neural dysfunction, RGC degeneration, and blood–retinal barrier breakdown. A role of mitochondrial sirtuins in retinal disease is supported by the finding that genetic knockout of *SIRT3*, a mitochondrial SIRT, mirrors NAD$^+$ deficiency and leads to early and rapid retinal degeneration [164].

The immediate consequence of an increased mitochondrial NADH/NAD$^+$ redox ratio is reductive stress (increased NADH) and NAD$^+$ deficiency, which is detrimental to photoreceptor integrity [153]. Mitochondrial production of ROS is largely governed by the NADH/NAD$^+$ ratio, as an increased [NADH] slows the ETC flux. The antioxidant defense is supported by the NADPH/NADP$^+$ redox ratio. NADPH is a potent reducing agent involved the regeneration of antioxidant compounds such as reduced glutathione. Importantly, the mitochondrial NADH/NAD$^+$ and NADPH/NADP$^+$ redox couples are linked by nicotinamide nucleotide transhydrogenase (NNT), an enzyme that leverages the proton-motive force in the oxidation of NADH and the simultaneous reduction of NADP$^+$ (Figure 4A). NNT maintains a NADPH/NADP$^+$ ratio several-fold higher than the NADH/NAD$^+$ ratio, and thus is a physiologically relevant source of NADPH that drives the reduction of H_2O_2 [179]. While NNT is reported to be expressed exclusively in cardiac tissue [180], we provide evidence here that the NNT protein is also expressed in the retina (Figure 4B). The role of NNT to maintain the mitochondrial redox state and antioxidant defense is yet to be determined.

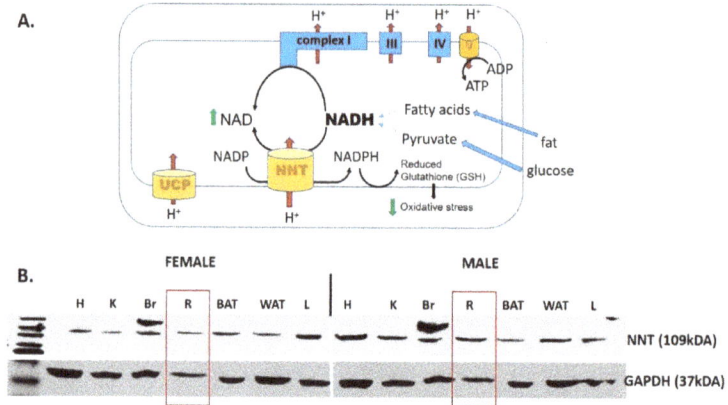

Figure 4. Nicotinamide nucleotide transhydrogenase (NNT). (**A**) NNT is a mitochondrial enzyme

that oxidizes NADH, and therefore supplements complex I in the process of regenerating NAD$^+$. In addition, the enzyme forms NADPH that is critical to maintain the antioxidant potency of mitochondria by maintaining the reduced glutathione (GSH) [181,182]. (**B**) Western blot analysis of the NNT protein expression in a variety of tissues in both male in female mice. Abbreviations: UCP, uncoupling protein; H, heart; K, kidney; Br, brain; R, retina; BAT, brown adipose tissue; WAT, white adipose tissue; L, liver.

8. Alterations in Mitochondrial Turnover

8.1. Mitochondrial Biogenesis and Mitophagy

The balance between mitochondrial formation and destruction regulates the cellular mitochondrial mass. Mitochondrial biogenesis is the cellular process to increase total mitochondrial content. This process relies on the coordinated action of cell signaling molecules, molecular chaperones, and transcription factors, all of which working in tandem to replicate the mitochondrial genome and proteome. One of the most upstream factors is the peroxisome proliferator-activated receptor gamma coactivator 1-α (PGC-1α), which has been referred to as the "master regulator" of mitochondrial biogenesis [183]. Among its many downstream targets is mitochondrial transcription factor A (TFAM), which is translocated to the mitochondrial matrix and initiates mitochondrial genome replication. In the past decade, a series of studies conducted by Santos et al. [127,129,184] have shown that mitochondrial biogenesis is altered in both experimental and human DR. Specifically, Santos et al. [129] found that nuclear-mitochondrial translocation of TFAM is impaired within 12 months of STZ-induced diabetes. Subsequent experiments by the same group determined that TFAM is ubiquitinated and targeted for proteasomal degradation, and its translocation to the matrix is impaired [128]. Overexpression of MnSOD or administration of the exogenous antioxidant lipoid acid had a positive impact on mitochondrial localization of TFAM and mtDNA copy number [127,129], further supporting a role of oxidative stress as an upstream regulator of mitochondrial biogenesis. An important limitation, however, is that most of these studies were performed in retinal homogenate or endothelial cells. Thus, whether these specific findings translate to specific cell populations within the neural retina is an important question that remains to be explored.

Mitophagy is a specialized form of macro-autophagy by which damaged or excessive mitochondria are selectively targeted for lysosomal degradation. Several groups have reported that Müller cells grown in high glucose exhibit enhanced mitophagy [119–121,124]. This phenomenon is thought to occur in part as a consequence of hyperglycemia-induced expression of thioredoxin-interacting protein (TXNIP), which binds to and inhibits the antioxidants thioredoxin 1 and thioredoxin 2. Hyperglycemia-induced expression of TXNIP is observed in the vasculature, pericytes, and the RPE [130,185], suggesting a conserved mechanism across cell types. Knockdown of TXNIP reduces oxidative stress, improves ATP synthesis, and restores mitophagic flux [119]. Some of these findings have since been validated in the db/db mouse model by Zhou et al. [124]. When considered together with the work of Santos et al. [114,127–129,186], these findings suggest that DR is characterized by a gradual decrease in mitochondrial content, both due to impaired biogenesis and enhanced mitophagy. Recent work by Hombrebueno et al. [121] suggests that these processes have a temporal relationship. Using the spontaneous $Ins2^{Akita}$ diabetic mouse model, Hombrebueno et al. [121] observed enhanced PTEN-induced kinase (PINK1)-dependent mitophagy in both Müller cells and photoreceptors within the first 2 months of diabetes. While increased mitochondrial biogenesis can compensate for enhanced mitophagy, compensatory mechanisms begin to fail at 8 months of diabetes, resulting in decreased mitochondrial mass.

8.2. Fusion–Fission Dynamics in the Retina

Mitochondria exist in a constant flux of fusion and fission, which is necessary to respond to the energy requirements of the cell (for a review, see [187]). This process is regulated by mitofusin-2 (Mfn2) and dynamin-related protein 1 (Drp1), two antagonistic GTPases that regulate fusion and fission, respectively. In human DR, Mfn2 protein levels are reduced, while Drp1 is increased, suggesting an imbalance between these two GTPases that favors mitochondrial fission, reduced mtDNA, and possibly decreased ATP synthesis [188]. These findings have also been observed in Müller cells and photoreceptors grown in high-glucose conditions [119]. Although the exact mechanism is largely unexplored, a shift toward mitochondrial fission may also be due to oxidative damage. In support of this hypothesis, administration of melatonin, which is well-known for its antioxidant properties, preserved mitochondrial fusion in photoreceptors both in vitro and in vivo [118]. Alternatively, enhanced mitochondrial fission may be due to increased methylation at the *MFN2* promoter site, as shown in endothelial cells [136]. However, this finding alone does not explain the reported increase in Drp1, which independently favors mitochondrial fission. This area of research is still in its preliminary stages, and subsequent studies will be necessary to confirm its significance in DR.

9. Consequences of Increased Oxidative Stress in the Neural Retina

9.1. Diabetic Milieu Alters Ion Channel Homeostasis in the Retina

Early in its course, diabetes causes a paradoxical closure of the L-type calcium ion channels (LTCCs) in the dark, as suggested by manganese-enhanced magnetic resonance imaging (MEMRI) studies that have shown that photoreceptor uptake of manganese (a calcium surrogate) is significantly reduced in the dark-adapted rodents [189]. Because these ion channels are essential for the regulated release of neurotransmitters at the photoreceptor synapses, paradoxically closed photoreceptor LTCCs in the dark have significant functional consequences. Alterations in ion channel homeostasis have also been reported at the level of the mitochondria. The expression of the mitochondrial calcium uniporter (MCU), which plays important roles in calcium buffering and ion channel homeostasis, is decreased in photoreceptors grown in high glucose conditions [190]. Retinal neurons cultured in high glucose exhibit increased mitochondrial calcium load, associated with depolarization of mitochondrial membrane and ROS generation. Similar observations were made in retinas from 9-week-old diabetic rats [191].

Long-term diabetes causes mitochondrial ETC defects and decreases mitochondrial respiration efficiency in the retina, with both being canonical causes of energy deficit. However, available data do not support the hypothesis that ATP deficit is responsible for the dysfunction in ion channels as retinal [ATP] is unchanged in diabetes [192]. Decreasing oxidative stress in diabetic rodents with copper/zinc superoxide dismutase (Cu/Zn SOD) overexpression or lipoic acid administration corrected the diabetes-induced ion flux abnormalities in photoreceptors in the dark [145,193], suggesting that abnormalities in ion homeostasis are induced by increased oxidative stress. Studies showing that diabetes elevates oxidative stress in the retina by both promoting ROS production and suppressing the antioxidant defense [117] also provide strong support for this hypothesis.

9.2. Apoptosis

The intrinsic (mitochondrial) pathway of apoptosis is initiated by increased permeabilization of the mitochondrial outer membrane and activation of the apoptotic signaling cascade. Notably, the intrinsic pathway is induced by increased oxidative stress [194], making this pathway highly relevant in DR, as virtually all cell types in the retina experience hyperglycemia-induced oxidative stress [116,123,164,195]. RGCs [133] and the retinal microvasculature in particular have been shown to undergo oxidative stress-induced apoptosis [114,160]. Several groups have reported that administration of exogenous antioxidants preserved mitochondrial integrity and prevent cell death in the diabetic retina [116,133]. These findings reiterate the concept that oxidative stress is an early event in the pathogenesis of DR, whereas cell death generally occurs as a later and secondary event.

10. Therapeutic Implications

10.1. Therapies Focused on Maintaining the Integrity of Retinal Mitochondria

The Diabetes Control and Complications Trial showed that intensive insulin replacement therapy reduces the incidence and slows the progression of DR [5]. However, the incidence of DR remains high, and many patients still progress to PDR despite advances in diabetes care. Accordingly, second-line treatments are frequently necessary to manage the later complications of DR. These therapies are highly effective in managing the sight-threatening complications of DR. Thus, it is critical to better understand the early stages of DR and develop new therapies to prevent its progression. The need for new therapies in early stages of DR is further highlighted by the "metabolic memory" phenomenon (for a review, see [2]), which may be a consequence of persistent mitochondrial damage and oxidative stress [142]. This hypothesis is consistent with the benefit of mitochondrial targeted therapy to preserve mitochondrial integrity and vision in experimental DR.

An important antioxidant therapy is the Szeto–Schiller (SS) tetra-peptide, SS-31 (elamipretide), which is concentrated in the inner mitochondrial membrane and selectively stabilizes cardiolipin [196], a phospholipid critical for mitochondrial integrity and function, which is prone to oxidative damage in diabetes [197]. SS-31 enhances the interaction between cytochrome c and cardiolipin to facilitate better electron transfer from complex III to complex IV, and reduces mitochondrial oxidative stress [198,199]. Evidence from animal studies suggests that SS-31 could reduce the risk of vascular disease in diabetes, as administration of SS-31 alleviated the microvascular retinal disease in rodent models of DR [200,201], and increased SIRT1 while ameliorating retinal inflammation in rodent and human subjects with T2D [202]. However, human studies have shown limited efficacy to date, and no studies have been performed in patients with DR.

Numerous studies have suggested that oxidative stress may be modulated by uncoupling proteins (UCPs), a family of proteins named for their ability to uncouple electron transport from ATP synthesis. These proteins decrease mitochondrial ROS production by decreasing the electrochemical gradient [203], a process called "mild uncoupling". The theory is based on the observation of Korshunov et al. [204] that ROS generation increases in an exponential manner when mitochondrial membrane potential exceeds a threshold that is higher than that corresponding to the mitochondrial energetic state in in vivo settings. The hypothesis is also based on the assumption that the diabetic milieu increases the availability of energetic substrates (glucose, FAs) to the retina, which are oxidized to increase mitochondrial membrane potential ("hyperpolarization"). This hypothesis is supported by the observation that *UCP2*-deficient mice exhibit increased ROS generation [205], whereas overexpression of the *UCP2* gene preserves mitochondrial function in human umbilical endothelial cells [206]. In the retina, UCP2 protein levels and activity are increased in retinal endothelial cells grown in high-glucose conditions [207], which may indicate a compensatory response to oxidative stress. However, administration of the uncoupling agent niclosamide ethanolamine has shown no benefit in the treatment of diabetes or its complications in db/db mice [208] indicating the lack of benefit of uncouplers in in vivo settings. A potential explanation is that Oxphos is a process regulated by energy demand rather than substrate availability. In diabetes, increased substrate availability does not increase oxidative metabolism that exceeds ATP synthesis [109], a mechanism that would lead to "hyperpolarization". While UCPs may be an important endogenous defense mechanism in the setting of oxidative stress, their therapeutic utility is unclear.

Improving the efficiency of electron flow within the defective mitochondrial ETC may be an optimal approach to relieve the increased electron density at specific ETC sites and eliminate the risk of oxygen univalent reduction and superoxide formation. Methylene blue, a redox compound that provides an alternative electron route between mitochondrial complex I and cytochrome c [209], preserves mitochondrial and photoreceptor integrity by preventing oxidative stress in a model of complex I defect [153] and experimental diabetes [34].

Idebenone, a synthetic benzoquinone that mediates electron transfer to complex III by bypassing complex I [210], is a free radical scavenger [211], reduces intracellular ROS and increases ATP production in complex I-defective cells [212–214], and promotes an increase in mitochondrial mass by regulating mitophagy [215]. Its mitochondrial protective effects have recently been investigated as a drug therapy for Leber's hereditary optic neuropathy, a rare genetic mitochondrial disease that causes rapid and progressive bilateral vision loss in young adults. A 24-week multi-center double-blind, randomized, placebo-controlled trial in patients with Leber's hereditary optic neuropathy show a mild benefit in visual acuity [216] that was confirmed when treatment started 5 years after the diagnosis [217]. The benefic outcomes are considered a result of idebenone to restore the bioenergetics in the remaining dysfunctional RGC. Evidence for efficacy of idebenone in human patients with primary or acquired mitochondrial defects are still limited, and restrict its use in DR.

10.2. Clinical Trials and the Role of Antioxidants in the Management of DR

Despite the evidence that antioxidants can slow the progression of DR, clinical trials have had mixed results. This topic was very recently reviewed by Garcia-Medina et al. [218], but is summarized here for completeness. The most successful interventions have been those that use combined antioxidant therapy (CAT). The Diabetes Visual Function Supplement Study showed that CAT may improve visual acuity and contrast sensitivity among participants with T1D and T2D without clinically detectable retinopathy or with mild non-proliferative diabetic retinopathy (NPDR) [219]. This finding is supported by the prior work of Hu et al. [220], who showed that patients with NPDR have lower levels of lutein and zeaxanthin, and further demonstrated that supplementation with these antioxidants reduces oxidative stress and may improve visual function. Although the previous two studies suggest a role of CAT in the management of DR, the conclusions are limited by the short study duration (6 and 3 months, respectively) relative to the chronicity of DR. To date, the longest trial that has been conducted was a 5-year follow-up of patients taking a commercially available multi-vitamin showing that antioxidants may slow the progression of DR as detected by ophthalmic examination [221]. However, in contrast to the above studies, the investigators did not observe a significant improvement in visual acuity. These discrepancies highlight the need for additional studies to find better therapeutic strategies that decrease the mitochondrial ROS generation by preserving mitochondrial function rather than scavenging the already generated ROS.

11. Conclusions

The pathogenesis of DR is complex and likely involves the simultaneous dysregulation of multiple metabolic and signaling pathways throughout the retinal neurovascular unit. Alterations in mitochondrial function has broader consequences than changes in ATP content. Increased oxidative stress and alterations in the redox balance are interrelated mechanisms that are altered by diabetes, and their effect on retinal structure and function in diabetes is yet to be explored. The benefit of maintaining retinal energetic flexibility and optimal fuel selection between plentiful competing substrates (glucose versus FA) in diabetes remains largely unexplored, and may represent a promising area of research. Although the present review focuses on the roles of mitochondrial dysfunction and oxidative stress, cellular dysfunction in the retina can take many forms, including neuroinflammation and blood–retinal barrier breakdown. These processes likely occur in parallel and thus future studies should adopt a comprehensive approach that appreciates the interconnectedness of the retina.

Author Contributions: Conceptualization, D.J.M., M.A.C., and M.G.R.; resources, D.J.M. and M.G.R.; writing—original draft preparation, D.J.M.; writing—review and editing, M.A.C. and M.G.R.; visualization, D.J.M. and M.G.R.; supervision, M.A.C. and M.G.R.; project administration, M.A.C. and M.G.R.; funding acquisition, M.G.R. All authors reviewed and edited the references. All authors have read and agreed to the published version of the manuscript.

Funding: This research was funded by the American Heart Association, grant number 18AIREA33990023. MGR and DJM were also funded by startup funds and a student research publication grant, respectively, provided by the Central Michigan University College of Medicine.

Acknowledgments: We thank Timothy Kern for his feedback during writing the manuscript. We apologize to authors of other important studies that were not included in this review because of space limitations.

Conflicts of Interest: The authors declare no conflict of interest.

References

1. Saeedi, P.; Petersohn, I.; Salpea, P.; Malanda, B.; Karuranga, S.; Unwin, N.; Colagiuri, S.; Guariguata, L.; Motala, A.A.; Ogurtsova, K.; et al. Global and regional diabetes prevalence estimates for 2019 and projections for 2030 and 2045: Results from the International Diabetes Federation Diabetes Atlas, 9th edition. *Diabetes Res. Clin. Pract.* **2019**, *157*, 107843. [CrossRef] [PubMed]
2. Yau, J.W.Y.; Rogers, S.L.; Kawasaki, R.; Lamoureux, E.L.; Kowalski, J.W.; Bek, T.; Chen, S.J.; Dekker, J.M.; Fletcher, A.; Grauslund, J.; et al. Global Prevalence and Major Risk Factors of Diabetic Retinopathy. *Diabetes Care* **2012**, *35*, 556–564. [CrossRef] [PubMed]
3. Klein, R.; Knudtson, M.D.; Lee, K.E.; Gangnon, R.; Klein, B.E.K. The Wisconsin Epidemiologic Study of Diabetic Retinopathy: XXII the twenty-five-year progression of retinopathy in persons with type 1 diabetes. *Ophthalmology* **2008**, *115*, 1859–1868. [CrossRef] [PubMed]
4. Hirsch, I.B.; Brownlee, M. Beyond Hemoglobin A1c—Need for Additional Markers of Risk for Diabetic Microvascular Complications. *JAMA* **2010**, *303*, 2291–2292. [CrossRef] [PubMed]
5. Royle, P.; Mistry, H.; Auguste, P.; Shyangdan, D.; Freeman, K.; Lois, N.; Waugh, N. Pan-retinal photocoagulation and other forms of laser treatment and drug therapies for non-proliferative diabetic retinopathy: Systematic review and economic evaluation. *Health Technol. Assess.* **2015**, *19*, 1–247. [CrossRef]
6. Antonetti, D.A.; Klein, R.; Gardner, T.W. Diabetic retinopathy. *N. Engl. J. Med.* **2012**, *366*, 1227–1239. [CrossRef]
7. Antonetti, D.A.; Barber, A.J.; Khin, S.; Lieth, E.; Tarbell, J.M.; Gardner, T.W. Vascular Permeability in Experimental Diabetes Is Associated With Reduced Endothelial Occludin Content: Vascular endothelial growth factor decreases occludin in retinal endothelial cells. Penn State Retina Research Group. *Diabetes* **1998**, *47*, 1953–1959. [CrossRef]
8. Roy, S.; Maiello, M.; Lorenzi, M. Increased expression of basement membrane collagen in human diabetic retinopathy. *J. Clin. Investig.* **1994**, *93*, 438–442. [CrossRef]
9. Biallosterski, C.; Van Velthoven, M.E.J.; Michels, R.P.J.; Schlingemann, R.O.; Devries, J.H.; Verbraak, F.D. Decreased optical coherence tomography-measured pericentral retinal thickness in patients with diabetes mellitus type 1 with minimal diabetic retinopathy. *Br. J. Ophthalmol.* **2007**, *91*, 1135–1138. [CrossRef]
10. Van Dijk, H.W.; Kok, P.H.B.; Garvin, M.; Sonka, M.; Devries, J.H.; Michels, R.P.J.; Van Velthoven, M.E.J.; Schlingemann, R.O.; Verbraak, F.D.; AbraMoff, M.D. Selective Loss of Inner Retinal Layer Thickness in Type 1 Diabetic Patients with Minimal Diabetic Retinopathy. *Investig. Opthalmol. Vis. Sci.* **2009**, *50*, 340–3409. [CrossRef]
11. Simo, R.; Hernandez, C.; European Consortium for the Early Treatment of Diabetic Retinopathy (EUROCONDOR). Neurodegeneration is an early event in diabetic retinopathy: Therapeutic implications. *Br. J. Ophthalmol.* **2012**, *96*, 1285–1290. [CrossRef] [PubMed]
12. Vujosevic, S.; Midena, E. Retinal Layers Changes in Human Preclinical and Early Clinical Diabetic Retinopathy Support Early Retinal Neuronal and Müller Cells Alterations. *J. Diabetes Res.* **2013**, *2013*, 905058. [CrossRef]
13. Yang, J.H.; Kwak, H.W.; Kim, T.G.; Han, J.; Moon, S.W.; Yu, S.Y. Retinal Neurodegeneration in Type II Diabetic Otsuka Long-Evans Tokushima Fatty Rats. *Investig. Opthalmol. Vis. Sci.* **2013**, *54*, 3844–3851. [CrossRef] [PubMed]
14. Wolter, J.R. Diabetic Retinopathy. *Am. J. Ophthalmol.* **1961**, *51*, 1123/1251–1141/1269. [CrossRef]
15. Barber, A.J.; Lieth, E.; Khin, S.A.; Antonetti, D.A.; Buchanan, A.G.; Gardner, T.W. Neural apoptosis in the retina during experimental and human diabetes. Early onset and effect of insulin. *J. Clin. Investig.* **1998**, *102*, 783–791. [CrossRef]
16. Sokol, S.; Moskowitz, A.; Skarf, B.; Evans, R.; Molitch, M.; Senior, B. Contrast Sensitivity in Diabetes with and Without Background Retinopathy. *Arch. Ophthalmol.* **1985**, *103*, 51–54. [CrossRef] [PubMed]
17. Roy, M.S.; Gunkel, R.D.; Podgor, M.J. Color Vision Defects in Early Diabetic Retinopathy. *Arch. Ophthalmol.* **1986**, *104*, 225–228. [CrossRef] [PubMed]

18. Cho, N.-C. Selective Loss of S-Cones in Diabetic Retinopathy. *Arch. Ophthalmol.* **2000**, *118*, 1393–1400. [CrossRef] [PubMed]
19. Wachtmeister, L. Oscillatory potentials in the retina: What do they reveal. *Prog. Retin Eye Res.* **1998**, *17*, 485–521. [CrossRef]
20. Bresnick, G.H.; Korth, K.; Groo, A.; Palta, M. Electroretinographic oscillatory potentials predict progression of diabetic retinopathy. Preliminary report. *Arch. Ophthalmol.* **1984**, *102*, 1307–1311. [CrossRef] [PubMed]
21. Coupland, S.G. A comparison of oscillatory potential and pattern electroretinogram measures in diabetic retinopathy. *Doc. Ophthalmol.* **1987**, *66*, 207–218. [CrossRef] [PubMed]
22. Iadecola, C. Neurovascular regulation in the normal brain and in Alzheimer's disease. *Nat. Rev. Neurosci.* **2004**, *5*, 347–360. [CrossRef] [PubMed]
23. Metea, M.R.; Newman, E.A. Signalling within the neurovascular unit in the mammalian retina. *Exp. Physiol.* **2007**, *92*, 635–640. [CrossRef]
24. Bilimoria, P.M.; Stevens, B. Microglia function during brain development: New insights from animal models. *Brain Res.* **2015**, *1617*, 7–17. [CrossRef]
25. Koehler, R.C.; Gebremedhin, D.; Harder, D.R. Role of astrocytes in cerebrovascular regulation. *J. Appl. Physiol.* **2006**, *100*, 307–317. [CrossRef]
26. Kurihara, T. Development and pathological changes of neurovascular unit regulated by hypoxia response in the retina. *Prog. Brain Res.* **2016**, *225*, 201–211. [CrossRef]
27. Gardner, T.W.; Davila, J.R. The neurovascular unit and the pathophysiologic basis of diabetic retinopathy. *Graefes Arch. Clin. Exp. Ophthalmol.* **2017**, *255*, 1–6. [CrossRef]
28. Kowluru, R.A.; Chan, P.S. Oxidative stress and diabetic retinopathy. *Exp. Diabetes Res.* **2007**, *2007*, 43603. [CrossRef]
29. Hammes, H.P. Diabetic retinopathy: Hyperglycaemia, oxidative stress and beyond. *Diabetologia* **2018**, *61*, 29–38. [CrossRef]
30. Kim, J.A.; Wei, Y.; Sowers, J.R. Role of mitochondrial dysfunction in insulin resistance. *Circ. Res.* **2008**, *102*, 401–414. [CrossRef] [PubMed]
31. Sivitz, W.I.; Yorek, M.A. Mitochondrial dysfunction in diabetes: From molecular mechanisms to functional significance and therapeutic opportunities. *Antioxid. Redox Signal.* **2010**, *12*, 537–577. [CrossRef]
32. Du, X.L.; Edelstein, D.; Rossetti, L.; Fantus, I.G.; Goldberg, H.; Ziyadeh, F.; Wu, J.; Brownlee, M. Hyperglycemia-induced mitochondrial superoxide overproduction activates the hexosamine pathway and induces plasminogen activator inhibitor-1 expression by increasing Sp1 glycosylation. *Proc. Natl. Acad. Sci. USA* **2000**, *97*, 12222–12226. [CrossRef] [PubMed]
33. Nishikawa, T.; Edelstein, D.; Du, X.L.; Yamagishi, S.-I.; Matsumura, T.; Kaneda, Y.; Yorek, M.A.; Beebe, D.; Oates, P.J.; Hammes, H.-P.; et al. Normalizing mitochondrial superoxide production blocks three pathways of hyperglycaemic damage. *Nature* **2000**, *404*, 787–790. [CrossRef] [PubMed]
34. Du, Y.; Veenstra, A.; Palczewski, K.; Kern, T.S. Photoreceptor cells are major contributors to diabetes-induced oxidative stress and local inflammation in the retina. *Proc. Natl. Acad. Sci. USA* **2013**, *110*, 16586–16591. [CrossRef] [PubMed]
35. Tonade, D.; Liu, H.; Kern, T.S. Photoreceptor Cells Produce Inflammatory Mediators That Contribute to Endothelial Cell Death in Diabetes. *Investig. Ophthalmol. Vis. Sci.* **2016**, *57*, 4264–4271. [CrossRef]
36. Arden, G.B. The absence of diabetic retinopathy in patients with retinitis pigmentosa: Implications for pathophysiology and possible treatment. *Br. J. Ophthalmol.* **2001**, *85*, 366–370. [CrossRef] [PubMed]
37. De Gooyer, T.E.; Stevenson, K.A.; Humphries, P.; Simpson, D.A.C.; Gardiner, T.A.; Stitt, A.W. Retinopathy Is Reduced during Experimental Diabetes in a Mouse Model of Outer Retinal Degeneration. *Investig. Opthalmol. Vis. Sci.* **2006**, *47*, 5561–5568. [CrossRef] [PubMed]
38. Jezek, P.; Holendova, B.; Plecita-Hlavata, L. Redox Signaling from Mitochondria: Signal Propagation and Its Targets. *Biomolecules* **2020**, *10*, 93. [CrossRef] [PubMed]
39. Bock, F.J.; Tait, S.W.G. Mitochondria as multifaceted regulators of cell death. *Nat. Rev. Mol. Cell Biol.* **2020**, *21*, 85–100. [CrossRef]
40. Yu-Wai-Man, P.; Newman, N.J. Inherited eye-related disorders due to mitochondrial dysfunction. *Hum. Mol. Genet.* **2017**, *26*, R12–R20. [CrossRef]
41. Hoegger, M.J.; Lieven, C.J.; Levin, L.A. Differential production of superoxide by neuronal mitochondria. *BMC Neurosci.* **2008**, *9*, 4. [CrossRef] [PubMed]

42. Remor, A.P.; de Matos, F.J.; Ghisoni, K.; da Silva, T.L.; Eidt, G.; Burigo, M.; de Bem, A.F.; Silveira, P.C.; de Leon, A.; Sanchez, M.C.; et al. Differential effects of insulin on peripheral diabetes-related changes in mitochondrial bioenergetics: Involvement of advanced glycosylated end products. *Biochim. Biophys. Acta* **2011**, *1812*, 1460–1471. [CrossRef]
43. Cogan, D.G.; Kuwabara, T. Capillary Shunts in the Pathogenesis of Diabetic Retinopathy. *Diabetes* **1963**, *12*, 293–300. [CrossRef] [PubMed]
44. Mizutani, M.; Kern, T.S.; Lorenzi, M. Accelerated death of retinal microvascular cells in human and experimental diabetic retinopathy. *J. Clin. Investig.* **1996**, *97*, 2883–2890. [CrossRef] [PubMed]
45. Franco, C.A.; Jones, M.L.; Bernabeu, M.O.; Geudens, I.; Mathivet, T.; Rosa, A.; Lopes, F.M.; Lima, A.P.; Ragab, A.; Collins, R.T.; et al. Dynamic Endothelial Cell Rearrangements Drive Developmental Vessel Regression. *PLoS Biol.* **2015**, *13*, e1002125. [CrossRef]
46. Lenard, A.; Daetwyler, S.; Betz, C.; Ellertsdottir, E.; Belting, H.-G.; Huisken, J.; Affolter, M. Endothelial Cell Self-fusion during Vascular Pruning. *PLoS Biol.* **2015**, *13*, e1002126. [CrossRef]
47. Cogan, D.G.; Kuwabara, T. The Mural Cell in Perspective. *Arch. Ophthalmol.* **1967**, *78*, 133–139. [CrossRef]
48. Pfister, F.; Feng, Y.; vom Hagen, F.; Hoffmann, S.; Molema, G.; Hillebrands, J.L.; Shani, M.; Deutsch, U.; Hammes, H.P. Pericyte migration: A novel mechanism of pericyte loss in experimental diabetic retinopathy. *Diabetes* **2008**, *57*, 2495–2502. [CrossRef]
49. Warmke, N.; Griffin, K.J.; Cubbon, R.M. Pericytes in diabetes-associated vascular disease. *J. Diabetes Complicat.* **2016**, *30*, 1643–1650. [CrossRef]
50. Valdez, C.N.; Arboleda-Velasquez, J.F.; Amarnani, D.S.; Kim, L.A.; D'Amore, P.A. Retinal Microangiopathy in a Mouse Model of Inducible Mural Cell Loss. *Am. J. Pathol.* **2014**, *184*, 2618–2626. [CrossRef]
51. Hammes, H.-P.; Feng, Y.; Pfister, F.; Brownlee, M. Diabetic Retinopathy: Targeting Vasoregression. *Diabetes* **2011**, *60*, 9–16. [CrossRef] [PubMed]
52. Santos, G.S.P.; Prazeres, P.; Mintz, A.; Birbrair, A. Role of pericytes in the retina. *Eye* **2018**, *32*, 483–486. [CrossRef] [PubMed]
53. Nilsson, M.; von Wendt, G.; Wanger, P.; Martin, L. Early detection of macular changes in patients with diabetes using Rarebit Fovea Test and optical coherence tomography. *Br. J. Ophthalmol.* **2007**, *91*, 1596–1598. [CrossRef] [PubMed]
54. Valverde, A.M.; Miranda, S.; García-Ramírez, M.; González-Rodriguez, Á.; Hernández, C.; Simó, R. Proapoptotic and survival signaling in the neuroretina at early stages of diabetic retinopathy. *Mol. Vis.* **2013**, *19*, 47–53.
55. Trudeau, K.; Molina, A.J.A.; Guo, W.; Roy, S. High Glucose Disrupts Mitochondrial Morphology in Retinal Endothelial Cells. *Am. J. Pathol.* **2010**, *177*, 447–455. [CrossRef]
56. Kern, T.S.; Barber, A.J. Retinal ganglion cells in diabetes. *J. Physiol.* **2008**, *586*, 4401–4408. [CrossRef] [PubMed]
57. Gastinger, M.J.; Singh, R.S.J.; Barber, A.J. Loss of Cholinergic and Dopaminergic Amacrine Cells in Streptozotocin-Diabetic Rat and Ins2Akita-Diabetic Mouse Retinas. *Investig. Opthalmol. Vis. Sci.* **2006**, *47*, 3143–3150. [CrossRef] [PubMed]
58. Szabo, K.; Enzsoly, A.; Dekany, B.; Szabo, A.; Hajdu, R.I.; Radovits, T.; Matyas, C.; Olah, A.; Laurik, L.K.; Somfai, G.M.; et al. Histological Evaluation of Diabetic Neurodegeneration in the Retina of Zucker Diabetic Fatty (ZDF) Rats. *Sci. Rep.* **2017**, *7*, 8891. [CrossRef]
59. Rodrigues, E.B.; Urias, M.G.; Penha, F.M.; Badaro, E.; Novais, E.; Meirelles, R.; Farah, M.E. Diabetes induces changes in neuroretina before retinal vessels: A spectral-domain optical coherence tomography study. *Int. J. Retina Vitreous* **2015**, *1*, 4. [CrossRef]
60. Barber, A.J.; Gardner, T.W.; Abcouwer, S.F. The Significance of Vascular and Neural Apoptosis to the Pathology of Diabetic Retinopathy. *Investig. Opthalmol. Vis. Sci.* **2011**, *52*, 1156–1163. [CrossRef]
61. Enzsoly, A.; Szabo, A.; Kantor, O.; David, C.; Szalay, P.; Szabo, K.; Szel, A.; Nemeth, J.; Lukats, A. Pathologic alterations of the outer retina in streptozotocin-induced diabetes. *Investig. Opthalmol. Vis. Sci.* **2014**, *55*, 3686–3699. [CrossRef] [PubMed]
62. Hombrebueno, J.R.; Chen, M.; Penalva, R.G.; Xu, H. Loss of synaptic connectivity, particularly in second order neurons is a key feature of diabetic retinal neuropathy in the Ins2Akita mouse. *PLoS ONE* **2014**, *9*, e97970. [CrossRef] [PubMed]

63. Zarebska, A.; Czerny, K.; Bakiera, K.; Cichacz-Kwiatkowska, B.; Lis-Sochocka, M.; Kis, G.; Wojtowicz, Z. Histological changes in the retina in experimental alloxan-induced diabetes in rabbits. *Ann. Univ. Mariae Curie Sklodowska Med.* **2001**, *56*, 81–84. [PubMed]
64. Alvarez, Y.; Chen, K.; Reynolds, A.L.; Waghorne, N.; O'Connor, J.J.; Kennedy, B.N. Predominant cone photoreceptor dysfunction in a hyperglycaemic model of non-proliferative diabetic retinopathy. *Dis. Model. Mech.* **2010**, *3*, 236–245. [CrossRef]
65. Shin, H.J.; Chung, H.; Kim, H.C. Association between integrity of foveal photoreceptor layer and visual outcome in retinal vein occlusion. *Acta Ophthalmol.* **2011**, *89*, e35–e40. [CrossRef]
66. Forooghian, F.; Stetson, P.F.; Meyer, S.A.; Chew, E.Y.; Wong, W.T.; Cukras, C.; Meyerle, C.B.; Ferris, F.L., 3rd. Relationship between photoreceptor outer segment length and visual acuity in diabetic macular edema. *Retina* **2010**, *30*, 63–70. [CrossRef]
67. Ito, S.; Miyamoto, N.; Ishida, K.; Kurimoto, Y. Association between external limiting membrane status and visual acuity in diabetic macular oedema. *Br. J. Ophthalmol.* **2013**, *97*, 228–232. [CrossRef]
68. Park, S.H.; Park, J.W.; Park, S.J.; Kim, K.Y.; Chung, J.W.; Chun, M.H.; Oh, S.J. Apoptotic death of photoreceptors in the streptozotocin-induced diabetic rat retina. *Diabetologia* **2003**, *46*, 1260–1268. [CrossRef]
69. Ottlecz, A.; Bensaoula, T. Captopril ameliorates the decreased Na+,K(+)-ATPase activity in the retina of streptozotocin-induced diabetic rats. *Investig. Ophthalmol. Vis. Sci.* **1996**, *37*, 1633–1641.
70. Ottlecz, A.; Garcia, C.A.; Eichberg, J.; Fox, D.A. Alterations in retinal Na+, K(+)-ATPase in diabetes: Streptozotocin-induced and Zucker diabetic fatty rats. *Curr. Eye Res.* **1993**, *12*, 1111–1121. [CrossRef]
71. Phipps, J.A.; Fletcher, E.L.; Vingrys, A.J. Paired-flash identification of rod and cone dysfunction in the diabetic rat. *Investig. Ophthalmol. Vis. Sci.* **2004**, *45*, 4592–4600. [CrossRef]
72. Kern, T.S.; Berkowitz, B.A. Photoreceptors in diabetic retinopathy. *J. Diabetes Investig.* **2015**, *6*, 371–380. [CrossRef] [PubMed]
73. Country, M.W. Retinal metabolism: A comparative look at energetics in the retina. *Brain Res.* **2017**, *1672*, 50–57. [CrossRef]
74. Tang, P.H.; Kono, M.; Koutalos, Y.; Ablonczy, Z.; Crouch, R.K. New insights into retinoid metabolism and cycling within the retina. *Prog. Retin Eye Res.* **2013**, *32*, 48–63. [CrossRef]
75. Kolesnikov, A.V.; Ala-Laurila, P.; Shukolyukov, S.A.; Crouch, R.K.; Wiggert, B.; Estevez, M.E.; Govardovskii, V.I.; Cornwall, M.C. Visual cycle and its metabolic support in gecko photoreceptors. *Vision Res.* **2007**, *47*, 363–374. [CrossRef] [PubMed]
76. LaVail, M.M. Rod outer segment disk shedding in rat retina: Relationship to cyclic lighting. *Science* **1976**, *194*, 1071–1074. [CrossRef] [PubMed]
77. Wang, X.; Iannaccone, A.; Jablonski, M.M. Contribution of Muller cells toward the regulation of photoreceptor outer segment assembly. *Neuron Glia Biol.* **2005**, *1*, 1–6. [CrossRef] [PubMed]
78. Jablonski, M.M.; Iannaccone, A. Targeted disruption of Muller cell metabolism induces photoreceptor dysmorphogenesis. *Glia* **2000**, *32*, 192–204. [CrossRef]
79. Hurley, J.B. Warburg's vision. *Elife* **2017**, *6*, e29217. [CrossRef]
80. Rueda, E.M.; Johnson, J.E., Jr.; Giddabasappa, A.; Swaroop, A.; Brooks, M.J.; Sigel, I.; Chaney, S.Y.; Fox, D.A. The cellular and compartmental profile of mouse retinal glycolysis, tricarboxylic acid cycle, oxidative phosphorylation, and ~P transferring kinases. *Mol. Vis.* **2016**, *22*, 847–885.
81. Mitchell, P. Chemiosmotic coupling in oxidative and photosynthetic phosphorylation. 1966. *Biochim. Biophys. Acta* **2011**, *1807*, 1507–1538. [CrossRef] [PubMed]
82. Du, J.; Rountree, A.; Cleghorn, W.M.; Contreras, L.; Lindsay, K.J.; Sadilek, M.; Gu, H.; Djukovic, D.; Raftery, D.; Satrústegui, J.; et al. Phototransduction Influences Metabolic Flux and Nucleotide Metabolism in Mouse Retina. *J. Biol. Chem.* **2016**, *291*, 4698–4710. [CrossRef] [PubMed]
83. Linsenmeier, R.A. Effects of light and darkness on oxygen distribution and consumption in the cat retina. *J. Gen. Physiol.* **1986**, *88*, 521–542. [CrossRef] [PubMed]
84. Ames, A., 3rd; Li, Y.Y.; Heher, E.C.; Kimble, C.R. Energy metabolism of rabbit retina as related to function: High cost of Na+ transport. *J. Neurosci.* **1992**, *12*, 840–853. [CrossRef]
85. Perezleon, J.A.; Osorio-Paz, I.; Francois, L.; Salceda, R. Immunohistochemical localization of glycogen synthase and GSK3beta: Control of glycogen content in retina. *Neurochem. Res.* **2013**, *38*, 1063–1069. [CrossRef]

86. Winkler, B.S.; Arnold, M.J.; Brassell, M.A.; Puro, D.G. Energy metabolism in human retinal Muller cells. *Investig. Ophthalmol. Vis. Sci.* **2000**, *41*, 3183–3190.
87. Toft-Kehler, A.K.; Skytt, D.M.; Svare, A.; Lefevere, E.; Van Hove, I.; Moons, L.; Waagepetersen, H.S.; Kolko, M. Mitochondrial function in Müller cells—Does it matter? *Mitochondrion* **2017**, *36*, 43–51. [CrossRef]
88. Tsacopoulos, M.; Poitry-Yamate, C.L.; MacLeish, P.R.; Poitry, S. Trafficking of molecules and metabolic signals in the retina. *Prog. Retin Eye Res.* **1998**, *17*, 429–442. [CrossRef]
89. Puchalska, P.; Crawford, P.A. Multi-dimensional Roles of Ketone Bodies in Fuel Metabolism, Signaling, and Therapeutics. *Cell Metab.* **2017**, *25*, 262–284. [CrossRef]
90. Bayeva, M.; Sawicki, K.T.; Ardehali, H. Taking diabetes to heart–deregulation of myocardial lipid metabolism in diabetic cardiomyopathy. *J. Am. Heart Assoc.* **2013**, *2*, e000433. [CrossRef]
91. Muoio, D.M. Metabolic inflexibility: When mitochondrial indecision leads to metabolic gridlock. *Cell* **2014**, *159*, 1253–1262. [CrossRef] [PubMed]
92. Joyal, J.S.; Sun, Y.; Gantner, M.L.; Shao, Z.; Evans, L.P.; Saba, N.; Fredrick, T.; Burnim, S.; Kim, J.S.; Patel, G.; et al. Retinal lipid and glucose metabolism dictates angiogenesis through the lipid sensor Ffar1. *Nat. Med.* **2016**, *22*, 439–445. [CrossRef] [PubMed]
93. Tyni, T.; Johnson, M.; Eaton, S.; Pourfarzam, M.; Andrews, R.; Turnbull, D.M. Mitochondrial fatty acid beta-oxidation in the retinal pigment epithelium. *Pediatr. Res.* **2002**, *52*, 595–600. [CrossRef] [PubMed]
94. Atsuzawa, K.; Nakazawa, A.; Mizutani, K.; Fukasawa, M.; Yamamoto, N.; Hashimoto, T.; Usuda, N. Immunohistochemical localization of mitochondrial fatty acid beta-oxidation enzymes in Muller cells of the retina. *Histochem. Cell. Biol.* **2010**, *134*, 565–579. [CrossRef] [PubMed]
95. Fletcher, A.L.; Pennesi, M.E.; Harding, C.O.; Weleber, R.G.; Gillingham, M.B. Observations regarding retinopathy in mitochondrial trifunctional protein deficiencies. *Mol. Genet. Metab.* **2012**, *106*, 18–24. [CrossRef]
96. Pearsall, E.A.; Cheng, R.; Matsuzaki, S.; Zhou, K.; Ding, L.; Ahn, B.; Kinter, M.; Humphries, K.M.; Quiambao, A.B.; Farjo, R.A.; et al. Neuroprotective effects of PPARalpha in retinopathy of type 1 diabetes. *PLoS ONE* **2019**, *14*, e0208399. [CrossRef]
97. Group, A.S.; Group, A.E.S.; Chew, E.Y.; Ambrosius, W.T.; Davis, M.D.; Danis, R.P.; Gangaputra, S.; Greven, C.M.; Hubbard, L.; Esser, B.A.; et al. Effects of medical therapies on retinopathy progression in type 2 diabetes. *N. Engl. J. Med.* **2010**, *363*, 233–244. [CrossRef]
98. Keech, A.C.; Mitchell, P.; Summanen, P.A.; O'Day, J.; Davis, T.M.; Moffitt, M.S.; Taskinen, M.R.; Simes, R.J.; Tse, D.; Williamson, E.; et al. Effect of fenofibrate on the need for laser treatment for diabetic retinopathy (FIELD study): A randomised controlled trial. *Lancet* **2007**, *370*, 1687–1697. [CrossRef]
99. Schoors, S.; Bruning, U.; Missiaen, R.; Queiroz, K.C.; Borgers, G.; Elia, I.; Zecchin, A.; Cantelmo, A.R.; Christen, S.; Goveia, J.; et al. Fatty acid carbon is essential for dNTP synthesis in endothelial cells. *Nature* **2015**, *520*, 192–197. [CrossRef]
100. Masser, D.R.; Otalora, L.; Clark, N.W.; Kinter, M.T.; Elliott, M.H.; Freeman, W.M. Functional changes in the neural retina occur in the absence of mitochondrial dysfunction in a rodent model of diabetic retinopathy. *J. Neurochem.* **2017**, *143*, 595–608. [CrossRef]
101. Lopaschuk, G.D. Fatty Acid Oxidation and Its Relation with Insulin Resistance and Associated Disorders. *Ann. Nutr. Metab.* **2016**, *68* (Suppl. 3), 15–20. [CrossRef]
102. Swarup, A.; Samuels, I.S.; Bell, B.A.; Han, J.Y.S.; Du, J.; Massenzio, E.; Abel, E.D.; Boesze-Battaglia, K.; Peachey, N.S.; Philp, N.J. Modulating GLUT1 expression in retinal pigment epithelium decreases glucose levels in the retina: Impact on photoreceptors and Muller glial cells. *Am. J. Physiol. Cell Physiol.* **2019**, *316*, C121–C133. [CrossRef]
103. Sanchez-Chavez, G.; Pena-Rangel, M.T.; Riesgo-Escovar, J.R.; Martinez-Martinez, A.; Salceda, R. Insulin stimulated-glucose transporter Glut 4 is expressed in the retina. *PLoS ONE* **2012**, *7*, e52959. [CrossRef] [PubMed]
104. Itoh, Y.; Kawamata, Y.; Harada, M.; Kobayashi, M.; Fujii, R.; Fukusumi, S.; Ogi, K.; Hosoya, M.; Tanaka, Y.; Uejima, H.; et al. Free fatty acids regulate insulin secretion from pancreatic beta cells through GPR40. *Nature* **2003**, *422*, 173–176. [CrossRef] [PubMed]
105. Falomir-Lockhart, L.J.; Cavazzutti, G.F.; Gimenez, E.; Toscani, A.M. Fatty Acid Signaling Mechanisms in Neural Cells: Fatty Acid Receptors. *Front. Cell Neurosci.* **2019**, *13*, 162. [CrossRef] [PubMed]

106. Pan, Y.; Mansfield, K.D.; Bertozzi, C.C.; Rudenko, V.; Chan, D.A.; Giaccia, A.J.; Simon, M.C. Multiple factors affecting cellular redox status and energy metabolism modulate hypoxia-inducible factor prolyl hydroxylase activity in vivo and in vitro. *Mol. Cell Biol.* **2007**, *27*, 912–925. [CrossRef] [PubMed]
107. Germer, A.; Biedermann, B.; Wolburg, H.; Schuck, J.; Grosche, J.; Kuhrt, H.; Reichelt, W.; Schousboe, A.; Paasche, G.; Mack, A.F.; et al. Distribution of mitochondria within Muller cells–I. Correlation with retinal vascularization in different mammalian species. *J. Neurocytol.* **1998**, *27*, 329–345. [CrossRef]
108. Stone, J.; van Driel, D.; Valter, K.; Rees, S.; Provis, J. The locations of mitochondria in mammalian photoreceptors: Relation to retinal vasculature. *Brain Res.* **2008**, *1189*, 58–69. [CrossRef]
109. Osorio-Paz, I.; Uribe-Carvajal, S.; Salceda, R. In the Early Stages of Diabetes, Rat Retinal Mitochondria Undergo Mild Uncoupling due to UCP2 Activity. *PLoS ONE* **2015**, *10*, e0122727. [CrossRef]
110. Han, W.H.; Gotzmann, J.; Kuny, S.; Huang, H.; Chan, C.B.; Lemieux, H.; Sauve, Y. Modifications in Retinal Mitochondrial Respiration Precede Type 2 Diabetes and Protracted Microvascular Retinopathy. *Investig. Ophthalmol. Vis. Sci.* **2017**, *58*, 3826–3839. [CrossRef]
111. Kowluru, R.A.; Mishra, M.; Kowluru, A.; Kumar, B. Hyperlipidemia and the development of diabetic retinopathy: Comparison between type 1 and type 2 animal models. *Metabolism* **2016**, *65*, 1570–1581. [CrossRef] [PubMed]
112. Kanwar, M.; Chan, P.S.; Kern, T.S.; Kowluru, R.A. Oxidative damage in the retinal mitochondria of diabetic mice: Possible protection by superoxide dismutase. *Investig. Ophthalmol. Vis. Sci.* **2007**, *48*, 3805–3811. [CrossRef] [PubMed]
113. Madsen-Bouterse, S.A.; Mohammad, G.; Kanwar, M.; Kowluru, R.A. Role of mitochondrial DNA damage in the development of diabetic retinopathy, and the metabolic memory phenomenon associated with its progression. *Antioxid. Redox Signal.* **2010**, *13*, 797–805. [CrossRef] [PubMed]
114. Santos, J.M.; Tewari, S.; Kowluru, R.A. A compensatory mechanism protects retinal mitochondria from initial insult in diabetic retinopathy. *Free Radic. Biol. Med.* **2012**, *53*, 1729–1737. [CrossRef] [PubMed]
115. Wang, H.; Zheng, Z.; Gong, Y.; Zhu, B.; Xu, X. U83836E inhibits retinal neurodegeneration in early-stage streptozotocin-induced diabetic rats. *Ophthalmic Res.* **2011**, *46*, 19–24. [CrossRef] [PubMed]
116. Fan, Y.; Lai, J.; Yuan, Y.; Wang, L.; Wang, Q.; Yuan, F. Taurine Protects Retinal Cells and Improves Synaptic Connections in Early Diabetic Rats. *Curr. Eye Res.* **2020**, *45*, 52–63. [CrossRef]
117. Li, X.; Zhang, M.; Zhou, H. The morphological features and mitochondrial oxidative stress mechanism of the retinal neurons apoptosis in early diabetic rats. *J. Diabetes Res.* **2014**, *2014*, 678123. [CrossRef]
118. Chang, J.Y.; Yu, F.; Shi, L.; Ko, M.L.; Ko, G.Y. Melatonin Affects Mitochondrial Fission/Fusion Dynamics in the Diabetic Retina. *J. Diabetes Res.* **2019**, *2019*, 8463125. [CrossRef]
119. Devi, T.S.; Lee, I.; Huttemann, M.; Kumar, A.; Nantwi, K.D.; Singh, L.P. TXNIP links innate host defense mechanisms to oxidative stress and inflammation in retinal Muller glia under chronic hyperglycemia: Implications for diabetic retinopathy. *Exp. Diabetes Res.* **2012**, *2012*, 438238. [CrossRef]
120. Devi, T.S.; Somayajulu, M.; Kowluru, R.A.; Singh, L.P. TXNIP regulates mitophagy in retinal Muller cells under high-glucose conditions: Implications for diabetic retinopathy. *Cell Death Dis.* **2017**, *8*, e2777. [CrossRef]
121. Hombrebueno, J.R.; Cairns, L.; Dutton, L.R.; Lyons, T.J.; Brazil, D.P.; Moynagh, P.; Curtis, T.M.; Xu, H. Uncoupled turnover disrupts mitochondrial quality control in diabetic retinopathy. *JCI Insight* **2019**, *4*, e129760. [CrossRef] [PubMed]
122. Krugel, K.; Wurm, A.; Pannicke, T.; Hollborn, M.; Karl, A.; Wiedemann, P.; Reichenbach, A.; Kohen, L.; Bringmann, A. Involvement of oxidative stress and mitochondrial dysfunction in the osmotic swelling of retinal glial cells from diabetic rats. *Exp. Eye Res.* **2011**, *92*, 87–93. [CrossRef] [PubMed]
123. Tien, T.; Zhang, J.; Muto, T.; Kim, D.; Sarthy, V.P.; Roy, S. High Glucose Induces Mitochondrial Dysfunction in Retinal Muller Cells: Implications for Diabetic Retinopathy. *Investig. Ophthalmol. Vis. Sci.* **2017**, *58*, 2915–2921. [CrossRef] [PubMed]
124. Zhou, P.; Xie, W.; Meng, X.; Zhai, Y.; Dong, X.; Zhang, X.; Sun, G.; Sun, X. Notoginsenoside R1 Ameliorates Diabetic Retinopathy through PINK1-Dependent Activation of Mitophagy. *Cells* **2019**, *8*, 213. [CrossRef] [PubMed]
125. Mishra, M.; Kowluru, R.A. DNA Methylation-a Potential Source of Mitochondria DNA Base Mismatch in the Development of Diabetic Retinopathy. *Mol. Neurobiol.* **2019**, *56*, 88–101. [CrossRef] [PubMed]
126. Mohammad, G.; Duraisamy, A.J.; Kowluru, A.; Kowluru, R.A. Functional Regulation of an Oxidative Stress Mediator, Rac1, in Diabetic Retinopathy. *Mol. Neurobiol.* **2019**, *56*, 8643–8655. [CrossRef]

127. Santos, J.M.; Kowluru, R.A. Role of mitochondria biogenesis in the metabolic memory associated with the continued progression of diabetic retinopathy and its regulation by lipoic acid. *Investig. Ophthalmol. Vis. Sci.* **2011**, *52*, 8791–8798. [CrossRef]
128. Santos, J.M.; Kowluru, R.A. Impaired transport of mitochondrial transcription factor A (TFAM) and the metabolic memory phenomenon associated with the progression of diabetic retinopathy. *Diabetes Metab.Res. Rev.* **2013**, *29*, 204–213. [CrossRef]
129. Santos, J.M.; Tewari, S.; Goldberg, A.F.; Kowluru, R.A. Mitochondrial biogenesis and the development of diabetic retinopathy. *Free Radic. Biol. Med.* **2011**, *51*, 1849–1860. [CrossRef]
130. Schulze, P.C.; Yoshioka, J.; Takahashi, T.; He, Z.; King, G.L.; Lee, R.T. Hyperglycemia promotes oxidative stress through inhibition of thioredoxin function by thioredoxin-interacting protein. *J. Biol. Chem.* **2004**, *279*, 30369–30374. [CrossRef]
131. Zou, Y.L.; Luo, W.B.; Xie, L.; Mao, X.B.; Wu, C.; You, Z.P. Targeting human 8-oxoguanine DNA glycosylase to mitochondria protects cells from high glucose-induced apoptosis. *Endocrine* **2018**, *60*, 445–457. [CrossRef] [PubMed]
132. Zhu, H.; Zhang, W.; Zhao, Y.; Shu, X.; Wang, W.; Wang, D.; Yang, Y.; He, Z.; Wang, X.; Ying, Y. GSK3beta-mediated tau hyperphosphorylation triggers diabetic retinal neurodegeneration by disrupting synaptic and mitochondrial functions. *Mol. Neurodegener.* **2018**, *13*, 62. [CrossRef] [PubMed]
133. Liu, W.Y.; Liou, S.S.; Hong, T.Y.; Liu, I.M. Protective Effects of Hesperidin (Citrus Flavonone) on High Glucose Induced Oxidative Stress and Apoptosis in a Cellular Model for Diabetic Retinopathy. *Nutrients* **2017**, *9*, 1312. [CrossRef] [PubMed]
134. Kowluru, R.A.; Mishra, M.; Kumar, B. Diabetic retinopathy and transcriptional regulation of a small molecular weight G-Protein, Rac1. *Exp. Eye Res.* **2016**, *147*, 72–77. [CrossRef] [PubMed]
135. Devi, T.S.; Hosoya, K.; Terasaki, T.; Singh, L.P. Critical role of TXNIP in oxidative stress, DNA damage and retinal pericyte apoptosis under high glucose: Implications for diabetic retinopathy. *Exp. Cell Res.* **2013**, *319*, 1001–1012. [CrossRef]
136. Duraisamy, A.J.; Mohammad, G.; Kowluru, R.A. Mitochondrial fusion and maintenance of mitochondrial homeostasis in diabetic retinopathy. *Biochim. Biophys. Acta Mol. Basis Dis.* **2019**, *1865*, 1617–1626. [CrossRef]
137. Leal, E.C.; Aveleira, C.A.; Castilho, A.F.; Serra, A.M.; Baptista, F.I.; Hosoya, K.; Forrester, J.V.; Ambrosio, A.F. High glucose and oxidative/nitrosative stress conditions induce apoptosis in retinal endothelial cells by a caspase-independent pathway. *Exp. Eye Res.* **2009**, *88*, 983–991. [CrossRef]
138. Madsen-Bouterse, S.A.; Zhong, Q.; Mohammad, G.; Ho, Y.S.; Kowluru, R.A. Oxidative damage of mitochondrial DNA in diabetes and its protection by manganese superoxide dismutase. *Free Radic. Res.* **2010**, *44*, 313–321. [CrossRef]
139. Xie, L.; Zhu, X.; Hu, Y.; Li, T.; Gao, Y.; Shi, Y.; Tang, S. Mitochondrial DNA oxidative damage triggering mitochondrial dysfunction and apoptosis in high glucose-induced HRECs. *Investig. Ophthalmol. Vis. Sci.* **2008**, *49*, 4203–4209. [CrossRef]
140. Van Meerloo, J.; Kaspers, G.J.; Cloos, J. Cell sensitivity assays: The MTT assay. *Methods Mol. Biol.* **2011**, *731*, 237–245. [CrossRef]
141. Betteridge, D.J. What is oxidative stress? *Metabolism* **2000**, *49*, 3–8. [CrossRef]
142. Kowluru, R.A. Diabetic retinopathy, metabolic memory and epigenetic modifications. *Vision Res.* **2017**, *139*, 30–38. [CrossRef] [PubMed]
143. Kowluru, R.A.; Tang, J.; Kern, T.S. Abnormalities of retinal metabolism in diabetes and experimental galactosemia. VII. Effect of long-term administration of antioxidants on the development of retinopathy. *Diabetes* **2001**, *50*, 1938–1942. [CrossRef]
144. Kowluru, R.; Kern, T.S.; Engerman, R.L. Abnormalities of retinal metabolism in diabetes or galactosemia. II. Comparison of gamma-glutamyl transpeptidase in retina and cerebral cortex, and effects of antioxidant therapy. *Curr. Eye Res.* **1994**, *13*, 891–896. [CrossRef] [PubMed]
145. Berkowitz, B.A.; Gradianu, M.; Bissig, D.; Kern, T.S.; Roberts, R. Retinal ion regulation in a mouse model of diabetic retinopathy: Natural history and the effect of Cu/Zn superoxide dismutase overexpression. *Investig. Ophthalmol. Vis. Sci.* **2009**, *50*, 2351–2358. [CrossRef] [PubMed]
146. Kowluru, R.A.; Abbas, S.N. Diabetes-induced mitochondrial dysfunction in the retina. *Investig. Ophthalmol. Vis. Sci.* **2003**, *44*, 5327–5334. [CrossRef]

147. Madsen-Bouterse, S.; Mohammad, G.; Kowluru, R.A. Glyceraldehyde-3-phosphate dehydrogenase in retinal microvasculature: Implications for the development and progression of diabetic retinopathy. *Investig. Ophthalmol. Vis. Sci.* **2010**, *51*, 1765–1772. [CrossRef]
148. Lott, M.E.; Slocomb, J.E.; Shivkumar, V.; Smith, B.; Gabbay, R.A.; Quillen, D.; Gardner, T.W.; Bettermann, K. Comparison of retinal vasodilator and constrictor responses in type 2 diabetes. *Acta Ophthalmol.* **2012**, *90*, e434–e441. [CrossRef]
149. Du, Y.; Miller, C.M.; Kern, T.S. Hyperglycemia increases mitochondrial superoxide in retina and retinal cells. *Free Radic. Biol. Med.* **2003**, *35*, 1491–1499. [CrossRef]
150. Adam-Vizi, V. Production of reactive oxygen species in brain mitochondria: Contribution by electron transport chain and non-electron transport chain sources. *Antioxid. Redox. Signal.* **2005**, *7*, 1140–1149. [CrossRef]
151. Murphy, M.P. How mitochondria produce reactive oxygen species. *Biochem. J.* **2009**, *417*, 1–13. [CrossRef] [PubMed]
152. Bek, T. Mitochondrial dysfunction and diabetic retinopathy. *Mitochondrion* **2017**, *36*, 4–6. [CrossRef]
153. Mekala, N.K.; Kurdys, J.; Depuydt, M.M.; Vazquez, E.J.; Rosca, M.G. Apoptosis inducing factor deficiency causes retinal photoreceptor degeneration. The protective role of the redox compound methylene blue. *Redox. Biol.* **2019**, *20*, 107–117. [CrossRef] [PubMed]
154. Austin, S.; Klimcakova, E.; St-Pierre, J. Impact of PGC-1alpha on the topology and rate of superoxide production by the mitochondrial electron transport chain. *Free Radic. Biol. Med.* **2011**, *51*, 2243–2248. [CrossRef] [PubMed]
155. St-Pierre, J.; Buckingham, J.A.; Roebuck, S.J.; Brand, M.D. Topology of superoxide production from different sites in the mitochondrial electron transport chain. *J. Biol. Chem.* **2002**, *277*, 44784–44790. [CrossRef] [PubMed]
156. Rosca, M.G.; Vazquez, E.J.; Chen, Q.; Kerner, J.; Kern, T.S.; Hoppel, C.L. Oxidation of fatty acids is the source of increased mitochondrial reactive oxygen species production in kidney cortical tubules in early diabetes. *Diabetes* **2012**, *61*, 2074–2083. [CrossRef]
157. Ji, L.L.; Gomez-Cabrera, M.C.; Vina, J. Exercise and hormesis: Activation of cellular antioxidant signaling pathway. *Ann. N. Y. Acad. Sci.* **2006**, *1067*, 425–435. [CrossRef]
158. Roy, S.; Kern, T.S.; Song, B.; Stuebe, C. Mechanistic Insights into Pathological Changes in the Diabetic Retina: Implications for Targeting Diabetic Retinopathy. *Am. J. Pathol.* **2017**, *187*, 9–19. [CrossRef]
159. Tang, J.; Kern, T.S. Inflammation in diabetic retinopathy. *Prog. Retin Eye Res.* **2011**, *30*, 343–358. [CrossRef]
160. Tewari, S.; Santos, J.M.; Kowluru, R.A. Damaged mitochondrial DNA replication system and the development of diabetic retinopathy. *Antioxid. Redox. Signal.* **2012**, *17*, 492–504. [CrossRef]
161. Tewari, S.; Zhong, Q.; Santos, J.M.; Kowluru, R.A. Mitochondria DNA replication and DNA methylation in the metabolic memory associated with continued progression of diabetic retinopathy. *Investig. Ophthalmol. Vis. Sci.* **2012**, *53*, 4881–4888. [CrossRef] [PubMed]
162. Smith, J.S.; Brachmann, C.B.; Celic, I.; Kenna, M.A.; Muhammad, S.; Starai, V.J.; Avalos, J.L.; Escalante-Semerena, J.C.; Grubmeyer, C.; Wolberger, C.; et al. A phylogenetically conserved NAD+-dependent protein deacetylase activity in the Sir2 protein family. *Proc. Natl. Acad. Sci. USA* **2000**, *97*, 6658–6663. [CrossRef] [PubMed]
163. Canto, C.; Sauve, A.A.; Bai, P. Crosstalk between poly(ADP-ribose) polymerase and sirtuin enzymes. *Mol. Aspects Med.* **2013**, *34*, 1168–1201. [CrossRef] [PubMed]
164. Lin, J.B.; Kubota, S.; Ban, N.; Yoshida, M.; Santeford, A.; Sene, A.; Nakamura, R.; Zapata, N.; Kubota, M.; Tsubota, K.; et al. NAMPT-Mediated NAD(+) Biosynthesis Is Essential for Vision In Mice. *Cell Rep.* **2016**, *17*, 69–85. [CrossRef]
165. Ido, Y.; Nyengaard, J.R.; Chang, K.; Tilton, R.G.; Kilo, C.; Mylari, B.L.; Oates, P.J.; Williamson, J.R. Early neural and vascular dysfunctions in diabetic rats are largely sequelae of increased sorbitol oxidation. *Antioxid. Redox. Signal.* **2010**, *12*, 39–51. [CrossRef]
166. Williamson, J.R.; Chang, K.; Frangos, M.; Hasan, K.S.; Ido, Y.; Kawamura, T.; Nyengaard, J.R.; van den Enden, M.; Kilo, C.; Tilton, R.G. Hyperglycemic pseudohypoxia and diabetic complications. *Diabetes* **1993**, *42*, 801–813. [CrossRef]
167. Lorenzi, M. The polyol pathway as a mechanism for diabetic retinopathy: Attractive, elusive, and resilient. *Exp. Diabetes Res.* **2007**, *2007*, 61038. [CrossRef]

168. Li, Q.; Hwang, Y.C.; Ananthakrishnan, R.; Oates, P.J.; Guberski, D.; Ramasamy, R. Polyol pathway and modulation of ischemia-reperfusion injury in Type 2 diabetic BBZ rat hearts. *Cardiovasc. Diabetol.* **2008**, *7*, 33. [CrossRef]
169. Obrosova, I.G.; Drel, V.R.; Kumagai, A.K.; Szabo, C.; Pacher, P.; Stevens, M.J. Early diabetes-induced biochemical changes in the retina: Comparison of rat and mouse models. *Diabetologia* **2006**, *49*, 2525–2533. [CrossRef]
170. Tang, J.; Du, Y.; Petrash, J.M.; Sheibani, N.; Kern, T.S. Deletion of aldose reductase from mice inhibits diabetes-induced retinal capillary degeneration and superoxide generation. *PLoS ONE* **2013**, *8*, e62081. [CrossRef]
171. Berthiaume, J.M.; Kurdys, J.G.; Muntean, D.M.; Rosca, M.G. Mitochondrial NAD(+)/NADH Redox State and Diabetic Cardiomyopathy. *Antioxid. Redox Signal.* **2019**, *30*, 375–398. [CrossRef]
172. Diederen, R.M.H.; Starnes, C.A.; Berkowitz, B.A.; Winkler, B.S. Reexamining the Hyperglycemic Pseudohypoxia Hypothesis of Diabetic Oculopathy. *Investig. Ophtal. Vis. Sci.* **2006**, *47*, 2726. [CrossRef] [PubMed]
173. Karamanlidis, G.; Lee, C.F.; Garcia-Menendez, L.; Kolwicz, S.C., Jr.; Suthammarak, W.; Gong, G.; Sedensky, M.M.; Morgan, P.G.; Wang, W.; Tian, R. Mitochondrial complex I deficiency increases protein acetylation and accelerates heart failure. *Cell Metab.* **2013**, *18*, 239–250. [CrossRef] [PubMed]
174. Sung, H.J.; Ma, W.; Wang, P.Y.; Hynes, J.; O'Riordan, T.C.; Combs, C.A.; McCoy, J.P., Jr.; Bunz, F.; Kang, J.G.; Hwang, P.M. Mitochondrial respiration protects against oxygen-associated DNA damage. *Nat. Commun.* **2010**, *1*, 5. [CrossRef] [PubMed]
175. Akie, T.E.; Liu, L.; Nam, M.; Lei, S.; Cooper, M.P. OXPHOS-Mediated Induction of NAD+ Promotes Complete Oxidation of Fatty Acids and Interdicts Non-Alcoholic Fatty Liver Disease. *PLoS ONE* **2015**, *10*, e0125617. [CrossRef]
176. Masutani, M.; Suzuki, H.; Kamada, N.; Watanabe, M.; Ueda, O.; Nozaki, T.; Jishage, K.; Watanabe, T.; Sugimoto, T.; Nakagama, H.; et al. Poly(ADP-ribose) polymerase gene disruption conferred mice resistant to streptozotocin-induced diabetes. *Proc. Natl. Acad. Sci. USA* **1999**, *96*, 2301–2304. [CrossRef]
177. Bai, P.; Canto, C.; Oudart, H.; Brunyanszki, A.; Cen, Y.; Thomas, C.; Yamamoto, H.; Huber, A.; Kiss, B.; Houtkooper, R.H.; et al. PARP-1 inhibition increases mitochondrial metabolism through SIRT1 activation. *Cell Metab.* **2011**, *13*, 461–468. [CrossRef]
178. Mishra, M.; Duraisamy, A.J.; Kowluru, R.A. Sirt1- A Guardian of the Development of Diabetic Retinopathy. *Diabetes* **2018**, *67*, 745–754. [CrossRef]
179. Rydstrom, J. Mitochondrial NADPH, transhydrogenase and disease. *Biochim. Biophys. Acta* **2006**, *1757*, 721–726. [CrossRef]
180. Nickel, A.G.; von Hardenberg, A.; Hohl, M.; Loffler, J.R.; Kohlhaas, M.; Becker, J.; Reil, J.C.; Kazakov, A.; Bonnekoh, J.; Stadelmaier, M.; et al. Reversal of Mitochondrial Transhydrogenase Causes Oxidative Stress in Heart Failure. *Cell Metab.* **2015**, *22*, 472–484. [CrossRef]
181. Fisher-Wellman, K.H.; Lin, C.T.; Ryan, T.E.; Reese, L.R.; Gilliam, L.A.; Cathey, B.L.; Lark, D.S.; Smith, C.D.; Muoio, D.M.; Neufer, P.D. Pyruvate dehydrogenase complex and nicotinamide nucleotide transhydrogenase constitute an energy-consuming redox circuit. *Biochem. J.* **2015**, *467*, 271–280. [CrossRef] [PubMed]
182. Ronchi, J.A.; Francisco, A.; Passos, L.A.; Figueira, T.R.; Castilho, R.F. The Contribution of Nicotinamide Nucleotide Transhydrogenase to Peroxide Detoxification Is Dependent on the Respiratory State and Counterbalanced by Other Sources of NADPH in Liver Mitochondria. *J. Biol. Chem.* **2016**, *291*, 20173–20187. [CrossRef]
183. Ventura-Clapier, R.; Garnier, A.; Veksler, V. Transcriptional control of mitochondrial biogenesis: The central role of PGC-1alpha. *Cardiovasc. Res.* **2008**, *79*, 208–217. [CrossRef] [PubMed]
184. Santos, J.M.; Mishra, M.; Kowluru, R.A. Posttranslational modification of mitochondrial transcription factor A in impaired mitochondria biogenesis: Implications in diabetic retinopathy and metabolic memory phenomenon. *Exp. Eye Res.* **2014**, *121*, 168–177. [CrossRef] [PubMed]
185. Devi, T.S.; Yumnamcha, T.; Yao, F.; Somayajulu, M.; Kowluru, R.A.; Singh, L.P. TXNIP mediates high glucose-induced mitophagic flux and lysosome enlargement in human retinal pigment epithelial cells. *Biol. Open* **2019**, *8*, bio038521. [CrossRef]
186. Santos, J.M.; Mohammad, G.; Zhong, Q.; Kowluru, R.A. Diabetic retinopathy, superoxide damage and antioxidants. *Curr. Pharm. Biotechnol.* **2011**, *12*, 352–361. [CrossRef]

187. Westermann, B. Mitochondrial fusion and fission in cell life and death. *Nat. Rev. Mol. Cell Biol.* **2010**, *11*, 872–884. [CrossRef]
188. Zhong, Q.; Kowluru, R.A. Diabetic retinopathy and damage to mitochondrial structure and transport machinery. *Investig. Ophthalmol. Vis. Sci.* **2011**, *52*, 8739–8746. [CrossRef]
189. Berkowitz, B.A.; Roberts, R.; Luan, H.; Bissig, D.; Bui, B.V.; Gradianu, M.; Calkins, D.J.; Vingrys, A.J. Manganese-enhanced MRI studies of alterations of intraretinal ion demand in models of ocular injury. *Investig. Ophthalmol. Vis. Sci.* **2007**, *48*, 3796–3804. [CrossRef]
190. Bangi, B.B.; Ginjupally, U.; Nadendla, L.K.; Mekala, M.R.; Lakshmi B, J.; Kakumani, A. Evaluation of Gustatory Function in Oral Submucous Fibrosis Patients and Gutka Chewers. *Asian Pac. J. Cancer Prev.* **2019**, *20*, 569–573. [CrossRef]
191. Haider, S.Z.; Sadanandan, N.P.; Joshi, P.G.; Mehta, B. Early Diabetes Induces Changes in Mitochondrial Physiology of Inner Retinal Neurons. *Neuroscience* **2019**, *406*, 140–149. [CrossRef]
192. Kern, T.S.; Kowluru, R.A.; Engerman, R.L. Abnormalities of retinal metabolism in diabetes or galactosemia: ATPases and glutathione. *Investig. Ophthalmol. Vis. Sci.* **1994**, *35*, 2962–2967.
193. Berkowitz, B.A.; Roberts, R.; Stemmler, A.; Luan, H.; Gradianu, M. Impaired apparent ion demand in experimental diabetic retinopathy: Correction by lipoic Acid. *Investig. Ophthalmol. Vis. Sci.* **2007**, *48*, 4753–4758. [CrossRef]
194. Kannan, K.; Jain, S.K. Oxidative stress and apoptosis. *Pathophysiology* **2000**, *7*, 153–163. [CrossRef]
195. Chen, C.; Peng, S.; Chen, F.; Liu, L.; Li, Z.; Zeng, G.; Huang, Q. Protective effects of pioglitazone on vascular endothelial cell dysfunction induced by high glucose via inhibition of IKKalpha/beta-NFkappaB signaling mediated by PPARgamma in vitro. *Can. J. Physiol. Pharmacol.* **2017**, *95*, 1480–1487. [CrossRef] [PubMed]
196. Birk, A.V.; Liu, S.; Soong, Y.; Mills, W.; Singh, P.; Warren, J.D.; Seshan, S.V.; Pardee, J.D.; Szeto, H.H. The mitochondrial-targeted compound SS-31 re-energizes ischemic mitochondria by interacting with cardiolipin. *J. Am. Soc. Nephrol.* **2013**, *24*, 1250–1261. [CrossRef] [PubMed]
197. Dudek, J. Role of Cardiolipin in Mitochondrial Signaling Pathways. *Front. Cell Dev. Biol.* **2017**, *5*, 90. [CrossRef]
198. Birk, A.V.; Chao, W.M.; Bracken, C.; Warren, J.D.; Szeto, H.H. Targeting mitochondrial cardiolipin and the cytochrome c/cardiolipin complex to promote electron transport and optimize mitochondrial ATP synthesis. *Br. J. Pharmacol.* **2014**, *171*, 2017–2028. [CrossRef]
199. Szeto, H.H.; Liu, S.; Soong, Y.; Birk, A.V. Improving mitochondrial bioenergetics under ischemic conditions increases warm ischemia tolerance in the kidney. *Am. J. Physiol. Renal Physiol.* **2015**, *308*, F11–F21. [CrossRef]
200. Alam, N.M.; Mills, W.C.t.; Wong, A.A.; Douglas, R.M.; Szeto, H.H.; Prusky, G.T. A mitochondrial therapeutic reverses visual decline in mouse models of diabetes. *Dis. Model. Mech.* **2015**, *8*, 701–710. [CrossRef]
201. Huang, J.; Li, X.; Li, M.; Li, J.; Xiao, W.; Ma, W.; Chen, X.; Liang, X.; Tang, S.; Luo, Y. Mitochondria-targeted antioxidant peptide SS31 protects the retinas of diabetic rats. *Curr. Mol. Med.* **2013**, *13*, 935–945. [CrossRef] [PubMed]
202. Escribano-Lopez, I.; Diaz-Morales, N.; Iannantuoni, F.; Lopez-Domenech, S.; de Maranon, A.M.; Abad-Jimenez, Z.; Banuls, C.; Rovira-Llopis, S.; Herance, J.R.; Rocha, M.; et al. The mitochondrial antioxidant SS-31 increases SIRT1 levels and ameliorates inflammation, oxidative stress and leukocyte-endothelium interactions in type 2 diabetes. *Sci. Rep.* **2018**, *8*, 15862. [CrossRef] [PubMed]
203. Brand, M.D.; Esteves, T.C. Physiological functions of the mitochondrial uncoupling proteins UCP2 and UCP3. *Cell Metab.* **2005**, *2*, 85–93. [CrossRef] [PubMed]
204. Korshunov, S.S.; Skulachev, V.P.; Starkov, A.A. High protonic potential actuates a mechanism of production of reactive oxygen species in mitochondria. *FEBS Lett.* **1997**, *416*, 15–18. [CrossRef]
205. Arsenijevic, D.; Onuma, H.; Pecqueur, C.; Raimbault, S.; Manning, B.S.; Miroux, B.; Couplan, E.; Alves-Guerra, M.C.; Goubern, M.; Surwit, R.; et al. Disruption of the uncoupling protein-2 gene in mice reveals a role in immunity and reactive oxygen species production. *Nat. Genet.* **2000**, *26*, 435–439. [CrossRef]
206. He, Y.; Luan, Z.; Fu, X.; Xu, X. Overexpression of uncoupling protein 2 inhibits the high glucose-induced apoptosis of human umbilical vein endothelial cells. *Int. J. Mol. Med.* **2016**, *37*, 631–638. [CrossRef]
207. Cui, Y.; Xu, X.; Bi, H.; Zhu, Q.; Wu, J.; Xia, X.; Qiushi, R.; Ho, P.C. Expression modification of uncoupling proteins and MnSOD in retinal endothelial cells and pericytes induced by high glucose: The role of reactive oxygen species in diabetic retinopathy. *Exp. Eye Res.* **2006**, *83*, 807–816. [CrossRef]

208. Hinder, L.M.; Sas, K.M.; O'Brien, P.D.; Backus, C.; Kayampilly, P.; Hayes, J.M.; Lin, C.M.; Zhang, H.; Shanmugam, S.; Rumora, A.E.; et al. Mitochondrial uncoupling has no effect on microvascular complications in type 2 diabetes. *Sci. Rep.* **2019**, *9*, 881. [CrossRef]
209. Wen, Y.; Li, W.; Poteet, E.C.; Xie, L.; Tan, C.; Yan, L.J.; Ju, X.; Liu, R.; Qian, H.; Marvin, M.A.; et al. Alternative mitochondrial electron transfer as a novel strategy for neuroprotection. *J. Biol. Chem.* **2011**, *286*, 16504–16515. [CrossRef]
210. Haefeli, R.H.; Erb, M.; Gemperli, A.C.; Robay, D.; Courdier Fruh, I.; Anklin, C.; Dallmann, R.; Gueven, N. NQO1-dependent redox cycling of idebenone: Effects on cellular redox potential and energy levels. *PLoS ONE* **2011**, *6*, e17963. [CrossRef]
211. Mordente, A.; Martorana, G.E.; Minotti, G.; Giardina, B. Antioxidant properties of 2,3-dimethoxy-5-methyl-6-(10-hydroxydecyl)-1,4-benzoquinone (idebenone). *Chem. Res. Toxicol.* **1998**, *11*, 54–63. [CrossRef] [PubMed]
212. Heitz, F.D.; Erb, M.; Anklin, C.; Robay, D.; Pernet, V.; Gueven, N. Idebenone protects against retinal damage and loss of vision in a mouse model of Leber's hereditary optic neuropathy. *PLoS ONE* **2012**, *7*, e45182. [CrossRef] [PubMed]
213. Erb, M.; Hoffmann-Enger, B.; Deppe, H.; Soeberdt, M.; Haefeli, R.H.; Rummey, C.; Feurer, A.; Gueven, N. Features of idebenone and related short-chain quinones that rescue ATP levels under conditions of impaired mitochondrial complex I. *PLoS ONE* **2012**, *7*, e36153. [CrossRef]
214. Yu-Wai-Man, P.; Soiferman, D.; Moore, D.G.; Burte, F.; Saada, A. Evaluating the therapeutic potential of idebenone and related quinone analogues in Leber hereditary optic neuropathy. *Mitochondrion* **2017**, *36*, 36–42. [CrossRef] [PubMed]
215. Dombi, E.; Diot, A.; Morten, K.; Carver, J.; Lodge, T.; Fratter, C.; Ng, Y.S.; Liao, C.; Muir, R.; Blakely, E.L.; et al. The m.13051G>A mitochondrial DNA mutation results in variable neurology and activated mitophagy. *Neurology* **2016**, *86*, 1921–1923. [CrossRef]
216. Klopstock, T.; Yu-Wai-Man, P.; Dimitriadis, K.; Rouleau, J.; Heck, S.; Bailie, M.; Atawan, A.; Chattopadhyay, S.; Schubert, M.; Garip, A.; et al. A randomized placebo-controlled trial of idebenone in Leber's hereditary optic neuropathy. *Brain* **2011**, *134*, 2677–2686. [CrossRef]
217. Pemp, B.; Kircher, K.; Reitner, A. Visual function in chronic Leber's hereditary optic neuropathy during idebenone treatment initiated 5 to 50 years after onset. *Graefes Arch. Clin. Exp. Ophthalmol.* **2019**, *257*, 2751–2757. [CrossRef]
218. Garcia-Medina, J.J.; Rubio-Velazquez, E.; Foulquie-Moreno, E.; Casaroli-Marano, R.P.; Pinazo-Duran, M.D.; Zanon-Moreno, V.; Del-Rio-Vellosillo, M. Update on the Effects of Antioxidants on Diabetic Retinopathy: In Vitro Experiments, Animal Studies and Clinical Trials. *Antioxidants* **2020**, *9*, 561. [CrossRef]
219. Chous, A.P.; Richer, S.P.; Gerson, J.D.; Kowluru, R.A. The Diabetes Visual Function Supplement Study (DiVFuSS). *Br. J. Ophthalmol.* **2016**, *100*, 227–234. [CrossRef]
220. Hu, B.J.; Hu, Y.N.; Lin, S.; Ma, W.J.; Li, X.R. Application of Lutein and Zeaxanthin in nonproliferative diabetic retinopathy. *Int. J. Ophthalmol.* **2011**, *4*, 303–306. [CrossRef]
221. Garcia-Medina, J.J.; Pinazo-Duran, M.D.; Garcia-Medina, M.; Zanon-Moreno, V.; Pons-Vazquez, S. A 5-year follow-up of antioxidant supplementation in type 2 diabetic retinopathy. *Eur. J. Ophthalmol.* **2011**, *21*, 637–643. [CrossRef] [PubMed]

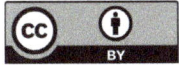

© 2020 by the authors. Licensee MDPI, Basel, Switzerland. This article is an open access article distributed under the terms and conditions of the Creative Commons Attribution (CC BY) license (http://creativecommons.org/licenses/by/4.0/).

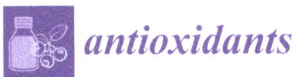

Review

Glyoxalase System as a Therapeutic Target against Diabetic Retinopathy

Gemma Aragonès [1], Sheldon Rowan [1,2,3], Sarah G Francisco [1], Wenxin Yang [1], Jasper Weinberg [1], Allen Taylor [1,2,3,*] and Eloy Bejarano [1,4,*]

1. Laboratory for Nutrition and Vision Research, USDA Human Nutrition Research Center on Aging, Tufts University, Boston, MA 02155, USA; gemma.aragones@tufts.edu (G.A.); sheldon.rowan@tufts.edu (S.R.); sarah.francisco@tufts.edu (S.G.F.); wenxiny7@brandeis.edu (W.Y.); jasper.weinberg@tufts.edu (J.W.)
2. Department of Ophthalmology, Tufts University School of Medicine, Boston, MA 02155, USA
3. Friedman School of Nutrition and Science Policy, Tufts University, Boston, MA 02155, USA
4. Universidad Cardenal Herrera-CEU, CEU Universities, 46115 Valencia, Spain
* Correspondence: allen.taylor@tufts.edu (A.T.); eloy.bejarano@tufts.edu (E.B.); Tel.: +617-556-3156 (A.T.)

Received: 25 September 2020; Accepted: 27 October 2020; Published: 30 October 2020

Abstract: Hyperglycemia, a defining characteristic of diabetes, combined with oxidative stress, results in the formation of advanced glycation end products (AGEs). AGEs are toxic compounds that have adverse effects on many tissues including the retina and lens. AGEs promote the formation of reactive oxygen species (ROS), which, in turn, boost the production of AGEs, resulting in positive feedback loops, a vicious cycle that compromises tissue fitness. Oxidative stress and the accumulation of AGEs are etiologically associated with the pathogenesis of multiple diseases including diabetic retinopathy (DR). DR is a devastating microvascular complication of diabetes mellitus and the leading cause of blindness in working-age adults. The onset and development of DR is multifactorial. Lowering AGEs accumulation may represent a potential therapeutic approach to slow this sight-threatening diabetic complication. To set DR in a physiological context, in this review we first describe relations between oxidative stress, formation of AGEs, and aging in several tissues of the eye, each of which is associated with a major age-related eye pathology. We summarize mechanisms of AGEs generation and anti-AGEs detoxifying systems. We specifically feature the potential of the glyoxalase system in the retina in the prevention of AGEs-associated damage linked to DR. We provide a comparative analysis of glyoxalase activity in different tissues from wild-type mice, supporting a major role for the glyoxalase system in the detoxification of AGEs in the retina, and present the manipulation of this system as a therapeutic strategy to prevent the onset of DR.

Keywords: diabetic retinopathy; oxidative stress; glycation; aging; glyoxalase

1. Oxidative Stress is Related to Many Age-Related Eye Diseases

Age-related eye diseases such as cataract, age-related macular degeneration (AMD), glaucoma, and diabetic retinopathy (DR) are the main causes of progressive and irreversible vision loss worldwide [1]. Loss of vision caused by these diseases diminishes quality of life [2–4]. The World Health Organization (WHO) reported that in 2010, there were 285 million people visually impaired, of which 39 million were blind, and that by 2050 it is estimated that the number will triple, exacerbating the enormous personal and public health burdens [5,6].

The pathogenesis of age-related eye diseases is complex and depends on many factors, some of which remain to be identified. However, it is clear that oxidative stress and the resultant dysfunctional cellular moieties are pathoetiologic for the development of age-related eye diseases [7–10].

Oxidative stress is defined as the generation of excess reactive oxygen species (ROS) beyond the capacity of the biological systems that detoxify these reactive free radicals [11]. Examples of ROS include hydrogen peroxide (H_2O_2), superoxide ($O_2^{\bullet-}$), and nitric oxide (NO). These imbalances lead to oxidative alterations of cellular macromolecular targets such as DNA, RNA, lipids, proteins, and carbohydrates, and eventually to dysfunction and degeneration of tissues [12–14]. In proteins, carbonyls are formed by the Fenton reaction of oxidants with lysine, arginine, proline, and threonine residues of the protein side chains [15]. Typical sequelae of oxidation are the formation of protein aggregates and impaired activity of many proteins, both structural and catalytic [16–19].

Although not the focus of this review, additional biological oxidation processes involve the formation of oxidized lipid metabolites such as hydroxynonenal, and the oxidation of lipids such as low-density lipoproteins in which both the protein and the lipids undergo oxidative changes that can cause cholesterol accumulation [20]. There is also oxidative damage to DNA resulting in several mutagenic lesions including 2-hydroxy adenine, 8-oxoadenine, 5-hydroxycytosine, cytosine glycol, thymine, and glycol [21].

A significant literature indicates that several eye tissues are particularly vulnerable to oxidative stress. Retinal photoreceptor cells and retinal ganglion cells have a large number of mitochondria, sustain high exposure to light and have a high rate of metabolism. As might be anticipated for a tissue in which light energy is transformed to chemical and then electrical impulses, which are chemically transmitted to the brain, retinal photoreceptor cells and retinal ganglion cells are susceptible to oxidative stress [8]. Outside the neurosensory retina, the retinal pigment epithelium (RPE) is also highly sensitive to photo-oxidative stress. The RPE is a single layer of cells located between photoreceptors and the choroid that plays key roles in the maintenance of photoreceptors. Oxidative stress is pathoetiologic in the RPE degeneration associated with the onset of AMD [9].

Oxidative stress is also pathoetiologic in other ocular tissues: (1) Damage to cell membrane fibers, lenticular proteins, photoreceptors, and DNA in most cells, (2) angiogenesis, endothelial dysfunction, and cell apoptosis, (3) loss of lens transparency by disrupting electrolyte balance homeostasis, and (4) increase of intraocular pressure and associated glaucoma [10]. Thus, it is not surprising that multiple ocular diseases have been linked to oxidative stress. These include retinitis pigmentosa, AMD, glaucoma, cataract, and others [12,22,23]. For example, intraocular pressure seems to increase with oxidative stress and accumulation of ROS in retinal ganglion cells [24]. In addition, glaucoma patients have diminished levels of antioxidant biomarkers such as vitamin E [23]. Crabb et al. using mass spectrometry, observed several oxidized proteins in drusen, extracellular deposits accumulated below the RPE on Bruch's membrane, from human AMD samples [25]. The accumulation of drusen is considered to be indicative of early AMD. Oxidative stress also plays a pathologic role in the onset and progression of cataracts. Crystallins, the major gene products in the eye lens, see sulfhydryls transformed to disulfides in cross-linked and aggregated cataractogenic moieties [26].

Based upon these associations between oxidative stress and the risk for cataract, AMD, glaucoma, and DR, many studies have tried to elucidate whether the dietary intake of nutrients with anti-oxidative properties could prevent different age-related eye diseases [27–30]. In the age-related eye diseases double-blinded placebo controlled study (AREDS), it was demonstrated that consumers of fruit and vegetable-rich diets, and people who consume supplements of vitamins C and E, as well as zinc and lutein (all involved in antioxidant function) are protected against AMD [27,31].

2. Advanced Glycation End Products: A Special Case of Oxidative Stress Found in Aged Eye Tissues and Throughout the Body

Advanced glycation end products (AGEs) are oxidation products of particular interest for this review because they are associated with multiple diseases of aging, including DR [32–37].

Dietary sugars or dicarbonyls generated from carbohydrate metabolism can be highly reactive and transform many biomolecules and structures through a process called glycation. This non-enzymatic process is initiated with the Maillard reaction, in which a reversible Schiff base is formed between the carbonyl group of reducing sugars and free amino groups of proteins (Figure 1). These precursors undergo additional oxidations and rearrangements, resulting in the biogenesis of Amadori products. Depending on pH, Amadori products can rearrange to different types of dicarbonyls including 1,2-dicarbonyls such as methylglyoxal (MG) or 3-deoxyglucosone (3-DG), or 2,3-dicarbonyls such as 1-deoxyglucosone. The major glycating biologic reagent is MG, formed by the degradation of dihydroxyacetone phosphate and glyceraldehyde 3-phosphate, both glycolytic metabolites, as well as by the metabolism of threonine, the oxidation of ketone bodies, and upon degradation of glycated proteins [38]. Glyoxal and 3-DG are also highly reactive dicarbonyls formed during sugar metabolism [32,33]. These dicarbonyls are maintained at low levels under homeostatic conditions. Subsequent reactions result in methylglyoxal-derived hydroimidazolone 1 (MG-H1), Nε-carboxy-methyl-lysine (CML), Nε-carboxy-ethyl-lysine (CEL), pentosidine, glucosepane, and other types of AGEs [39] (Figure 1). As discussed later, AGE accumulation boosts the formation of ROS, resulting in increased production of AGEs. This vicious cycle of the oxidative formation of AGEs impacts cellular metabolism and contributes to hyperglycemia-induced tissue injury.

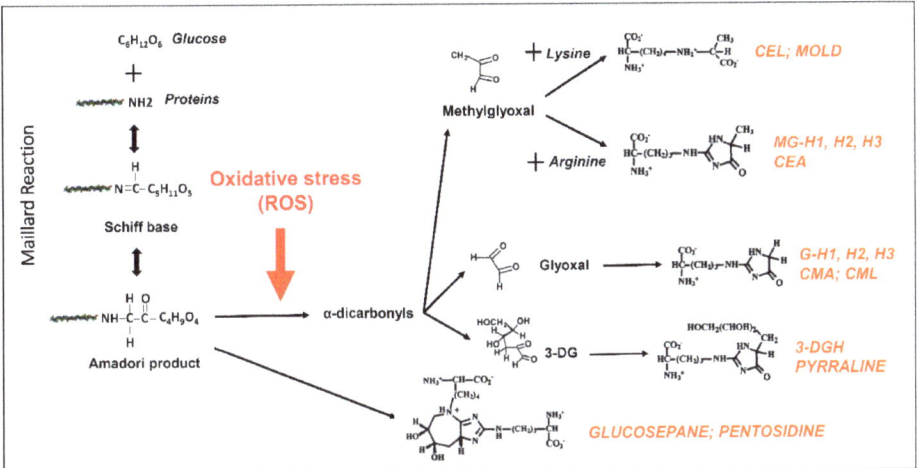

Figure 1. Production of advanced glycation end-products (AGEs) is accelerated under oxidative stress. AGEs are derived from sugars or dicarbonyls generated from carbohydrate metabolism through different chemical routes including the Maillard reaction. The excess of reactive oxidative species (ROS) promotes the production of different AGEs from dicarbonyls (methylglyoxal, glyoxal, or 3-deoxyglucosone (3-DG). AGEs are highlighted in orange. CML: Nε-(carboxymethyl)-lysine; CMA: Nε-(carboxymethyl)-arginine; 3-DG: 3-deoxyglucosone; 3-DGH: GH-1,2,3: Glyoxal-derived hydroimidazolone; MGH-1,2,3: Methylglyoxal-derived hydroimidazolone; CEL: Nε-(carboxyethyl)-lysine; CEA: Nε-(carboxyethyl)-arginine; MOLD: Methylglyoxal-derived lysine dimer.

AGEs are accumulated throughout the body upon aging and particularly in diabetic patients. Three decades ago, different studies reported higher levels of different AGEs in diabetic tissues [40–43]. One of the best examples of glycation with aging is the extracellular matrix. Examination of interstitial collagen shows a gradual increase in AGEs upon aging [44] (Figure 2A). Another example of the relation between AGEs accumulation and aging occurs in eye tissues. Cataracts are perhaps the earliest example of pathobiology of AGEs in aged tissues [45]. Human lens crystallins become progressively yellow-brown pigmented with age as a result of the accumulation of Maillard products [46] (Figure 2B,C). The extensive modification of crystallins by glycation alters the dynamic state of crystallins, promotes their aggregation, and disrupts their chaperone function, contributing to cataractogenesis.

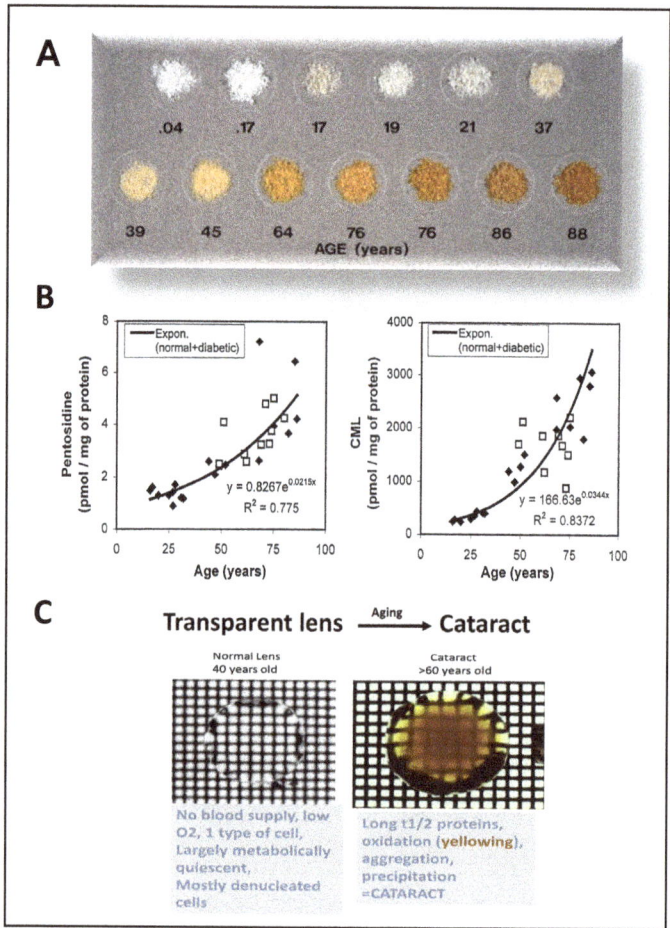

Figure 2. Aging promotes the accumulation of AGEs throughout the body. (**A**) Age-dependent changes in costal cartilage isolated at autopsy from donors of various ages (reprinted with permission of Dr. Baynes) [44]. (**B**) Level of pentosidine (left) and Nε-(carboxymethyl)-lysine (CML) (right) in lens crystallins from diabetic (■) and non-diabetic (♦) subjects as a function of age (reprinted with permission of Dr. Monnier) [46]. (**C**) Transillumination of isolated lenses: Normal lens from young donor (left) and cataractous lens from older donor (right). Lenses were placed in a culture dish that had a grid etched in its bottom surface. The dish was placed on the stage of a dissecting microscope and viewed with transmitted light. Note the degree of yellowing and opacity in the cataractous lens.

The deleterious effect of glycative damage is cell-type dependent and the molecular consequences of AGEs accumulation occur at different levels in eye tissues [47]. Regarding DR, the involvement of AGEs in the pathogenesis of the disease is complex. Glycation of the extracellular matrix results in decreased elasticity and increased vascular stiffness, leading to abnormal vascular function due to rigidity of the vessel wall. AGEs can also exert an indirect effect by binding to different cellular receptors in the plasma membrane, triggering intracellular pathways such as NF-κB activation via Ras-MAPK or RhoA/ROCK pathways [48]. As a result, changes in intracellular signaling cascades and cytopathological responses are triggered that include releases of pro-inflammatory cytokines and pro-angiogenic factors. This also leads to ROS generation, pericyte apoptosis, vascular inflammation, angiogenesis, changes in vasopermeability, and compromised blood–retinal barrier [47] (Figure 3).

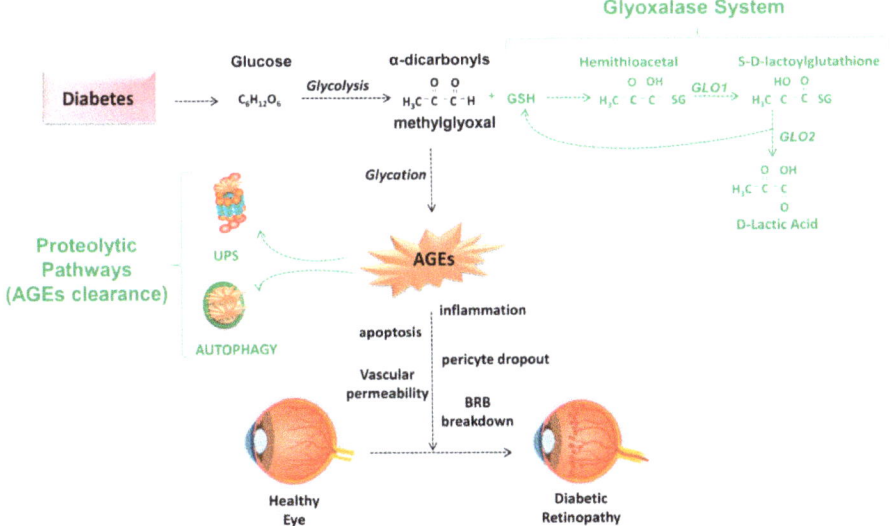

Figure 3. Schematic overview of detoxifying pathways against AGEs-derived damage in diabetic retinopathy (DR). Hyperglycemia-associated diabetes involves the abnormal formation of highly reactive α-dicarbonyls such as methylglyoxal which leads to accelerated AGEs formation. The glyoxalase system is a protective mechanism that slows down the synthesis of AGEs by limiting formation of dicarbonyls. Once formed, AGEs can be cleared by two proteolytic pathways: The ubiquitin-proteasome (UPS) system and autophagy. These protective mechanisms (highlighted in green) decline under diabetic conditions and with age. AGEs are pathologic features in the early stages of DR, impacting the function of neuroglial and vascular cells. AGEs-derived damage results in cellular and tissue dysfunction contributing to the onset of DR. BRB: Blood–retina barrier; GLO1: Glyoxalase 1; GLO2: Glyoxalase 2; GSH: Glutathione.

3. Role of Advanced Glycation End Products in the Pathogenesis of DR

Among the best studied pathologies related to oxidative stress are diabetes and DR, which occur in about 15% of those with long-lasting diabetes mellitus. DR is characterized by high levels of circulating sugars, high levels of oxidative stress, accumulation of AGEs, and microvascular damage [49]. DR is a leading cause of blindness in adults. During the early stage of DR, there is a loss of pericytes from capillaries, leading to the formation of acellular capillaries and retinal microaneurysms, along with thickening of the capillary basement membrane. Oxidative stress enhances damage to tight-junction complexes, causing vascular permeability, and blood–retinal barrier damage [50]. Together, these pathological changes result in irreversible damage to the blood–retinal barrier. Once the disease progresses to a late stage, neovascularization and bleeding can occur along with retinal detachment and macular edema, ultimately resulting in vision loss [51].

Several lines of evidence point to a relationship between oxidative stress and glycation-derived damage. Urinary 8-hydroxy-2′-deoxyguanosine, a marker for oxidative stress, was positively associated with glycated albumin levels in patients with type 2 diabetes, whereas improved glycemic control was associated with decreased levels of oxidative stress [52]. *In vitro* experiments showed that glycated human serum albumin protein promoted sustained ROS production in human endothelial cells. These findings support the hypotheses that there is a vicious cycle of oxidative stress, formation of AGEs, and production of more ROS. Furthermore, long-term oxidative stress induced by AGEs results in endothelial dysfunction which is associated with DR [53]. Indeed, oral administration of AGEs through a diet highly enriched in AGEs promoted oxidative stress, increasing inflammation and insulin resistance [54]. In addition, it has been shown that levels of H_2O_2 and $O_2^{\bullet-}$ are increased in the retinas of diabetic rats, consistent with oxidative stress as a component of the pathobiology of DR [55,56]. Together, this experimental evidence indicates a relationship between elevated levels of ROS, AGEs, and DR.

Glycation is a critical biological process in the retina given that this ocular tissue has high metabolic activity whose activity depends on glucose demand. Such is the case in other neural tissues with the same embryological origin such as the cerebral cortex. The retina and cerebral cortex are exposed to comparable levels of blood glucose; however, the retina is more vulnerable to microvascular lesions derived from hyperglycemia. For example, in diabetic rats, intracellular concentrations of glucose increased significantly in the retina but not in the cerebral cortex, suggesting that a differential response of glucose uptake might contribute to the higher susceptibility of the retina to diabetes-induced microvascular complications [57].

The reasons for the high vulnerability of the retina to glycative stress remain unclear but some evidence indicates that the regulation of glucose uptake could be key. In the retina, the glucose delivery from systemic circulation occurs across retinal capillaries and the RPE. Glucose transport is mainly mediated by the sodium-independent glucose transporters (GLUTs). There are fourteen GLUTs, of which five are well characterized [58]. GLUT1 and GLUT3 are expressed in all cell types (including retina, lens, brain, vascular endothelium). GLUT2 is mainly expressed in the liver, kidney, intestine, and in beta cells of the pancreas. GLUT4 is found in the heart, adipose, and skeletal muscle. Transport of glucose via GLUT1 is insulin independent, thus GLUT1 is always "open", allowing unimpeded transport of glucose. GLUT1 is expressed in retina and retinal capillaries, although the highest levels are found in the RPE. Thus, the RPE appears to be the major route for glucose delivery from the choriocapillaris to the neural retina [59]. Changes in the levels of this glucose transporter have been associated with the development of DR [60]. Levels of GLUT1 decreased in the retina of diabetic-induced rats; however, the expression of GLUT1 in the RPE was not affected by diabetes, suggesting that the trans-epithelial transport of glucose was not compromised [61–63]. The limited capacity of retinal endothelial cells to modulate glucose uptake makes them highly sensitive to the detrimental consequences of hyperglycemia in diabetes.

There are several plasma membrane proteins with the capacity to bind AGEs. The best studied receptor for AGEs in the context of DR is the receptor for advanced glycation end products (RAGE), also called AGER [64]. The binding of AGEs to RAGE is engaged in vital cellular processes such as inflammation, apoptosis, or proliferation and associated with the development of different human diseases. It is reported that RAGE-dependent signaling plays a major role in microvascular diabetic complications. In the eye, RAGE is expressed in multiple cells including pericytes, endothelial cells, microglia, Müller glia, and retinal pigmented epithelium cells, and expression of RAGE is increased under diabetic conditions [65,66]. This would appear to exacerbate the influx of glucose. Consistent with RAGE function, upon diabetes induction, *RAGE* knockout mice had reduced acellular capillary formation and showed less retinal vasopermeability, microglial activation, and Müller cell gliosis [67].

A vast amount of literature associates glycation and AGEs with the progression of DR. AGEs found in skin were shown to predict the risk of DR progression [68,69]. Intravenous administration of AGEs increased retinal vascular leakage *in vivo* by stimulating the expression of vascular endothelial growth factor (VEGF) and decreasing levels of the antiangiogenic pigment epithelium-derived factor (PEDF) [70].

Compounds that inhibit the formation of AGEs are reportedly effective against DR in preclinical settings [71]. An inhibitor of AGEs formation, aminoguanidine, significantly reduced serum AGEs and prevented the development of diabetes-induced basement membrane expansion in retinal capillaries of diabetic rats [72]. Aminoguanidine also reportedly reduced the number of acellular capillaries and abnormal microthrombus formations [73–75]. In addition, two different randomized, double-blind placebo-controlled trials reported that two different AGEs inhibitors, aminoguanidine and pimagedine, slow the progression of diabetic complications including DR [76,77]. Unfortunately, adverse side-effects of these AGEs inhibitors preclude their use in humans, and clinical trials for most of AGEs inhibitors have been discontinued. There is, therefore, a need to identify other means of lowering toxic AGEs.

4. Protective Mechanisms against Glycation-Derived Damage

4.1. Antioxidant Enzymes, Antioxidants, and Signaling

Since the biogenesis of AGEs involves oxidative stress, it might be anticipated that an ability to scavenge ROS would provide a first line of defense. Such enzymatic capacities are provided by antioxidant enzymes such as catalases, H_2O_2-detoxifying enzymes, and superoxide dismutases, as well as glutathione recycling enzymes, glutathione reductases, and glutathione peroxidases [78]. There are also non-enzymatic antioxidants, the most prevalent and most potent of which are ascorbate and glutathione (GSH). In the eye, these are present at mM concentrations, many times the levels in the blood [79–82]. GSH provides a reducing cellular environment. However, it is also a critical component of the glyoxalase system. It also regulates the ubiquitin proteolytic pathway (discussed later in the review). The GSH/GSSG ratio establishes cellular redox status, with consequences for many metabolic processes. Thus, scavenging ROS might be a useful strategy to diminish the production of AGEs in our tissues.

In addition to ascorbate, other non-enzymatic ROS-scavengers, albeit less effective on a per molecule basis, include vitamin E, carotenoids, and flavonoids. Several natural compounds with antioxidant properties have attracted attention with regard to DR, including multiple polyphenols, some of which have anti-glycating potential. For example, administration of curcumin to streptozotocin-induced diabetic rats enhanced the antioxidant capacity in the retina [55] and there was a protective effect on the glycation and crosslinking of collagen [83]. In addition, flavonols such as quercetin, catechin, or kaempferol were shown to diminish AGEs formation [84–86]. Treatment of hepatic cells with a hydroxytyrosol-enriched extract from olive leaves reduced protein carbonylation and the formation of AGEs [87]. Several studies also showed attenuating effects for resveratrol on the production of AGEs or the RAGE receptor in cell culture, animal models, and human studies (reviewed in [88]).

Among the pathobiological mechanisms by which AGEs enhance ROS production are perturbations in cellular signaling associated with the interaction between AGEs and RAGE. The production of free radicals by NADPH-oxidase and the mitochondrial electron transport system was shown to involve the AGEs–RAGE axis. The stimulation of the AGEs–RAGE signaling generates ROS by activating NADPH oxidases, augmenting the intracellular levels of H_2O_2, $O_2^{\bullet-}$, and NO [89–91]. Interestingly, AGEs-induced upregulation of H_2O_2 production, along with mitochondrial dysfunction, resulted in apoptosis in ARPE-19, an RPE-derived cell line from normal eyes [92].

Several studies found that the upregulation of AGE-Receptor 1 (AGER1) inhibited the activity of NADPH oxidase, thereby weakening ROS production [93,94]. AGER1 is linked to sirtuin1 (SIRT1) [54,95]. In this context, deacetylation of NFκB by SIRT1 reduced the NFκB-mediated proinflammatory response [54]. However, long-term exposure to AGEs reduced AGER1 and SIRT1 expression, causing oxidative stress, inflammation, and insulin resistance in several tissues [54]. Another study showed that the dietary limitation of AGEs in type 2 diabetes mellitus patients diminished insulin resistance and increased expression of SIRT1 and AGER1 [94].

In sum, glycative stress contributes to the pathogenesis of different human diseases, including DR, through the interaction of oxidative stress and AGE accumulation.

4.2. Detoxifying Mechanisms against AGEs: Glyoxalase System, Aldehyde Dehydrogenases (ALDH), Aldoketoreductases (AKR), DJ-1/Park7, and Aldol Condensations

There are also specific protective pathways with the capacity to detoxify reactive dicarbonyls formed during sugar metabolism [96–98]. Once AGEs are formed, most are irreversible, so these protective mechanisms diminish the accumulation of AGEs in our tissues through the clearance of AGEs intermediates.

The primary mechanism for detoxifying these reactive dicarbonyls is the glyoxalase system. This converts highly reactive MG into far less reactive D-lactate [99] (Figure 3). This process involves the sequential activity of two enzymes, glyoxalase 1 (GLO1) and glyoxalase 2 (GLO2), and a catalytic amount of GSH. First, GSH reacts spontaneously with the aldehyde of the dicarbonyl to form a hemithioacetal adduct. Then, GLO1 catalyzes the formation of S-D-lactoylglutathione. In the second enzymatic step, GLO2 catalyzes the reaction of S-D-lactoylglutathione into D-lactate, regenerating GSH. It is important to note that GLO1 activity is proportional to GSH levels, and that its activity decreases if cellular cytosolic GSH is diminished, as upon oxidative stress [100]. Unfortunately, such diminution of GSH also compromises the function of the ubiquitin proteasome system, diminishing the cellular capacity to degrade AGEs and cope with glycation-derived damage [19]. There are additional substrates metabolized via this pathway, including glyoxal, phenylglyoxal, and hydroxypyruvaldehyde [101]. Of note, GLO1 is the rate-limiting enzyme, catalyzing the first detoxification step in the glyoxalase system, and its activity is required to prevent the accumulation of these reactive α-oxoaldehydes [102]. Thus, GLO1 has a key protective role against glycative stress-induced AGEs formation.

The structure of glyoxalase is informative. Briefly, the human GLO1 translation product contains 184 amino acids. It is a dimeric protein of molecular mass 42 kDa and contains one zinc ion per subunit. Its structure has two domains per subunit and there are two active sites per protein formed by amino acid residues from the apposed subunit such that the monomer is inactive. The human *GLO1* gene is diallelic (on 6p21.2) and encodes two similar subunits in heterozygotes that result in the dimeric holoenzyme. The two alleles, *GLO1* and *GLO2*, give two similar subunits and three dimers: allozymes GLO 1-1, GLO 1-2, and GLO 2-2. The only amino acid difference between the expression products of the two *GLO1* alleles is at position 111 (Ala^{111} or Glu^{111}). Some studies showed association of this polymorphism with the variations of diabetes and its vascular complications [103]. In addition, in stage 5 renal failure patients on hemodialysis, the Glu111Glu homozygote was associated with increased prevalence of cardiovascular disease and peripheral vascular disease [104].

Transcriptional regulation of *GLO1* is only partially understood, but it is known that the *GLO1* sequence contains multiple regulatory elements. These include a metal-response element (MRE), insulin-response element (IRE), and early gene 2 factor isoform (E2F4) and activating enhancer-binding protein 2α (AP-2α) binding sites [98,105]. IRE and MRE functionalities were validated in reporter assays where insulin and zinc chloride exposure produced a 2-fold increased transcriptional response [105]. Similar functional activities were shown for E2F and AP-2α [106,107]. As discussed later, an antioxidant-response element (ARE) in exon 1 of *Glo1* enhances its transcription through the nuclear factor erythroid 2-related factor 2 (NRF2) oxidative stress-responsive transcriptional system [108].

Several systems appear to operate in the absence of glyoxalase activity, albeit their biological importance is largely unexplored. Other alternative routes for detoxification of dicarbonyls are aldehyde dehydrogenases (ALDHs), aldo-keto reductases (AKRs), the Parkinson-associated protein DJ-1, and scavenging by acetoacetate to form 3-hydroxyhexane-2,5-dione (3-HHD) [97,109].

AKRs are a large protein superfamily that is responsible for the reduction of aldehydes and ketones into primary and secondary alcohols. AKRs metabolize MG to hydroxyacetone or lactaldehyde. Transgenic expression of both human (*AKR7A2*) and mouse (*Akr7a5*) AKR in hamster fibroblasts cells protected against MG-induced cytotoxicity, suggesting that AKRs are able to detoxify MG and decrease AGE levels [110–112]. The role of AKR1B3 has also been studied in the hearts of induced diabetic *Akr1b3*-null mice, and it was observed that these mice had increased levels of MG and AGEs [112]. Human studies showed that aldose reductase activity (AKR1B1) contributed to the detoxification of MG in tissues where the protein was overexpressed and the levels of GSH were low [113]. An increase of AKR1B3 activity was observed in Schwann cells lacking glyoxalase activity, suggesting a compensatory relationship between these systems [114]. The theme of compensatory relationships between GLO1 activity and levels of various glycolytic metabolites will be noted in other systems, below.

ALDHs also metabolize MG, by oxidation to pyruvate. MG treatment induced ALDH expression in wild-type mouse Schwann cells [114]. Additionally, in both zebrafish and mouse models lacking glyoxalase activity, ALDH activity was induced, apparently as a compensatory mechanism [115,116].

3-deoxyglucosone (3-DG) is another highly reactive dicarbonyl formed during sugar metabolism. Although the physiological relevance of 3-deoxyglucosone (3-DG) in DR remains to be established, the 3-DG metabolite formed by ALDH1A1, 2-keto-3-deoxygluconic acid, was elevated in plasma and erythrocytes of diabetic patients [117]. High ALDH1A1 activity was also found in lung, testis and liver but is negligible in other tissues [118]. Interestingly, aldehyde detoxifying capacity is found in retina, however ALDHs were found to be downregulated in diabetic conditions [119].

Another protein with anti-glycation activity is DJ-1, also known as Parkinson's disease protein 7 (PARK7) [120,121]. DJ-1 was shown to have glyoxalase activity *in vitro*, converting MG into lactic acid, in the absence of GSH, and preventing MG-induced tissue damage in *C. elegans* [122]. In addition, DJ-1 was shown to repair methylglyoxal- and glyoxal-glycated proteins in vitro. This deglycase activity removes early-stage MG adducts from protein side chains and prevents the formation of irreversible AGEs [123]. However, no contribution of DJ-1 to MG accumulation was observed in DJ-1 knockdown Drosophila cells and DJ-1 knockout flies [124]. A recent finding shows that DJ-1 may function as a relevant DNA deglycase [125] and recent studies observed a similar deglycase function for DJ-1 on DNA-wrapped histone proteins [126,127].

It was also reported that the ketone body acetoacetate decreased MG via a non-enzymatic conversion during diabetic and dietary ketosis [128]. Indeed, acetoacetate was able to scavenge endogenous MG in a non-enzymatic aldol reaction [129]. This has great importance since physiological ketosis produces high levels of acetoacetate and this condition may prevent diabetes progression [130].

4.3. Proteolytic Pathways: The Last Line of Defense against Glycation-Derived Damage

Which other mechanisms limit the accumulation of AGEs-modified proteins? Although AGEs are irreversible adducts and cross-links in our tissues, these can be removed through different proteolytic capacities. AGEs are substrates of intracellular protein degradation pathways and two major proteolytic capacities are suggested to contribute to the clearance of AGEs: the ubiquitin proteasome system (UPS) and autophagy [96,131–135] (Figure 3).

As for other cargos, AGEs-modified proteins were shown to be ubiquitinated [132]. Ubiquitin is a 76 amino acid protein that when conjugated to a protein substrate can facilitate degradation of that substrate by the proteasome. Obsolete or damaged proteins are tagged with ubiquitin and these ubiquitinated substrates are degraded by the proteasome. The ubiquitin proteolytic system operates mainly on soluble substrates. Several lines of evidence point to a relevant role for the UPS in the clearance of AGEs. Pharmacological proteasomal inhibition boosts the accumulation of AGEs *in vitro* in RPE-derived cells [132]. However, excessive glycative stress decreases proteasomal capacity via the formation of intermolecular crosslinks that, consequently, lead to accelerated accumulation of AGEs [136–138].

Autophagy targets cargos for degradation and can operate on insoluble substrates, including organelles such as mitochondria. Autophagy requires macromolecular assemblies and organelles to identify, sequester, and eventually degrade substrates via the lysosome. Both proteolytic routes, autophagy and UPS, are functionally cooperative and a deficiency of one of these pathways triggers the upregulation of the other [139,140]. Several reports support a vital role for autophagy in the removal of AGEs. Pharmacological blockade of autophagy *in vitro* induced higher accumulation of AGEs in RPE cells [132]. Accumulation of AGEs was observed in kidney tubules of diabetic autophagy-deficient mice [131]. Importantly, mice lacking autophagy in the RPE showed increased levels of oxidized and glycated proteins and were predisposed to develop AMD-phenotypes and retinal degeneration [133].

In sum, a significant literature supports a critical role for the UPS and autophagy in maintaining non-toxic, homeostatic levels of AGEs. Unfortunately, the function of both proteolytic pathways declines with extensive glycative stress and upon aging in many tissues [141], resulting in intracellular accumulation of protein aggregates (also glycated conjugates) and dysfunctional organelles in aged tissues [132,142,143]. We propose that deficits of these pathways in diabetic conditions could contribute to the accumulation and deposition of AGE-modified proteins in the retina, thereby contributing to DR. To date, there is scarce information about how these proteolytic pathways remove AGEs. This thwarts development of strategies to lower AGEs accumulation by boosting proteolytic capacities (Figure 4).

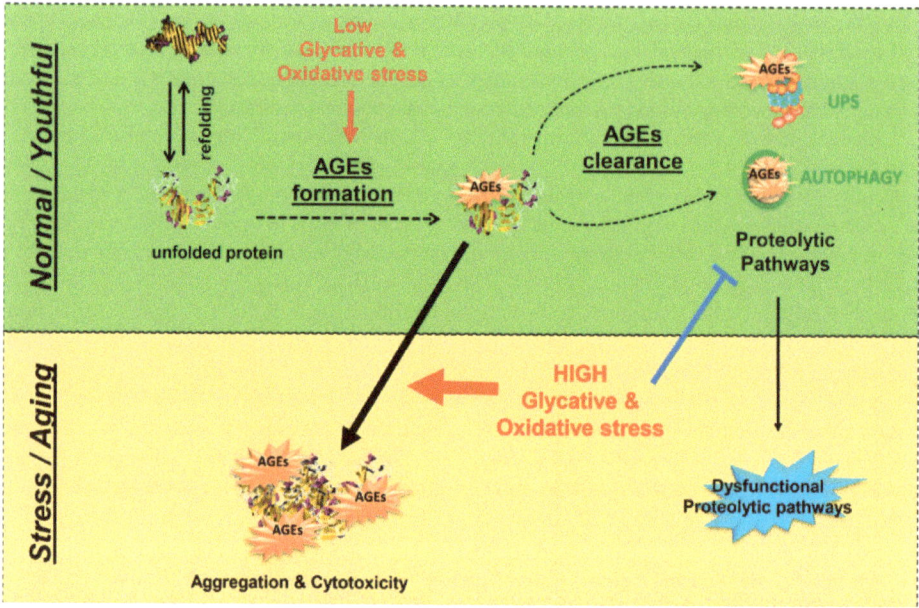

Figure 4. Proteolytic pathways are the last line of defense against AGE-derived proteotoxicity. Under homeostatic conditions (green box), different proteolytic pathways (UPS and autophagy) act to avoid the accumulation of toxic AGEs. Under high levels of glycative and oxidative stress and/or aging (orange box), the production of AGEs is boosted and tissue fitness is compromised as result of glycation-derived protein aggregation and cytotoxicity. Proteolytic capacities are insufficient to lower AGEs levels because of age-related changes in UPS and autophagy along with the inhibitory effect of glycative stress on proteolytic function.

4.4. Protective Role of NRF2 against Glycation-Derived Damage and Modulation of GLO1

NRF2 is an essential transcription factor for genes encoding a number of detoxification enzymes that contain one or more antioxidant response elements (AREs) in their regulatory regions. Examples of genes with AREs include glutathione S-transferases, UDP-glucuronosyltransferases, aldo-keto reductases, and NAD(P)H:quinone oxidoreductase 1. NRF2 acts indirectly by upregulating genes that metabolize and excrete the causative agents and byproducts of oxidative stress [144].

NRF2 is highly conserved from mammalian species to chicken and zebrafish, particularly within six regions designated the Neh1–6 domains [145]. The Neh1 domain contains the cnc-bZIP region, which dictates dimerization partners and confers DNA binding specificity. The Neh4 and Neh5 domains act cooperatively to bind the coactivator CREB-binding protein, thereby activating transcription [146].

Under physiological conditions, NRF2 is in the cytoplasm in a complex with KEAP1, a substrate adaptor protein for the cullin-3-dependent E3 ubiquitin ligase complex. This directs NRF2 for degradation by the 26S proteasome [147,148]. Under oxidative stress, the complex dissociates and NRF2 translocates into the nucleus and upregulates several antioxidant genes, including those related to MG metabolism, as well as genes required for glutathione synthesis [149–151].

Several studies investigated the effect of NRF2 activators on MG and AGEs formation and deposition. Hepatic, brain, heart, kidney, and lung Glo1 mRNA and protein were decreased in *Nrf2*-knockout mice [108]. Compounds that increase *GLO1* expression and activity, such as sulforaphane or trans-resveratrol, decreased cellular and extracellular concentrations of MG and MG-derived protein adducts [152–156]. In addition, the binding of NRF2 to the *Glo1*-ARE increases expression of *Glo1*; however, the inflammatory activation of NF-κB (nuclear factor κB) by NRF2 could diminish *Glo1* expression [157]. Of note, NF-kB directly can also downregulate GLO1 activity, and the inhibition thus takes place at both functional and transcriptional levels [158].

Other transcription factors can modulate the expression of *Glo1*. Under hypoxia conditions, *Glo1* expression is inversely regulated by HIF1α (hypoxia-inducible factor 1α), an important physiological driver of dicarbonyl stress [159]. In addition, *Glo1* is acetylated and probably deacetylated by cytosolic sirtuin-2 [160,161], and its expression may be decreased by activation of the RAGE [127,162].

Several additional observations regarding the above control pathways and GLO1 are noteworthy. GLO1 downregulation is linked to activation of the RAGE receptor that is involved in pro-inflammatory signaling and the development of vascular complications of diabetes [127,162]. Upon glycative stress, there is increased GLO1 ubiquitination and degradation in high glucose concentration media *in vitro* [163]. Downregulation of NRF2 signaling is linked to decreased expression of *Glo1* and reduction of NRF2-antioxidant pathway signaling is associated with inflammation [108,157]. Nevertheless, even in Nrf2-knockout mice, GLO1 protein is still present in the retina and can even be moderately increased through dietary treatment, suggesting that NRF2 is just one of many different regulatory nodes for *Glo1*, at least in this specific ocular tissue [164]. The molecular mechanisms behind the increased retinal GLO1 stability in mice lacking NRF2 remain unknown.

5. The Use of Glyoxalase 1 in Animal Models

As previously explained, AGEs precursors are mainly detoxified by the glyoxalase system and, given the impact of AGEs on age-related pathologies, there is a need to develop strategies to counteract the accumulation of these toxic compounds. In the last few years, the manipulation of GLO1 activity in both animals and cell lines has demonstrated the causal involvement of MG and AGEs in several diseases.

In *Glo1* knockdown cell culture and animal models, an increase in free MG and toxic AGEs was described, but compensatory mechanisms were also observed [165,166]. Giacco et al. showed that in non-diabetic mice, knockdown of *Glo1* increased MG modification of glomerular proteins and oxidative stress to diabetic levels, causing alterations in kidney morphology indistinguishable from those caused by diabetes [167]. Surprisingly, in cell culture and animal models where *Glo1* was knocked out using CRISPR-Cas9 technology, there was no observed increase in MG accumulation [114,116,126,168]. In addition, these healthy *Glo1* knockout animal models did not present defects during development, while genetic deletion of *Glo1* was shown to be embryonically lethal in mice [169]. MGO treatment of cells lacking *Glo1* also revealed a decreased median lethal concentration for exogenous MG [114,126], indicating compensatory mechanisms for the loss of *Glo1*. Indeed, the authors demonstrated in this study that the deglycase protein DJ-1 may play a role in limiting the accumulation of MG-H1 on chromatin in cells lacking *Glo1*. Conversely, *Drosophila melanogaster* and *Danio rerio Glo1* knockout models showed an increase in tissue MG [115,170]. Moraru et al. observed increased MG levels, lipid accumulation in tissues, increased blood glucose, and decreased insulin sensitivity in *Drosophila melanogaster Glo1* knockout [170]. Consistent with these observations, Lodd et al. found under high nutrient intake increased MG levels driving insulin resistance and hyperglycemia in *Danio rerio Glo1* knockout [115].

Other studies have used the gene overexpression of *Glo1* in order to evaluate the biological impact of the glyoxalase system. The overexpression of *Glo1* reduced basal MG concentration, prevented mitochondrial protein modification, and enhanced lifespan in worms [171]. Similarly, *Glo1* overexpression reduced baseline MG concentration in the brain of mice [172]. In diabetic mice, *Glo1* overexpression also prevented diabetes-induced increases in MG modification of glomerular proteins, reduced oxidative stress, and prevented the development of diabetic kidney pathology, despite unchanged levels of hyperglycemia [165]. In agreement with mouse studies, rat models overexpressing human *GLO1* led decreased MG levels, less AGEs formation, and reduced renal and endothelial dysfunction in response to induced diabetes compared with wild-type littermates [173–175]. Recently, GLO1 and aldose reductase were found to be upregulated in patients protected against diabetic nephropathy [176], suggesting that the manipulation of the glyoxalase system could be a potential therapeutic strategy to prevent the onset of AGEs-related diseases.

In addition, diabetes and its microvascular complications (nephropathy, retinopathy, and neuropathy), are associated with elevated levels of MG and reduced levels of GLO1 expression and activity. Some studies showed that overexpression of *Glo1* in transgenic rats and mice could prevent the development of nephropathy, retinopathy, and neuropathy [167,174,175]. In vitro studies showed increased levels of MG and decreased GLO1 activity in endothelial cells when cultured in high glucose concentration media [102,177,178]. In contrast, overexpression of *Glo1* in endothelial cells under the same conditions prevented increased formation of AGEs [102]. Additionally, microvascular complications of diabetes linked to high glucose concentration in retinal pericytes were prevented by overexpression of *Glo1* [179]. In animal models, *Glo1* expression was decreased in the kidney of obese (db/db) diabetic mice, in the kidney and the sciatic nerve of streptozotocin-induced diabetic mice, in the kidney and liver of streptozotocin-induced diabetic Sprague–Dawley rats, in streptozotocin-induced diabetic Wistar rats, and in streptozotocin-induced rats overexpressing the renin-angiotensin system in extra-renal tissues [180–184]. By contrast, GLO1 activity was increased in red blood cells of streptozotocin-induced diabetic C57BL/6 mice, compared to non-diabetic controls [185] and GLO1 activity was increased in the red blood cells of patients with type 1 diabetes and type 2 diabetes, compared to healthy control subjects [186]. Patients with diabetes and microvascular complications had significantly higher GLO1 activity in red blood cells compared to patients without complications. These findings suggest a compensatory increase in GLO1 activity in response to elevated MG concentration [186] and that the response of GLO1 under diabetic conditions may be cell- and tissue-dependent.

5.1. The Decline of Glyoxalase 1 Activity with Age

Aging is characterized by a reduction in the functional properties of cells, tissues, and whole organs, starting with the impairment of major cellular homeostatic processes, including mitochondrial function, proteostasis, and stress-scavenging systems [166,187,188].

GLO1 expression and activity are modified upon aging and in age-related diseases including diabetes and its microvascular complications such as DR. Dicarbonyl stress contributes to aging through the age-related decline in GLO1 activity [171,186,189–196]. The first study that showed a causal link between aging and GLO1 was presented by Morcos et al. [171]. They found a marked decline of GLO1 expression and activity in *C. elegans* with age. Moreover, overexpression of *Glo1* was associated with prolonged lifespan, whereas *Glo1* silencing decreased lifespan, demonstrating that a decrease in GLO1 activity increases mitochondrial ROS production, thereby limiting lifespan [171]. In mice, Sharma–Luthra et al. found tissue specific differences. They showed that GLO1 activity diminished in liver and spleen with age, but increased in kidneys to maximum levels at 24 months [191]. GLO1 activity in rat tissues was decreased with age, as well as by hypoxia in young rats [192]. In humans, several studies have been conducted to investigate the impact of aging on GLO1. Most of them reported a decline of GLO1 activity in multiple tissues, such as arterial tissues, lens, brain, and red blood cells, with age [186,193–196].

5.2. Glyoxalase 1 Activity in Ocular Tissues

In spite of the vast literature on non-ocular tissues, there is scarce information about the role of the glyoxalase system in ocular tissues. However, increasing evidence points to a link between alteration of the glyoxalase system and the development of DR. A polymorphism that alters *GLO1* promoter activity has been linked to retinopathy in type 2 diabetic patients [197]. Expression of *GLO1* and *GLO2* are downregulated in patients with DR, indicating that a failure of this detoxifying system in humans may be involved in retinopathy [198,199]. Glyoxalase activity is reported *in vitro* to promote pericyte survival under hyperglycemic conditions [179] and retinal extracts from a mouse model protected from hyperglycemia-evoked vasoregression showed higher GLO1 activity [200]. Interestingly, a transgenic rat model overexpressing Glo1 inhibits retinal AGE formation and prevents

DR lesions [174]. In sum, upregulation of GLO1 appears to reduce retinal AGEs in diabetic rats and ameliorate AGEs-related pathologies.

In order to explore the role of the glyoxalase system in the eye, we dissected retina, RPE/choroid, and lens, along with other non-ocular tissues from 2-month-old wild-type C57BL/6J mice. We quantified the GLO1 activity in cytosolic extracts of tissues, as previously reported [201]. As expected, we found activity in all tissues analyzed and the relative order of GLO1 activity was retina > liver > kidney > brain > heart > RPE/choroid > lens (Figure 5A). These results are consistent with previous publications in non-ocular tissues [116,184]. Regarding ocular tissues, we observed the highest activity of GLO1 in the retina of mice compared to the lens or RPE/choroid (Figure 5B). Glyoxalase activity is clearly tissue-dependent and retinal activity was about 9-fold and 13-fold greater than in the RPE/choroid and lens, respectively (Figure 5C,D). Clearly, there is even region-specific localization within tissues. This finding is highly relevant because avoiding the formation and accumulation of AGEs is especially important in highly differentiated tissues such as the retina or lens where the glycation damage cannot be diluted by cellular division [96,132]. Of note, when compared to non-ocular tissues, the retinal rate of detoxification was about 2-fold, 8.5-fold, 3.5-fold, and 4.5-fold greater than liver, heart, kidney, and brain, respectively (Figure 5E–H). From a teleological perspective, the high level of retinal GLO1 activity suggests an important protective role against AGE-derived damage in retina.

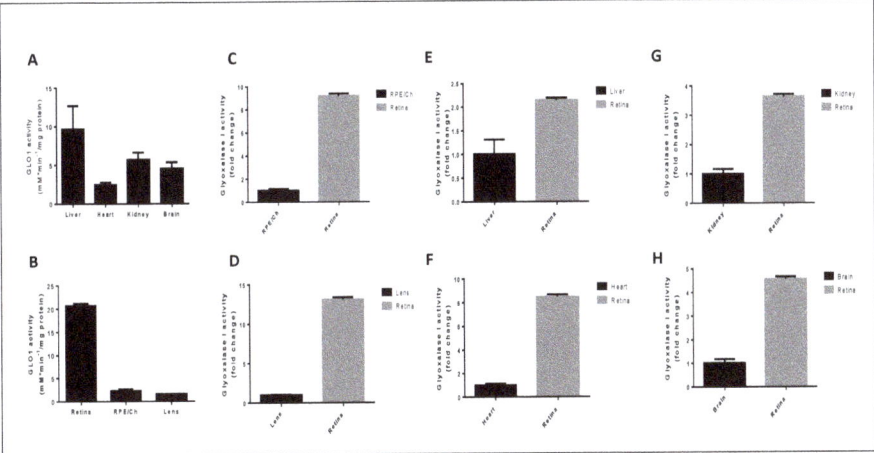

Figure 5. Evaluation of glyoxalase system activity in ocular and non-ocular tissues. Glyoxalase I activity was determined spectrophotometrically using 1 mL quartz cuvettes by following the initial rate of formation of S-D-lactoylglutathione. The assay mixture containing the glycating reagent MG and reduced GSH was equilibrated at room temperature for 10 min, to ensure hemithioacetal formation. The reaction was initiated by the addition of 20 µg of cytosolic extract and the A240 was monitored immediately and over the course of 5 min. The reaction rate was determined by following the increase in absorbance at 240 nm for which $\Delta\varepsilon 240 = 2.86$ mM^{-1} cm^{-1}. (**A,B**) Glyoxalase I activity was assayed in (**A**) non-ocular tissues and (**B**) ocular tissues and activity was expressed as milliunits per milligram of protein where one unit of GLO1 activity was the amount of enzyme which catalyzes the formation of 1 µmol S-D-lactoylglutathione per min under assay conditions. (**C–H**) Retinal glyoxalase I activity was compared to (**C**) RPE/choroid, (**D**) lens, (**E**) liver, (**F**) heart, (**G**) kidney, and (**H**) brain. Fold change was calculated relative to each tissue and values represent the mean ± standard error of the mean of 4 independent experiments from the GLO1 activity assay.

Several cautions are appropriate with regard to expectations of GLO1 overexpression, particularly in the lens. GLO1 may be found and function primarily in the epithelial layers where glucose is received from the aqueous or vitreous humors that nurture the lens. The epithelial layers comprise a minority of lens tissue; thus, the concentration of GLO1 might be significantly higher in the lens epithelium. This may explain glycation-related browning of lenses, particularly in the lens core, upon aging (Figure 2C). Given that the glyoxalase system declines in efficacy with age [189], enhancement of GLO1 activity might represent a therapeutic strategy to counteract the accumulation of these toxic compounds in the lens and retina.

The use of transcriptional modulators of GLO1 has been proposed as a potential intervention to support healthy aging and fight AGEs-related diseases. Metformin, an oral glucose-lowering agent for type 2 diabetes, increases GLO1 activity and was shown to lower circulating MG levels in patients with type 2 diabetes [202]. Candesartan, a synthetic drug that stimulates glyoxalase activity, reduced retinal acellular capillaries and attenuated inflammation and diabetic retinal vascular pathology [182]. In addition, dietary compounds including trans-resveratrol, fisetin, mangiferin, cyanidin, hesperetin, or sulforaphane possess stimulating GLO1-properties and lower MG and MG-derived adducts [152–156,203–208]. Proteomic analysis identified GLO1 as a protein differentially expressed in cells treated with sulforaphane [209]. Sulforaphane inhibited AGEs-derived pericyte damage [210] and delayed diabetes-induced retinal photoreceptor cell degeneration in streptozotocin-injected mice [211]. In addition, pyridoxamine, an MG scavenger that inhibits AGEs formation but also increases GLO1 activity [212], prevented the development of retinopathy in streptozotocin-induced diabetic rats [213]. There is a growing interest in drug discovery and high-throughput screening systems will identify novel regulators and small molecules with GLO1-stimulating properties [214], opening a possibility to treat DR. Clearly, further research is required to define nutritional and pharmacological approaches to overcome the progression of DR associated with glycative stress.

6. Conclusions

Currently there is no cure for DR. Modern therapies include anti-angiogenic strategies or surgery for retinal detachment, which cannot restore vision but only ameliorate further deterioration of the retina. A vast amount of literature stresses the pathogenic role of glycation and AGEs in the molecular basis of this eye-related disease. Based on this literature, lowering AGEs might be a potential therapeutic strategy against DR. Despite enormous effort to date, no AGEs inhibitors have reached clinical use. Exploiting the glyoxalase system and the discovery of compounds that enhance this detoxifying activity represent a therapeutic alternative to fight glycation-derived damage, under diabetic and non-diabetic conditions. As documented here, glyoxalase activity is highest in the retina, suggesting a significant role in eye physiology. The capacity of this detoxifying route is thought to decline with age. We propose that targeting the glyoxalase system through nutritional or pharmacological enhancers might be an alternative to fight this sight-threatening diabetic complication, aiming to reduce the economic burden caused by DR.

Author Contributions: G.A. carried out biochemical assays, analyzed the data, and wrote the paper; S.G.F., S.R., and W.Y. provided technical assistance for the optimization of glyoxalase activity assay, dissection of ocular tissues, and contributed to revision of the paper; J.W. edited the manuscript. E.B. and A.T. designed the experiments, analyzed the data, coordinated the study, and wrote the paper. All authors have read and agreed to the published version of the manuscript.

Funding: Funding was provided by NIH RO1EY028559, RO1EY026979 (to A.T.), USDA NIFA 2016–08885 (to A.T. and S.R.), USDA 8050-51000-089-01S (to A.T.), Kamada (to A.T.), Thome Memorial Foundation (to A.T.), BrightFocus Foundation (to S.R.), and a grant from the Human Nutrition Research Center on Aging (to E.B.). This material is based upon work supported by the US Department of Agriculture—Agricultural Research Service (ARS), under Agreement No. 58-1950-4-003.

Conflicts of Interest: The authors declare no conflict of interest.

References

1. Stevens, G.A.; White, R.A.; Flaxman, S.R.; Price, H.; Jonas, J.B.; Keeffe, J.; Leasher, J.; Naidoo, K.; Pesudovs, K.; Resnikoff, S.; et al. Global prevalence of vision impairment and blindness: Magnitude and temporal trends, 1990–2010. *Ophthalmology* **2013**, *120*, 2377–2384. [CrossRef] [PubMed]

2. Eckert, K.A.; Carter, M.J.; Lansingh, V.C.; Wilson, D.A.; Furtado, J.M.; Frick, K.D.; Resnikoff, S. A Simple Method for Estimating the Economic Cost of Productivity Loss Due to Blindness and Moderate to Severe Visual Impairment. *Ophthalmic Epidemiol.* **2015**, *22*, 349–355. [CrossRef] [PubMed]
3. Ramrattan, R.S.; Wolfs, R.C.; Panda-Jonas, S.; Jonas, J.B.; Bakker, D.; Pols, H.A.; Hofman, A.; de Jong, P.T. Prevalence and causes of visual field loss in the elderly and associations with impairment in daily functioning: The Rotterdam Study. *Arch. Ophthalmol.* **2001**, *119*, 1788–1794. [CrossRef] [PubMed]
4. Köberlein, J.; Beifus, K.; Schaffert, C.; Finger, R.P. The economic burden of visual impairment and blindness: A systematic review. *BMJ Open* **2013**, *3*, e003471. [CrossRef]
5. WHO. Draft action plan for the prevention of avoidable blindness and visual impairment 2014–2019. In *Universal Eye Health: A Global Action Plan 2014–2019*; World Health Organization: Geneva, Switzerland, 2013.
6. Bourne, R.R.A.; Flaxman, S.R.; Braithwaite, T.; Cicinelli, M.V.; Das, A.; Jonas, J.B.; Keeffe, J.; Kempen, J.H.; Leasher, J.; Limburg, H.; et al. Magnitude, temporal trends, and projections of the global prevalence of blindness and distance and near vision impairment: A systematic review and meta-analysis. *Lancet. Glob. Health* **2017**, *5*, e888–e897. [CrossRef]
7. Williams, D.L. Oxidative stress and the eye. *Vet. Clin. N. Am. Small Anim. Pract.* **2008**, *38*, 179–192. [CrossRef] [PubMed]
8. Domènech, E.B.; Marfany, G. The Relevance of Oxidative Stress in the Pathogenesis and Therapy of Retinal Dystrophies. *Antioxidants* **2020**, *9*, 347. [CrossRef] [PubMed]
9. Datta, S.; Cano, M.; Ebrahimi, K.; Wang, L.; Handa, J.T. The impact of oxidative stress and inflammation on RPE degeneration in non-neovascular AMD. *Prog. Retin. Eye Res.* **2017**, *60*, 201–218. [CrossRef]
10. Bungau, S.; Abdel-Daim, M.M.; Tit, D.M.; Ghanem, E.; Sato, S.; Maruyama-Inoue, M.; Yamane, S.; Kadonosono, K. Health Benefits of Polyphenols and Carotenoids in Age-Related Eye Diseases. *Oxidative Med. Cell. Longev.* **2019**, *2019*, 9783429. [CrossRef]
11. Abdel-Daim, M.M.; El-Tawil, O.S.; Bungau, S.G.; Atanasov, A.G. Applications of Antioxidants in Metabolic Disorders and Degenerative Diseases: Mechanistic Approach. *Oxidative Med. Cell. Longev.* **2019**, *2019*, 4179676. [CrossRef]
12. Kowluru, R.A.; Chan, P.S. Oxidative stress and diabetic retinopathy. *Exp. Diabetes Res.* **2007**, *2007*, 43603. [CrossRef]
13. Cabrera, M.P.; Chihuailaf, R.H. Antioxidants and the integrity of ocular tissues. *Vet. Med. Int.* **2011**, *2011*, 905153. [CrossRef] [PubMed]
14. Mitra, R.N.; Conley, S.M.; Naash, M.I. Therapeutic Approach of Nanotechnology for Oxidative Stress Induced Ocular Neurodegenerative Diseases. *Adv. Exp. Med. Biol.* **2016**, *854*, 463–469. [CrossRef] [PubMed]
15. Barreiro, E. Role of Protein Carbonylation in Skeletal Muscle Mass Loss Associated with Chronic Conditions. *Proteomes* **2016**, *4*, 18. [CrossRef]
16. Jahngen-Hodge, J.; Cyr, D.; Laxman, E.; Taylor, A. Ubiquitin and ubiquitin conjugates in human lens. *Exp. Eye Res.* **1992**, *55*, 897–902. [CrossRef]
17. Dudek, E.J.; Shang, F.; Valverde, P.; Liu, Q.; Hobbs, M.; Taylor, A. Selectivity of the ubiquitin pathway for oxidatively modified proteins: Relevance to protein precipitation diseases. *FASEB J. Off. Publ. Fed. Am. Soc. Exp. Biol.* **2005**, *19*, 1707–1709. [CrossRef] [PubMed]
18. Obin, M.; Shang, F.; Gong, X.; Handelman, G.; Blumberg, J.; Taylor, A. Redox regulation of ubiquitin-conjugating enzymes: Mechanistic insights using the thiol-specific oxidant diamide. *FASEB J. Off. Publ. Fed. Am. Soc. Exp. Biol.* **1998**, *12*, 561–569. [CrossRef]
19. Jahngen-Hodge, J.; Obin, M.S.; Gong, X.; Shang, F.; Nowell, T.R., Jr.; Gong, J.; Abasi, H.; Blumberg, J.; Taylor, A. Regulation of ubiquitin-conjugating enzymes by glutathione following oxidative stress. *J. Biol. Chem.* **1997**, *272*, 28218–28226. [CrossRef]
20. Trpkovic, A.; Resanovic, I.; Stanimirovic, J.; Radak, D.; Mousa, S.A.; Cenic-Milosevic, D.; Jevremovic, D.; Isenovic, E.R. Oxidized low-density lipoprotein as a biomarker of cardiovascular diseases. *Crit. Rev. Clin. Lab. Sci.* **2015**, *52*, 70–85. [CrossRef]
21. Jacob, K.D.; Noren Hooten, N.; Trzeciak, A.R.; Evans, M.K. Markers of oxidant stress that are clinically relevant in aging and age-related disease. *Mech. Ageing Dev.* **2013**, *134*, 139–157. [CrossRef]
22. Chen, J.; Patil, S.; Seal, S.; McGinnis, J.F. Rare earth nanoparticles prevent retinal degeneration induced by intracellular peroxides. *Nat. Nanotechnol.* **2006**, *1*, 142–150. [CrossRef]

23. Martínez-Fernández de la Cámara, C.; Salom, D.; Sequedo, M.D.; Hervás, D.; Marín-Lambíes, C.; Aller, E.; Jaijo, T.; Díaz-Llopis, M.; Millán, J.M.; Rodrigo, R. Altered antioxidant-oxidant status in the aqueous humor and peripheral blood of patients with retinitis pigmentosa. *PLoS ONE* **2013**, *8*, e74223. [CrossRef]
24. Liu, Q.; Ju, W.K.; Crowston, J.G.; Xie, F.; Perry, G.; Smith, M.A.; Lindsey, J.D.; Weinreb, R.N. Oxidative stress is an early event in hydrostatic pressure induced retinal ganglion cell damage. *Investig. Ophthalmol. Vis. Sci.* **2007**, *48*, 4580–4589. [CrossRef]
25. Crabb, J.W.; Miyagi, M.; Gu, X.; Shadrach, K.; West, K.A.; Sakaguchi, H.; Kamei, M.; Hasan, A.; Yan, L.; Rayborn, M.E.; et al. Drusen proteome analysis: An approach to the etiology of age-related macular degeneration. *Proc. Natl. Acad. Sci. USA* **2002**, *99*, 14682–14687. [CrossRef]
26. Serebryany, E.; Yu, S.; Trauger, S.A.; Budnik, B.; Shakhnovich, E.I. Dynamic disulfide exchange in a crystallin protein in the human eye lens promotes cataract-associated aggregation. *J. Biol. Chem.* **2018**, *293*, 17997–18009. [CrossRef]
27. Weikel, K.A.; Chiu, C.J.; Taylor, A. Nutritional modulation of age-related macular degeneration. *Mol. Asp. Med.* **2012**, *33*, 318–375. [CrossRef] [PubMed]
28. Saccà, S.C.; Corazza, P.; Gandolfi, S.; Ferrari, D.; Sukkar, S.; Iorio, E.L.; Traverso, C.E. Substances of Interest That Support Glaucoma Therapy. *Nutrients* **2019**, *11*, 239. [CrossRef]
29. Perez, C.I.; Singh, K.; Lin, S. Relationship of lifestyle, exercise, and nutrition with glaucoma. *Curr. Opin. Ophthalmol.* **2019**, *30*, 82–88. [CrossRef] [PubMed]
30. Weikel, K.A.; Garber, C.; Baburins, A.; Taylor, A. Nutritional modulation of cataract. *Nutr. Rev.* **2014**, *72*, 30–47. [CrossRef]
31. Lutein + zeaxanthin and omega-3 fatty acids for age-related macular degeneration: The Age-Related Eye Disease Study 2 (AREDS2) randomized clinical trial. *JAMA* **2013**, *309*, 2005–2015. [CrossRef]
32. Thornalley, P.J.; Langborg, A.; Minhas, H.S. Formation of glyoxal, methylglyoxal and 3-deoxyglucosone in the glycation of proteins by glucose. *Biochem. J.* **1999**, *344*, 109–116.
33. Rabbani, N.; Thornalley, P.J. Dicarbonyl stress in cell and tissue dysfunction contributing to ageing and disease. *Biochem. Biophys. Res. Commun.* **2015**, *458*, 221–226. [CrossRef]
34. Rabbani, N.; Thornalley, P.J. Dicarbonyl proteome and genome damage in metabolic and vascular disease. *Biochem. Soc. Trans.* **2014**, *42*, 425–432. [CrossRef]
35. Bejarano, E.; Taylor, A. Too sweet: Problems of protein glycation in the eye. *Exp. Eye Res.* **2019**, *178*, 255–262. [CrossRef]
36. Kandarakis, S.A.; Piperi, C.; Topouzis, F.; Papavassiliou, A.G. Emerging role of advanced glycation-end products (AGEs) in the pathobiology of eye diseases. *Prog. Retin. Eye Res.* **2014**, *42*, 85–102. [CrossRef]
37. Lapolla, A.; Flamini, R.; Dalla Vedova, A.; Senesi, A.; Reitano, R.; Fedele, D.; Basso, E.; Seraglia, R.; Traldi, P. Glyoxal and methylglyoxal levels in diabetic patients: Quantitative determination by a new GC/MS method. *Clin. Chem. Lab. Med.* **2003**, *41*, 1166–1173. [CrossRef]
38. Allaman, I.; Bélanger, M.; Magistretti, P.J. Methylglyoxal, the dark side of glycolysis. *Front. Neurosci.* **2015**, *9*, 23. [CrossRef]
39. Cepas, V.; Collino, M.; Mayo, J.C.; Sainz, R.M. Redox Signaling and Advanced Glycation Endproducts (AGEs) in Diet-Related Diseases. *Antioxidants* **2020**, *9*, 142. [CrossRef]
40. Miyata, S.; Monnier, V. Immunohistochemical detection of advanced glycosylation end products in diabetic tissues using monoclonal antibody to pyrraline. *J. Clin. Investig.* **1992**, *89*, 1102–1112. [CrossRef]
41. Sell, D.R.; Nagaraj, R.H.; Grandhee, S.K.; Odetti, P.; Lapolla, A.; Fogarty, J.; Monnier, V.M. Pentosidine: A molecular marker for the cumulative damage to proteins in diabetes, aging, and uremia. *Diabetes Metab. Rev.* **1991**, *7*, 239–251. [CrossRef]
42. Schleicher, E.D.; Wagner, E.; Nerlich, A.G. Increased accumulation of the glycoxidation product N(epsilon)-(carboxymethyl)lysine in human tissues in diabetes and aging. *J. Clin. Investig.* **1997**, *99*, 457–468. [CrossRef] [PubMed]
43. Stitt, A.W.; Moore, J.E.; Sharkey, J.A.; Murphy, G.; Simpson, D.A.; Bucala, R.; Vlassara, H.; Archer, D.B. Advanced glycation end products in vitreous: Structural and functional implications for diabetic vitreopathy. *Investig. Ophthalmol. Vis. Sci.* **1998**, *39*, 2517–2523.
44. Dyer, D.G.; Blackledge, J.A.; Katz, B.M.; Hull, C.J.; Adkisson, H.D.; Thorpe, S.R.; Lyons, T.J.; Baynes, J.W. The Maillard reaction in vivo. *Z. Fur Ernahr.* **1991**, *30*, 29–45. [CrossRef]

45. Pescosolido, N.; Barbato, A.; Giannotti, R.; Komaiha, C.; Lenarduzzi, F. Age-related changes in the kinetics of human lenses: Prevention of the cataract. *Int. J. Ophthalmol.* **2016**, *9*, 1506–1517. [CrossRef] [PubMed]
46. Tessier, F.; Obrenovich, M.; Monnier, V.M. Structure and mechanism of formation of human lens fluorophore LM-1. Relationship to vesperlysine A and the advanced Maillard reaction in aging, diabetes, and cataractogenesis. *J. Biol. Chem.* **1999**, *274*, 20796–20804. [CrossRef]
47. Xu, J.; Chen, L.J.; Yu, J.; Wang, H.J.; Zhang, F.; Liu, Q.; Wu, J. Involvement of Advanced Glycation End Products in the Pathogenesis of Diabetic Retinopathy. *Cell. Physiol. Biochem. Int. J. Exp. Cell. Physiol. Biochem. Pharmacol.* **2018**, *48*, 705–717. [CrossRef]
48. Okamoto, T.; Yamagishi, S.; Inagaki, Y.; Amano, S.; Koga, K.; Abe, R.; Takeuchi, M.; Ohno, S.; Yoshimura, A.; Makita, Z. Angiogenesis induced by advanced glycation end products and its prevention by cerivastatin. *FASEB J. Off. Publ. Fed. Am. Soc. Exp. Biol.* **2002**, *16*, 1928–1930. [CrossRef]
49. Baynes, J.W.; Thorpe, S.R. Role of oxidative stress in diabetic complications: A new perspective on an old paradigm. *Diabetes* **1999**, *48*, 1–9. [CrossRef]
50. Frey, T.; Antonetti, D.A. Alterations to the blood-retinal barrier in diabetes: Cytokines and reactive oxygen species. *Antioxid Redox Signal* **2011**, *15*, 1271–1284. [CrossRef]
51. Klaassen, I.; Van Noorden, C.J.; Schlingemann, R.O. Molecular basis of the inner blood-retinal barrier and its breakdown in diabetic macular edema and other pathological conditions. *Prog. Retin. Eye Res.* **2013**, *34*, 19–48. [CrossRef]
52. Nojima, H.; Watanabe, H.; Yamane, K.; Kitahara, Y.; Sekikawa, K.; Yamamoto, H.; Yokoyama, A.; Inamizu, T.; Asahara, T.; Kohno, N. Effect of aerobic exercise training on oxidative stress in patients with type 2 diabetes mellitus. *Metab. Clin. Exp.* **2008**, *57*, 170–176. [CrossRef] [PubMed]
53. Rodiño-Janeiro, B.K.; González-Peteiro, M.; Ucieda-Somoza, R.; González-Juanatey, J.R.; Alvarez, E. Glycated albumin, a precursor of advanced glycation end-products, up-regulates NADPH oxidase and enhances oxidative stress in human endothelial cells: Molecular correlate of diabetic vasculopathy. *Diabetes Metab. Res. Rev.* **2010**, *26*, 550–558. [CrossRef] [PubMed]
54. Cai, W.; Ramdas, M.; Zhu, L.; Chen, X.; Striker, G.E.; Vlassara, H. Oral advanced glycation endproducts (AGEs) promote insulin resistance and diabetes by depleting the antioxidant defenses AGE receptor-1 and sirtuin 1. *Proc. Natl. Acad. Sci. USA* **2012**, *109*, 15888–15893. [CrossRef] [PubMed]
55. Kowluru, R.A.; Kanwar, M. Effects of curcumin on retinal oxidative stress and inflammation in diabetes. *Nutr. Metab.* **2007**, *4*, 8. [CrossRef] [PubMed]
56. Rodríguez, M.L.; Pérez, S.; Mena-Mollá, S.; Desco, M.C.; Ortega, Á.L. Oxidative Stress and Microvascular Alterations in Diabetic Retinopathy: Future Therapies. *Oxidative Med. Cell. Longev.* **2019**, *2019*, 4940825. [CrossRef]
57. Tang, J.; Zhu, X.W.; Lust, W.D.; Kern, T.S. Retina accumulates more glucose than does the embryologically similar cerebral cortex in diabetic rats. *Diabetologia* **2000**, *43*, 1417–1423. [CrossRef]
58. Thorens, B.; Mueckler, M. Glucose transporters in the 21st Century. *Am. J. Physiol. Endocrinol. Metab.* **2010**, *298*, E141–E145. [CrossRef]
59. Sugasawa, K.; Deguchi, J.; Okami, T.; Yamamoto, A.; Omori, K.; Uyama, M.; Tashiro, Y. Immunocytochemical analyses of distributions of Na, K-ATPase and GLUT1, insulin and transferrin receptors in the developing retinal pigment epithelial cells. *Cell Struct. Funct.* **1994**, *19*, 21–28. [CrossRef]
60. You, Z.-P.; Zhang, Y.-L.; Shi, K.; Shi, L.; Zhang, Y.-Z.; Zhou, Y.; Wang, C.-y. Suppression of diabetic retinopathy with GLUT1 siRNA. *Sci. Rep.* **2017**, *7*, 7437. [CrossRef]
61. Ulas, M.; Orhan, C.; Tuzcu, M.; Ozercan, I.H.; Sahin, N.; Gencoglu, H.; Komorowski, J.R.; Sahin, K. Anti-diabetic potential of chromium histidinate in diabetic retinopathy rats. *BMC Complement. Altern. Med.* **2015**, *15*, 16. [CrossRef]
62. Badr, G.A.; Tang, J.; Ismail-Beigi, F.; Kern, T.S. Diabetes downregulates GLUT1 expression in the retina and its microvessels but not in the cerebral cortex or its microvessels. *Diabetes* **2000**, *49*, 1016–1021. [CrossRef] [PubMed]
63. Rajah, T.T.; Olson, A.L.; Grammas, P. Differential glucose uptake in retina- and brain-derived endothelial cells. *Microvasc. Res.* **2001**, *62*, 236–242. [CrossRef]
64. Nass, N.; Bartling, B.; Navarrete Santos, A.; Scheubel, R.J.; Börgermann, J.; Silber, R.E.; Simm, A. Advanced glycation end products, diabetes and ageing. *Z. Fur. Gerontol. Und Geriatr.* **2007**, *40*, 349–356. [CrossRef] [PubMed]

65. Stitt, A.W.; Li, Y.M.; Gardiner, T.A.; Bucala, R.; Archer, D.B.; Vlassara, H. Advanced glycation end products (AGEs) co-localize with AGE receptors in the retinal vasculature of diabetic and of AGE-infused rats. *Am. J. Pathol.* **1997**, *150*, 523–531.
66. Chen, M.; Curtis, T.M.; Stitt, A.W. Advanced glycation end products and diabetic retinopathy. *Curr. Med. Chem.* **2013**, *20*, 3234–3240. [CrossRef]
67. McVicar, C.M.; Ward, M.; Colhoun, L.M.; Guduric-Fuchs, J.; Bierhaus, A.; Fleming, T.; Schlotterer, A.; Kolibabka, M.; Hammes, H.P.; Chen, M.; et al. Role of the receptor for advanced glycation endproducts (RAGE) in retinal vasodegenerative pathology during diabetes in mice. *Diabetologia* **2015**, *58*, 1129–1137. [CrossRef]
68. Genuth, S.; Sun, W.; Cleary, P.; Sell, D.R.; Dahms, W.; Malone, J.; Sivitz, W.; Monnier, V.M. Glycation and carboxymethyllysine levels in skin collagen predict the risk of future 10-year progression of diabetic retinopathy and nephropathy in the diabetes control and complications trial and epidemiology of diabetes interventions and complications participants with type 1 diabetes. *Diabetes* **2005**, *54*, 3103–3111. [CrossRef]
69. Genuth, S.; Sun, W.; Cleary, P.; Gao, X.; Sell, D.R.; Lachin, J.; Monnier, V.M. Skin advanced glycation end products glucosepane and methylglyoxal hydroimidazolone are independently associated with long-term microvascular complication progression of type 1 diabetes. *Diabetes* **2015**, *64*, 266–278. [CrossRef] [PubMed]
70. Yamagishi, S.; Nakamura, K.; Matsui, T.; Inagaki, Y.; Takenaka, K.; Jinnouchi, Y.; Yoshida, Y.; Matsuura, T.; Narama, I.; Motomiya, Y.; et al. Pigment epithelium-derived factor inhibits advanced glycation end product-induced retinal vascular hyperpermeability by blocking reactive oxygen species-mediated vascular endothelial growth factor expression. *J. Biol. Chem.* **2006**, *281*, 20213–20220. [CrossRef]
71. Borg, D.J.; Forbes, J.M. Targeting advanced glycation with pharmaceutical agents: Where are we now? *Glycoconj. J.* **2016**, *33*, 653–670. [CrossRef]
72. Gardiner, T.A.; Anderson, H.R.; Stitt, A.W. Inhibition of advanced glycation end-products protects against retinal capillary basement membrane expansion during long-term diabetes. *J. Pathol.* **2003**, *201*, 328–333. [CrossRef] [PubMed]
73. Hammes, H.P.; Martin, S.; Federlin, K.; Geisen, K.; Brownlee, M. Aminoguanidine treatment inhibits the development of experimental diabetic retinopathy. *Proc. Natl. Acad. Sci. USA* **1991**, *88*, 11555–11558. [CrossRef] [PubMed]
74. Hammes, H.P.; Brownlee, M.; Edelstein, D.; Saleck, M.; Martin, S.; Federlin, K. Aminoguanidine inhibits the development of accelerated diabetic retinopathy in the spontaneous hypertensive rat. *Diabetologia* **1994**, *37*, 32–35. [CrossRef] [PubMed]
75. Hammes, H.P.; Strödter, D.; Weiss, A.; Bretzel, R.G.; Federlin, K.; Brownlee, M. Secondary intervention with aminoguanidine retards the progression of diabetic retinopathy in the rat model. *Diabetologia* **1995**, *38*, 656–660. [CrossRef]
76. Freedman, B.I.; Wuerth, J.P.; Cartwright, K.; Bain, R.P.; Dippe, S.; Hershon, K.; Mooradian, A.D.; Spinowitz, B.S. Design and baseline characteristics for the aminoguanidine Clinical Trial in Overt Type 2 Diabetic Nephropathy (ACTION II). *Control. Clin. Trials* **1999**, *20*, 493–510. [CrossRef]
77. Bolton, W.K.; Cattran, D.C.; Williams, M.E.; Adler, S.G.; Appel, G.B.; Cartwright, K.; Foiles, P.G.; Freedman, B.I.; Raskin, P.; Ratner, R.E.; et al. Randomized trial of an inhibitor of formation of advanced glycation end products in diabetic nephropathy. *Am. J. Nephrol.* **2004**, *24*, 32–40. [CrossRef]
78. Nowotny, K.; Jung, T.; Höhn, A.; Weber, D.; Grune, T. Advanced glycation end products and oxidative stress in type 2 diabetes mellitus. *Biomolecules* **2015**, *5*, 194–222. [CrossRef]
79. Berger, J.; Shephard, D.; Morrow, F.; Sadowski, J.; Haire, T.; Taylor, A. Reduced and total ascorbate in guinea pig eye tissues in response to dietary intake. *Curr. Eye Res.* **1988**, *7*, 681–686. [CrossRef]
80. Berger, J.; Shepard, D.; Morrow, F.; Taylor, A. Relationship between dietary intake and tissue levels of reduced and total vitamin C in the nonscorbutic guinea pig. *J. Nutr.* **1989**, *119*, 734–740. [CrossRef]
81. Taylor, A.; Jacques, P.F.; Nowell, T.; Perrone, G.; Blumberg, J.; Handelman, G.; Jozwiak, B.; Nadler, D. Vitamin C in human and guinea pig aqueous, lens and plasma in relation to intake. *Curr. Eye Res.* **1997**, *16*, 857–864. [CrossRef]
82. Yeum, K.J.; Shang, F.M.; Schalch, W.M.; Russell, R.M.; Taylor, A. Fat-soluble nutrient concentrations in different layers of human cataractous lens. *Curr. Eye Res.* **1999**, *19*, 502–505. [CrossRef]
83. Sajithlal, G.B.; Chithra, P.; Chandrakasan, G. Effect of curcumin on the advanced glycation and cross-linking of collagen in diabetic rats. *Biochem. Pharmacol.* **1998**, *56*, 1607–1614. [CrossRef]

84. Li, X.; Zheng, T.; Sang, S.; Lv, L. Quercetin inhibits advanced glycation end product formation by trapping methylglyoxal and glyoxal. *J. Agric. Food Chem.* **2014**, *62*, 12152–12158. [CrossRef] [PubMed]
85. Sampath, C.; Rashid, M.R.; Sang, S.; Ahmedna, M. Green tea epigallocatechin 3-gallate alleviates hyperglycemia and reduces advanced glycation end products via nrf2 pathway in mice with high fat diet-induced obesity. *Biomed. Pharm.* **2017**, *87*, 73–81. [CrossRef]
86. Kishore, L.; Kaur, N.; Singh, R. Effect of Kaempferol isolated from seeds of Eruca sativa on changes of pain sensitivity in Streptozotocin-induced diabetic neuropathy. *Inflammopharmacology* **2018**, *26*, 993–1003. [CrossRef]
87. Navarro, M.; Morales, F.J.; Ramos, S. Olive leaf extract concentrated in hydroxytyrosol attenuates protein carbonylation and the formation of advanced glycation end products in a hepatic cell line (HepG2). *Food Funct.* **2017**, *8*, 944–953. [CrossRef]
88. Hajizadeh-Sharafabad, F.; Sahebkar, A.; Zabetian-Targhi, F.; Maleki, V. The impact of resveratrol on toxicity and related complications of advanced glycation end products: A systematic review. *Biofactors* **2019**, *45*, 651–665. [CrossRef]
89. Basta, G.; Lazzerini, G.; Del Turco, S.; Ratto, G.M.; Schmidt, A.M.; De Caterina, R. At least 2 distinct pathways generating reactive oxygen species mediate vascular cell adhesion molecule-1 induction by advanced glycation end products. *Arterioscler. Thromb. Vasc. Biol.* **2005**, *25*, 1401–1407. [CrossRef]
90. Nam, M.H.; Son, W.R.; Lee, Y.S.; Lee, K.W. Glycolaldehyde-derived advanced glycation end products (glycol-AGEs)-induced vascular smooth muscle cell dysfunction is regulated by the AGES-receptor (RAGE) axis in endothelium. *Cell Commun. Adhes.* **2015**, *22*, 67–78. [CrossRef]
91. Dobi, A.; Bravo, S.B.; Veeren, B.; Paradela-Dobarro, B.; Álvarez, E.; Meilhac, O.; Viranaicken, W.; Baret, P.; Devin, A.; Rondeau, P. Advanced glycation end-products disrupt human endothelial cells redox homeostasis: New insights into reactive oxygen species production. *Free Radic. Res.* **2019**, *53*, 150–169. [CrossRef]
92. Wang, X.L.; Yu, T.; Yan, Q.C.; Wang, W.; Meng, N.; Li, X.J.; Luo, Y.H. AGEs Promote Oxidative Stress and Induce Apoptosis in Retinal Pigmented Epithelium Cells RAGE-dependently. *J. Mol. Neurosci.* **2015**, *56*, 449–460. [CrossRef] [PubMed]
93. Cai, W.; Torreggiani, M.; Zhu, L.; Chen, X.; He, J.C.; Striker, G.E.; Vlassara, H. AGER1 regulates endothelial cell NADPH oxidase-dependent oxidant stress via PKC-delta: Implications for vascular disease. *Am. J. Physiol. Cell Physiol.* **2010**, *298*, C624–C634. [CrossRef]
94. Vlassara, H.; Cai, W.; Goodman, S.; Pyzik, R.; Yong, A.; Chen, X.; Zhu, L.; Neade, T.; Beeri, M.; Silverman, J.M.; et al. Protection against loss of innate defenses in adulthood by low advanced glycation end products (AGE) intake: Role of the antiinflammatory AGE receptor-1. *J. Clin. Endocrinol. Metab.* **2009**, *94*, 4483–4491. [CrossRef] [PubMed]
95. Uribarri, J.; Cai, W.; Ramdas, M.; Goodman, S.; Pyzik, R.; Chen, X.; Zhu, L.; Striker, G.E.; Vlassara, H. Restriction of advanced glycation end products improves insulin resistance in human type 2 diabetes: Potential role of AGER1 and SIRT1. *Diabetes Care* **2011**, *34*, 1610–1616. [CrossRef] [PubMed]
96. Taylor, A. Mechanistically linking age-related diseases and dietary carbohydrate via autophagy and the ubiquitin proteolytic systems. *Autophagy* **2012**, *8*, 1404–1406. [CrossRef]
97. Rowan, S.; Bejarano, E.; Taylor, A. Mechanistic targeting of advanced glycation end-products in age-related diseases. *Biochim. Et Biophys. Acta. Mol. Basis Dis.* **2018**, *1864*, 3631–3643. [CrossRef]
98. Antognelli, C.; Talesa, V.N. Glyoxalases in Urological Malignancies. *Int. J. Mol. Sci.* **2018**, *19*, 415. [CrossRef]
99. Thornalley, P.J. The glyoxalase system: New developments towards functional characterization of a metabolic pathway fundamental to biological life. *Biochem. J.* **1990**, *269*, 1–11. [CrossRef]
100. Abordo, E.A.; Minhas, H.S.; Thornalley, P.J. Accumulation of alpha-oxoaldehydes during oxidative stress: A role in cytotoxicity. *Biochem. Pharmacol.* **1999**, *58*, 641–648. [CrossRef]
101. Clelland, J.D.; Thornalley, P.J. S-2-hydroxyacylglutathione-derivatives: Enzymatic preparation, purification and characterisation. *J. Chem. Soc. Perkin Trans. 1* **1991**, 3009–3015. [CrossRef]
102. Shinohara, M.; Thornalley, P.J.; Giardino, I.; Beisswenger, P.; Thorpe, S.R.; Onorato, J.; Brownlee, M. Overexpression of glyoxalase-I in bovine endothelial cells inhibits intracellular advanced glycation endproduct formation and prevents hyperglycemia-induced increases in macromolecular endocytosis. *J. Clin. Investig.* **1998**, *101*, 1142–1147. [CrossRef] [PubMed]
103. McCann, V.J.; Davis, R.E.; Welborn, T.A.; Constable, I.J.; Beale, D.G. Glyoxalase phenotypes in patients with diabetes mellitus. *Aust. N. Z. J. Med.* **1981**, *11*, 380–382. [CrossRef]

104. Kalousová, M.; Germanová, A.; Jáchymová, M.; Mestek, O.; Tesar, V.; Zima, T. A419C (E111A) polymorphism of the glyoxalase I gene and vascular complications in chronic hemodialysis patients. *Ann. N. Y. Acad. Sci.* **2008**, *1126*, 268–271. [CrossRef] [PubMed]
105. Ranganathan, S.; Ciaccio, P.J.; Walsh, E.S.; Tew, K.D. Genomic sequence of human glyoxalase-I: Analysis of promoter activity and its regulation. *Gene* **1999**, *240*, 149–155. [CrossRef]
106. Conboy, C.M.; Spyrou, C.; Thorne, N.P.; Wade, E.J.; Barbosa-Morais, N.L.; Wilson, M.D.; Bhattacharjee, A.; Young, R.A.; Tavaré, S.; Lees, J.A.; et al. Cell cycle genes are the evolutionarily conserved targets of the E2F4 transcription factor. *PLoS ONE* **2007**, *2*, e1061. [CrossRef] [PubMed]
107. Orso, F.; Corà, D.; Ubezio, B.; Provero, P.; Caselle, M.; Taverna, D. Identification of functional TFAP2A and SP1 binding sites in new TFAP2A-modulated genes. *Bmc Genom.* **2010**, *11*, 355. [CrossRef] [PubMed]
108. Xue, M.; Rabbani, N.; Momiji, H.; Imbasi, P.; Anwar, M.M.; Kitteringham, N.; Park, B.K.; Souma, T.; Moriguchi, T.; Yamamoto, M.; et al. Transcriptional control of glyoxalase 1 by Nrf2 provides a stress-responsive defence against dicarbonyl glycation. *Biochem. J.* **2012**, *443*, 213–222. [CrossRef]
109. Kold-Christensen, R.; Johannsen, M. Methylglyoxal Metabolism and Aging-Related Disease: Moving from Correlation toward Causation. *Trends Endocrinol. Metab.* **2020**, *31*, 81–92. [CrossRef]
110. Li, D.; Ferrari, M.; Ellis, E.M. Human aldo-keto reductase AKR7A2 protects against the cytotoxicity and mutagenicity of reactive aldehydes and lowers intracellular reactive oxygen species in hamster V79-4 cells. *Chem. Biol. Interact.* **2012**, *195*, 25–34. [CrossRef]
111. Li, D.; Ellis, E.M. Aldo-keto reductase 7A5 (AKR7A5) attenuates oxidative stress and reactive aldehyde toxicity in V79-4 cells. *Toxicol. Vitr. Int. J. Publ. Assoc. Bibra* **2014**, *28*, 707–714. [CrossRef]
112. Baba, S.P.; Barski, O.A.; Ahmed, Y.; O'Toole, T.E.; Conklin, D.J.; Bhatnagar, A.; Srivastava, S. Reductive metabolism of AGE precursors: A metabolic route for preventing AGE accumulation in cardiovascular tissue. *Diabetes* **2009**, *58*, 2486–2497. [CrossRef] [PubMed]
113. Vander Jagt, D.L.; Hunsaker, L.A. Methylglyoxal metabolism and diabetic complications: Roles of aldose reductase, glyoxalase-I, betaine aldehyde dehydrogenase and 2-oxoaldehyde dehydrogenase. *Chem. Biol. Interact.* **2003**, *143-144*, 341–351. [CrossRef]
114. Morgenstern, J.; Fleming, T.; Schumacher, D.; Eckstein, V.; Freichel, M.; Herzig, S.; Nawroth, P. Loss of Glyoxalase 1 Induces Compensatory Mechanism to Achieve Dicarbonyl Detoxification in Mammalian Schwann Cells. *J. Biol. Chem.* **2017**, *292*, 3224–3238. [CrossRef]
115. Lodd, E.; Wiggenhauser, L.M.; Morgenstern, J.; Fleming, T.H.; Poschet, G.; Büttner, M.; Tabler, C.T.; Wohlfart, D.P.; Nawroth, P.P.; Kroll, J. The combination of loss of glyoxalase1 and obesity results in hyperglycemia. *JCI Insight* **2019**, *4*. [CrossRef] [PubMed]
116. Schumacher, D.; Morgenstern, J.; Oguchi, Y.; Volk, N.; Kopf, S.; Groener, J.B.; Nawroth, P.P.; Fleming, T.; Freichel, M. Compensatory mechanisms for methylglyoxal detoxification in experimental & clinical diabetes. *Mol. Metab.* **2018**, *18*, 143–152. [CrossRef]
117. Fujii, E.; Iwase, H.; Ishii-Karakasa, I.; Yajima, Y.; Hotta, K. The presence of 2-keto-3-deoxygluconic acid and oxoaldehyde dehydrogenase activity in human erythrocytes. *Biochem. Biophys. Res. Commun.* **1995**, *210*, 852–857. [CrossRef] [PubMed]
118. Collard, F.; Vertommen, D.; Fortpied, J.; Duester, G.; Van Schaftingen, E. Identification of 3-deoxyglucosone dehydrogenase as aldehyde dehydrogenase 1A1 (retinaldehyde dehydrogenase 1). *Biochimie* **2007**, *89*, 369–373. [CrossRef]
119. McDowell, R.E.; McGahon, M.K.; Augustine, J.; Chen, M.; McGeown, J.G.; Curtis, T.M. Diabetes Impairs the Aldehyde Detoxifying Capacity of the Retina. *Investig. Ophthalmol. Vis. Sci.* **2016**, *57*, 4762–4771. [CrossRef] [PubMed]
120. Bonifati, V.; Rizzu, P.; van Baren, M.J.; Schaap, O.; Breedveld, G.J.; Krieger, E.; Dekker, M.C.; Squitieri, F.; Ibanez, P.; Joosse, M.; et al. Mutations in the DJ-1 gene associated with autosomal recessive early-onset parkinsonism. *Science* **2003**, *299*, 256–259. [CrossRef]
121. Lev, N.; Roncevic, D.; Ickowicz, D.; Melamed, E.; Offen, D. Role of DJ-1 in Parkinson's disease. *J. Mol. Neurosci.* **2006**, *29*, 215–225. [CrossRef]
122. Lee, J.Y.; Song, J.; Kwon, K.; Jang, S.; Kim, C.; Baek, K.; Kim, J.; Park, C. Human DJ-1 and its homologs are novel glyoxalases. *Hum. Mol. Genet.* **2012**, *21*, 3215–3225. [CrossRef]

123. Richarme, G.; Mihoub, M.; Dairou, J.; Bui, L.C.; Leger, T.; Lamouri, A. Parkinsonism-associated protein DJ-1/Park7 is a major protein deglycase that repairs methylglyoxal- and glyoxal-glycated cysteine, arginine, and lysine residues. *J. Biol. Chem.* **2015**, *290*, 1885–1897. [CrossRef] [PubMed]
124. Pfaff, D.H.; Fleming, T.; Nawroth, P.; Teleman, A.A. Evidence Against a Role for the Parkinsonism-associated Protein DJ-1 in Methylglyoxal Detoxification. *J. Biol. Chem.* **2017**, *292*, 685–690. [CrossRef]
125. Richarme, G.; Liu, C.; Mihoub, M.; Abdallah, J.; Leger, T.; Joly, N.; Liebart, J.C.; Jurkunas, U.V.; Nadal, M.; Bouloc, P.; et al. Guanine glycation repair by DJ-1/Park7 and its bacterial homologs. *Science* **2017**, *357*, 208–211. [CrossRef]
126. Galligan, J.J.; Wepy, J.A.; Streeter, M.D.; Kingsley, P.J.; Mitchener, M.M.; Wauchope, O.R.; Beavers, W.N.; Rose, K.L.; Wang, T.; Spiegel, D.A.; et al. Methylglyoxal-derived posttranslational arginine modifications are abundant histone marks. *Proc. Natl. Acad. Sci. USA* **2018**, *115*, 9228–9233. [CrossRef]
127. Zheng, Q.; Omans, N.D.; Leicher, R.; Osunsade, A.; Agustinus, A.S.; Finkin-Groner, E.; D'Ambrosio, H.; Liu, B.; Chandarlapaty, S.; Liu, S.; et al. Reversible histone glycation is associated with disease-related changes in chromatin architecture. *Nat. Commun.* **2019**, *10*, 1289. [CrossRef]
128. Kalapos, M.P. On the mammalian acetone metabolism: From chemistry to clinical implications. *Biochim. Biophys. Acta* **2003**, *1621*, 122–139. [CrossRef]
129. Salomón, T.; Sibbersen, C.; Hansen, J.; Britz, D.; Svart, M.V.; Voss, T.S.; Møller, N.; Gregersen, N.; Jørgensen, K.A.; Palmfeldt, J.; et al. Ketone Body Acetoacetate Buffers Methylglyoxal via a Non-enzymatic Conversion during Diabetic and Dietary Ketosis. *Cell Chem. Biol.* **2017**, *24*, 935–943.e937. [CrossRef]
130. Barnosky, A.R.; Hoddy, K.K.; Unterman, T.G.; Varady, K.A. Intermittent fasting vs daily calorie restriction for type 2 diabetes prevention: A review of human findings. *Transl. Res. J. Lab. Clin. Med.* **2014**, *164*, 302–311. [CrossRef] [PubMed]
131. Takahashi, A.; Takabatake, Y.; Kimura, T.; Maejima, I.; Namba, T.; Yamamoto, T.; Matsuda, J.; Minami, S.; Kaimori, J.Y.; Matsui, I.; et al. Autophagy Inhibits the Accumulation of Advanced Glycation End Products by Promoting Lysosomal Biogenesis and Function in the Kidney Proximal Tubules. *Diabetes* **2017**, *66*, 1359–1372. [CrossRef]
132. Uchiki, T.; Weikel, K.A.; Jiao, W.; Shang, F.; Caceres, A.; Pawlak, D.; Handa, J.T.; Brownlee, M.; Nagaraj, R.; Taylor, A. Glycation-altered proteolysis as a pathobiologic mechanism that links dietary glycemic index, aging, and age-related disease (in nondiabetics). *Aging Cell* **2012**, *11*, 1–13. [CrossRef] [PubMed]
133. Zhang, Y.; Cross, S.D.; Stanton, J.B.; Marmorstein, A.D.; Le, Y.Z.; Marmorstein, L.Y. Early AMD-like defects in the RPE and retinal degeneration in aged mice with RPE-specific deletion of Atg5 or Atg7. *Mol. Vis.* **2017**, *23*, 228–241. [PubMed]
134. Chai, P.; Ni, H.; Zhang, H.; Fan, X. The Evolving Functions of Autophagy in Ocular Health: A Double-edged Sword. *Int. J. Biol. Sci.* **2016**, *12*, 1332–1340. [CrossRef] [PubMed]
135. Rosa, M.D.; Distefano, G.; Gagliano, C.; Rusciano, D.; Malaguarnera, L. Autophagy in Diabetic Retinopathy. *Curr. Neuropharmacol.* **2016**, *14*, 810–825. [CrossRef]
136. Grimm, S.; Ernst, L.; Grötzinger, N.; Höhn, A.; Breusing, N.; Reinheckel, T.; Grune, T. Cathepsin D is one of the major enzymes involved in intracellular degradation of AGE-modified proteins. *Free Radic. Res.* **2010**, *44*, 1013–1026. [CrossRef]
137. Bulteau, A.L.; Verbeke, P.; Petropoulos, I.; Chaffotte, A.F.; Friguet, B. Proteasome inhibition in glyoxal-treated fibroblasts and resistance of glycated glucose-6-phosphate dehydrogenase to 20 S proteasome degradation in vitro. *J. Biol. Chem.* **2001**, *276*, 45662–45668. [CrossRef]
138. Raupbach, J.; Ott, C.; Koenig, J.; Grune, T. Proteasomal degradation of glycated proteins depends on substrate unfolding: Preferred degradation of moderately modified myoglobin. *Free Radic. Biol. Med.* **2020**, *152*, 516–524. [CrossRef]
139. Gavilán, E.; Pintado, C.; Gavilan, M.P.; Daza, P.; Sánchez-Aguayo, I.; Castaño, A.; Ruano, D. Age-related dysfunctions of the autophagy lysosomal pathway in hippocampal pyramidal neurons under proteasome stress. *Neurobiol. Aging* **2015**, *36*, 1953–1963. [CrossRef]
140. Kwon, Y.T.; Ciechanover, A. The Ubiquitin Code in the Ubiquitin-Proteasome System and Autophagy. *Trends Biochem. Sci.* **2017**, *42*, 873–886. [CrossRef]
141. Cuervo, A.M. Autophagy and aging: Keeping that old broom working. *Trends Genet.* **2008**, *24*, 604–612. [CrossRef]

142. Shang, F.; Taylor, A. Ubiquitin Conjugates: A Sensitive Marker of Oxidative Stress. In *Biomarkers for Antioxidant Defense and Oxidative Damage: Principles and Practical Applications*; Wiley: Hoboken, NJ, USA, 2010; pp. 219–228. [CrossRef]
143. Shang, F.; Taylor, A. Roles for the ubiquitin-proteasome pathway in protein quality control and signaling in the retina: Implications in the pathogenesis of age-related macular degeneration. *Mol. Asp. Med.* **2012**, *33*, 446–466. [CrossRef] [PubMed]
144. Itoh, K.; Ishii, T.; Wakabayashi, N.; Yamamoto, M. Regulatory mechanisms of cellular response to oxidative stress. *Free Radic. Res.* **1999**, *31*, 319–324. [CrossRef] [PubMed]
145. Kobayashi, M.; Itoh, K.; Suzuki, T.; Osanai, H.; Nishikawa, K.; Katoh, Y.; Takagi, Y.; Yamamoto, M. Identification of the interactive interface and phylogenic conservation of the Nrf2-Keap1 system. *Genes Cells Devoted Mol. Cell. Mech.* **2002**, *7*, 807–820. [CrossRef]
146. Katoh, Y.; Itoh, K.; Yoshida, E.; Miyagishi, M.; Fukamizu, A.; Yamamoto, M. Two domains of Nrf2 cooperatively bind CBP, a CREB binding protein, and synergistically activate transcription. *Genes Cells Devoted Mol. Cell. Mech.* **2001**, *6*, 857–868. [CrossRef]
147. Cullinan, S.B.; Gordan, J.D.; Jin, J.; Harper, J.W.; Diehl, J.A. The Keap1-BTB protein is an adaptor that bridges Nrf2 to a Cul3-based E3 ligase: Oxidative stress sensing by a Cul3-Keap1 ligase. *Mol. Cell. Biol.* **2004**, *24*, 8477–8486. [CrossRef]
148. Nguyen, T.; Sherratt, P.J.; Nioi, P.; Yang, C.S.; Pickett, C.B. Nrf2 controls constitutive and inducible expression of ARE-driven genes through a dynamic pathway involving nucleocytoplasmic shuttling by Keap1. *J. Biol. Chem.* **2005**, *280*, 32485–32492. [CrossRef]
149. Antognelli, C.; Trapani, E.; Delle Monache, S.; Perrelli, A.; Daga, M.; Pizzimenti, S.; Barrera, G.; Cassoni, P.; Angelucci, A.; Trabalzini, L.; et al. KRIT1 loss-of-function induces a chronic Nrf2-mediated adaptive homeostasis that sensitizes cells to oxidative stress: Implication for Cerebral Cavernous Malformation disease. *Free Radic. Biol. Med.* **2018**, *115*, 202–218. [CrossRef]
150. Antognelli, C.; Trapani, E.; Delle Monache, S.; Perrelli, A.; Fornelli, C.; Retta, F.; Cassoni, P.; Talesa, V.N.; Retta, S.F. Data in support of sustained upregulation of adaptive redox homeostasis mechanisms caused by KRIT1 loss-of-function. *Data Brief* **2018**, *16*, 929–938. [CrossRef]
151. Gambelunghe, A.; Giovagnoli, S.; Di Michele, A.; Boncompagni, S.; Dell'Omo, M.; Leopold, K.; Iavicoli, I.; Talesa, V.N.; Antognelli, C. Redox-Sensitive Glyoxalase 1 Up-Regulation Is Crucial for Protecting Human Lung Cells from Gold Nanoparticles Toxicity. *Antioxidants* **2020**, *9*, 697. [CrossRef]
152. James, D.; Devaraj, S.; Bellur, P.; Lakkanna, S.; Vicini, J.; Boddupalli, S. Novel concepts of broccoli sulforaphanes and disease: Induction of phase II antioxidant and detoxification enzymes by enhanced-glucoraphanin broccoli. *Nutr. Rev.* **2012**, *70*, 654–665. [CrossRef]
153. Angeloni, C.; Malaguti, M.; Rizzo, B.; Barbalace, M.C.; Fabbri, D.; Hrelia, S. Neuroprotective effect of sulforaphane against methylglyoxal cytotoxicity. *Chem. Res. Toxicol.* **2015**, *28*, 1234–1245. [CrossRef]
154. Alfarano, M.; Pastore, D.; Fogliano, V.; Schalkwijk, C.G.; Oliviero, T. The Effect of Sulforaphane on Glyoxalase I Expression and Activity in Peripheral Blood Mononuclear Cells. *Nutrients* **2018**, *10*, 1773. [CrossRef] [PubMed]
155. Pereira, A.; Fernandes, R.; Crisóstomo, J.; Seiça, R.M.; Sena, C.M. The Sulforaphane and pyridoxamine supplementation normalize endothelial dysfunction associated with type 2 diabetes. *Sci. Rep.* **2017**, *7*, 14357. [CrossRef]
156. Nishimoto, S.; Koike, S.; Inoue, N.; Suzuki, T.; Ogasawara, Y. Activation of Nrf2 attenuates carbonyl stress induced by methylglyoxal in human neuroblastoma cells: Increase in GSH levels is a critical event for the detoxification mechanism. *Biochem. Biophys. Res. Commun.* **2017**, *483*, 874–879. [CrossRef]
157. Liu, G.H.; Qu, J.; Shen, X. NF-kappaB/p65 antagonizes Nrf2-ARE pathway by depriving CBP from Nrf2 and facilitating recruitment of HDAC3 to MafK. *Biochim. Biophys. Acta* **2008**, *1783*, 713–727. [CrossRef] [PubMed]
158. Antognelli, C.; Gambelunghe, A.; Muzi, G.; Talesa, V.N. Peroxynitrite-mediated glyoxalase I epigenetic inhibition drives apoptosis in airway epithelial cells exposed to crystalline silica via a novel mechanism involving argpyrimidine-modified Hsp70, JNK, and NF-κB. *Free Radic. Biol. Med.* **2015**, *84*, 128–141. [CrossRef] [PubMed]
159. Zhang, H.; Li, H.; Xi, H.S.; Li, S. HIF1α is required for survival maintenance of chronic myeloid leukemia stem cells. *Blood* **2012**, *119*, 2595–2607. [CrossRef]

160. Rauh, D.; Fischer, F.; Gertz, M.; Lakshminarasimhan, M.; Bergbrede, T.; Aladini, F.; Kambach, C.; Becker, C.F.; Zerweck, J.; Schutkowski, M.; et al. An acetylome peptide microarray reveals specificities and deacetylation substrates for all human sirtuin isoforms. *Nat. Commun.* **2013**, *4*, 2327. [CrossRef]
161. Lundby, A.; Lage, K.; Weinert, B.T.; Bekker-Jensen, D.B.; Secher, A.; Skovgaard, T.; Kelstrup, C.D.; Dmytriyev, A.; Choudhary, C.; Lundby, C.; et al. Proteomic analysis of lysine acetylation sites in rat tissues reveals organ specificity and subcellular patterns. *Cell Rep.* **2012**, *2*, 419–431. [CrossRef]
162. Reiniger, N.; Lau, K.; McCalla, D.; Eby, B.; Cheng, B.; Lu, Y.; Qu, W.; Quadri, N.; Ananthakrishnan, R.; Furmansky, M.; et al. Deletion of the receptor for advanced glycation end products reduces glomerulosclerosis and preserves renal function in the diabetic OVE26 mouse. *Diabetes* **2010**, *59*, 2043–2054. [CrossRef]
163. Irshad, Z.; Xue, M.; Ashour, A.; Larkin, J.R.; Thornalley, P.J.; Rabbani, N. Activation of the unfolded protein response in high glucose treated endothelial cells is mediated by methylglyoxal. *Sci. Rep.* **2019**, *9*, 7889. [CrossRef] [PubMed]
164. Rowan, S.; Jiang, S.; Chang, M.L.; Volkin, J.; Cassalman, C.; Smith, K.M.; Streeter, M.D.; Spiegel, D.A.; Moreira-Neto, C.; Rabbani, N.; et al. A low glycemic diet protects disease-prone Nrf2-deficient mice against age-related macular degeneration. *Free Radic. Biol. Med.* **2020**, *150*, 75–86. [CrossRef] [PubMed]
165. Stratmann, B.; Goldstein, B.; Thornalley, P.J.; Rabbani, N.; Tschoepe, D. Intracellular Accumulation of Methylglyoxal by Glyoxalase 1 Knock Down Alters Collagen Homoeostasis in L6 Myoblasts. *Int. J. Mol. Sci.* **2017**, *18*, 480. [CrossRef]
166. Nigro, C.; Leone, A.; Fiory, F.; Prevenzano, I.; Nicolò, A.; Mirra, P.; Beguinot, F.; Miele, C. Dicarbonyl Stress at the Crossroads of Healthy and Unhealthy Aging. *Cells* **2019**, *8*. [CrossRef] [PubMed]
167. Giacco, F.; Du, X.; D'Agati, V.D.; Milne, R.; Sui, G.; Geoffrion, M.; Brownlee, M. Knockdown of glyoxalase 1 mimics diabetic nephropathy in nondiabetic mice. *Diabetes* **2014**, *63*, 291–299. [CrossRef] [PubMed]
168. Jang, S.; Kwon, D.M.; Kwon, K.; Park, C. Generation and characterization of mouse knockout for glyoxalase 1. *Biochem. Biophys. Res. Commun.* **2017**, *490*, 460–465. [CrossRef] [PubMed]
169. Shafie, A.; Xue, M.; Barker, G.; Zehnder, D.; Thornalley, P.J.; Rabbani, N. Reappraisal of putative glyoxalase 1-deficient mouse and dicarbonyl stress on embryonic stem cells in vitro. *Biochem. J.* **2016**, *473*, 4255–4270. [CrossRef]
170. Moraru, A.; Wiederstein, J.; Pfaff, D.; Fleming, T.; Miller, A.K.; Nawroth, P.; Teleman, A.A. Elevated Levels of the Reactive Metabolite Methylglyoxal Recapitulate Progression of Type 2 Diabetes. *Cell Metab.* **2018**, *27*, 926–934. [CrossRef]
171. Morcos, M.; Du, X.; Pfisterer, F.; Hutter, H.; Sayed, A.A.; Thornalley, P.; Ahmed, N.; Baynes, J.; Thorpe, S.; Kukudov, G.; et al. Glyoxalase-1 prevents mitochondrial protein modification and enhances lifespan in Caenorhabditis elegans. *Aging Cell* **2008**, *7*, 260–269. [CrossRef]
172. Distler, M.G.; Plant, L.D.; Sokoloff, G.; Hawk, A.J.; Aneas, I.; Wuenschell, G.E.; Termini, J.; Meredith, S.C.; Nobrega, M.A.; Palmer, A.A. Glyoxalase 1 increases anxiety by reducing GABAA receptor agonist methylglyoxal. *J. Clin. Investig.* **2012**, *122*, 2306–2315. [CrossRef]
173. Brouwers, O.; Niessen, P.M.; Ferreira, I.; Miyata, T.; Scheffer, P.G.; Teerlink, T.; Schrauwen, P.; Brownlee, M.; Stehouwer, C.D.; Schalkwijk, C.G. Overexpression of glyoxalase-I reduces hyperglycemia-induced levels of advanced glycation end products and oxidative stress in diabetic rats. *J. Biol. Chem.* **2011**, *286*, 1374–1380. [CrossRef] [PubMed]
174. Berner, A.K.; Brouwers, O.; Pringle, R.; Klaassen, I.; Colhoun, L.; McVicar, C.; Brockbank, S.; Curry, J.W.; Miyata, T.; Brownlee, M.; et al. Protection against methylglyoxal-derived AGEs by regulation of glyoxalase 1 prevents retinal neuroglial and vasodegenerative pathology. *Diabetologia* **2012**, *55*, 845–854. [CrossRef] [PubMed]
175. Brouwers, O.; Niessen, P.M.; Miyata, T.; Østergaard, J.A.; Flyvbjerg, A.; Peutz-Kootstra, C.J.; Sieber, J.; Mundel, P.H.; Brownlee, M.; Janssen, B.J.; et al. Glyoxalase-1 overexpression reduces endothelial dysfunction and attenuates early renal impairment in a rat model of diabetes. *Diabetologia* **2014**, *57*, 224–235. [CrossRef]
176. Qi, W.; Keenan, H.A.; Li, Q.; Ishikado, A.; Kannt, A.; Sadowski, T.; Yorek, M.A.; Wu, I.H.; Lockhart, S.; Coppey, L.J.; et al. Pyruvate kinase M2 activation may protect against the progression of diabetic glomerular pathology and mitochondrial dysfunction. *Nat. Med.* **2017**, *23*, 753–762. [CrossRef]
177. Yao, D.; Brownlee, M. Hyperglycemia-induced reactive oxygen species increase expression of the receptor for advanced glycation end products (RAGE) and RAGE ligands. *Diabetes* **2010**, *59*, 249–255. [CrossRef]

178. Dobler, D.; Ahmed, N.; Song, L.; Eboigbodin, K.E.; Thornalley, P.J. Increased dicarbonyl metabolism in endothelial cells in hyperglycemia induces anoikis and impairs angiogenesis by RGD and GFOGER motif modification. *Diabetes* **2006**, *55*, 1961–1969. [CrossRef] [PubMed]
179. Miller, A.G.; Smith, D.G.; Bhat, M.; Nagaraj, R.H. Glyoxalase I is critical for human retinal capillary pericyte survival under hyperglycemic conditions. *J. Biol. Chem.* **2006**, *281*, 11864–11871. [CrossRef]
180. Barati, M.T.; Merchant, M.L.; Kain, A.B.; Jevans, A.W.; McLeish, K.R.; Klein, J.B. Proteomic analysis defines altered cellular redox pathways and advanced glycation end-product metabolism in glomeruli of db/db diabetic mice. *Am. J. Physiol. Ren. Physiol.* **2007**, *293*, F1157–F1165. [CrossRef]
181. Palsamy, P.; Subramanian, S. Resveratrol protects diabetic kidney by attenuating hyperglycemia-mediated oxidative stress and renal inflammatory cytokines via Nrf2-Keap1 signaling. *Biochim. Et Biophys. Acta* **2011**, *1812*, 719–731. [CrossRef]
182. Miller, A.G.; Tan, G.; Binger, K.J.; Pickering, R.J.; Thomas, M.C.; Nagaraj, R.H.; Cooper, M.E.; Wilkinson-Berka, J.L. Candesartan attenuates diabetic retinal vascular pathology by restoring glyoxalase-I function. *Diabetes* **2010**, *59*, 3208–3215. [CrossRef]
183. Phillips, S.A.; Mirrlees, D.; Thornalley, P.J. Modification of the glyoxalase system in streptozotocin-induced diabetic rats. Effect of the aldose reductase inhibitor Statil. *Biochem. Pharmacol.* **1993**, *46*, 805–811. [CrossRef]
184. Bierhaus, A.; Fleming, T.; Stoyanov, S.; Leffler, A.; Babes, A.; Neacsu, C.; Sauer, S.K.; Eberhardt, M.; Schnölzer, M.; Lasitschka, F.; et al. Methylglyoxal modification of Nav1.8 facilitates nociceptive neuron firing and causes hyperalgesia in diabetic neuropathy. *Nat. Med.* **2012**, *18*, 926–933. [CrossRef]
185. Atkins, T.W.; Thornally, P.J. Erythrocyte glyoxalase activity in genetically obese (ob/ob) and streptozotocin diabetic mice. *Diabetes Res.* **1989**, *11*, 125–129. [PubMed]
186. McLellan, A.C.; Thornalley, P.J. Glyoxalase activity in human red blood cells fractioned by age. *Mech. Ageing Dev.* **1989**, *48*, 63–71. [CrossRef]
187. López-Otín, C.; Blasco, M.A.; Partridge, L.; Serrano, M.; Kroemer, G. The hallmarks of aging. *Cell* **2013**, *153*, 1194–1217. [CrossRef]
188. Schalkwijk, C.G.; Stehouwer, C.D.A. Methylglyoxal, a Highly Reactive Dicarbonyl Compound, in Diabetes, Its Vascular Complications, and Other Age-Related Diseases. *Physiol. Rev.* **2020**, *100*, 407–461. [CrossRef] [PubMed]
189. Xue, M.; Rabbani, N.; Thornalley, P.J. Glyoxalase in ageing. *Semin. Cell Dev. Biol.* **2011**, *22*, 293–301. [CrossRef]
190. Rabbani, N.; Xue, M.; Thornalley, P.J. Methylglyoxal-induced dicarbonyl stress in aging and disease: First steps towards glyoxalase 1-based treatments. *Clin. Sci.* **2016**, *130*, 1677–1696. [CrossRef]
191. Sharma-Luthra, R.; Kale, R.K. Age related changes in the activity of the glyoxalase system. *Mech. Ageing Dev.* **1994**, *73*, 39–45. [CrossRef]
192. Amicarelli, F.; Di Ilio, C.; Masciocco, L.; Bonfigli, A.; Zarivi, O.; D'Andrea, M.R.; Di Giulio, C.; Miranda, M. Aging and detoxifying enzymes responses to hypoxic or hyperoxic treatment. *Mech. Ageing Dev.* **1997**, *97*, 215–226. [CrossRef]
193. Kirk, J.E. The glyoxalase I activity of arterial tissue in individuals of various ages. *J. Gerontol.* **1960**, *15*, 139–141. [CrossRef]
194. Haik, G.M., Jr.; Lo, T.W.; Thornalley, P.J. Methylglyoxal concentration and glyoxalase activities in the human lens. *Exp. Eye Res.* **1994**, *59*, 497–500. [CrossRef] [PubMed]
195. Mailankot, M.; Padmanabha, S.; Pasupuleti, N.; Major, D.; Howell, S.; Nagaraj, R.H. Glyoxalase I activity and immunoreactivity in the aging human lens. *Biogerontology* **2009**, *10*, 711–720. [CrossRef] [PubMed]
196. Kuhla, B.; Boeck, K.; Lüth, H.J.; Schmidt, A.; Weigle, B.; Schmitz, M.; Ogunlade, V.; Münch, G.; Arendt, T. Age-dependent changes of glyoxalase I expression in human brain. *Neurobiol. Aging* **2006**, *27*, 815–822. [CrossRef] [PubMed]
197. Wu, J.C.; Li, X.H.; Peng, Y.D.; Wang, J.B.; Tang, J.F.; Wang, Y.F. Association of two glyoxalase I gene polymorphisms with nephropathy and retinopathy in Type 2 diabetes. *J. Endocrinol. Investig.* **2011**, *34*, e343–e348. [CrossRef]
198. Rasul, A.; Rashid, A.; Waheed, P.; Khan, S.A. Expression analysis of glyoxalase I gene among patients of diabetic retinopathy. *Pak. J. Med. Sci.* **2018**, *34*, 139–143. [CrossRef] [PubMed]
199. Zaidi, A.; Waheed, P.; Rashid, A.; Khan, S.A. Gene Expression of Glyoxalase II in Diabetic Retinopathy. *J. Coll. Physicians Surg. Pak.* **2018**, *28*, 523–526. [CrossRef]

200. Sachdeva, R.; Schlotterer, A.; Schumacher, D.; Matka, C.; Mathar, I.; Dietrich, N.; Medert, R.; Kriebs, U.; Lin, J.; Nawroth, P.; et al. TRPC proteins contribute to development of diabetic retinopathy and regulate glyoxalase 1 activity and methylglyoxal accumulation. *Mol. Metab.* **2018**, *9*, 156–167. [CrossRef]
201. Arai, M.; Nihonmatsu-Kikuchi, N.; Itokawa, M.; Rabbani, N.; Thornalley, P.J. Measurement of glyoxalase activities. *Biochem. Soc. Trans.* **2014**, *42*, 491–494. [CrossRef]
202. Peters, A.S.; Wortmann, M.; Fleming, T.H.; Nawroth, P.P.; Bruckner, T.; Böckler, D.; Hakimi, M. Effect of metformin treatment in patients with type 2 diabetes with respect to glyoxalase 1 activity in atherosclerotic lesions. *Vasa. Z. Fur Gefasskrankh.* **2019**, *48*, 186–192. [CrossRef]
203. Cheng, A.S.; Cheng, Y.H.; Chiou, C.H.; Chang, T.L. Resveratrol upregulates Nrf2 expression to attenuate methylglyoxal-induced insulin resistance in Hep G2 cells. *J. Agric. Food Chem.* **2012**, *60*, 9180–9187. [CrossRef] [PubMed]
204. Maher, P.; Dargusch, R.; Ehren, J.L.; Okada, S.; Sharma, K.; Schubert, D. Fisetin lowers methylglyoxal dependent protein glycation and limits the complications of diabetes. *PLoS ONE* **2011**, *6*, e21226. [CrossRef] [PubMed]
205. Liu, Y.W.; Zhu, X.; Zhang, L.; Lu, Q.; Wang, J.Y.; Zhang, F.; Guo, H.; Yin, J.L.; Yin, X.X. Up-regulation of glyoxalase 1 by mangiferin prevents diabetic nephropathy progression in streptozotocin-induced diabetic rats. *Eur. J. Pharmacol.* **2013**, *721*, 355–364. [CrossRef]
206. Liu, Y.W.; Cheng, Y.Q.; Liu, X.L.; Hao, Y.C.; Li, Y.; Zhu, X.; Zhang, F.; Yin, X.X. Mangiferin Upregulates Glyoxalase 1 Through Activation of Nrf2/ARE Signaling in Central Neurons Cultured with High Glucose. *Mol. Neurobiol.* **2017**, *54*, 4060–4070. [CrossRef] [PubMed]
207. Suantawee, T.; Thilavech, T.; Cheng, H.; Adisakwattana, S. Cyanidin Attenuates Methylglyoxal-Induced Oxidative Stress and Apoptosis in INS-1 Pancreatic β-Cells by Increasing Glyoxalase-1 Activity. *Nutrients* **2020**, *12*, 1319. [CrossRef]
208. Xue, M.; Weickert, M.O.; Qureshi, S.; Kandala, N.B.; Anwar, A.; Waldron, M.; Shafie, A.; Messenger, D.; Fowler, M.; Jenkins, G.; et al. Improved Glycemic Control and Vascular Function in Overweight and Obese Subjects by Glyoxalase 1 Inducer Formulation. *Diabetes* **2016**, *65*, 2282–2294. [CrossRef]
209. Angeloni, C.; Turroni, S.; Bianchi, L.; Fabbri, D.; Motori, E.; Malaguti, M.; Leoncini, E.; Maraldi, T.; Bini, L.; Brigidi, P.; et al. Novel targets of sulforaphane in primary cardiomyocytes identified by proteomic analysis. *PLoS ONE* **2013**, *8*, e83283. [CrossRef]
210. Maeda, S.; Matsui, T.; Ojima, A.; Takeuchi, M.; Yamagishi, S. Sulforaphane inhibits advanced glycation end product-induced pericyte damage by reducing expression of receptor for advanced glycation end products. *Nutr. Res.* **2014**, *34*, 807–813. [CrossRef]
211. Lv, J.; Bao, S.; Liu, T.; Wei, L.; Wang, D.; Ye, W.; Wang, N.; Song, S.; Li, J.; Chudhary, M.; et al. Sulforaphane delays diabetes-induced retinal photoreceptor cell degeneration. *Cell Tissue Res.* **2020**. [CrossRef]
212. Oh, S.; Ahn, H.; Park, H.; Lee, J.I.; Park, K.Y.; Hwang, D.; Lee, S.; Son, K.H.; Byun, K. The attenuating effects of pyridoxamine on adipocyte hypertrophy and inflammation differ by adipocyte location. *J. Nutr. Biochem.* **2019**, *72*, 108173. [CrossRef]
213. Stitt, A.; Gardiner, T.A.; Alderson, N.L.; Canning, P.; Frizzell, N.; Duffy, N.; Boyle, C.; Januszewski, A.S.; Chachich, M.; Baynes, J.W.; et al. The AGE inhibitor pyridoxamine inhibits development of retinopathy in experimental diabetes. *Diabetes* **2002**, *51*, 2826–2832. [CrossRef] [PubMed]
214. He, Y.; Zhou, C.; Huang, M.; Tang, C.; Liu, X.; Yue, Y.; Diao, Q.; Zheng, Z.; Liu, D. Glyoxalase system: A systematic review of its biological activity, related-diseases, screening methods and small molecule regulators. *Biomed Pharm.* **2020**, *131*, 110663. [CrossRef] [PubMed]

Publisher's Note: MDPI stays neutral with regard to jurisdictional claims in published maps and institutional affiliations.

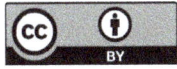

© 2020 by the authors. Licensee MDPI, Basel, Switzerland. This article is an open access article distributed under the terms and conditions of the Creative Commons Attribution (CC BY) license (http://creativecommons.org/licenses/by/4.0/).

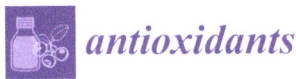

Review

Eicosanoids and Oxidative Stress in Diabetic Retinopathy

Mong-Heng Wang [1,*], George Hsiao [2,3] and Mohamed Al-Shabrawey [4,5,6,*]

1. Department of Physiology, Augusta University, Augusta, GA 30912, USA
2. Graduate Institute of Medical Sciences, College of Medicine, Taipei Medical University, Taipei 110, Taiwan; geohsiao@tmu.edu.tw
3. Department of Pharmacology, School of Medicine, College of Medicine, Taipei Medical University, Taipei 110, Taiwan
4. Department of Oral Biology and Diagnostic Sciences, Augusta University, Augusta, GA 30912, USA
5. Department of Cellular Biology and Anatomy, Augusta University, Augusta, GA 30912, USA
6. Culver Vision Discovery Institute and Ophthalmology, Augusta University, Augusta, GA 30912, USA
* Correspondence: mwang@augusta.edu (M.-H.W.); malshabrawey@augusta.edu (M.A.-S.); Tel.: +706-721-3830 (M.-H.W.); +706-721-2991 (M.A.-S.); Fax: +706-721-7299 (M.-H.W.); +706-721-9415 (M.A.-S.)

Received: 12 May 2020; Accepted: 10 June 2020; Published: 12 June 2020

Abstract: Oxidative stress is an important factor to cause the pathogenesis of diabetic retinopathy (DR) because the retina has high vascularization and long-time light exposition. Cyclooxygenase (COX), lipoxygenase (LOX), and cytochrome P450 (CYP) enzymes can convert arachidonic acid (AA) into eicosanoids, which are important lipid mediators to regulate DR development. COX-derived metabolites appear to be significant factors causative to oxidative stress and retinal microvascular dysfunction. Several elegant studies have unraveled the importance of LOX-derived eicosanoids, including LTs and HETEs, to oxidative stress and retinal microvascular dysfunction. The role of CYP eicosanoids in DR is yet to be explored. There is clear evidence that CYP-derived epoxyeicosatrienoic acids (EETs) have detrimental effects on the retina. Our recent study showed that the renin-angiotensin system (RAS) activation augments retinal soluble epoxide hydrolase (sEH), a crucial enzyme degrading EETs. Our findings suggest that EETs blockade can enhance the ability of RAS blockade to prevent or mitigate microvascular damage in DR. This review will focus on the critical information related the function of these eicosanoids in the retina, the interaction between eicosanoids and reactive oxygen species (ROS), and the involvement of eicosanoids in DR. We also identify potential targets for the treatment of DR.

Keywords: eicosanoids; oxidative stress; diabetic retinopathy; cyclooxygenase; lipoxygenase; Cytochrome P450

---

1. Introduction

Diabetes can be divided into type 1 (T1DM) and type 2 diabetes mellitus (T2DM). T1DM is mainly due to the autoimmune destruction of β cells [1,2]. Eventually, circulating insulin levels are negligible or completely absent in patients with T1DM [3]. T2DM is mainly associated with obesity, which affects one in three Americans [4,5]. Diabetic retinopathy (DR), a severe microvascular complication of T1DM and T2DM, is a disease that affects 7.7 million working-age adults in the U.S. DR-related blindness costs approximately $500 million annually in the U.S. [6] By 2050 more than a third of the U.S. population is expected to be diabetic; thus, the incidence of DR will increase dramatically [6]. The lack of productivity, high treatment costs, and diminished quality of life in patients with DR cause a pronounced socioeconomic burden.

In the retina, microvessels are vulnerable to oxidative stress because of chronic hyperglycemia, leading to increased reactive oxygen species (ROS) production. It has been observed that ROS imbalance is involved in DR [7]. The primary ROS species includes superoxide anion, hydroxyl anion, hydrogen peroxide (H_2O_2), and peroxynitrite [8]. Superoxide anion can be rapidly reduced to H_2O_2, which, due to its lipid-soluble properties, can modify cellular proteins, RNA, and DNA [9]. Hydroxide anion can oxidize DNA nucleotides and lipids. Superoxide anion may also react with NO to rapidly form peroxynitrite, which influences the properties of a variety of proteins, including inducible NO synthase (iNOS) and eNOS [10]. The endogenous antioxidant enzymes, including superoxide dismutase, glutathione peroxidase, and catalase, are involved in reducing these ROS. Of note, ROS play an essential role in the retinal pathological processes of DR, including inflammation and angiogenesis [11].

Since retinal microvascular dysfunction and damage are the key events in the onset and progression of DR, this review will focus on how arachidonic acid (AA; 20:4 n-6)-derived eicosanoids affect retinal microvascular function, and the role of these eicosanoids in DR. Our daily diets contain AA, which is the polyunsaturated fatty acid (PUFA). For example, AA is found in meat, including both red and white meat, organ meats, including kidney, liver, and brain, and eggs [12,13]. It is estimated that our mean daily AA intakes are about 100 to 350 mg in developed countries [12,13]. Additionally, humans can synthesize AA from linoleic acid (LA; 18:2 n-6), which is the principal PUFA in most western diets, including many nuts and seeds, vegetable oils, and products made from vegetable oils such as margarine [13]. AA is incorporated at the sn-2 position of the glycerol component of membrane phospholipids or other compound lipids. When the cell membrane is subjected to inflammatory stimuli, AA is released from the endogenous lipid pool by the action of phospholipase A2 (PLA2) (Figure 1). It is well-established that AA is converted by COX, LOX, and CYP pathway into eicosanoids (Figure 1) [14–17]. These lipid mediators can contribute considerably to oxidative stress, inflammation [15,18], and vascular function [19,20]. These three eicosanoid pathways are essential therapeutic targets for inflammatory and cardiovascular diseases because many receptors and metabolites of these three pathways are well defined. This review will provide valuable information related to the function of these lipid mediators in the retina and the involvement of these mediators in DR.

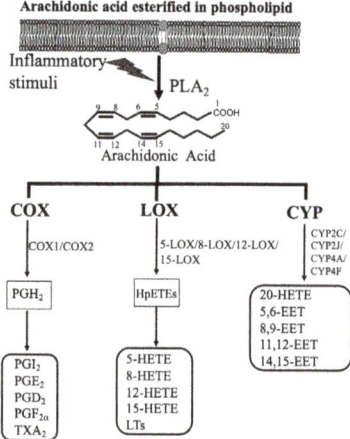

Figure 1. Bioactive eicosanoids derived from arachidonic acid (AA) cascade. After trigging by inflammatory conditions such as the presence of cytokines and growth factors, AA-containing phospholipids are hydrolyzed by phospholipase A2 (PLA2), resulting in the release of free AA. AA can be further metabolized by three pathways, i.e., the cyclooxygenase (COX), lipoxygenase (LOX), and cytochrome P450 (CYP) pathways. AA cascade generates prostaglandins (PGs), thromboxane A2 (TXA2), and a series of hydroxyeicosatetraenoic acids (HETEs), leukotrienes (LTs), and epoxyeicosatrienoic acids (EETs).

2. Functions of Eicosanoids in the Retina and Their Interaction with ROS

2.1. COX-Derived Eicosanoids

The major COX-derived eicosanoids include prostaglandins (PGs) and thromboxane (TX). COX enzymes catalyze the first two steps of the enzymatic reaction, including cyclooxygenase (dioxygenase) and peroxidase activity, to convert AA into PGH2 [21]. Of note, PGH2 is not stable, and it is the precursor for the production of PGs and TX, which is depending on the differential expression of isomerases and PG synthases in different tissues [22]. COX enzymes include two isozymes, COX-1 and COX-2. COX-1 is the constitutive isoform, which is responsible for the low PGs synthesis required for cell homeostasis, whereas COX-2 is inducible by many extracellular stimuli, including cytokines and growth factors, during chronic inflammation [17,23]. The major PGs are PGD2, PGE2, PGI2, and PGF2α, and the central TX is TXA2. The function of these PGs and TXA2 is mediated via the binding of DP, EPs (EP1 to EP4), IP, FP, and TP receptors.

It is well established that PGs are produced in retinal and choroidal blood vessels [24–26]. Several studies [27,28] have demonstrated that PGs play a vital role in the regulation of retinal blood flow (RBF) and choroidal blood flow (ChBF) [27,28]. Of note, RBF supplies the inner layers of the retina, whereas ChBF nourishes the outer layers (retinal pigment epithelium (RPE) and the photoreceptors) of the retina with nutrition and oxygen. During a rise in perfusion pressure, PGE2 and PGF2α are amply released in retinal and choroidal blood vessels, and these PGs cause vasoconstriction [29]. On the other hand, the release of PGI2 and PGD2 in retinal and choroidal blood vessels during perfusion causes vasorelaxation [29]. Notably, several studies [27,30] have suggested that PGs are involved in the inability of autoregulation of RBF and ChBF in newborn animals, which results in excess delivery of oxygen to the retina, and causes retinal microvascular damage in retinopathy of prematurity (ROP). Moreover, PGE2 has detrimental effects on the blood vessels, including increased oxidative stress, increased vasodilation, increased vascular permeability, and increased production of proinflammatory cytokines [16].

As mentioned above, PGs are produced from AA released from the phospholipids of the cell membrane by COXs by generating PGG2 and PGH2. The reaction for the generation of PGG2 by COXs needs peroxides as critical components in COX activation. Thus, several studies [31–33] have reported that in the blood vessels, ROS can affect both the activity and expression of COXs. For example, H_2O_2 increases COX-2 expression in endothelial or vascular smooth muscle cells (VSMCs) [31–33]. Moreover, there is some evidence that PGs can directly regulate the production of ROS in the blood vessels. For example, TXA2 up-regulates the expression and activity of NADPH oxidase, a crucial enzyme to produce ROS in all blood vessel wall cells [34]. PGE2 promotes ROS formation via the EP1 receptor, which is associated with hypertension and endothelial dysfunction [35,36].

2.2. LOX-Derived Eicosanoids

The major components in LOX-derived eicosanoids are hydroxyeicosatetraenoic acids (HETEs), including 5-HETE, 8-HETE, 12-HETE, and 15-HETE, as well as leukotrienes (LTs), containing LTA4, LTB4, LTC4, LTD4, LTE4, and LTF4 (Figure 1). Under the catalysis of lipoxygenases (5-LOX, 8-LOX, 12-LOX, and 15-LOX), which are non-heme iron-containing enzymes, AA is metabolized into hydroperoxyeicosatetraenoic acid (HpETE). 12-HpETE and 15-HpETE are reduced into 12-HETE and 15-HETE. 5-HETE is generated from 5-LOX, and 8-HETE is generated from 8-LOX. 5-HETE induces the degranulation of neutrophils, and 8-HETE is involved in skin inflammation. 5-LOX metabolizes AA into 5-HpETE, which is the precursor for the synthesis of proinflammatory LTA4. LTA4 is metabolized to LTB4 by leukotriene A4 hydrolase, and LTB4 binds to its receptors (BLT1 or BLT2) for its action [37]. LTA4 is unstable, and it can be merged with glutathione to form cysteinyl-LTs (cysLTs), which include LTC4, LTD4, LTE4, and LTF4 [38,39]. The function of LTs is mediated through the binding of these LTs to their receptors, including BLT, cysLT, and LTE4 receptors.

LOX-derived eicosanoids are implicated in several critical inflammatory conditions, and LTs (LTC4, LTD4, and LTE4) are mostly synthesized by neutrophils, macrophages, and mast cells [38]. As LTs have a relatively short half-life, these lipid mediators act as autacoids near their synthesizing sites [40]. LTC4, LTD4, and LTE4 were named slow-reacting substances of anaphylaxis because these products cause contractions in the smooth muscles of guinea pig ileum [41]. A substantial body of evidence indicates that LTB4 promotes leukocyte chemotaxis, adhesion and degranulation, and enhances oxidative stress, vascular permeability, and the production of proinflammatory cytokines [40,42]. 12-HETE and 15-HETE are generated in the microvessels. Several studies [43,44] indicate that 12-HETE is a potent vasodilator, whereas 15-HETE causes vasoconstriction. Notably, 5-LOX-derived products act as potent chemotactic agents for the recruitment of several proinflammatory cells, namely neutrophils, eosinophils, and monocytes in the blood vessels [40,45]. Accordingly, most investigators consider 5-LOX products to be detrimental factors in pathological conditions, including asthma [41], rheumatoid arthritis [41], DR [46], and cardiovascular diseases [40,45]. Leukotriene antagonists are clinically beneficial to treat asthma because leukotriene induces bronchoconstriction [41].

Although the mechanisms that LOX-derived metabolites promote ROS have not been well established, these metabolites are reported to act as the upstream of NADPH oxidase (NOX) pathways in cancer research [47]. For example, 12-HETE stimulates NOX1-mediated ROS production and migration in colon adenocarcinoma cells [48]. Besides 12-HETE, some evidence suggests that 15-HETE induces apoptosis in K-562 cells (myeloid leukemia) through NOX-mediated ROS production [49]. Of note, several studies have reported that BLT2, the LTB4 receptor, is involved in cancer cell growth and proliferation via NOX-mediated ROS production [50,51].

2.3. CYP-Derived Eicosanoids

The CYP-derived eicosanoids contain epoxyeicosatrienoic acids (EETs) (5,6-EET, 8,9-EET, 11,12-EET, and 14,15-EET) and 20-HETE (Figure 1). The CYP enzymes, about 45–55 kDa, are heme-containing proteins [52]. In the presence of NADPH and oxygen, AA is oxidized by the CYP enzyme system into EETs and HETEs. Among HETEs, 20-HETE, the ω-hydroxylation product of AA, is the major lipid metabolite in blood vessels and the kidneys [53]. CYP4A and CYP4F isoforms are the major enzymes for 20-HETE synthesis [16]. Production of EETs is less specific, and several CYP isoforms are involved, including CYP1A, 2B, 2C, 2D, 2E, and 2J [16]. It is well established that the major CYP epoxygenases for EETs synthesis in the kidneys and the microvasculature are CYP2C and CYP2J [15]. For example, CYP2C11, a rat isoform, has the highest epoxygenase activity, whereas CYP2C24 has the lowest activity [15]. Similarly, CYP2J isoforms are involved in EETs synthesis [54,55]. These CYP-derived eicosanoids are essential to regulate cardiovascular and renal function [15,16]. 20-HETE and EETs have been connected to regulate vascular function [15]. 20-HETE causes vasoconstriction in the microvasculature, and it is a vital regulator of the myogenic tone [17]. Notably, EETs elicit relaxation in the microvasculature, and they are the endothelium-derived hyperpolarizing factors [56,57]. Importantly, EETs can act as angiogenic factors [15,58]. EETs are readily hydrolyzed by soluble epoxide hydrolase (sEH) to form 5,6-dihydroxyepoxyeicosatrienoic acids (DHETs), 8,9-DHET, 11,12-DHET, and 14,15-DHET, which possess less biologically active than are EETs [15,58]. It is well established that sEH is the crucial enzyme in the metabolism of EETs, and blockades and deletion of sEH can change the level of EETs in vivo [15,58].

It has been demonstrated that EETs are generated in the retina [59], retinal endothelial cells [60], and significant EETs levels are evident in vitreous samples from diabetic patients [61]. Although it has been demonstrated that CYP2C and CYP2J isoforms are responsible for EET production in the kidneys [62,63], the major CYP enzymes for retinal EETs production are still unclear. Our recent study [64] has determined the expression of retinal CYP2C and CYP2J in mice compared with renal tissues as a positive control. We showed that CYP2J expression is absent, and CYP2C isoforms are the major epoxygenases in mouse retina [64]. Interestingly, these findings suggest that the blockade of CYP2C could be a target to reduce ROS production in the diabetic retina because CYP2C generates detrimental ROS in the heart [65]. Notably, a recent study by Park et al. has demonstrated that GPR40 is an EET receptor in vascular cells, and GPR40 plays a role in endothelial proliferation and tube formation that can contribute to angiogenesis [66]. To address whether EET receptor (GPR40) is expressed in the retina, we determined the expression of GPR40 in retinal samples isolated from mice and in human retinal endothelial cells (HRECs). The animal protocol was approved by the Institutional Animal Care and Use Committee. It was in accord with the requirements of the National Research Council Guide for the Care and Use of Laboratory Animals. Using the pancreas as a positive control [66], the expression of GPR40 is shown in the mouse retina and HRECs (Figure 2A). Notably, GPR40 is also highly expressed in the retinal blood vessels (Figure 2B). These results suggest that GPR40 could be a target to modulate the action of EETs in the retina. To determine the physiological function of 20-HETE and EETs in the retina, Metea et al. [67] investigated the role of HET0016 (a 20-HETE-selective blocker [53]) and MS-PPOH (an EETs-selective blocker [53]) in the function of retinal arterioles. This study [67] showed that glial-evoked vasodilation was blocked by MS-PPOH, whereas HET0016 blocked vasoconstriction. These results support the hypothesis that glial stimulation elicits vasodilation via EETs, whereas glial stimulation results in vasoconstriction mediated by 20-HETE in the retina.

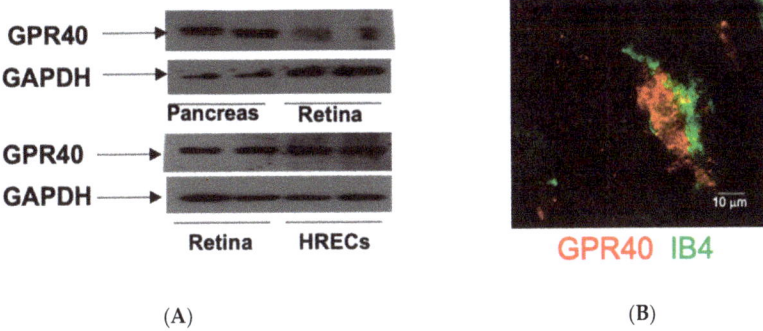

Figure 2. (**A**) EET receptor (GPR40) protein is expressed in the retina and human retinal endothelial cells (HRECs). The samples from the pancreas were used as a positive control. (**B**) GPR40 (red) and IB4 (green; a marker of the retinal blood vessel) in the retina. The retinal and pancreatic samples were isolated from male mice.

As mentioned above, CYP enzymes are involved in the synthesis of EETs and 20-HETE. Several studies [68,69] suggested that CYP catalytic cycle's poor coupling results in the continuous production of ROS, which affects different signaling pathways and other cellular functions. Edin et al. [69] determined the effects of increased endothelial expression of CYP2C8 (Tie2-CYP2C8) and CYP2J2 (Tie2-CYP2J2) transgenic mice to ischemia/reperfusion (I/R) injury in the isolated heart. They showed that infarct size was unchanged in Tie2-CYP2J2 mice after I/R, whereas Tie2-CYP2C8 mouse hearts had significantly increased infarct size after I/R. The reason for increasing the infarct size of Tie2-CYP2C8 hearts is because of increased ROS production. These results support the notion that CYP2J2 generates cardioprotective EETs, whereas another isozyme in the heart, CYP2C, generates EETs as well as detrimental ROS [65]. Some evidence suggests that hepatic fibrosis may be mediated in liver disease is through CYP2E1-dependent release of ROS from hepatocytes, which then may stimulate collagen production in stellate cells [70].

3. Diabetic Retinopathy

The retina is an extension of the central nervous system and highly metabolic active organ. It is made of several layers, and the retinal layers from inside to outside are nerve fiber (NF), ganglion cell (GC), inner plexiform (IPL), inner nuclear (INL), outer plexiform (OPL), outer nuclear (ONL), and RPE (Figure 3A) [11]. The retina is related anteriorly to the vitreous, lens, and cornea, which are avascular transparent media. The development of abnormal blood vessels in the vitreous such as in DR causes interruption of light and vision deterioration. Retinal vessels are localized in the inner neural retina, where they are distributed in the nerve fiber, inner and outer plexiform layers (Figure 3B) [11]. However, the photoreceptor layer lacks retinal vessels and receives its nutrition by diffusion from choroidal blood vessels. The flow of nutrients materials, metabolites, ions, proteins, and water flux to and from the retina is regulated by two blood-retinal barriers (BRB), inner and outer. The inner barrier is made of endothelial cells, pericytes, and glial cells; however, the outer barrier is made of RPE and choroidal endothelial cells. Disruption of inner and outer barriers is a characteristic feature of retinal diseases such as DR and age-related macular degeneration.

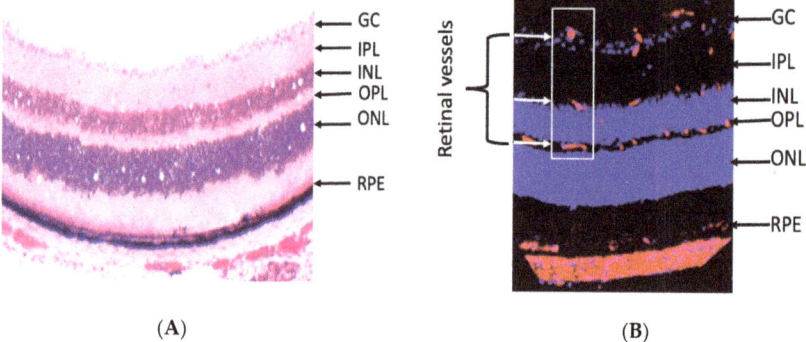

Figure 3. (**A**) Retinal section, which was isolated from mice, stained with hematoxylin and eosin showing different retinal layers as seen under the microscope from inside to outside are the ganglion cell (GC), inner plexiform (IPL), inner nuclear (INL), outer plexiform (OPL), outer nuclear (ONL), and retinal pigment epithelium (RPE). (**B**) Immunostaining of retinal section (mouse) with the vascular marker (isolectin-B4, red) and nuclear marker (DAPI, blue), showing that retinal blood vessels (inside the white box) are primarily localized in the inner retinal layers (the nerve fiber and ganglion cell layer and plexiform layer). The arrow in B is pointing to inner retinal layers that contain blood vessels (red).

DR, a neurovascular complication, remains one of the most common causes of blindness worldwide. World Health Organization (WHO) has placed DR on the top list of eye conditions that should be treated [11,71]. The microvascular dysfunction in DR is characterized by apoptosis of retinal pericytes and endothelial cells, leading to BRB breakdown, capillary degeneration, and development of retinal ischemia. BRB breakdown causes retinal hyperpermeability and development of diabetic macular edema (DME), which is a leading cause of vision loss in DR. Capillary degeneration leads to the development of relative retinal ischemia and subsequently VEGF-dependent retinal neovascularization, a cardinal sign of proliferative DR (PDR). Current methods for treating diabetic retinopathy (DR), including laser photocoagulation and anti-vascular endothelial growth factor (VEGF), are limited by significant side effects and do not eliminate the risk of blindness. Thus, there is a critical need to identify new therapeutic targets for the treatment of DR [72,73].

The retina comprises a high content of PUFA, and it also has high oxygen and glucose uptake as compared with other tissues. Thus, the retina is more prone to oxidative stress [11]. Chronic hyperglycemia is related to the development of DR, although the underlying mechanisms of this association are still not clear. Several biochemical pathways and molecular mechanisms have been implicated in the possible links, including activation of the renin-angiotensin system (RAS), increased advanced glycation end products, dysregulation of the polyol pathway, activation of PKC, and chronic inflammation [11]. Of note, many of these pathways are leading to ROS production and the burden of oxidative stress in retinal tissues [11]. DR is mostly a disease of the retinal microvasculature, although damage to neurons and glia also occurs [11]. This review will focus on the role of eicosanoids in oxidative stress, retinal microvascular dysfunction, and neovascularization to DR. The following section will provide

4. Eicosanoids and Diabetic Retinopathy

4.1. Role of COX-Eicosanoids in Diabetic Retinopathy

In DR, vascular leakiness and proliferation are two important factors to cause vision impairment [74,75]. Patients with diabetes are usually vulnerable to DR, and retinal neovascularization (NV) in the late stage of DR could lead to blindness. Of note, in DR, ischemia is the common precursor to NV, and it is well established that early proinflammatory genes are generally expressed in ischemic retina [76]. One of these genes expressed at high levels in the early stages of DR is COX-2, which is induced by inflammatory cytokines [16,17]. Moreover, increased PGs in DR have been found in the vitreous cavity in both animal and clinical studies [77,78]. Thus, a lot of research effort has focused on the role of COX-2 and PGE2 in the pathogenesis of DR. VEGF is a proinflammatory molecule that plays an essential role in the development of vascular leakage and retinal NV in DR [79]. A previous study [80] has shown that PGE2 increases VEGF expression in cultured Müller cells. Interestingly, Yanni et al. [81] have reported that in Müller cells, activation of the EP4 receptor, the receptor of PGE2, increases VEGF production. In contrast, a blockade of EP4 receptors decreases VEGF production in a concentration-dependent manner. An EP4 blockade by L-161982 significantly reduced pathologic NV in oxygen-induced retinopathy (OIR). Noteworthy, earlier work by Ayalasomayajula et al. [82] has demonstrated that celecoxib (a selective COX-2 inhibitor) inhibited VEGF expression without any significant effect in COX-2 expression. Moreover, the COX-2 blockade significantly decreased vitreous to plasma protein ratio, which is an index of the retinal vascular leakage in diabetic rats. These results support the hypothesis that COX-2 and EP4 could be valuable therapeutic targets for the early stages of DR and proliferative DR.

NF-κB is a family of highly conserved transcription factors that regulate many genes involved in the inflammatory response [79]. Thus, NF-κB is a proinflammatory transcription factor. NF-κB is composed of homodimers and heterodimers, and the most abundant forms are the p65 and p50 subunits [79]. The NF-κB proteins are typically sequestered in the cytoplasm by IκB. The primary mechanism for NF-κB activation is the inducible degradation of IκB triggered through its site-specific phosphorylation by the IκB kinase (IKK) complex, resulting in IκB degradation [79]. The degradation of IκB releases the NF-κB heterodimers to translocate to the nucleus where they bind to nuclear DNA, leading to activation of inflammatory mediators, including tumor necrosis factor α (TNFα), ICAM-1, and interleukin-1β. Of note, NF-κB activation induces inflammatory mediators and increases oxidative stress, which is involved in the pathogenesis of DR [83–86]. Notably, Zheng et al. [87] have reported that treatment with aspirin (a COX inhibitor) not only inhibited NF-κB activation, but also inhibited the expression of iNOS, ICAM-1, VCAM, and capillary degeneration and capillary cell death in the diabetic retina. Moreover, NF-κB activation contributes to ROS generation [11]. These results provide substantial evidence that aspirin-mediated inhibition of capillary degeneration in the early stage of DR is mediated via inhibition of NF-κB and the subsequent oxidative stress and inflammatory response.

Several studies have determined the effects of COX blockade in clinical studies [88–91]. In the Early Treatment Diabetic Retinopathy Study (ETDRS), researchers examined the effects of aspirin (650 mg per day) or placebo in 3711 patients with mild-to-severe nonproliferative DR (NPDR) or early proliferative DR (PDR) [88]. They found that aspirin did not prevent high-risk PDR development and did not reduce the risk of visual loss in these DR patients. This study suggests that the COX blockade does not have beneficial effects in advanced DR patients. The reason that aspirin did not provide protective effects in advanced DR patients is still not clear. It could be due to the dose of aspirin because, in a previous study, Zheng et al. [87] used the dose of 26 mg/kg/day, which is about 1820 mg per day based on the bodyweight of 70 kg of healthy persons, to inhibit the early lesion of DR in diabetic rats. Thus, a higher dose of aspirin is needed to provide beneficial effects in DR patients.

Interestingly, in the Dipyridamole Aspirin Microangiopathy Diabetes Study (DAMAD) trial, a higher dose of aspirin (990 mg per day) has a significant protective effect of slowing the development of retinal microaneurysms [89]. Moreover, a pilot study in Japan [90], researchers investigated the effects of sulindac (a non-specific COX-2 inhibitor; 200 mg/day, 100 mg twice a day; $n = 16$) on DR progression in patients with T2DM as compared to controls (24 patients) for three years. They found that patients in the sulindac group did not develop DR, nor was there the progression of pathology in those who began the study with mild NPDR. On the other hand, six patients progressed to mild NPDR in the control group. Subsequently, a prospective randomized study [91] showed that treatment with celecoxib caused the reduction of fluorescein leakage in patients with diabetic macular edema. These clinical studies [88–91] support the notion that COX blockade might have beneficial effects in the development of DR in patients with the early stages of DR.

4.2. Role of LOX-Eicosanoids in Diabetic Retinopathy

It is well established that inflammatory insults to the retina are essential factors in the development of the early stages of DR. 5-LOX-derived metabolites, including LTB4 and cysteinyl leukotrienes (LTC4, LTD4, and LTE4), play an important role in the inflammatory processes. To determine the role of 5-LOX in the pathogenesis of DR, a study by Gubitosi-Klug et al. [37] has evaluated the role of 5-LOX knockout (KO) and wild-type (WT) mice in the development of DR. They found that diabetic WT mice developed degeneration of retinal capillaries and pericyte at nine months post-streptozotocin (STZ) treatment and increases in both leukostasis and superoxide production at three months post-STZ treatment. Diabetic 5-LOX KO mice developed less capillary degeneration and loss of pericytes and less leukostasis, less superoxide production, and less activation of NF-κB, which contributes to ROS generation [11]. These results provide substantial evidence that 5-LOX-derived metabolites promote proinflammatory mediators and oxidative stress, and play a role in DR's pathogenesis. Moreover, using STZ-induced diabetic mouse model and cultured retinal cells, Talahalli et al. [46] showed that bone marrow-derived cells from diabetic mice synthesize more LTB4 than do those from WT mice; the mouse retina, retinal glial cells, and retinal endothelial cells (mREC) need LTA4 for the synthesis of LTB4 by transcellular metabolism; and high-glucose conditions increase BLT1 receptor expression in retinal glial cells and mREC, which then cause retinal microvascular endothelial cell death. These results support the notion that transcellular delivery of LTA4 from bone marrow-derived cells to retinal cells results in the production of LTB4, which can contribute to chronic inflammation and the development of DR. Retinal angiogenesis, the formation of new blood vessels in the retinal vasculature, is one the most damaging pathological events occurring during advanced DR. Several studies [92–94] have demonstrated that 5-LOX-derived leukotrienes promote retinal NF-κB expression and its subsequent downstream target pathways, including ROS production, cytokine molecules, and adhesion molecules; these lipid mediators cause leukostasis and degeneration of retinal capillaries; they increase retinal microvascular permeability leading to retinal edema; they activate NADPH oxidase, thereby increasing oxidative stress; and they promote retinal endothelial cell proliferation and migration. All of these pathological actions can contribute to the retinal angiogenesis in advanced DR.

Extensive research activities have focused on the effect of 12/15-LOX products in the pathogenesis of DM. 12/15-LOX is found in the retinal cells, including endothelial cells and glial cells [95]. The primary 12/15-LOX-derived products from AA are 12-HETE and 15-HETE. 12-HETE has a role in various biological processes, including atherogenesis, cancer cell growth, and neuronal apoptosis. Moreover, 12-HETE has proinflammatory effects [96,97] and has been implicated in diabetic vascular complications [98]. To determine the role of 12/15-LOX in PDR, we showed that 12-HETE and 15-HETE production were significantly increased in oxygen-induced ischemic retinopathy (OIR), a model of PDR [95]. We then found that 12-HETE and 15-HEHE levels were elevated in the vitreous of diabetic patients with PDR. Interestingly, the blockade or deletion of 12/15-LOX attenuated retinal NV. Additionally, 12-HETE administration augmented VEGF expression in Müller cells and astrocytes. These results support the hypothesis that 12-HETE and 15-HETE production by 12/15-LOX are essential regulators of retinal NV through modulation of VEGF expression and could provide a new therapeutic target to prevent and treat ischemic retinopathy. Our research group then determined the effect of 12/15-LOX metabolites on endothelial cell barrier function in the presence or absence of NADPH oxidase, an important enzyme to produce ROS, inhibitors. Our previous study [99] showed that activation of 12/15-LOX is a contributing factor to the vascular hyperpermeability during DR and that NADPH oxidase plays a role in this process via activating VEGF receptor 2 (VEGF-R2)-signal pathway. Interestingly, our another study [100] showed that the products of the 12/15-LOX pathway were significantly up-regulated under hyperglycemic conditions with 15-HETE exhibiting the most significant increase; 15-HETE activates retinal endothelial cells through the NOX system leading to increases in leukocyte adhesion, hyperpermeability, and finally NV, the cardinal signs of DR. Based on these previous studies [95,99,100], we proposed a hypothesis that hyperglycemia activates PLA2 to release AA from the retinal cell membrane. AA is then converted to 12-HETE or 15-HETE that generates ROS through NOX, creating a status of oxidative stress. Oxidative stress leads to the activation of retinal endothelial cells through various inflammatory signaling pathways, leading to leukocyte adhesion, hyperpermeability, and ultimately NV, which is the pathogenesis of advanced DR (Figure 4).

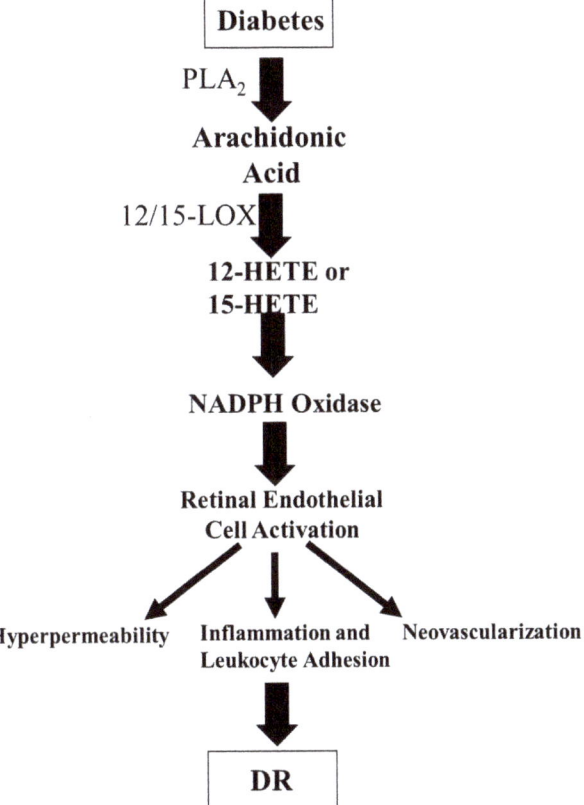

Figure 4. Cascade events involved in the pathogenesis of DR: Hyperglycemia activates the PLA2 to release AA from the retinal cell membrane. AA is converted to 12- or 15-HETE that generates ROS through NOX, creating a status of oxidative stress. This oxidative stress leads to the activation of retinal endothelial cells through various inflammatory signaling pathways, leading to leukocyte adhesion, hyperpermeability, and ultimately NV (the cardinal signs of DR).

To study the biological effects of 12/15-LOX in DR, our previous study [99] determined the effects of baicalein, 12/15-LOX inhibitor, in diabetic mice. Treatment of diabetic mice with baicalein significantly decreased retinal HETE, intercellular adhesion molecule 1 (ICAM-1), vascular cell adhesion molecule 1 (VCAM-1), interleukin 6 (IL-6), ROS generation, and NOX2 expression. Baicalein also reduced VEGF-R2 levels in the diabetic retina. Our findings suggest that 12/15-LOX contributes to vascular hyperpermeability during DR via the NADPH oxidase-dependent mechanism, which involves the suppression of protein tyrosine phosphatase and activation of VEGF-R2 signal pathway [99]. Besides baicalein, several pharmacological inhibitors, including nordihydroguaiaretic acid (NDGA), cinnamyl-3,4-dihydroxy-cyanocinnamate (CDC), have been developed. However, these 12/15-LOX inhibitors did not show a clear isoform specificity [101,102]. Moreover, these inhibitors display a species-specificity, and they have off-target effects. For example, these inhibitors have anti-oxidative properties, and they affect the cellular redox homeostasis. Thus, it is hard to determine which of the two functions, LOX inhibition or redox homeostasis, is the main reason for the detected biological result [103]. Consequently, results obtained from these inhibitors must be interpreted with caution. To address this issue, the inhibitor studies should always be confirmed by another approach, for example, 12/15-LOX KO [11].

4.3. Role of CYP-Eicosanoids in Diabetic Retinopathy

As compared to COX and LOX pathways, the role of the CYP pathway in retinopathy and DR is less documented. Although it has been reported that EETs are involved in neurovascular coupling [67], little is known about retinal angiogenesis. A previous publication by Michaelis et al. [60] is the first to determine the role of CYP2C-derived EETs in hypoxia-induced cell migration and angiogenesis. They showed that CYP2C isoforms are expressed, and EETs are generated in cultured retinal endothelial cells. Additionally, hypoxia-induced CYP2C protein expression and EET formation. Moreover, the CYP2C blockade attenuated the effects of EETs on endothelial cell migration and endothelial tube formation. These results support the notion that endothelial EETs are implicated in retinal angiogenesis, especially under hypoxia conditions. Future study is needed to investigate whether CYP2C-induced ROS production [65] contributes to retinal angiogenesis under hypoxia. Importantly, another previous study showed that 11,12-EET has a proangiogenic activity in the retina following hypoxia [104], which supports the notion that EETs blockade could be a therapeutic target for retinal NV. EETs have been shown to promote retinal NV in OIR [105], and the CYP2C blockade provides the protective effects on pathological retinal NV in OIR [106]. To determine lipidomic profiles of various PUFA, which including LA, AA, eicosapentaenoic acid (EPA, 20:5 n-3), and docosahexaenoic acid (DHA, 22:6 n-3), we used LC/MS/MS to measure the levels of 12/15-LOX-, COX-, and CYP-derived metabolites in diabetic (STZ model) and control mice. Among the 107 lipid metabolites screened, only a few lipids were significantly increased in diabetic mice. Notably, we found that 5,6-DHET, 11,12-DHET, and 14,15-DHET levels are significantly elevated in diabetic mice [107]. These results suggest that retinal sEH levels and activity are elevated in diabetes.

A robust body of literature has established the role of RAS in DR [108–115]. In RAS, prorenin is activated to form renin [108–112], which converts angiotensinogen to Angiotensin I (Ang I) [108,109,116]. Ang I is then hydrolyzed by angiotensin-converting enzyme (ACE) to produce Angiotensin II (Ang II) [108,109]. Ang II is the major bioactive product of RAS, and Ang II receptor type 1 (AT1 receptor) is the primary receptor to mediate the function of Ang II [117–120]. Several clinical studies are designed to determine the effects of RAS blockade in the development of DR because RAS activation is implicated in DR development in animal studies [108–112]. EUCLID trial demonstrates that ACE blockade by lisinopril attenuated the progress of DR to proliferative DR [121]. The DIRECT trial was divided into the DIRECT-Prevent group ($n > 1400$) and the DIRECT-Protect group ($n > 1900$) [108,122]. While AT1 blockade by candesartan decreased the incidence of DR, AT1 blockade did not attenuate the progression of established DR [122]. Thus, a lack of understanding of the molecular mechanism of retinal microvascular damage induced by RAS is a critical barrier to the use of RAS blockade to prevent or treat DR. To address the disappointing results of the DIRECT trial, our recent study [64] shows that Ang II increases retinal sEH expression, which is blunted by an AT1 blocker; 11,12-EET exacerbates Ang II-retinal vascular leakage; diabetes (STZ model) induces retinal angiotensinogen and AT1 expression (RAS activation), which is associated with increased retinal sEH expression; and sEH KO (increasing EETs) exacerbates diabetes-induced retinal vascular leakage. Based on these results, we propose a hypothesis that during diabetes, RAS activation augments retinal sEH, via AT1, which decreases EETs (pro-permeability and pro-angiogenesis factors) to counterbalance the effects of RAS on retinal microvascular damage (Figure 5).

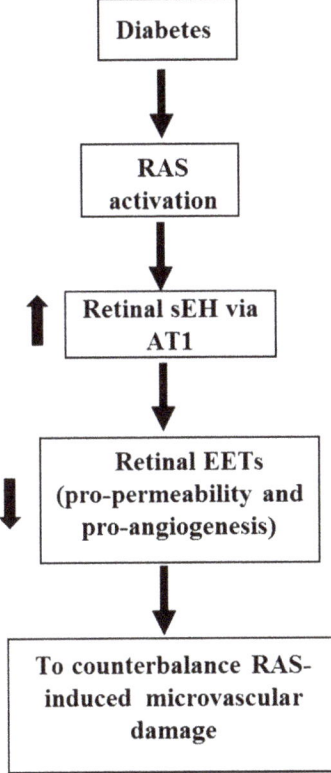

Figure 5. The hypothesis about the interaction of sEH/EETs and RAS in DR. During diabetes, RAS activation augments retinal sEH, via AT1, which decreases EETs (pro-permeability and pro-angiogenesis factors) to counterbalance the effects of RAS on retinal microvascular damage.

4.4. Role of Omega 3-Derived Metabolites in Diabetic Retinopathy

Besides generating from omega 6 (ω-6) PUFAs, such as AA, eicosanoids can also be produced from ω-3 PUFA, such as EPA and DHA. Several studies have reported that COX- and LOX-derived products generated from ω-3 PUFAs inhibit inflammation and angiogenesis, and may possess protective effects in the development of retinopathy and DR [105,123]. To determine the role of ω-3 PUFA COX-derived PGs on angiogenesis, Szymczak et al. investigated the modulation of proangiogenic activation of human endothelial cells (ECs) by ω-3 PUFA [123]. They showed that ω-6 PUFAs stimulate, but ω-3 PUFAs inhibit major proangiogenic processes in human ECs, including the induction of angiopoietin-2 (Ang2), endothelial invasion, and tube formation, that are usually activated by the major ω-6 PUFA AA [123]. Importantly, they found that PGE3 (ω-3 PUFA-derived PG) suppressed the induction of Ang2, a vital factor in the angiogenic differentiation of ECs, by growth factors in human ECs, which is the opposite to the effects of PGE2. These results support the notion that ω-3 PUFA-derived PG protects against NV as compared with the detrimental effects of ω-6 PUFA-derived PG. Furthermore, resolvins, produced from ω-3 PUFAs via COX-2, have potent anti-inflammatory properties by blocking the production of pro-inflammatory factors [124]. To determine the role of ω-3 PUFA-derived metabolites in NV, Sapieha et al. [125] fed ω-3 PUFA diets into COX-1 KO, COX-2 KO, 5-LOX KO, 12/15-LOX KO, and WT mice, and then retinopathy was induced by oxygen exposure (OIR). They showed that only 5-LOX KO mice, but not COX-1 KO, COX-2 KO, or 12/15-LOX KO, abrogated the protection against OIR by dietary ω-3 PUFAs. This study identified 4-hydroxydocosahexaenoic acid (4-HDHA), a product of ω-3 PUFA via 5-LOX, which regulates NV in OIR modeling ROP and advanced DR [125].

To determine the role of ω-3 and ω-6 PUFA-derived metabolites via CYP in NV, Shao et al. [126] fed ω-3 or ω-6 PUFA diets into Tie2-CYP2C8, Tie2-sEH, and WT mice in the OIR model. They found that in OIR, there is increased NV in Tie2-CYP2C8 mice fed a diet with either ω-3 or ω-6 PUFAs, whereas there is reduced NV in Tie2-sEH mice. These results support the hypothesis that both of ω-3 and ω-6 PUFA lipid products of CYP2C promote NV in the retina and advanced DR. Recently, an exciting study by Fleming and colleagues [59] has demonstrated that sEH is involved in the metabolism of 19, 20-epoxydocosapentaenoic acid (19, 20-EDP; DHA-CYP-derived product) to 19,20-dihydroxydocosapentaenoic acid (19, 20-DHDP). They also showed that the accumulation of 19, 20-DHDP, and overexpression of sEH in the retinal Müller glial cells causes retinopathy [59]. Although these findings support the importance of sEH and 19, 20-DHDP in the Müller glial cells, the same research group (Fleming and colleagues) [127,128] has shown that increasing EETs levels in the retinal endothelial cells causes retinopathy, which supports our hypothesis indicating in Figure 5. These studies [59,105] suggest that regarding CYP-mediated ω-3 PUFA products in angiogenesis could be cell- or tissue-dependent.

5. Conclusions and Perspectives

It is well established that PGs play a vital role in the regulation of retinal blood flow and choroidal blood flow. Overproduction of TXA2 and PGE2 promotes ROS formation, which is associated with cardiovascular diseases. COX blockade decreases retinal VEGF and inhibits NF-κB activation, which regulates the production of inflammatory mediators and ROS production in the retina. Clinical studies suggest that high dose of aspirin might have beneficial effects in the development of DR in patients with early stages of DR. Since PGE2 promotes the production of retinal VEGF via EP4 receptor, the development of novel pharmacological agents targeting EP4 receptors could be an important area for clinical studies in patients with DR.

12-HETE, one of the LOX-derived eicosanoids, is a potent vasodilator, whereas 15-HETE causes vasoconstriction. Deletion of the 5-LOX gene decreases capillary degeneration, leukostasis, and activation of NF-κB in diabetic animals, suggesting that 5-LOX-derived proinflammatory metabolites play a role in the pathogenesis of DR. There is a significant elevation of 12-HETE and 15-HETE levels in the vitreous of diabetic patients with PDR. There is some evidence that 12-HETE or 15-HETE generates ROS through NOX, creating a status of oxidative stress, which is an important factor in the development of DR. More research is needed to determine whether 12/15-LOX blockade can prevent the development of DR in clinical studies.

EETs and 20-HETE, the CYP-derived eicosanoids, are produced in the retinal circulation. There is some evidence that glial stimulation elicited vasodilation via EETs, whereas glial stimulation results in vasoconstriction mediated by 20-HETE in the retina. Less research is known about the role of EETs in the development of DR. Several studies indicate that EETs are implicated in retinal angiogenesis, especially under hypoxia conditions. RAS activation contributes to retinal hyperpermeability and retinal neovascularization in DR. Although the blockade of RAS with an AT1 receptor blocker has reduced the incidence of DR in clinical studies, the AT1 blockade did not reduce the progression of DR in diabetic patients. Our recent publication [64] shows that in DR, RAS activation augments retinal levels of sEH, degrading EETs to compensate RAS-induced retinal microvascular damage. In the future study, it is needed to test whether EETs or EET receptor (Figure 2) blockade can optimize RAS blockade to prevent or reduce DR-induced microvascular damage.

Growing evidence support that ω-3 PUFA metabolites via COX- and LOX-pathway inhibit inflammation and retinal angiogenesis. On the other hand, the ω-3 and ω-6 PUFA metabolites via CYP2C promote neovascularization in the retina. Thus, more research is needed to determine whether ω-3 PUFA supplementation along with the CYP2C blockade can prevent the development of advanced DR.

In conclusion, although anti-VEGF and photocoagulation therapy have improved care in DR patients, these therapies still cause significant side effects. Thus, there is a critical need to identify new therapeutic targets to treat or prevent DR progression. COX-derived, LOX-derived, and CYP-derived eicosanoids regulate oxidative stress, retinal VEGF levels, and inflammatory cytokines, as well as being involved in the pathophysiology of DR. There are many available approaches, including selective blockers, transgenic mice, and knockout mice, to permit researchers to study the functions of these lipid mediators in the retina as well as their role in the pathophysiology of DR. These lipid mediators are essential therapeutic targets for DR because many receptors and these three eicosanoid pathways are well defined. Thus, we propose that COX blockers (aspirin and celecoxib), EET blockers (montelukast (a selective CYP2C inhibitor [129,130]) and DC260126(an EET receptor antagonist [131,132])), and 12/15-LOX blockers (baicalein, NDGA, and CDC) could be the potential therapeutic methods to prevent the development of early-stage DR (Figure 6). We also propose that EP4 receptor blocker (L-161982), ω-3 PUFA diet + EET blockers (montelukast and DC260126), AT1 blockers + EET blockers (montelukast and DC260126), and 12/15-LOX blockers (baicalein, NDGA, and CDC) could be the potential therapeutic methods to prevent the development of proliferative DR (Figure 6). Finally, since oxidative stress represents a vital regulator of eicosanoids-mediated microvascular dysfunction in DR and other diseases, antioxidants could be a therapeutic approach to interrupt eicosanoid signaling and in turn improving visual outcome in DR.

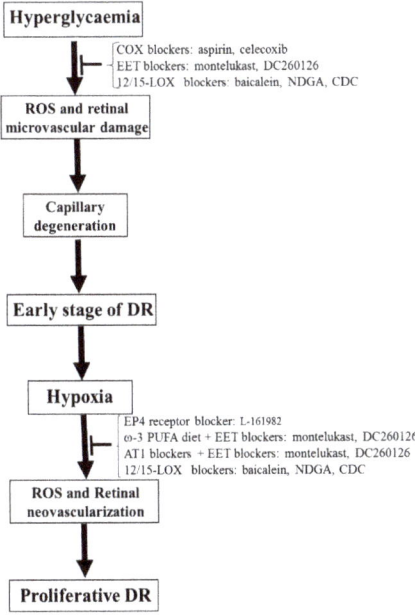

Figure 6. General mechanisms for the development of the early stage of DR and proliferative DR. We also indicate the potential therapeutic methods of the eicosanoid pathways to prevent the development of the early stage of DR and proliferative DR.

Author Contributions: Conceptualization, M.-H.W., G.H. and M.A.-S.; methodology, M.-H.W. and M.A.-S.; software, M.-H.W., G.H. and M.A.-S.; validation, M.-H.W., G.H. and M.A.-S.; formal analysis, M.-H.W., G.H. and M.A.-S.; investigation, M.-H.W.; resources, M.A.-S.; data curation, M.-H.W.; writing—original draft preparation, M.-H.W.; writing—review and editing, M.-H.W., G.H. and M.A.-S.; visualization, M.-H.W. and M.A.-S.; supervision, M.-H.W. and M.A.-S.; project administration, M.-H.W.; funding acquisition, M.A.-S. All authors have read and agreed to the published version of the manuscript.

Funding: The following grants support this study: AHA Grant-in-Aid grant (AHASE00144) to M.-H W. and (NIH R01EY023315) and (NIH 1R01 EY030054) to M. A.-S.

Conflicts of Interest: The authors declare no conflict of interest.

References

1. Yoon, J.W.; Jun, H.S. Autoimmune destruction of pancreatic beta cells. *Am. J. Ther.* **2005**, *12*, 580–591. [CrossRef]
2. Cnop, M.; Welsh, N.; Jonas, J.C.; Jorns, A.; Lenzen, S.; Eizirik, D.L. Mechanisms of pancreatic beta-cell death in type 1 and type 2 diabetes: Many differences, few similarities. *Diabetes* **2005**, *54* (Suppl. 2), S97–S107. [CrossRef] [PubMed]
3. Eizirik, D.L.; Colli, M.L.; Ortis, F. The role of inflammation in insulitis and beta-cell loss in type 1 diabetes. *Nat. Rev. Endocrinol.* **2009**, *5*, 219–226. [CrossRef] [PubMed]
4. Boden, G. Obesity, insulin resistance and free fatty acids. *Curr. Opin. Endocrinol. Diabetes Obes.* **2011**, *18*, 139. [CrossRef] [PubMed]
5. Eckardt, K.; Taube, A.; Eckel, J. Obesity-associated insulin resistance in skeletal muscle: Role of lipid accumulation and physical inactivity. *Rev. Endocr. Metab. Disord.* **2011**, *12*, 163–172. [CrossRef]
6. Wilkinson-Berka, J.L.; Rana, I.; Armani, R.; Agrotis, A. Reactive oxygen species, nox and angiotensin II in angiogenesis: Implications for retinopathy. *Clin. Sci.* **2013**, *124*, 597–615. [CrossRef]
7. Nishikawa, T.; Edelstein, D.; Du, X.L.; Yamagishi, S.; Matsumura, T.; Kaneda, Y.; Yorek, M.A.; Beebe, D.; Oates, P.J.; Hammes, H.P.; et al. Normalizing mitochondrial superoxide production blocks three pathways of hyperglycaemic damage. *Nature* **2000**, *404*, 787–790. [CrossRef]
8. Ohno, Y.; Gallin, J.I. Diffusion of extracellular hydrogen peroxide into intracellular compartments of human neutrophils. Studies utilizing the inactivation of myeloperoxidase by hydrogen peroxide and azide. *J. Biol. Chem.* **1985**, *260*, 8438–8446.
9. Weyemi, U.; Dupuy, C. The emerging role of ROS-generating NADPH oxidase NOX4 in DNA-damage responses. *Mutat. Res.* **2012**, *751*, 77–81. [CrossRef]
10. White, C.R.; Brock, T.A.; Chang, L.Y.; Crapo, J.; Briscoe, P.; Ku, D.; Bradley, W.A.; Gianturco, S.H.; Gore, J.; Freeman, B.A.; et al. Superoxide and peroxynitrite in atherosclerosis. *Proc. Natl. Acad. Sci. USA* **1994**, *91*, 1044–1048. [CrossRef]
11. Elmasry, K.; Ibrahim, A.S.; Abdulmoneim, S.; Al-Shabrawey, M. Bioactive lipids and pathological retinal angiogenesis. *Br. J. Pharmacol.* **2019**, *176*, 93–109. [CrossRef] [PubMed]
12. Forsyth, S.; Gautier, S.; Salem, N., Jr. Global estimates of dietary intake of docosahexaenoic acid and arachidonic acid in developing and developed countries. *Ann. Nutr. Metab.* **2016**, *68*, 258–267. [CrossRef] [PubMed]
13. Innes, J.K.; Calder, P.C. Omega-6 fatty acids and inflammation. Prostaglandins leukot essent fatty acids. *Curr. Pharm. Biotechnol.* **2018**, *132*, 41–48. [CrossRef]
14. Roman, R.J. P-450 metabolites of arachidonic acid in the control of cardiovascular function. *Physiol. Rev.* **2002**, *82*, 131–185. [CrossRef] [PubMed]
15. Imig, J.D.; Hammock, B.D. Soluble epoxide hydrolase as a therapeutic target for cardiovascular diseases. *Nat. Rev. Drug Discov.* **2009**, *8*, 794–805. [CrossRef]
16. Huang, H.; Al-Shabrawey, M.; Wang, M.H. Cyclooxygenase-and cytochrome P450-derived eicosanoids in stroke. *Prostag. Other Lipid Mediat.* **2016**, *122*, 45–53. [CrossRef]
17. Luo, P.; Wang, M.H. Eicosanoids, beta-cell function, and diabetes. *Prostag. Other Lipid Mediat.* **2011**, *95*, 1–10. [CrossRef]
18. Dobrian, A.D.; Lieb, D.C.; Cole, B.K.; Taylor-Fishwick, D.A.; Chakrabarti, S.K.; Nadler, J.L. Functional and pathological roles of the 12-and 15-lipoxygenases. *Prog. Lipid Res.* **2011**, *50*, 115–131. [CrossRef]

19. Feletou, M.; Huang, Y.; Vanhoutte, P.M. Vasoconstrictor prostanoids. *Pflugers Arch.* **2010**, *459*, 941–950. [CrossRef] [PubMed]
20. Wong, M.S.; Vanhoutte, P.M. COX-mediated endothelium-dependent contractions: From the past to recent discoveries. *Acta Pharmacol. Sin.* **2010**, *31*, 1095–1102. [CrossRef]
21. Vane, J.R.; Bakhle, Y.S.; Botting, R.M. Cyclooxygenases 1 and 2. *Annu. Rev. Pharmacol. Toxicol.* **1998**, *38*, 97–120. [CrossRef] [PubMed]
22. Harris, R.C. COX-2 and the kidney. *J. Cardiovasc. Pharmacol.* **2006**, *47* (Suppl. 1), S37–S42. [CrossRef] [PubMed]
23. Cheng, H.F.; Harris, R.C. Cyclooxygenases, the kidney, and hypertension. *Hypertension* **2004**, *43*, 525–530. [CrossRef] [PubMed]
24. Birkle, D.L.; Bazan, N.G. Lipoxygenase and cyclooxygenase reaction products and incorporation into glycerolipids of arachidonic acid in the bovine retina. *Prostaglandins* **1984**, *27*, 203–216. [CrossRef]
25. Bhattacherjee, P. The role of arachidonate metabolites in ocular inflammation. In *The Ocular Effects of Prostaglandins and Other Eicosanoids*; Bito, L.Z., Stjernschantz, J., Alan, R., Eds.; Liss: New York, NY, USA, 1989; pp. 211–228.
26. Kass, M.A.; Holmberg, N.J. Prostaglandin and thromboxane synthesis by microsomes of rabbit ocular tissues. *Investig. Ophthalmol. Vis. Sci.* **1979**, *18*, 166–171.
27. Hardy, P.; Peri, K.G.; Lahaie, I.; Varma, D.R.; Chemtob, S. Increased nitric oxide synthesis and action preclude choroidal vasoconstriction to hyperoxia in newborn pigs. *Circ. Res.* **1996**, *79*, 504–511. [CrossRef]
28. Abran, D.; Li, D.Y.; Varma, D.R.; Chemtob, S. Characterization and ontogeny of PGE2 and PGF2 alpha receptors on the retinal vasculature of the pig. *Prostaglandins* **1995**, *50*, 253–267. [CrossRef]
29. Abran, D.; Varma, D.R.; Chemtob, S. Regulation of prostanoid vasomotor effects and receptors in choroidal vessels of newborn pigs. *Am. J. Physiol.* **1997**, *272*, R995–R1001. [CrossRef]
30. Chemtob, S.; Beharry, K.; Rex, J.; Chatterjee, T.; Varma, D.R.; Aranda, J.V. Ibuprofen enhances retinal and choroidal blood flow autoregulation in newborn piglets. *Investig. Ophthalmol. Vis. Sci.* **1991**, *32*, 1799–1807.
31. Martin, A.; Perez-Giron, J.V.; Hernanz, R.; Palacios, R.; Briones, A.M.; Fortuno, A.; Zalba, G.; Salaices, M.; Alonso, M.J. Peroxisome proliferator-activated receptor-gamma activation reduces cyclooxygenase-2 expression in vascular smooth muscle cells from hypertensive rats by interfering with oxidative stress. *J. Hypertens.* **2012**, *30*, 315–326. [CrossRef]
32. Karaa, A.; Kamoun, W.S.; Xu, H.; Zhang, J.; Clemens, M.G. Differential effects of oxidative stress on hepatic endothelial and Kupffer cell eicosanoid release in response to endothelin-1. *Microcirculation* **2006**, *13*, 457–466. [CrossRef] [PubMed]
33. Li, Y.B.; Han, J.Y.; Jiang, W.; Wang, J. Selenium inhibits high glucose-induced cyclooxygenase-2 and P-selectin expression in vascular endothelial cells. *Mol. Biol. Rep.* **2011**, *38*, 2301–2306. [CrossRef] [PubMed]
34. Muzaffar, S.; Shukla, N.; Lobo, C.; Angelini, G.D.; Jeremy, J.Y. Iloprost inhibits superoxide formation and gp91phox expression induced by the thromboxane A2 analogue U46619, 8-isoprostane F2alpha, prostaglandin F2alpha, cytokines and endotoxin in the pig pulmonary artery. *Br. J. Pharmacol.* **2004**, *141*, 488–496. [CrossRef] [PubMed]
35. Capone, C.; Faraco, G.; Anrather, J.; Zhou, P.; Iadecola, C. Cyclooxygenase 1-derived prostaglandin E2 and EP1 receptors are required for the cerebrovascular dysfunction induced by angiotensin II. *Hypertension* **2010**, *55*, 911–917. [CrossRef]
36. Cao, X.; Peterson, J.R.; Wang, G.; Anrather, J.; Young, C.N.; Guruju, M.R.; Burmeister, M.A.; Iadecola, C.; Davisson, R.L. Angiotensin II-dependent hypertension requires cyclooxygenase 1-derived prostaglandin E2 and EP1 receptor signaling in the subfornical organ of the brain. *Hypertension* **2012**, *59*, 869–876. [CrossRef]
37. Gubitosi-Klug, R.A.; Talahalli, R.; Du, Y.; Nadler, J.L.; Kern, T.S. 5-Lipoxygenase, but not 12/15-lipoxygenase, contributes to degeneration of retinal capillaries in a mouse model of diabetic retinopathy. *Diabetes* **2008**, *57*, 1387–1393. [CrossRef]
38. Camara, N.O.; Martins, J.O.; Landgraf, R.G.; Jancar, S. Emerging roles for eicosanoids in renal diseases. *Curr. Opin. Nephrol. Hypertens.* **2009**, *18*, 21–27. [CrossRef]
39. Baba, T.; Black, K.L.; Ikezaki, K.; Chen, K.N.; Becker, D.P. Intracarotid infusion of leukotriene C4 selectively increases blood-brain barrier permeability after focal ischemia in rats. *J. Cereb. Blood Flow Metab.* **1991**, *11*, 638–643. [CrossRef]

40. Poeckel, D.; Funk, C.D. The 5-lipoxygenase/leukotriene pathway in preclinical models of cardiovascular disease. *Cardiovasc. Res.* **2010**, *86*, 243–253. [CrossRef]
41. Behl, T.; Kaur, I.; Kotwani, A. Role of leukotrienes in diabetic retinopathy. *Prostag. Other Lipid. Mediat.* **2016**, *122*, 1–9. [CrossRef]
42. McMurdo, L.; Stephenson, A.H.; Baldassare, J.J.; Sprague, R.S.; Lonigro, A.J. Biosynthesis of sulfidopeptide leukotrienes via the transfer of leukotriene A4 from polymorphonuclear cells to bovine retinal pericytes. *J. Pharmacol. Exp. Ther.* **1998**, *285*, 1255–1259. [PubMed]
43. Tang, D.G.; Renaud, C.; Stojakovic, S.; Diglio, C.A.; Porter, A.; Honn, K.V. 12(S)-HETE is a mitogenic factor for microvascular endothelial cells: Its potential role in angiogenesis. *Biochem. Biophys. Res. Commun.* **1995**, *211*, 462–468. [CrossRef]
44. Takayama, H.; Gimbrone, M.A., Jr.; Schafer, A.I. Vascular lipoxygenase activity: Synthesis of 15-hydroxyeicosatetraenoic acid from arachidonic acid by blood vessels and cultured vascular endothelial cells. *Thromb Res.* **1987**, *45*, 803–816. [CrossRef]
45. Mochizuki, N.; Kwon, Y.G. 15-lipoxygenase-1 in the vasculature: Expanding roles in angiogenesis. *Circ. Res.* **2008**, *102*, 143–145. [CrossRef]
46. Talahalli, R.; Zarini, S.; Sheibani, N.; Murphy, R.C.; Gubitosi-Klug, R.A. Increased synthesis of leukotrienes in the mouse model of diabetic retinopathy. *Investig. Ophthalmol. Vis. Sci.* **2010**, *51*, 1699–1708. [CrossRef]
47. De Carvalho, D.D.; Sadok, A.; Bourgarel-Rey, V.; Gattacceca, F.; Penel, C.; Lehmann, M.; Kovacic, H. Nox1 downstream of 12-lipoxygenase controls cell proliferation but not cell spreading of colon cancer cells. *Int. J. Cancer* **2008**, *122*, 1757–1764. [CrossRef]
48. Sadok, A.; Bourgarel-Rey, V.; Gattacceca, F.; Penel, C.; Lehmann, M.; Kovacic, H. Nox1-dependent superoxide production controls colon adenocarcinoma cell migration. *Biochim. Biophys. Acta* **2008**, *1783*, 23–33. [CrossRef] [PubMed]
49. Mahipal, S.V.; Subhashini, J.; Reddy, M.C.; Reddy, M.M.; Anilkumar, K.; Roy, K.R.; Reddy, G.V.; Reddanna, P. Effect of 15-lipoxygenase metabolites, 15-(S)-HPETE and 15-(S)-HETE on chronic myelogenous leukemia cell line K-562: Reactive oxygen species (ROS) mediate caspase-dependent apoptosis. *Biochem. Pharmacol.* **2007**, *74*, 202–214. [CrossRef]
50. Choi, J.A.; Kim, E.Y.; Song, H.; Kim, C.; Kim, J.H. Reactive oxygen species are generated through a BLT2-linked cascade in Ras-transformed cells. *Free Radic. Biol. Med.* **2008**, *44*, 624–634. [CrossRef]
51. Kim, E.Y.; Seo, J.M.; Cho, K.J.; Kim, J.H. Ras-induced invasion and metastasis are regulated by a leukotriene B4 receptor BLT2-linked pathway. *Oncogene* **2010**, *29*, 1167–1178. [CrossRef]
52. White, R.E. The involvement of free radicals in the mechanisms of monooxygenases. *Pharmacol. Ther.* **1991**, *49*, 21–42. [CrossRef]
53. Wang, M.-H. Renal cytochrome P450-derived eicosanoids and hypertension. *Curr. Hypertens. Rev.* **2006**, *2*, 227–236. [CrossRef]
54. Ma, J.; Qu, W.; Scarborough, P.E.; Tomer, K.B.; Moomaw, C.R.; Maronpot, R.; Davis, L.S.; Breyer, M.D.; Zeldin, D.C. Molecular cloning, enzymatic characterization, developmental expression, and cellular localization of a mouse cytochrome P450 highly expressed in kidney. *J. Biol. Chem.* **1999**, *274*, 17777–17788. [CrossRef]
55. Wu, S.; Moomaw, C.R.; Tomer, K.B.; Falck, J.R.; Zeldin, D.C. Molecular cloning and expression of CYP2J2, a human cytochrome P450 arachidonic acid epoxygenase highly expressed in heart. *J. Biol. Chem.* **1996**, *271*, 3460–3468. [CrossRef] [PubMed]
56. Imig, J.D.; Navar, L.G.; Roman, R.J.; Reddy, K.K.; Falck, J.R. Actions of epoxygenase metabolites on the preglomerular vasculature. *J. Am. Soc. Nephrol.* **1996**, *7*, 2364–2370. [PubMed]
57. Campbell, W.B.; Gebremedhin, D.; Pratt, P.F.; Harder, D.R. Identification of epoxyeicosatrienoic acids as endothelium-derived hyperpolarizing factors. *Circ. Res.* **1996**, *78*, 415–423. [CrossRef] [PubMed]
58. Imig, J.D. Epoxide hydrolase and epoxygenase metabolites as therapeutic targets for renal diseases. *Am. J. Physiol. Renal Physiol.* **2005**, *289*, F496–F503. [CrossRef] [PubMed]
59. Hu, J.; Dziumbla, S.; Lin, J.; Bibli, S.I.; Zukunft, S.; de Mos, J.; Awwad, K.; Fromel, T.; Jungmann, A.; Devraj, K.; et al. Inhibition of soluble epoxide hydrolase prevents diabetic retinopathy. *Nature* **2017**, *552*, 248–252. [CrossRef]

60. Michaelis, U.R.; Xia, N.; Barbosa-Sicard, E.; Falck, J.R.; Fleming, I. Role of cytochrome P450 2C epoxygenases in hypoxia-induced cell migration and angiogenesis in retinal endothelial cells. *Investig. Ophthalmol. Vis. Sci.* **2008**, *49*, 1242–1247. [CrossRef]
61. Schwartzman, M.L.; Iserovich, P.; Gotlinger, K.; Bellner, L.; Dunn, M.W.; Sartore, M.; Grazia Pertile, M.; Leonardi, A.; Sathe, S.; Beaton, A.; et al. Profile of lipid and protein autacoids in diabetic vitreous correlates with the progression of diabetic retinopathy. *Diabetes* **2010**, *59*, 1780–1788. [CrossRef]
62. Fang, X.; Hu, S.; Watanabe, T.; Weintraub, N.L.; Snyder, G.D.; Yao, J.; Liu, Y.; Shyy, J.Y.; Hammock, B.D.; Spector, A.A. Activation of peroxisome proliferator-activated receptor alpha by substituted urea-derived soluble epoxide hydrolase inhibitors. *J. Pharmacol. Exp. Ther.* **2005**, *314*, 260–270. [CrossRef] [PubMed]
63. Imig, J.D. Epoxyeicosatrienoic acids, 20-hydroxyeicosatetraenoic acid, and renal microvascular function. *Prostag. Other Lipid Mediat.* **2013**, *104*, 2–7. [CrossRef] [PubMed]
64. Wang, M.H.; Ibrahimb, A.S.; Hsiao, G.; Tawfik, A.; Al-Shabrawe, M. A novel interaction between soluble epoxide hydrolase and the AT1 receptor in retinal microvascular damage. *Prostag. Other Lipid Mediat.* **2020**. [CrossRef] [PubMed]
65. Sato, M.; Yokoyama, U.; Fujita, T.; Okumura, S.; Ishikawa, Y. The roles of cytochrome p450 in ischemic heart disease. *Curr. Drug Metab.* **2011**, *12*, 526–532. [CrossRef]
66. Park, S.K.; Herrnreiter, A.; Pfister, S.L.; Gauthier, K.M.; Falck, B.A.; Falck, J.R.; Campbell, W.B. GPR40 is a low-affinity epoxyeicosatrienoic acid receptor in vascular cells. *J. Biol. Chem.* **2018**, *293*, 10675–10691. [CrossRef]
67. Metea, M.R.; Newman, E.A. Glial cells dilate and constrict blood vessels: A mechanism of neurovascular coupling. *J. Neurosci.* **2006**, *26*, 2862–2870. [CrossRef]
68. Zangar, R.C.; Davydov, D.R.; Verma, S. Mechanisms that regulate production of reactive oxygen species by cytochrome P450. *Toxicol. Appl. Pharmacol.* **2004**, *199*, 316–331. [CrossRef]
69. Edin, M.L.; Wang, Z.; Bradbury, J.A.; Graves, J.P.; Lih, F.B.; DeGraff, L.M.; Foley, J.F.; Torphy, R.; Ronnekleiv, O.K.; Tomer, K.B.; et al. Endothelial expression of human cytochrome P450 epoxygenase CYP2C8 increases susceptibility to ischemia-reperfusion injury in isolated mouse heart. *FASEB J.* **2011**, *25*, 3436–3447. [CrossRef]
70. Nieto, N.; Friedman, S.L.; Cederbaum, A.I. Stimulation and proliferation of primary rat hepatic stellate cells by cytochrome P450 2E1-derived reactive oxygen species. *Hepatology* **2002**, *35*, 62–73. [CrossRef]
71. Lee, R.; Wong, T.Y.; Sabanayagam, C. Epidemiology of diabetic retinopathy, diabetic macular edema and related vision loss. *Eye Vis.* **2015**, *2*, 17. [CrossRef]
72. Phipps, J.A.; Jobling, A.I.; Greferath, U.; Fletcher, E.L.; Vessey, K.A. Alternative pathways in the development of diabetic retinopathy: The renin-angiotensin and kallikrein-kinin systems. *Clin. Exp. Optom.* **2012**, *95*, 282–289. [CrossRef] [PubMed]
73. Shah, A.R.; Gardner, T.W. Diabetic retinopathy: Research to clinical practice. *Clin. Diabetes Endocrinol.* **2017**, *3*, 9. [CrossRef] [PubMed]
74. Gibson, D.M. Diabetic retinopathy and age-related macular degeneration in the U.S. *Am. J. Prev. Med.* **2012**, *43*, 48–54. [CrossRef] [PubMed]
75. Caldwell, R.B.; Bartoli, M.; Behzadian, M.A.; El-Remessy, A.E.; Al-Shabrawey, M.; Platt, D.H.; Caldwell, R.W. Vascular endothelial growth factor and diabetic retinopathy: Pathophysiological mechanisms and treatment perspectives. *Diabetes Metab. Res. Rev.* **2003**, *19*, 442–455. [CrossRef] [PubMed]
76. Aiello, L.P.; Avery, R.L.; Arrigg, P.G.; Keyt, B.A.; Jampel, H.D.; Shah, S.T.; Pasquale, L.R.; Thieme, H.; Iwamoto, M.A.; Park, J.E.; et al. Vascular endothelial growth factor in ocular fluid of patients with diabetic retinopathy and other retinal disorders. *N. Engl. J. Med.* **1994**, *331*, 1480–1487. [CrossRef]
77. Lane, L.S.; Jansen, P.D.; Lahav, M.; Rudy, C. Circulating prostacyclin and thromboxane levels in patients with diabetic retinopathy. *Ophthalmology* **1982**, *89*, 763–766. [CrossRef]
78. Zhou, J.; Wang, S.; Xia, X. Role of intravitreal inflammatory cytokines and angiogenic factors in proliferative diabetic retinopathy. *Curr. Eye Res.* **2012**, *37*, 416–420. [CrossRef]
79. Kern, T.S. Contributions of inflammatory processes to the development of the early stages of diabetic retinopathy. *Exp. Diabetes Res.* **2007**, *2007*, 95103. [CrossRef]
80. Cheng, T.; Cao, W.; Wen, R.; Steinberg, R.H.; LaVail, M.M. Prostaglandin E2 induces vascular endothelial growth factor and basic fibroblast growth factor mRNA expression in cultured rat Muller cells. *Investig. Ophthalmol. Vis. Sci.* **1998**, *39*, 581–591.

81. Yanni, S.E.; Barnett, J.M.; Clark, M.L.; Penn, J.S. The role of PGE2 receptor EP4 in pathologic ocular angiogenesis. *Investig. Ophthalmol. Vis. Sci.* **2009**, *50*, 5479–5486. [CrossRef] [PubMed]
82. Ayalasomayajula, S.P.; Kompella, U.B. Celecoxib, a selective cyclooxygenase-2 inhibitor, inhibits retinal vascular endothelial growth factor expression and vascular leakage in a streptozotocin-induced diabetic rat model. *Eur. J. Pharmacol.* **2003**, *458*, 283–289. [CrossRef]
83. Du, Y.; Sarthy, V.P.; Kern, T.S. Interaction between NO and COX pathways in retinal cells exposed to elevated glucose and retina of diabetic rats. *Am. J. Physiol. Regul. Integr. Comp. Physiol.* **2004**, *287*, R735–R741. [CrossRef] [PubMed]
84. Zheng, L.; Szabo, C.; Kern, T.S. Poly(ADP-ribose) polymerase is involved in the development of diabetic retinopathy via regulation of nuclear factor-kappaB. *Diabetes* **2004**, *53*, 2960–2967. [CrossRef] [PubMed]
85. Joussen, A.M.; Poulaki, V.; Mitsiades, N.; Kirchhof, B.; Koizumi, K.; Dohmen, S.; Adamis, A.P. Nonsteroidal anti-inflammatory drugs prevent early diabetic retinopathy via TNF-alpha suppression. *FASEB J.* **2002**, *16*, 438–440. [CrossRef] [PubMed]
86. Kowluru, R.A.; Odenbach, S. Role of interleukin-1beta in the development of retinopathy in rats: Effect of antioxidants. *Investig. Ophthalmol. Vis. Sci.* **2004**, *45*, 4161–4166. [CrossRef]
87. Zheng, L.; Howell, S.J.; Hatala, D.A.; Huang, K.; Kern, T.S. Salicylate-based anti-inflammatory drugs inhibit the early lesion of diabetic retinopathy. *Diabetes* **2007**, *56*, 337–345. [CrossRef] [PubMed]
88. Early Treatment Diabetic Retinopathy Study Research Group. Effects of aspirin treatment on diabetic retionopathy: ETDRS Report number 8. *Ophthalmology* **1991**, *98*, 757–765.
89. The Damad Study Group. Effect of aspirin alone and aspirin plus dipyridamole in early diabetic retinopathy. A multicenter randomized controlled clinical trial. *Diabetes* **1989**, *38*, 491–498. [CrossRef]
90. Hattori, Y.; Hashizume, K.; Nakajima, K.; Nishimura, Y.; Naka, M.; Miyanaga, K. The effect of long-term treatment with sulindac on the progression of diabetic retinopathy. *Curr. Med. Res. Opin.* **2007**, *23*, 1913–1917. [CrossRef]
91. Chew, E.Y.; Kim, J.; Coleman, H.R.; Aiello, L.P.; Fish, G.; Ip, M.; Haller, J.A.; Figueroa, M.; Martin, D.; Callanan, D.; et al. Preliminary assessment of celecoxib and microdiode pulse laser treatment of diabetic macular edema. *Retina* **2010**, *30*, 459–467. [CrossRef]
92. Kim, G.Y.; Lee, J.W.; Ryu, H.C.; Wei, J.D.; Seong, C.M.; Kim, J.H. Proinflammatory cytokine IL-1beta stimulates IL-8 synthesis in mast cells via a leukotriene B4 receptor 2-linked pathway, contributing to angiogenesis. *J. Immunol.* **2010**, *184*, 3946–3954. [CrossRef] [PubMed]
93. Ichiyama, T.; Kajimoto, M.; Hasegawa, M.; Hashimoto, K.; Matsubara, T.; Furukawa, S. Cysteinyl leukotrienes enhance tumour necrosis factor-alpha-induced matrix metalloproteinase-9 in human monocytes/macrophages. *Clin. Exp. Allergy* **2007**, *37*, 608–614. [CrossRef] [PubMed]
94. Thompson, C.; Cloutier, A.; Bosse, Y.; Thivierge, M.; Gouill, C.L.; Larivee, P.; McDonald, P.P.; Stankova, J.; Rola-Pleszczynski, M. CysLT1 receptor engagement induces activator protein-1- and NF-kappaB-dependent IL-8 expression. *Am. J. Respir. Cell. Mol. Biol.* **2006**, *35*, 697–704. [CrossRef]
95. Al-Shabrawey, M.; Mussell, R.; Kahook, K.; Tawfik, A.; Eladl, M.; Sarthy, V.; Nussbaum, J.; El-Marakby, A.; Park, S.Y.; Gurel, Z.; et al. Increased expression and activity of 12-lipoxygenase in oxygen-induced ischemic retinopathy and proliferative diabetic retinopathy: Implications in retinal neovascularization. *Diabetes* **2011**, *60*, 614–624. [CrossRef]
96. Bolick, D.T.; Orr, A.W.; Whetzel, A.; Srinivasan, S.; Hatley, M.E.; Schwartz, M.A.; Hedrick, C.C. 12/15-lipoxygenase regulates intercellular adhesion molecule-1 expression and monocyte adhesion to endothelium through activation of RhoA and nuclear factor-kappaB. *Arterioscler. Thromb. Vasc. Biol.* **2005**, *25*, 2301–2307. [CrossRef] [PubMed]
97. Li, S.L.; Dwarakanath, R.S.; Cai, Q.; Lanting, L.; Natarajan, R. Effects of silencing leukocyte-type 12/15-lipoxygenase using short interfering RNAs. *J. Lipid. Res.* **2005**, *46*, 220–229. [CrossRef]
98. Natarajan, R.; Gerrity, R.G.; Gu, J.L.; Lanting, L.; Thomas, L.; Nadler, J.L. Role of 12-lipoxygenase and oxidant stress in hyperglycaemia-induced acceleration of atherosclerosis in a diabetic pig model. *Diabetologia* **2002**, *45*, 125–133. [CrossRef] [PubMed]
99. Othman, A.; Ahmad, S.; Megyerdi, S.; Mussell, R.; Choksi, K.; Maddipati, K.R.; Elmarakby, A.; Rizk, N.; Al-Shabrawey, M. 12/15-Lipoxygenase-derived lipid metabolites induce retinal endothelial cell barrier dysfunction: Contribution of NADPH oxidase. *PLoS ONE* **2013**, *8*, e57254. [CrossRef]

100. Ibrahim, A.S.; Elshafey, S.; Sellak, H.; Hussein, K.A.; El-Sherbiny, M.; Abdelsaid, M.; Rizk, N.; Beasley, S.; Tawfik, A.M.; Smith, S.B.; et al. A lipidomic screen of hyperglycemia-treated HRECs links 12/15-Lipoxygenase to microvascular dysfunction during diabetic retinopathy via NADPH oxidase. *J. Lipid Res.* **2015**, *56*, 599–611. [CrossRef]
101. Rai, G.; Kenyon, V.; Jadhav, A.; Schultz, L.; Armstrong, M.; Jameson, J.B.; Hoobler, E.; Leister, W.; Simeonov, A.; Holman, T.R.; et al. Discovery of potent and selective inhibitors of human reticulocyte 15-lipoxygenase-1. *J. Med. Chem.* **2010**, *53*, 7392–7404. [CrossRef]
102. Kenyon, V.; Rai, G.; Jadhav, A.; Schultz, L.; Armstrong, M.; Jameson, J.B.; Perry, S.; Joshi, N.; Bougie, J.M.; Leister, W.; et al. Discovery of potent and selective inhibitors of human platelet-type 12-lipoxygenase. *J. Med. Chem.* **2011**, *54*, 5485–5497. [CrossRef] [PubMed]
103. Goswami, S.K. Cellular redox, epigenetics and diseases. *Subcell Biochem.* **2013**, *61*, 527–542. [CrossRef] [PubMed]
104. Capozzi, M.E.; McCollum, G.W.; Penn, J.S. The role of cytochrome P450 epoxygenases in retinal angiogenesis. *Investig. Ophthalmol. Vis. Sci.* **2014**, *55*, 4253–4260. [CrossRef] [PubMed]
105. Gong, Y.; Fu, Z.; Liegl, R.; Chen, J.; Hellstrom, A.; Smith, L.E. omega-3 and omega-6 long-chain PUFAs and their enzymatic metabolites in neovascular eye diseases. *Am. J. Clin. Nutr.* **2017**, *106*, 16–26. [CrossRef]
106. Gong, Y.; Fu, Z.; Edin, M.L.; Liu, C.H.; Wang, Z.; Shao, Z.; Fredrick, T.W.; Saba, N.J.; Morss, P.C.; Burnim, S.B.; et al. Cytochrome P450 oxidase 2C inhibition adds to omega-3 long-chain polyunsaturated fatty acids protection against retinal and choroidal neovascularization. *Arterioscler. Thromb. Vasc. Biol.* **2016**, *36*, 1919–1927. [CrossRef]
107. Ibrahim, A.S.; Saleh, H.; El-Shafey, M.; Hussein, K.A.; El-Masry, K.; Baban, B.; Sheibani, N.; Wang, M.H.; Tawfik, A.; Al-Shabrawey, M. Targeting of 12/15-Lipoxygenase in retinal endothelial cells, but not in monocytes/macrophages, attenuates high glucose-induced retinal leukostasis. *Biochim. Biophys. Acta* **2017**, *1862*, 636–645. [CrossRef]
108. Fouda, A.Y.; Artham, S.; El-Remessy, A.B.; Fagan, S.C. Renin-angiotensin system as a potential therapeutic target in stroke and retinopathy: Experimental and clinical evidence. *Clin. Sci.* **2016**, *130*, 221–238. [CrossRef]
109. Bender, S.B.; McGraw, A.P.; Jaffe, I.Z.; Sowers, J.R. Mineralocorticoid receptor-mediated vascular insulin resistance: An early contributor to diabetes-related vascular disease? *Diabetes* **2013**, *62*, 313–319. [CrossRef]
110. Phipps, J.A.; Clermont, A.C.; Sinha, S.; Chilcote, T.J.; Bursell, S.E.; Feener, E.P. Plasma kallikrein mediates angiotensin II type 1 receptor-stimulated retinal vascular permeability. *Hypertension* **2009**, *53*, 175–181. [CrossRef]
111. Wright, A.D.; Dodson, P.M. Diabetic retinopathy and blockade of the renin-angiotensin system: New data from the DIRECT study programme. *Eye* **2010**, *24*, 1–6. [CrossRef]
112. Marin Garcia, P.J.; Marin-Castano, M.E. Angiotensin II-related hypertension and eye diseases. *World J. Cardiol.* **2014**, *6*, 968–984. [CrossRef] [PubMed]
113. Duan, Y.; Beli, E.; Li Calzi, S.; Quigley, J.L.; Miller, R.C.; Moldovan, L.; Feng, D.; Salazar, T.E.; Hazra, S.; Al-Sabah, J.; et al. Loss of angiotensin-converting enzyme 2 exacerbates diabetic retinopathy by promoting bone marrow dysfunction. *Stem. Cells* **2018**. [CrossRef] [PubMed]
114. Dominguez, J.M.; Hu, P.; Caballero, S.; Moldovan, L.; Verma, A.; Oudit, G.Y.; Li, Q.; Grant, M.B. Adeno-Associated virus overexpression of angiotensin-converting enzyme-2 reverses diabetic retinopathy in type 1 Diabetes in mice. *Am. J. Pathol.* **2016**, *186*, 1688–1700. [CrossRef]
115. Verma, A.; Shan, Z.; Lei, B.; Yuan, L.; Liu, X.; Nakagawa, T.; Grant, M.B.; Lewin, A.S.; Hauswirth, W.W.; Raizada, M.K.; et al. ACE2 and Ang-(1-7) confer protection against development of diabetic retinopathy. *Mol. Ther.* **2012**, *20*, 28–36. [CrossRef]
116. Sun, Z.; Cade, R.; Zhang, Z.; Alouidor, J.; Van, H. Angiotensinogen gene knockout delays and attenuates cold-induced hypertension. *Hypertension* **2003**, *41*, 322–327. [CrossRef]
117. Sun, Z.; Wang, X.; Wood, C.E.; Cade, J.R. Genetic AT1A receptor deficiency attenuates cold-induced hypertension. *Am. J. Physiol. Regul. Integr. Comp. Physiol.* **2005**, *288*, R433–R439. [CrossRef] [PubMed]
118. Pires, P.W.; Ko, E.A.; Pritchard, H.A.T.; Rudokas, M.; Yamasaki, E.; Earley, S. The angiotensin II receptor type 1b is the primary sensor of intraluminal pressure in cerebral artery smooth muscle cells. *J. Physiol.* **2017**, *595*, 4735–4753. [CrossRef] [PubMed]

119. Marques-Lopes, J.; Lynch, M.K.; Van Kempen, T.A.; Waters, E.M.; Wang, G.; Iadecola, C.; Pickel, V.M.; Milner, T.A. Female protection from slow-pressor effects of angiotensin II involves prevention of ROS production independent of NMDA receptor trafficking in hypothalamic neurons expressing angiotensin 1A receptors. *Synapse* **2015**, *69*, 148–165. [CrossRef]
120. Patel, D.; Alhawaj, R.; Kelly, M.R.; Accarino, J.J.; Lakhkar, A.; Gupte, S.A.; Sun, D.; Wolin, M.S. Potential role of mitochondrial superoxide decreasing ferrochelatase and heme in coronary artery soluble guanylate cyclase depletion by angiotensin II. *Am. J. Physiol. Heart Circ. Physiol.* **2016**, *310*, H1439–H1447. [CrossRef]
121. Chaturvedi, N.; Sjolie, A.K.; Stephenson, J.M.; Abrahamian, H.; Keipes, M.; Castellarin, A.; Rogulja-Pepeonik, Z.; Fuller, J.H. Effect of lisinopril on progression of retinopathy in normotensive people with type 1 diabetes. The EUCLID study group. EURODIAB controlled trial of lisinopril in insulin-dependent Diabetes mellitus. *Lancet* **1998**, *351*, 28–31. [CrossRef]
122. Chaturvedi, N.; Porta, M.; Klein, R.; Orchard, T.; Fuller, J.; Parving, H.H.; Bilous, R.; Sjolie, A.K. Effect of candesartan on prevention (DIRECT-Prevent 1) and progression (DIRECT-Protect 1) of retinopathy in type 1 diabetes: Randomised, placebo-controlled trials. *Lancet* **2008**, *372*, 1394–1402. [CrossRef]
123. Szymczak, M.; Murray, M.; Petrovic, N. Modulation of angiogenesis by omega-3 polyunsaturated fatty acids is mediated by cyclooxygenases. *Blood* **2008**, *111*, 3514–3521. [CrossRef] [PubMed]
124. Serhan, C.N. Resolution phase of inflammation: Novel endogenous anti-inflammatory and proresolving lipid mediators and pathways. *Annu. Rev. Immunol.* **2007**, *25*, 101–137. [CrossRef] [PubMed]
125. Sapieha, P.; Stahl, A.; Chen, J.; Seaward, M.R.; Willett, K.L.; Krah, N.M.; Dennison, R.J.; Connor, K.M.; Aderman, C.M.; Liclican, E.; et al. 5-Lipoxygenase metabolite 4-HDHA is a mediator of the antiangiogenic effect of omega-3 polyunsaturated fatty acids. *Sci. Transl. Med.* **2011**, *3*. [CrossRef]
126. Shao, Z.; Fu, Z.; Stahl, A.; Joyal, J.S.; Hatton, C.; Juan, A.; Hurst, C.; Evans, L.; Cui, Z.; Pei, D.; et al. Cytochrome P450 2C8 omega3-long-chain polyunsaturated fatty acid metabolites increase mouse retinal pathologic neovascularization-brief report. *Arterioscler. Thromb. Vasc. Biol.* **2014**, *34*, 581–586. [CrossRef] [PubMed]
127. Michaelis, U.R.; Fisslthaler, B.; Barbosa-Sicard, E.; Falck, J.R.; Fleming, I.; Busse, R. Cytochrome P450 epoxygenases 2C8 and 2C9 are implicated in hypoxia-induced endothelial cell migration and angiogenesis. *J. Cell Sci.* **2005**, *118*, 5489–5498. [CrossRef] [PubMed]
128. Webler, A.C.; Michaelis, U.R.; Popp, R.; Barbosa-Sicard, E.; Murugan, A.; Falck, J.R.; Fisslthaler, B.; Fleming, I. Epoxyeicosatrienoic acids are part of the VEGF-activated signaling cascade leading to angiogenesis. *Am. J. Physiol. Cell Physiol.* **2008**, *295*, C1292–C1301. [CrossRef]
129. Walsky, R.L.; Gaman, E.A.; Obach, R.S. Examination of 209 drugs for inhibition of cytochrome P450 2C8. *J. Clin. Pharmacol.* **2005**, *45*, 68–78. [CrossRef]
130. Walsky, R.L.; Obach, R.S.; Gaman, E.A.; Gleeson, J.P.; Proctor, W.R. Selective inhibition of human cytochrome P4502C8 by montelukast. *Drug Metab. Dispos.* **2005**, *33*, 413–418. [CrossRef]
131. Zhang, X.; Yan, G.; Li, Y.; Zhu, W.; Wang, H. DC260126, a small-molecule antagonist of GPR40, improves insulin tolerance but not glucose tolerance in obese Zucker rats. *Biomed. Pharmacother.* **2010**, *64*, 647–651. [CrossRef]
132. Sun, P.; Wang, T.; Zhou, Y.; Liu, H.; Jiang, H.; Zhu, W.; Wang, H. DC260126: A small-molecule antagonist of GPR40 that protects against pancreatic beta-Cells dysfunction in db/db mice. *PLoS ONE* **2013**, *8*, e66744. [CrossRef] [PubMed]

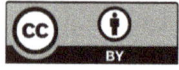

© 2020 by the authors. Licensee MDPI, Basel, Switzerland. This article is an open access article distributed under the terms and conditions of the Creative Commons Attribution (CC BY) license (http://creativecommons.org/licenses/by/4.0/).

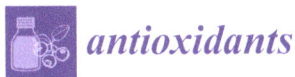

Review

The Complex Relationship between Diabetic Retinopathy and High-Mobility Group Box: A Review of Molecular Pathways and Therapeutic Strategies

Marcella Nebbioso [1], Alessandro Lambiase [1,*], Marta Armentano [1], Giosuè Tucciarone [1], Vincenza Bonfiglio [2], Rocco Plateroti [1] and Ludovico Alisi [1]

[1] Department of Sense Organs, Faculty of Medicine and Odontology, Policlinico Umberto I, Sapienza University of Rome, p. le A. Moro 5, 00185 Rome, Italy; marcella.nebbioso@uniroma1.it (M.N.); marta.armentano@uniroma1.it (M.A.); giosue.tucciarone@uniroma1.it (G.T.); rocco.plateroti@uniroma1.it (R.P.); ludovico.alisi@uniroma1.it (L.A.)

[2] Department of Ophthalmology, University of Catania, Via S. Sofia 76, 95100 Catania, Italy; vincenzamariaelena.bonfiglio@unipa.it

* Correspondence: alessandro.lambiase@uniroma1.it; Tel.: +39-06-4997-5357; Fax: +39-06-4997-5425

Received: 19 June 2020; Accepted: 22 July 2020; Published: 26 July 2020

Abstract: High-mobility group box 1 (HMGB1) is a protein that is part of a larger family of non-histone nuclear proteins. HMGB1 is a ubiquitary protein with different isoforms, linked to numerous physiological and pathological pathways. HMGB1 is involved in cytokine and chemokine release, leukocyte activation and migration, tumorigenesis, neoangiogenesis, and the activation of several inflammatory pathways. HMGB1 is, in fact, responsible for the trigger, among others, of nuclear factor-κB (NF-κB), tumor necrosis factor-α (TNF-α), toll-like receptor-4 (TLR-4), and vascular endothelial growth factor (VEGF) pathways. Diabetic retinopathy (DR) is a common complication of diabetes mellitus (DM) that is rapidly growing in number. DR is an inflammatory disease caused by hyperglycemia, which determines the accumulation of oxidative stress and cell damage, which ultimately leads to hypoxia and neovascularization. Recent evidence has shown that hyperglycemia is responsible for the hyperexpression of HMGB1. This protein activates numerous pathways that cause the development of DR, and HMGB1 levels are constantly increased in diabetic retinas in both proliferative and non-proliferative stages of the disease. Several molecules, such as glycyrrhizin (GA), have proven effective in reducing diabetic damage to the retina through the inhibition of HMGB1. The main focus of this review is the growing amount of evidence linking HMGB1 and DR as well as the new therapeutic strategies involving this protein.

Keywords: antioxidants; diabetes mellitus; diabetic retinopathy; free radicals; high-mobility group box 1 (HMGB1); inflammatory pathways; novel therapies; oxidative stress

---

1. Introduction to Diabetic Retinopathy (DR)

Diabetes mellitus (DM) is a well-known metabolic disease that causes numerous chronic complications. To this day, the number of patients affected by type one and type two DM is estimated to be 463 million. This number will rise to 700 million by 2045 (around 10.9% of the global population) [1]. The most common complications, such as diabetic retinopathy (DR), are caused by microvascular damages. Nowadays, the number of patients affected by DR is calculated as around 93 million [2]. These numbers place DR as the fifth most common cause of severe visual impairment in the world [3]. From a clinical point of view, DR is characterized by typical vascular and macular abnormalities. In non-proliferative DR (N-PDR), the most common findings are microaneurysms, cotton wool spots, hemorrhages, hard exudates, and venous dilatation. The progression toward the stage of PDR is defined by the development of neovascularization that may lead to retinal and vitreous hemorrhages, fibrovascular proliferation, and tractive retinal detachment. Other complications of DR are neovascular glaucoma, steaming from iris neovascularization, and macular edema (Figures 1 and 2) [4,5].

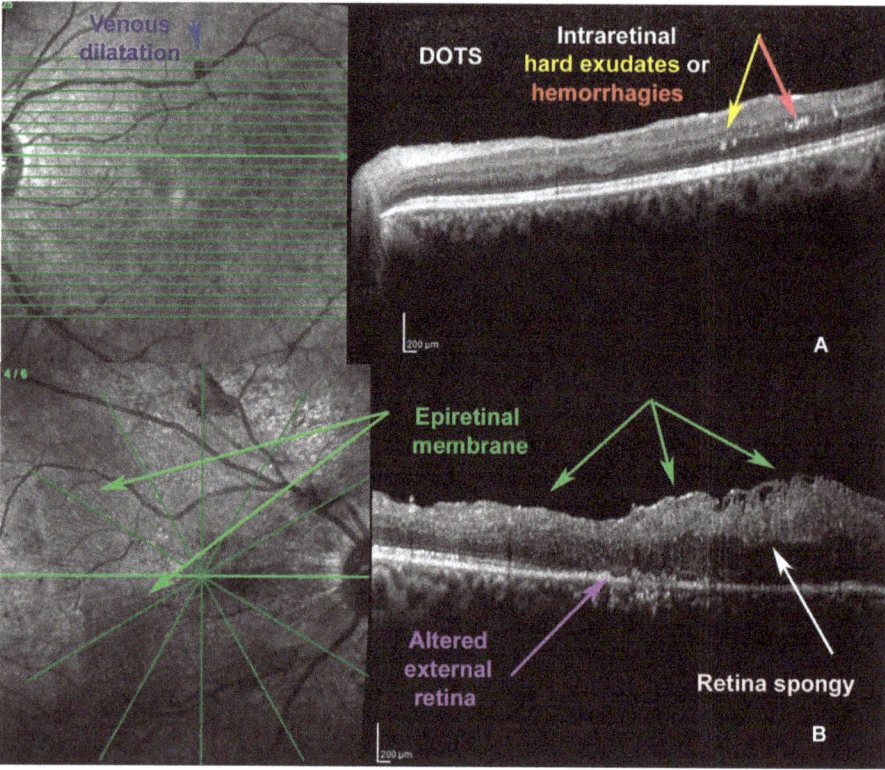

Figure 1. Spectral-domain optical coherence tomography exam of two patients. Patient (**A**). Initial diabetic retinopathy (DR) characterized by typical vascular and retinal abnormalities: microaneurysms, hemorrhages (hyperreflective dots), hard exudates (hyperreflective dots), and venous dilatation (blue arrow). Patient (**B**). Preproliferating ischemic-exudative DR to the posterior pole with epiretinal membrane (green arrows), retina spongy (white arrow), and altered layers of photoreceptors and retinal pigment epithelium (external retina).

The pathogenesis of DR is an extremely complex mechanism that involves numerous biochemical and inflammatory pathways triggered by long exposition to hyperglycemia. The development of DR is characterized by the concomitant participation of vascular endothelial dysfunction, pericyte loss, and neurodegeneration, which ultimately leads to hypoxia and neovascularization [6]. Interestingly, neuronal degeneration appears to precede vascular disease and develop as an independent mechanism [7].

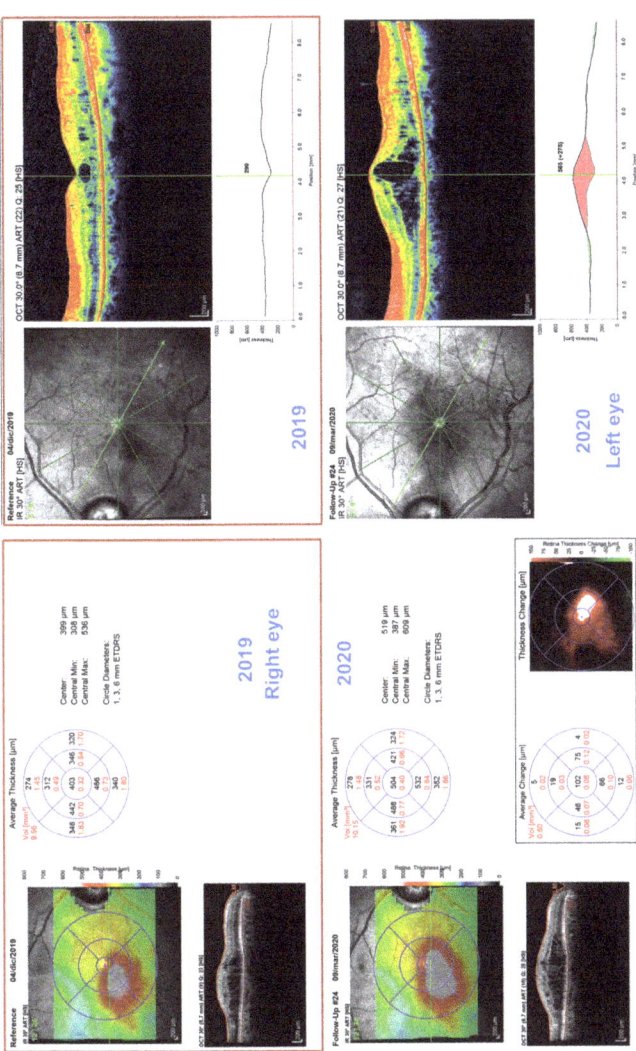

Figure 2. Spectral-domain optical coherence tomography (SD-OCT) of a diabetic patient right and left eye. The progression of the disease toward the stage of proliferative diabetic retinopathy (PDR) is defined by the development of persistent/chronic macular edema with flower petal cysts, important retinal and vitreous hemorrhages, marked fibrovascular proliferation, tractive retinal detachment, and, finally, vitreoretinal neovascularization with retinal detachment. SD-OCT exam: above 4 December 2019 and under 9 March 2020.

The persistence of high levels of blood glucose is determinant for the activation of inflammatory mechanisms, the enhancement of oxidative stress, and, consequently, the production of advanced glycation end-products (AGEs) [4]. The inflammation determines the local accumulation of cytokines, such as vascular endothelial growth factor (VEGF), tumor necrosis factor-alpha (TNF-α), and inducible nitric oxide synthase (iNOS), that favor the establishment of hypoxia in the diabetic retina [8]. Inflammation leads also to the accumulation of chemokines and adhesion molecules such as intercellular adhesion molecule-1 (ICAM-1). This mechanism causes the migration of leukocytes towards the retinal endothelium, increased vascular permeability, and the breakdown of the blood–retinal barrier (BRB) that ultimately leads to edema [9].

Hyperglycemia determines the production of AGEs. The binding of AGEs to their receptors (RAGE) allows for the activation of nuclear factor-κB (NF-κB) pathways, which ultimately leads to the production of reactive oxygen species (ROS) and the reduction of antioxidant defense systems [10]. Oxidative stress conducts to the metabolic memory phenomenon in mitochondria. This phenomenon is deemed responsible for the persistence of vascular damage, even when glycemic control is perfectly achieved [11]. Moreover, hyperglycemia determines the production of sorbitol through the activation of the polyol pathway. High volumes of sorbitol lead to the depletion of reduced glutathione (GSH) and the accumulation of ROS [12].

Hyperglycemia is also able to activate different isoforms of protein kinase C (PKC). This enzyme participates in the retinal vascular damage through its efficiency in the induction of nicotinamide adenine dinucleotide phosphate oxidase (NOX). The resulting O_2^- contributes to the worsening of endothelial dysfunction [13,14]. PKC is also involved in the increase of endothelial cell death and pericyte loss via the accumulation of oxidative and nitrosative products, contributing to the development of microaneurysms and the recruitment of leukocytes [15].

Another pathway heavily affected by chronic exposition to hyperglycemia is the hexosamine pathway. The alternative cycle to glycolysis is needed to convert the excess of fructose 6-phosphate that cannot be metabolized by classic glycolysis. This leads to the production of N-acetyl glucosamine and the overexpression of transforming growth factor-β1 (TGF-β1) and plasminogen activator inhibitor-1 (PAI-1), increasing the apoptotic rate of endothelial cells (EC) and pericytes [16,17]. Moreover, AGE accumulation activates the hexosamine pathway, determining the production of angiopoietin-2 and the development of neovascularization [18,19]. Lastly, it has been recently demonstrated that the activation of the innate immune response facilitates the development of inflammation and therefore DR. Specifically, concentrations of toll-like receptor (TLR)–4 and –2 as well as their downstream inflammatory cytokines TNF-α, interleukin (IL)-1β, and interferon (IFN)-β were found to be significantly increased in murine models of DM [20,21].

Current therapeutic approaches, such as anti-angiogenic agents or corticosteroids intravitreal injections and laser therapy, only target the manifestations of DR. The complexity of the metabolic pathways activated during DR shows how single-target therapies have limited success [22–24]. The lack of preventive treatments and the increasing number of patients show the need for the development of new specific agents targeting the metabolic pathways that lead to DR (Scheme 1).

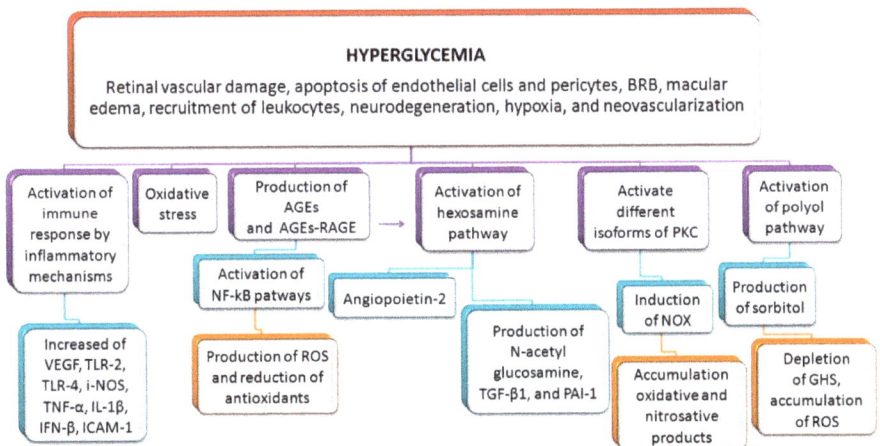

Scheme 1. Predominant biochemical alterations in diabetes mellitus (DM) patients and related dysfunctions caused by hyperglycemia. HMGB1: high-mobility group box 1; DR: diabetic retinopathy; BRB: blood–retinal barrier; AGEs: advanced glycation end-products; RAGE: receptors for AGEs; PKC: protein kinase C; NF-κB: nuclear factor-κB; TGF-β1: transforming growth factor-β1; PAI-1: plasminogen activator inhibitor-1; NOX: nicotinamide adenine dinucleotide phosphate oxidase; VEGF: vascular endothelial growth factor; TLR: toll-like receptor; iNOS: inducible nitric oxide synthase; TNF-α: tumor necrosis factor-α; IL-1β: interleukin-1β; IFN-β: interferon-β; ICAM-1: intercellular adhesion molecule-1; ROS: reactive oxygen species; GSH: reduced glutathione.

2. Introduction to High-Mobility Group Box 1 (HMGB1)

High-mobility group (HMG) proteins are a group of non-histone nuclear proteins discovered in 1973 in the calf thymus, including three families, named HMGB, HMGN, and HMGA [25]. This group of proteins owes their name to their high electrophoretic mobility [26]. The high-mobility group box (HMGB) family contains several different proteins unified by the constant presence of at least one HMGB. The most studied and ubiquitary protein of this family is HMGB1 [27]. HMGB1 is an evolutionary conserved chromatin-binding protein composed of 215 amino acids and characterized by two DNA binding domains named Box-A and Box-B and a C-terminal acidic domain [28]. Initially considered a nuclear protein, HMGB1 has subsequently shown a cytosolic location inside several cell organelles and structures, such as mitochondria and the cellular membrane as well as extracellular space [29].

HMGB1 may be present in a reduced, oxidized, or disulfide form. Its actions appear to be largely dependent on the redox state [30]. The reduced form is characterized by the reduction of specific cysteine residues. In this configuration, HMGB1 can recruit leukocyte independently from the release of cytokines or chemokines [31]. The oxidized configuration determines the loss of the immunogenic properties of HMGB1 [32]. Lastly, the disulfide form activates the NF-κB inflammatory pathway, determining the production of IL- 6, -8, and TNF-α [31].

HMGB1, due to its ubiquitous location in the cell, performs numerous activities (Figure 3).

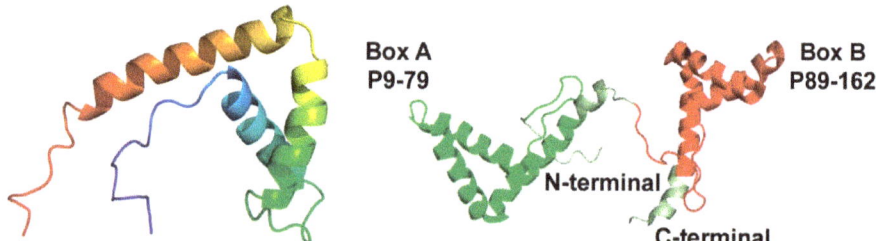

Figure 3. Structure of high-mobility group box 1 (HMGB1) protein. HMGB1 is a protein consisting of 216 residues, 30 kD, highly conserved among mammals. The protein contains three alpha-helices, connected together by loops. It consists of two homologous DNA-binding domains of the HMG-box type: Box A (and Box B) and segment C-terminal, a negatively charged "tail". There are two nuclear localization sequences. Green marks the linker and terminal regions of HMGB1. Box A (P9–79) is colored in green and Box B (P89–162) in red.

Inside the nucleus, HMGB1 controls chromatin stability and replication, nucleosome release from damaged cells, gene recombination, and transcription, DNA repair, and replication [27,33].

Cytosolic HMGB1 is usually secondary to the shuttling of nuclear HMGB1 in response to hypoxia, chemokines, cytokines, and ROS. In the cytosol, HMGB1 acts as a positive regulator of autophagia [34]. HMGB1 expression on the surface of cellular membranes is responsible for the activation of innate immunity and mediates cellular adhesion [35,36].

Extracellular HMGB1 is involved in numerous activities such as the regulation of T-cells [37], stem cells [38], and neoplastic cell differentiation [39]. This protein is also involved in the management of the inflammatory response, through the activation of numerous different immune cells [40,41], and the promotion of cytokine release [42,43]. HMGB1's extracellular functions consist of cellular proliferation [44] and migration [45], including vascular growth during inflammatory or neoplastic diseases and tissue repair [46,47]. During the inflammatory response, HMGB1 is secreted by macrophages, platelets, EC, and monocytes, as well as necrotic or damaged cells [48]. Disulfide HMGB1 binds together with myeloid differentiation factor-2 and TLR-4, determining the formation of a complex that triggers the inflammatory response [49,50]. In addition, HMGB1 deficient cellular lines show a reduced capacity to induce cytokines [51]. The binding of HMGB1 to RAGEs determines the formation of a complex responsible for the activation, among others, of NF-κB, phosphatidylinositol 3-kinase (PI3K)/PKB, mitogen-activated protein kinase (MAPK), and TNF-α pathways [52–54]. Thus, HMGB1 is involved in myriad diseases, such as hypoxia-induced injury [55], microglial damage and neuroinflammation [56], vascular barrier damage [57], and inflammatory heart diseases [58]. Moreover, ROS, through the activation of the NF-κB pathway, are responsible for the passive and active secretion of HMGB1 in monocytes and macrophages [59]. HMGB1 is recognized to be a direct angiogenic molecule as it induces a pro-angiogenic phenotype in EC [60,61]. It can, moreover, stimulate angiogenesis through the activation of the MAPK/extracellular signal-regulated kinase (ERK) 1/2 pathway. The bond between HMGB1 and RAGE results in the stimulation of NF-κB signaling in leukocytes, which leads to the production of proinflammatory and angiogenic molecules [62]. HMGB1 in conjunction with TLR-4 can influence the development of neovasis in proliferative and metabolic diseases [63,64]. Moreover, it has been demonstrated that HMGB1 can mediate angiogenesis through the activation of hypoxia-induced factor-1α (HIF-1α) [65].

In conclusion, HMGB1 shows a wide range of interactions in both physiological and pathological mechanisms. The next section of the review will focus on the growing amount of evidence linking HMGB1 expression and the development of DR. The main focus of this review is the growing amount of evidence linking HMGB1 and DR as well as the new therapeutic strategies involving this protein.

3. HMGB1 and DR

At the moment, information regarding the function of HMGB1 in DR is mostly limited to murine models and in vitro studies. DM upregulates the expression of HMGB1, leading to the activation of inflammatory signaling pathways such as the RAGE-mediated activation of ERK1/2-NF-κB. Intravitreal injection of HMGB1 mimics the effects of diabetes and increases RAGE, ERK1/2, NF-κB, and proinflammatory biomarkers such as ICAM-1 and soluble ICAM-1 (Scheme 2). These mechanisms decrease TLR-2 and occludin expression, increasing retinal vascular permeability and disrupting the stability of tight junction complex between adjacent retinal microvascular EC [66].

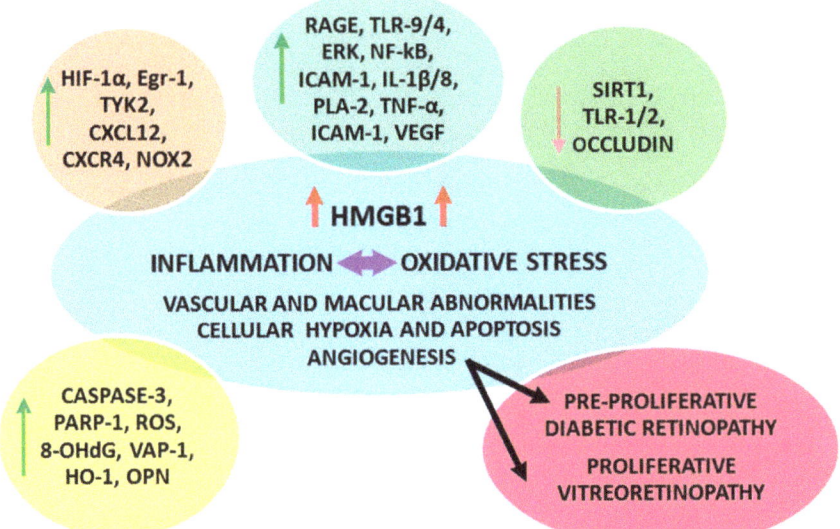

Scheme 2. High-mobility group box 1 (HMGB1) levels increased in diabetic retinopathy (DR). HMGB1 promotes angiogenesis directly and indirectly. Multiple functions of HMGB1 in DR are limited to murine models and in vitro studies. HIF-1α: hypoxia induced factor-1α; Egr-1: early growth response protein 1; TYK2: tyrosine kinase 2; CXCL12/CXCR4: chemokine; NOX2: nicotinamide adenine dinucleotide phosphate oxidase; RAGE: receptors for advanced glycation end-products; TLR-1/2/9/4: toll like receptor-1/2/9/4; ERK: extracellular signal-regulated kinase; NF-kB: nuclear factor-κB; ICAM-1: intercellular adhesion molecule-1; IL-1β/8: interleukin-1β/8; PLA-2: phospholipases A2; TNF-α: tumor necrosis factor-α; VEGF: vascular endothelial growth factor; SIRT1: sirtuin; PARP-1: poly ADP-ribose polymerase; ROS: reactive oxygen species; 8-OHdG: 8-hydroxydeoxyguanosine; VAP-1: vascular adhesion protein-1; HO-1: heme oxygenase-1; OPN: osteopontin.

High glucose stimulates the translocation of HMGB1 into the cytoplasm of retinal pericytes. RAGEs act as receptors for HMGB1 and, in diabetes, their expression is enhanced. HMGB1 is involved in the induction of DR through the activation of this receptor. HMGB1, through the binding of RAGEs, enhances the transcriptional activity of NF-κB in retinal pericytes in in vitro and in vivo models. Hyperglycemia also increases the binding of NF-κB to the RAGE promoter, inducing the overexpression of RAGEs and therefore establishing a vicious cycle [67].

HMGB1 is strictly related to the signal transducer and activator of transcription-3 (STAT-3). Constant intake of HMGB1 inhibitor glycyrrhizin (GA) attenuates the upregulation of phosphorylated STAT-3 (pSTAT-3). The inhibition of STAT-3 blocks HMGB1-induced VEGF upregulation and human retinal microvascular endothelial cell (HRMECs) migration, suggesting the role of STAT-3 in mediating HMGB1-induced angiogenesis in DR [68].

HMGB1 induces the significant upregulation of IL-1β and ROS and the expression of NOX2, caspase-3, and poly ADP-ribose polymerase-1 (PARP-1) in HRMECs [69].

HMGB1 may have a role in the alteration of BRB HMGB1 expression, which is enhanced in the retinas of diabetic rats, and BRB permeability is significantly increased [70].

Sirtuin 1 (SIRT1) is a member of the SIRT family of proteins with deacetylase activity. Many studies report its role in DNA repair, oxidative stress, angiogenesis, inflammation, and senescence. There is a strong link between SIRT1 expression and the development of DR and PDR. In particular, hyperglycemia and diabetes cause the downregulation of SIRT1, thus resulting in inflammation, angiogenesis, an increase in oxidative stress, and vascular permeability, all of which are hallmarks of diabetic damage [71]. There is a functional link between HMGB1 and SIRT1 in the regulation of the diabetes-induced breakdown of the BRB. Intravitreal injection of HMGB1 in normal rats results in the downregulation of SIRT1. The HMGB1 inhibitor GA attenuates the downregulation of and normalizes retinal SIRT1 expression. Moreover, treatment with the SIRT1 activator resveratrol attenuates the diabetes-induced downregulation of SIRT1, accompanied by reduced expression of HMGB1 and RAGEs. Resveratrol may confer protection against the diabetes-induced breakdown of BRB through SIRT1 upregulation and HMGB1 downregulation [72]. HMGB1, insulin-like growth factor-binding protein 3 (IGFBP-3), SIRT1, and protein kinase A (PKA) are strictly related. IGFBP-3 increases SIRT1 and decreases HMGB1. PKA mediates the reduction in cytoplasmic HMGB1 by increasing IGFBP-3 and SIRT1 activities [73].

Chen et al. found increased expression of HMGB1 and its receptor RAGEs TLR-2 and TLR-4 in the retinas of type 2 diabetic rats and human retinal pigment epithelial cell line-19 (ARPE-19) exposed to high glucose. The NF-κB activity was found to be increased as well. The blockage of HMGB1 downregulated NF-κB hyperactivation and VEGF production in high glucose cultured ARPE-19 cells [74].

High levels of HMGB1 expression are due to both gene transcription and protein synthesis. The specific mechanism by which HMGB1 leads to DR is unclear. It may exert its function via the TLR-9 pathway. The expression of TLR-9 was increased and positively related to the expression of HMGB1 [75].

A high glucose environment could promote HMGB1 expression and activate TLR-4 and NF-κB overexpression in retinal ganglion cells (RGC), thus leading to the inhibition of cell survival and growth. TLR-4 is an important receptor for HGMB-1 that is largely expressed in the nervous system and can regulate neuron growth and proliferation. When HMGB1 binds to TLR-4, it activates several signaling pathways such as NF-κB with the release of inflammatory cytokines, chemokines, and colony-stimulating factors, leading to leukocyte adhesion and inflammation [76]. Yu et al. showed a higher expression of HMGB1 in diabetic rats associated with the upregulation of phospholipases A2 (PLA-2), TNF-κ, VEGF, and ICAM-1. Regarding HMGB1 receptors, RAGEs protein was increased, whereas TLR-1 was reduced, suggesting that HMGB1 effects are RAGE-mediated [77].

Injury and death of the retinal pericytes and EC in DR might be due to the HMGB1/PLA2 induced cytotoxic activity of glial cells as well as the direct effect of HMGB1 on EC. HMGB1 could mediate EC death directly and pericyte death indirectly through the HMGB1-induced cytotoxic activity of glial cells. Regarding PLA2 it seems to be a positive regulator of VEGF-induced angiogenesis [78].

HMGB1 has an important role in angiogenesis. It can act directly through RAGEs and TLR-4 with EC activation, proliferation, and migration. HMGB1 also promotes angiogenesis indirectly through the production of proangiogenic cytokines, such as VEGF, TNF-κ, and IL-8 from EC and activated macrophages [79]. The same role of HMGB1 was also demonstrated by Santos et al. The authors suggest that HMGB1 is not able to mediate angiogenesis in the retina by itself [80].

According to Lee et al., AGEs cause a rise in intracellular ROS, inducing the release of HMGB1 into extracellular space. HMGB1 augments the signal via RAGEs or TLR and mediates the secretion of VEGF-A through the c-Jun N-terminal kinases signaling pathway that was blocked by HMGB1 inhibitor GA. This could be a possible way through which HMGB1 upregulates VEGF [81].

HMGB1 and VEGF-A expression are upregulated in serum samples of DR patients and are positively associated. The in vitro up-regulation of HMGB1 inhibits the retinal pigmented epithelium (RPE) cell viability and induces apoptosis. HMGB1 administration to RPE cells in high glucose conditions up-regulates the expression of VEGF-A [82].

The silencing of HMGB1 inhibits the activation of MAPK and NF-κB signaling pathway; modulates the levels of VEGF, ICAM-1 and vascular cell adhesion molecule-1 (VCAM-1), therefore influencing endothelial permeability; attenuates cell apoptosis, BRB damage, and the inflammatory response induced by high concentration of glucose [83].

HMGB1 may inhibit the expression of NF-κB light polypeptide gene enhancer in B-cell inhibitor-α, a protein capable of inhibiting NF-κB by binding to its promoter region. This determines the activation of the NF-κB pathway, influencing inflammation and angiogenic processes, thus leading to DR. High levels of HMGB1 stimulate apoptosis and inhibit the proliferation of human retinal endothelial cells (HRECs). HMGB1 may determine apoptosis through the NF-κB pathway thanks to an alternate mechanism of non-perfusion and neovascularization [84].

There is a potential link among HMGB1, vascular adhesion protein-1 (VAP-1), oxidative stress, and heme oxygenase-1 (HO-1) in the pathogenesis of inflammation and angiogenesis associated with PDR. HMGB1 levels are consistently increased in the vitreous of patients with PDR, particularly higher in patients with active PDR. Exogenous HMGB1 activates HRMECs to upregulate the adhesion molecule ICAM-1.

Increased levels of the oxidative marker 8-hydroxydeoxyguanosine (8-OHdG) in the vitreous of PDR patients, particularly in active PDR, have been found. The positive correlation between vitreous levels of HMGB1 and 8-OHdG in HRMECs suggests that HMGB1 is associated with oxidative stress.

Regarding VAP-1, there was a significant correlation between the levels of sVAP-1, HMGB1 concentration, and 8-OHdG in vitreous. Expression of VAP-1 was higher in diabetic patients compared to controls in the RPE, whereas no significant difference was found in the neuroretina.

Stimulation with HMGB1 caused the upregulation of HO-1 in HRMECs. HO-1 levels were significantly higher in eyes with active neovascularization compared with eyes with involuted PDR. These findings suggest that HO-1 might contribute to PDR angiogenesis and progression. Moreover, VEGF can induce the expression of HO-1 that stimulates the synthesis of VEGF in a positive feedback loop [85].

Vascular EC and stromal cells in diabetic epiretinal membranes express HMGB1, RAGE, osteopontin (OPN), and early growth response protein-1 (Egr-1). In diabetic epiretinal membranes, these proteins and receptors are specifically localized in myofibroblasts. This suggests that HMGB1/RAGE/OPN/Egr-1 signaling pathway is involved in the inflammatory, angiogenic, and fibrotic responses in proliferative vitreoretinopathy (PVR) and may contribute to the instauration of PDR and its most dangerous complications [86].

OPN, HMGB1, and connective tissue growth factor (CTGF) were upregulated in the vitreous of patients with PVR, particularly in their active form, whereas increased levels of pigment epithelium-derived factor (PEDF) may be a response designed to counteract the activity of the angiogenic and fibrogenic factors during the progression of PDR and PVR [87].

There is a relationship between the activity of PDR, the presence of vitreous hemorrhages, and levels of HMGB1. In fact, HMGB1 is higher in patients with active PDR compared with inactive PDR and is higher in PDR patients with vitreous hemorrhages compared with patients without it [88].

Shen et al. found that HMGB1, VEGF, RAGE, and IL-1β levels were significantly elevated in the vitreous and serum of patients with PDR, suggesting that the upregulation of HMGB1 might contribute to the initiation and progression of angiogenesis in PDR and that the HMGB1/RAGE signaling axis has a role in the progression of PDR [89].

The upregulation of HMGB1 can induce the downregulation of brain-derived neurotrophic factor (BDNF), a neurotrophin with a neurogenetic function, and also of synaptophysin, an integral membrane protein of synaptic vesicles involved in neurotransmission. HMGB1 upregulates cleaved caspase-3 in vitreous fluid and serum from patients with PDR, as well as in the retinas of diabetic rats. HMGB1 inhibitor GA is able to revert the downregulation of BDNF.

RAGEs and ICAMs levels are upregulated in the serum of patients with PDR. RAGEs bind its ligands, preventing their link to RAGE, therefore blocking the inflammatory cascade. Elevated levels of RAGEs in the serum of patients with PDR could negatively regulate inflammation and limit diabetes-induced retinal vascular and neuronal dysfunction [90].

HMGB1 and VEGF levels were higher in vitreous from PDR patients. Moreover, there were increased levels of soluble vascular endothelial-cadherin that could be a marker of EC activation or injury associated with angiogenesis, inflammation, and the breakdown of the inner BRB. Finally, there was lower angiogenic activity in patients with higher levels of soluble endoglin, suggesting that it could be protective against pathological angiogenesis [91].

The intravitreal injection of HMGB1 in normal rats mimics the effect of DM, with increased expression of HMGB1 protein and mRNA, caspase 3, and levels of glutamate (responsible for excitotoxic neuronal death). HMGB1 inhibitor glycyrrhizic acid attenuates all of these effects. The early retinal neuropathy induced by diabetes is, at least in part, attributable to the diabetes-induced upregulation of HMGB1. Inhibiting the release of HMGB1 with a constant intake of GA results in the reduction of diabetes-induced retinal neuropathy. This could be a novel therapeutic approach to DR [92].

The induction of DM and intravitreal injection of HMGB1 in normal rats resulted in the significant upregulation of HIF-1α, Egr-1, tyrosine kinase 2 (TYK2), and the CXCL12/CXCR4 chemokine axis. HIF-1α is associated with retinal inflammation induced by diabetes, Egr-1 may play a role in the development of vascular complications of DM, and the CXCL12/CXCR4 chemokine axis contributes to neovascularization. All these upregulations are mediated by the interaction of HMGB1 with RAGE. Inhibition of the release of HMGB1, for example with GA, attenuates the upregulation of all these molecules [93].

Exposure to hypoxia is able to release HMGB1 from RPE cells. HMGB1 may stimulate the overproduction of angiogenic and fibrogenic factors such as VEGF and CTGF in RPE cells. HMGB1 is involved in DR pathogenesis through binding to TLR-4, RAGE, and their signaling cascades such as PI3K, p38/MAPK, and NF-κB [94,95].

4. Future Therapeutic Approaches

Numerous molecules have been studied as inhibitors of HMGB1 in recent years for the treatment and prevention of DR and its complications (Table 1).

4.1. Glycyrrhizin (GA)

GA is a triterpene glycoconjugate naturally extracted from licorice root (*Glycyrrhiza glabra*). It is composed of two molecules of glucuronic acid and glycyrrhetinic acid aglycone [96]. This molecule inhibits the chemotactic and pathogenic functions of HMGB1 by binding directly the A and B boxes [97].

GA shows a wide range of effects such as antibacterial, hepatoprotective, antiproliferative, antiallergic, and antiviral [98].

As a result of recent studies on ARPE cells, it has been demonstrated that HMGB1 is connected to the increase in angiogenesis and fibrosis during the course of DR [94]. Oral administration of GA in diabetic mice strongly inhibited HMGB1 concentration in retinas. This result led to a reduction in vascular and neuronal damage related to DR. The anti-inflammatory effects of GA were mediated by the inhibition of TNF-κ, IL-1β, and the cleavage of caspase-3 in retinal EC. GA, through the inhibition of HMGB1, reduces ROS concentrations and blood circulating glucose [99]. In another work, GA reduced TLR-4 concentrations and ischemia-reperfusion damage as well as increasing the expression of insulin receptors, partially preserving the anatomical integrity of the retina [100]. In a recent study, Liu et al. demonstrated that exchange protein for cAMP1, an inflammatory molecule involved in leukostasis, acts in synergy with GA. The combination of these two proteins strongly inhibits HMGB1 through the activation of SIRT1. SIRT1 deacetylates HMGB1, exerting a protective role in the diabetic retina [101]. GA also suppresses the proangiogenic effects of HMGB1 as it blocks AGE-induced upregulation of VEGF [81]. Abu El-Asrar and Mohammad's workgroup demonstrated, in a diabetic murine model, that GA can inhibit HMGB1's cytokine-like activities. Specifically, oral GA determines a reduction in HIF-1α, transcription factor Egr-1, TYK2, CXCL12, and CXCR4 [93]. Moreover, the same authors demonstrated that GA can inhibit the upregulation of STAT-3 induced by HMGB1 and its translocation in retinal Müller cells [68], upregulate BDNF expression in experimental mice [90], attenuate the expression of NOX2, caspase-3, and PARP-1 in the retinas as well as lowering the concentrations of ROS [69] and cleave caspase-3 glutamate and downregulating neurodegeneration mediators and markers in murine retinas [92] and attenuating the expression of retinal ICAM-1 [84]; lastly, it inhibits HMGB1 mediated activation of NF-κB. [66]. GA in association with resveratrol shows the ability to replenish retinal SIRT1 expression [72].

All this evidence points in the direction of the potential use of GA in the prevention of DR and its complications. It is worth mentioning that, in human studies on male patients affected by chronic hepatitis and type 2 diabetes, the administration of GA reduced serum testosterone aggravating insulin resistance, atherosclerosis, and sexual dysfunctions [102]. Further studies, especially on human subjects, are needed in order to confirm the pathways and molecules involved and their efficacy and safety.

4.2. Small Interfering RNAs/Short Hairpin RNA (siRNA/shRNA)

Small interfering RNAs (siRNAs) are a class of double-strand RNA usually constituted by 21–25 nucleotides that are gaining importance as therapeutic tools in numerous diseases. SiRNAs are capable of selectively binding specific genomic sequences, silencing them and therefore inhibiting the protein expression [103,104].

SiRNA HMGB1 transfection can repress HMGB1 RNA overexpression, determining the suppression of TLR-4 and NF-κB mRNA in RGCs. The downregulation of these inflammatory pathways can promote the survival and growth rates of RGCs [76]. A similar study conducted by Jiang and Chen confirmed these results in both in vivo and in vitro models. HMGB1 suppression, mediated by intravitreal injections of siRNA, is capable, in diabetic rats, of reducing retinal apoptosis rates as well as improving retinal function. In HRECs exposed to high glucose concentrations, siRNA HMGB1 improved cell viability and reduced the oxidative damage lowering ROS production [105]. The same study group demonstrated the protective role of HMGB1 inhibition in murine DR models. Retinal cells isolated from 8-year-old rats were incubated with a recombinant lentivirus containing short hairpin RNA (shRNA) for HMGB1. Through this mechanism, the authors obtained the silencing of HMGB1 gene expression. The results showed the downregulation of both MAPK and NF-κB, contributing to the reduction of inflammation, cell death, and BRB breakdown [83].

4.3. Polygonum Cuspidatum (PCE)

P. cuspidatum, also known as "Hojang-geun" in Korea, is a commonly employed herbal medicine in East Asia. The plant shows anti-inflammatory and anti-diabetic effects [106]. Recent works have explored the potential role, as a preventive treatment, of *P. cuspidatum* extract in diabetic nephropathy [107]. PCE is rich in resveratrol, polidatyn, and emodin compounds, with strong anti-inflammatory properties [108]. Sohn et al. suggested a beneficial effect of the ethanol extract of the root in a DR murine model. It prevents diabetic-induced retinal vascular hyperpermeability, attenuating the HMGB1 signaling pathway through the downregulation of the RAGE-mediated activation of NF-κB. It directly blocks the binding of HMGB1 to RAGE, thus preventing retinal vascular inflammation. Moreover, fluorescein angiography demonstrated that PCE markedly inhibits fluorescein leakage, suggesting that it may prevent the breakdown of the BRB. PCE reduces the expression of HMGB1 in diabetic rat retinal tissue and inhibits the binding of NF-κB to the RAGE promoter, with considerable anti-inflammatory activity. It is worth mentioning that the oral administration of PCE showed no positive effects on glycemic and body weight control in the murine model [109].

4.4. Paeoniflorin

Paeoniflorin is a monoterpene glucoside extracted from the root of the *Paeonia Lactiflora*. Paeoniflorin shows anti-inflammatory properties and it is already used in traditional Chinese medicine for a wide range of pathologies [110,111]. Moreover, paeoniflorin shows immunomodulatory effects on microglial cells through the enhancement of the suppressor of cytokine signaling 3 (SOCS3) pathways [112]. Zhu et al. demonstrated, in an in vitro study on BV2 microglial cells exposed to high concentrations of glucose, that treatment with paeoniflorin reduces the expression of metalloproteinases-9 (MMP-9) through the inhibition of p38/NF-κB. In addition, paeoniflorin activates SOCS3, which blocks the TLR-4 pathway [112,113]. The repression of TLR-4 determines the reduction of HMGB1 mediated inflammation in retinal microglial cells [114].

4.5. Salicin

Salicin is the main component of the willow bark extract, commonly used in traditional medicine for its anti-inflammatory and antipyretic effects [115]. Salicin is metabolized to salicylic acid in vivo; therefore, it is also known as "nature's aspirin". Previous studies showed that salicin exerts protective effects on EC, both inhibiting angiogenesis [116] and reducing ROS production [117]. Song et al. demonstrated that the treatment of HRECs with salicin led to a reduction in HMGB1 release and the prevention of cellular apoptosis. Moreover, the authors demonstrated that salicin can suppress the production of IL-1β and its related cytokines, such as TNF-κ and IL-6, responsible for retinal toxicity. Salicin is also able to block the release of the adhesion molecules ICAM-1 and VCAM-1 and the NF-κB inflammatory pathway [118].

4.6. Ethyl Pyruvate (EP)

Ethyl pyruvate is a pyruvate derivative with the addition of an aliphatic ester group. EP is considered to be safer and more effective than pyruvate in inhibiting ROS and inflammation [119]. EP is a strong HMGB1 inhibitor. Treatment with EP promotes stable vascular growth and blocks retinal pathological neovascularization by preventing the overexpression of HMGB1. Moreover, EP can inhibit the expression of IL-6, TNF-κ, and NF-kB, exerting a protective role in chronic inflammatory diseases such as DR [120].

4.7. Bradykinin (BK)

BK is a vasoactive peptide part of the kinins family. BK participates in several processes such as inflammation, pain, and cell proliferation [121]. Zhu et al. studied the effects of BK in HRECs exposed to high concentrations of glucose. Results show that BK can suppress oxidative stress and the release of inflammatory mediators. It can also control the process of neovascularization, downregulating the expression of VEGF. Lastly, BK inhibits the HMGB1/NF-κB signaling pathway, therefore controlling the growth and proliferation of HRECs [122].

4.8. Kallistatin

Kallistatin is an endogenous serine proteinase that plays numerous physiological and pathological roles like tumorigenesis, vasodilation, inhibition of neovascularization, inflammation, oxidative stress, cellular death, and fibrosis [123]. It stimulates the expression of eNOS, SIRT1, and SOCS3, while it inhibits VEGF, HMGB1, TNF-κ, and NF-κB [124]. It has been demonstrated that vitreous humor levels of kallistatin in patients with PDR are lower when compared to healthy controls [125]. Xing et al. established that kallistatin is a strong inhibitor of angiogenesis and therefore may act as a potent drug in the prevention of PDR [126].

4.9. Compound 49b

Compound 49b is a recently discovered β-adrenergic receptor agonist that has already demonstrated efficacy in preventing apoptosis in in vitro models of EC and Müller cells exposed to high glucose [127,128]. Recent evidence shows that compound 49b can inhibit HMGB1 expression, TLR-4 downstream signaling, and, therefore, NF-κB in both EC and Müller cells. This leads to the idea that this agonist may preserve vascular and neuronal integrity in the diabetic retina [126,129].

4.10. Cyclosporine A (CyA)

Cyclosporine A is a polypeptide derived from the fungi *Beauveria nevus* and *Tolypocladium inflatum*, and it is well known for its anti-inflammatory and immunosuppressive effects [130]. Wang et al. demonstrated that CyA attenuates the enhanced expression of IL-1β and TNF-κ in the retinas of diabetic rats, probably via the suppression of HMGB1. The intravitreal injection of CyA may represent a novel therapeutic strategy to treat DR [131].

CyA is also involved in the reduction of BRB permeability in diabetic rats. In particular, it reduces the levels of IL-1β, nitric oxide (through a decreased expression of iNOS), and IL-1β-induced cyclooxygenase-2 (COX-2) expression. Moreover, CyA decreases vitreous protein concentration in diabetic rats. The authors suggest that this reduction in vitreous protein concentration can be linked to the reduction of BRB permeability [132].

Table 1. Summary of direct and indirect high-mobility group box (HMGB1) inhibitors with therapeutic potential in diabetic retinopathy. HRECs = human retinal endothelial cells; TLR = toll like receptor; TNF-α = tumor necrosis factor-α; GCL = ganglion cell layer; STZ = streptozotocin; SIRT1 = sirtuin 1; BDNF = brain-derived neurotrophic factor; ROS = reactive oxygen species; ICAM-1 = intercellular adhesion molecule-1; NF-κB = nuclear factor-κB; HIF-1α = hypoxia induced factor-1α; pSTAT-3 = phosphorylated signal transducer and activator of transcription-3; VEGF = vascular endothelial growth factor; siRNA = small interfering RNAs; shRNA = short hairpin RNA; RAGE = receptors for AGEs; MMP = metalloproteinases; IL = interleukin; SOCS3 = suppressor of cytokine signaling 3; ROP = Retinopathy of prematurity; SOD = superoxide dismutase; IGFBP-3 = insulin-like growth factor-binding protein-3; iNOS = inducible nitric oxide synthase; COX-2 = cyclooxygenase; BRB = blood retinal barrier.

Drug	Target Test	Diabetic Inducement	Mechanism of Action	Results	Reference
Glycyrrhizin	HRECs	High glucose concentrations	Inhibition of TLR-4 and TNF-α; cleavage of caspase 3 through inactivation of HMGB1	Increased insulin receptor signal transduction	[99,100]
	Mice	Ischemia/reperfusion damage	Block of the loss of retinal thickness	Protects GCL and retinal capillaries	[99,100]
	Mice	STZ	Upregulation of SIRT1, inhibition of inflammatory factors. Attenuates BDNF downregulation, reduces ROS, ICAM-1, NF-κB, and HIF-1α	Reduced vascular permeability, increased retinal thickness. Protection from diabetes-induced retinal damages and inflammation	[101] [67,88,95,90] [93]
	Retinal Muller Cells	High glucose concentrations	Attenuates p-STAT3 expression	Inhibition of VEGF expression	[69]
Small interfering RNAs	Mice	STZ	Intravitreal injection of HMGB1 siRNA	Protected morphological changes, and improved the function of the retina	[105]
	Retinal ganglion cells	High glucose concentrations	Transfection with HMGB1 siRNA reduced the expression of TLR-4 and NF-κB	Increased cell survival rate	[77]
	HRECs	High glucose concentrations	Transfection with HMGB1 siRNA reduced the expression of caspase 3	Inhibition the early stage of apoptosis	[105]
Short hairpin RNAs	Rat retinas	High glucose concentrations	Transfection with HMGB1 shRNA reduced the expression TNF-α and NF-κB	Increased cell survival rate and vascular permeability	[83]
Polygonum cuspidatum	Mice	STZ	Reduced RAGE and NF-κB expression	Reduced vascular permeability	[104]
Paeoniflorin	Mice	High glucose concentrations	Inhibition of MMP-9 and IL-1β	Alleviated microglial activation	[113]
	BV2 modified microglial cells	Incubated with IL-1β (inflammatory response)	Inhibition of NF-κB expression and SOCS3	Reduced MMP-9 and TLR-4 concentrations	[113]
Salicin	HRECs	Induction of ROP through exposition to hyperoxia	Suppression of NF-κB pathway and the release of MMP	Inhibition of IL-1β mediated inflammatory pathways	[18]
Ethyl pyruvate	Mice	High glucose concentrations	Reduction of ROS, NF-κB, IL-6, VEGF and TNF-α	Reduction of neoangiogenesis and areas of ischemic retina	[120]
Bradykinin	HRECs	High glucose concentrations	Suppression of NF-κB, caspase 3, VEGF, TNF-α, IL-1β. Increase in SOD activity	Promotion of retinal cells survival/inhibition of apoptosis. Reduction of vascular permeability	[122]
Kallistatin	HRECs	High glucose concentrations	Suppression of VEGF expression	Reduction of neoangiogenesis	[124]
Compound 49b	HRECs and rat retinal Muller cells	High glucose concentrations	Increase of IGFBP-3 levels and inhibition of TLR-4 pathway	Prevention of cellular apoptosis	[127,129]
	Mice	SZT	Increase of IGFBP-3 levels	Prevention of the decrease in retinal thickness and loss of cells in GCL	[127]
Cyclosporine A	Mice	STZ	Reduction of TNF-α and IL-1β	Amelioration of retinal thickness, regression of retinal edema	[131]
	Mice	STZ	Reduction of iNOS, IL-1β and COX-2	Reduction of BRB permeability	[132]

5. Conclusions

The purpose of this review is to show the role of HMGB1 in DR. Many studies have demonstrated that DM, and then hyperglycemia, upregulate the expression of and increase in the levels of HMGB1. This situation activates several pathways and involves a large number of molecules, such as ERK, NF-κB, ICAM, RAGE, VEGF, and TLR. The final result is the activation and increase of inflammation, angiogenesis, oxidative stress, and, ultimately, retinal damage to the patients. At the same time, the involvement of this great number of molecules can provide a hint of new therapeutic approaches to be developed and studied.

Author Contributions: Conceptualization, M.N. and A.L.; writing—original draft preparation, M.A., L.A., and G.T.; writing—review and editing, M.N., M.A., L.A., and G.T.; supervision, A.L., R.P., and V.B. All authors have read and agreed to the published version of the manuscript.

Funding: This research received no external funding.

Conflicts of Interest: The authors declare no conflict of interest.

Abbreviations

8-OHdG	8-hydroxydeoxyguanosine
AGE	advanced glycation end-products
ARPE-19	adult retinal pigment epithelial cell line-19
BDNF	brain-derived neurotrophic factor
BK	bradykinin
BRB	blood–retinal barrier
COX-2	cyclooxygenase
CTGF	connective tissue growth factor
CyA	cyclosporine A
DM	diabetes mellitus
DR	diabetic retinopathy
EC	endothelial cells
Egr-1	early growth response protein 1
eNOS	endothelial nitric oxide synthase
EP	ethyl pyruvate
ERK	extracellular signal-regulated kinase
GA	glycyrrhizin
GSH	reduced glutathione
HIF-1α	hypoxia induced factor-1α
HMGB	high-mobility group box
HO-1	heme oxygenase-1
HRECs	human retinal endothelial cells
HRMEC	human retinal microvascular endothelial cells
ICAM-1	intercellular adhesion molecule-1
IFN	interferon
IGFBP-3	insulin-like growth factor-binding protein-3
IL	interleukin
iNOS	inducible nitric oxide synthase
MAPK	mitogen-activated protein kinase
MMP-9	metalloproteinases-9
NF-κB	nuclear factor-κB
NOX	nicotinamide adenine dinucleotide phosphate oxidase
NPDR	non proliferative diabetic retinopathy

OPN	osteopontin
PAI-1	plasminogen activator inhibitor-1
PARP	poly ADP-ribose polymerase
PCE	polygonum cuspidatum
PDR	proliferative diabetic retinopathy
PEDF	pigment epithelium-derived factor
PI3K	phosphatidylinositol 3-kinase
PK	protein kinase
PLA-2	phospholipases A2
PVR	proliferative vitreoretinopathy
RAGE	receptors for AGEs
RGC	retinal ganglion cells
ROP	retinopathy of prematurity
ROS	reactive oxygen species
RPE	retinal pigmented epithelium
shRNA	short hairpin RNA
siRNA	small interfering RNAs
SIRT	sirtuin
SOCS3	suppressor of cytokine signaling 3
SOD	superoxide dismutase
STAT-3	signal transducer and activator of transcription-3
pSTAT-3	phosphorylated STAT-3
STZ	streptozotocin
TGF-β1	transforming growth factor-β1
TLR	toll like receptor
TNF-α	tumor necrosis factor-α
TYK2	tyrosine kinase 2
VAP-1	vascular adhesion protein-1
VCAM-1	vascular cell adhesion molecule-1
VEGF	vascular endothelial growth factor

References

1. International Diabetes Federation. *IDF Diabetes Atlas*, 9th ed.; International Diabetes Federation: Brussels, Belgium, 2019.
2. Yau, J.W.; Rogers, S.L.; Kawasaki, R.; Lamoureux, E.L.; Kowalski, J.W.; Bek, T.; Chen, S.J.; Dekker, J.M.; Fletcher, A.; Grauslund, J.; et al. Global prevalence and major risk factors of diabetic retinopathy. *Diabetes Care* **2012**, *35*, 556–564. [CrossRef] [PubMed]
3. Flaxman, S.R.; Bourne, R.R.A.; Resnikoff, S.; Ackland, P.; Braithwaite, T.; Cicinelli, M.V.; Das, A.; Jonas, J.B.; Keeffe, J.; Kempen, J.H.; et al. Global causes of blindness and distance vision impairment 1990–2020: A systematic review and meta-analysis. *Lancet Glob. Health* **2017**, *5*, e1221–e1234. [CrossRef]
4. Cheung, N.; Mitchell, P.; Wong, T.Y. Diabetic retinopathy. *Lancet* **2010**, *376*, 124–136. [CrossRef]
5. Hendrick, A.M.; Gibson, M.V.; Kulshreshtha, A. Diabetic Retinopathy. *Prim. Care* **2015**, *42*, 451–464. [CrossRef]
6. Robles-Rivera, R.R.; Castellanos-González, J.A.; Olvera-Montaño, C.; Flores-Martin, R.A.; López-Contreras, A.K.; Arevalo-Simental, D.E.; Cardona-Muñoz, E.G.; Roman-Pintos, L.M.; Rodríguez-Carrizalez, A.D. Adjuvant Therapies in Diabetic Retinopathy as an Early Approach to Delay Its Progression: The Importance of Oxidative Stress and Inflammation. *Oxid. Med. Cell. Longev.* **2020**, *2020*, 3096470. [CrossRef]
7. Sohn, E.H.; van Dijk, H.W.; Jiao, C.; Kok, P.H.; Jeong, W.; Demirkaya, N.; Garmager, A.; Wit, F.; Kucukevcilioglu, M.; van Velthoven, M.E.; et al. Retinal neurodegeneration may precede microvascular changes characteristic of diabetic retinopathy in diabetes mellitus. *Proc. Natl. Acad. Sci. USA* **2016**, *113*, E2655–E2664. [CrossRef]

8. Bandello, F.; Lattanzio, R.; Zucchiatti, I.; Del Turco, C. Pathophysiology and treatment of diabetic retinopathy. *Acta Diabetol.* **2013**, *50*, 1–20. [CrossRef]
9. Semeraro, F.; Morescalchi, F.; Cancarini, A.; Russo, A.; Rezzola, S.; Costagliola, C. Diabetic retinopathy, a vascular and inflammatory disease: Therapeutic implications. *Diabetes Metab.* **2019**. [CrossRef]
10. Stitt, A.W. AGEs and Diabetic Retinopathy. *Investig. Ophthalmol. Vis. Sci.* **2010**, *51*, 4867–4874. [CrossRef]
11. Testa, R.; Bonfigli, A.R.; Prattichizzo, F.; La Sala, L.; De Nigris, V.; Ceriello, A. The "Metabolic Memory" Theory and the Early Treatment of Hyperglycemia in Prevention of Diabetic Complications. *Nutrients* **2017**, *9*, 437. [CrossRef]
12. Rodríguez, M.L.; Pérez, S.; Mena-Mollá, S.; Desco, M.C.; Ortega, Á.L. Oxidative Stress and Microvascular Alterations in Diabetic Retinopathy: Future Therapies. *Oxid. Med. Cell. Longev.* **2019**, *2019*, 4940825. [CrossRef]
13. Kowluru, R.A.; Abbas, S.N. Diabetes-induced mitochondrial dysfunction in the retina. *Investig. Ophthalmol. Vis. Sci.* **2003**, *44*, 5327–5334. [CrossRef]
14. Chalupsky, K.; Cai, H. Endothelial dihydrofolate reductase: Critical for nitric oxide bioavailability and role in angiotensin II uncoupling of endothelial nitric oxide synthase. *Proc. Natl. Acad. Sci. USA* **2005**, *102*, 9056–9061. [CrossRef]
15. Geraldes, P.; Hiraoka-Yamamoto, J.; Matsumoto, M.; Clermont, A.; Leitges, M.; Marette, A.; Aiello, L.P.; Kern, T.S.; King, G.L. Activation of PKC-δ and SHP-1 by hyperglycemia causes vascular cell apoptosis and diabetic retinopathy. *Nat. Med.* **2009**, *15*, 1298–1306. [CrossRef]
16. Brownlee, M. The pathobiology of diabetic complications: A unifying mechanism. *Diabetes* **2005**, *54*, 1615–1625. [CrossRef]
17. Kowluru, R.A.; Mishra, M. Oxidative stress, mitochondrial damage and diabetic retinopathy. *Biochim. Biophys. Acta* **2015**, *1852*, 2474–2483. [CrossRef] [PubMed]
18. Hammes, H.P. Diabetic retinopathy: Hyperglycemia, oxidative stress and beyond. *Diabetologia* **2018**, *61*, 29–38. [CrossRef]
19. Yao, D.; Taguchi, T.; Matsumura, T.; Pestell, R.; Edelstein, D.; Giardino, I.; Suske, G.; Rabbani, N.; Thornalley, P.J.; Sarthy, V.P.; et al. High glucose increases angiopoietin-2 transcription in microvascular endothelial cells through methylglyoxal modification of mSin3A. *J. Biol. Chem.* **2007**, *282*, 31038–31045. [CrossRef]
20. Rajamani, U.; Jialal, I. Hyperglycemia induces Toll-like receptor-2 and -4 expression and activity in human microvascular retinal endothelial cells: Implications for diabetic retinopathy. *J. Diabetes Res.* **2014**, *2014*, 790902. [CrossRef]
21. Wang, Y.L.; Wang, K.; Yu, S.J.; Li, Q.; Li, N.; Lin, P.Y.; Li, M.M.; Guo, J.Y. Association of the TLR4 signaling pathway in the retina of streptozotocin-induced diabetic rats. *Graefes Arch. Clin. Exp. Ophthalmol.* **2015**, *253*, 389–398. [CrossRef]
22. PKC-DRS Study Group. The effect of ruboxistaurin on visual loss in patients with moderately severe to very severe nonproliferative diabetic retinopathy: Initial results of the Protein Kinase C beta Inhibitor Diabetic Retinopathy Study (PKC-DRS) multicenter randomized clinical trial. *Diabetes* **2005**, *54*, 2188–2197. [CrossRef]
23. Wang, W.; Lo, A.C.Y. Diabetic Retinopathy: Pathophysiology and Treatments. *Int. J. Mol. Sci.* **2018**, *19*, 1816. [CrossRef]
24. Lee, R.; Wong, T.Y.; Sabanayagam, C. Epidemiology of diabetic retinopathy, diabetic macular edema and related vision loss. *Eye Vis. (Lond.)* **2015**, *2*, 17. [CrossRef]
25. Goodwin, G.H.; Sanders, C.; Johns, E.W. A new group of chromatin-associated proteins with a high content of acidic and basic amino acids. *Eur. J. Biochem.* **1973**, *38*, 14–19. [CrossRef]
26. Tripathi, A.; Shrinet, K.; Kumar, A. HMGB1 protein as a novel target for cancer. *Toxicol. Rep.* **2019**, *6*, 253–261. [CrossRef] [PubMed]
27. Kang, R.; Chen, R.; Zhang, Q.; Hou, W.; Wu, S.; Cao, L.; Huang, J.; Yu, Y.; Fan, X.G.; Yan, Z.; et al. HMGB1 in health and disease. *Mol. Aspects Med.* **2014**, *40*, 1–116. [CrossRef]
28. Yang, H.; Antoine, D.J.; Andersson, U.; Tracey, K.J. The many faces of HMGB1: Molecular structure-functional activity in inflammation, apoptosis, and chemotaxis. *J. Leukoc. Biol.* **2013**, *93*, 865–873. [CrossRef]
29. Stumbo, A.C.; Cortez, E.; Rodrigues, C.A.; Henriques, M.D.; Porto, L.C.; Barbosa, H.S.; Carvalho, L. Mitochondrial localization of non-histone protein HMGB1 during human endothelial cell-Toxoplasma gondii infection. *Cell Biol. Int.* **2008**, *32*, 235–238. [CrossRef]

30. Tang, D.; Kang, R.; Zeh, H.J., 3rd; Lotze, M.T. High-mobility group box 1, oxidative stress, and disease. *Antioxid. Redox Signal.* **2011**, *14*, 1315–1335. [CrossRef]
31. Venereau, E.; Casalgrandi, M.; Schiraldi, M.; Antoine, D.J.; Cattaneo, A.; De Marchis, F.; Liu, J.; Antonelli, A.; Preti, A.; Raeli, L.; et al. Mutually exclusive redox forms of HMGB1 promote cell recruitment or proinflammatory cytokine release. *J. Exp. Med.* **2012**, *209*, 1519–1528. [CrossRef]
32. Kazama, H.; Ricci, J.E.; Herndon, J.M.; Hoppe, G.; Green, D.R.; Ferguson, T.A. Induction of immunological tolerance by apoptotic cells requires caspase-dependent oxidation of high-mobility group box-1 protein. *Immunity* **2008**, *29*, 21–32. [CrossRef] [PubMed]
33. Mandke, P.; Vasquez, K.M. Interactions of high mobility group box protein 1 (HMGB1) with nucleic acids: Implications in DNA repair and immune responses. *DNA Repair (Amst.)* **2019**, *83*, 102701. [CrossRef] [PubMed]
34. Tang, D.; Kang, R.; Livesey, K.M.; Cheh, C.W.; Farkas, A.; Loughran, P.; Hoppe, G.; Bianchi, M.E.; Tracey, K.J.; Zeh, H.J., 3rd; et al. Endogenous HMGB1 regulates autophagy. *J. Cell Biol.* **2010**, *190*, 881–892. [CrossRef] [PubMed]
35. Tadie, J.M.; Bae, H.B.; Jiang, S.; Park, D.W.; Bell, C.P.; Yang, H.; Pittet, J.F.; Tracey, K.; Thannickal, V.J.; Abraham, E.; et al. HMGB1 promotes neutrophil extracellular trap formation through interactions with Toll-like receptor 4. *Am. J. Physiol. Lung Cell. Mol. Physiol.* **2013**, *304*, L342–L349. [CrossRef] [PubMed]
36. Ciucci, A.; Gabriele, I.; Percario, Z.A.; Affabris, E.; Colizzi, V.; Mancino, G. HMGB1 and cord blood: Its role as immuno-adjuvant factor in innate immunity. *PLoS ONE* **2011**, *6*, e23766. [CrossRef]
37. Li, R.; Wang, J.; Zhu, F.; Li, R.; Liu, B.; Xu, W.; He, G.; Cao, H.; Wang, Y.; Yang, J. HMGB1 regulates T helper 2 and T helper17 cell differentiation both directly and indirectly in asthmatic mice. *Mol. Immunol.* **2018**, *97*, 45–55. [CrossRef]
38. Lee, G.; Espirito Santo, A.I.; Zwingenberger, S.; Cai, L.; Vogl, T.; Feldmann, M.; Horwood, N.J.; Chan, J.K.; Nanchahal, J. Fully reduced HMGB1 accelerates the regeneration of multiple tissues by transitioning stem cells to GAlert. *Proc. Natl. Acad. Sci. USA* **2018**, *115*, E4463–E4472. [CrossRef]
39. Andersson, U.; Erlandsson-Harris, H.; Yang, H.; Tracey, K.J. HMGB1 as a DNA-binding cytokine. *J. Leukoc. Biol.* **2002**, *72*, 1084–1091.
40. Park, J.S.; Arcaroli, J.; Yum, H.K.; Yang, H.; Wang, H.; Yang, K.Y.; Choe, K.H.; Strassheim, D.; Pitts, T.M.; Tracey, K.J.; et al. Activation of gene expression in human neutrophils by high mobility group box 1 protein. *Am. J. Physiol. Cell. Physiol.* **2003**, *284*, C870–C879. [CrossRef]
41. He, Q.; You, H.; Li, X.M.; Liu, T.H.; Wang, P.; Wang, B.E. HMGB1 promotes the synthesis of pro-IL-1β and pro-IL-18 by activation of p38 MAPK and NF-κB through receptors for advanced glycation end-products in macrophages. *Asian Pac. J. Cancer Prev.* **2012**, *13*, 1365–1370. [CrossRef]
42. Wu, X.; Mi, Y.; Yang, H.; Hu, A.; Zhang, Q.; Shang, C. The activation of HMGB1 as a progression factor on inflammation response in normal human bronchial epithelial cells through RAGE/JNK/NF-κB pathway. *Mol. Cell. Biochem.* **2013**, *380*, 249–257. [CrossRef] [PubMed]
43. Andersson, U.; Wang, H.; Palmblad, K.; Aveberger, A.C.; Bloom, O.; Erlandsson-Harris, H.; Janson, A.; Kokkola, R.; Zhang, M.; Yang, H.; et al. High mobility group 1 protein (HMG-1) stimulates proinflammatory cytokine synthesis in human monocytes. *J. Exp. Med.* **2000**, *192*, 565–570. [CrossRef] [PubMed]
44. Sundberg, E.; Fasth, A.E.; Palmblad, K.; Harris, H.E.; Andersson, U. High mobility group box chromosomal protein 1 acts as a proliferation signal for activated T lymphocytes. *Immunobiology* **2009**, *214*, 303–309. [CrossRef] [PubMed]
45. Degryse, B.; de Virgilio, M. The nuclear protein HMGB1, a new kind of chemokine? *FEBS Lett.* **2003**, *553*, 11–17. [CrossRef]
46. Schlueter, C.; Weber, H.; Meyer, B.; Rogalla, P.; Röser, K.; Hauke, S.; Bullerdiek, J. Angiogenetic signaling through hypoxia: HMGB1: An angiogenetic switch molecule. *Am. J. Pathol.* **2005**, *166*, 1259–1263. [CrossRef]
47. Yang, S.; Xu, L.; Yang, T.; Wang, F. High-mobility group box-1 and its role in angiogenesis. *J. Leukoc. Biol.* **2014**, *95*, 563–574. [CrossRef]
48. Harris, H.E.; Andersson, U.; Pisetsky, D.S. HMGB1: A multifunctional alarmin driving autoimmune and inflammatory disease. *Nat. Rev. Rheumatol.* **2012**, *8*, 195–202. [CrossRef]

49. Yang, H.; Wang, H.; Ju, Z.; Ragab, A.A.; Lundbäck, P.; Long, W.; Valdes-Ferrer, S.I.; He, M.; Pribis, J.P.; Li, J.; et al. MD-2 is required for disulfide HMGB1-dependent TLR4 signaling. *J. Exp. Med.* **2015**, *212*, 5–14. [CrossRef]
50. Yang, H.; Wang, H.; Andersson, U. Targeting Inflammation Driven by HMGB1. *Front. Immunol.* **2020**, *11*, 484. [CrossRef]
51. Scaffidi, P.; Misteli, T.; Bianchi, M.E. Release of chromatin protein HMGB1 by necrotic cellstriggers inflammation. *Nature* **2002**, *418*, 191–195. [CrossRef]
52. Hofmann, M.A.; Drury, S.; Fu, C.; Qu, W.; Taguchi, A.; Lu, Y.; Avila, C.; Kambham, N.; Bierhaus, A.; Nawroth, P.; et al. RAGE mediates a novel proinflammatory axis: A central cell surface receptor for S100/calgranulin polypeptides. *Cell* **1999**, *97*, 889–901. [CrossRef]
53. Toure, F.; Zahm, J.M.; Garnotel, R.; Lambert, E.; Bonnet, N.; Schmidt, A.M.; Vitry, F.; Chanard, J.; Gillery, P.; Rieu, P. Receptor for advanced glycationend-products (RAGE) modulates neutrophil adhesion and migration on glycoxidated extracellular matrix. *Biochem. J.* **2008**, *416*, 255–261. [CrossRef] [PubMed]
54. Sims, G.P.; Rowe, D.C.; Rietdijk, S.T.; Herbst, R.; Coyle, A.J. HMGB1 and RAGE in inflammation and cancer. *Annu. Rev. Immunol.* **2010**, *28*, 367–388. [CrossRef] [PubMed]
55. Zhang, C.; Dong, H.; Chen, F.; Wang, Y.; Ma, J.; Wang, G. The HMGB1-RAGE/TLR-TNF-α signaling pathway may contribute to kidney injury induced by hypoxia. *Exp. Ther. Med.* **2019**, *17*, 17–26. [CrossRef]
56. Massey, N.; Puttachary, S.; Bhat, S.M.; Kanthasamy, A.G.; Charavaryamath, C. HMGB1-RAGE Signaling Plays a Role in Organic Dust-Induced Microglial Activation and Neuroinflammation. *Toxicol. Sci.* **2019**, *169*, 579–592. [CrossRef]
57. Wolfson, R.K.; Chiang, E.T.; Garcia, J.G. HMGB1 induces human lung endothelial cell cytoskeletal rearrangement and barrier disruption. *Microvasc. Res.* **2011**, *81*, 189–197. [CrossRef]
58. Bangert, A.; Andrassy, M.; Müller, A.M.; Bockstahler, M.; Fischer, A.; Volz, C.H.; Leib, C.; Göser, S.; Korkmaz-Icöz, S.; Zittrich, S.; et al. Critical role of RAGE and HMGB1 in inflammatory heart disease. *Proc. Natl. Acad. Sci. USA* **2016**, *113*, E155–E164. [CrossRef]
59. Tang, D.; Shi, Y.; Kang, R.; Li, T.; Xiao, W.; Wang, H.; Xiao, X. Hydrogen peroxide stimulates macrophages and monocytes to actively release HMGB1. *J. Leukoc. Biol.* **2007**, *81*, 741–747. [CrossRef]
60. Mitola, S.; Belleri, M.; Urbinati, C.; Coltrini, D.; Sparatore, B.; Pedrazzi, M.; Melloni, E.; Presta, M. Cutting edge: Extracellular high mobility group box-1 protein is a proangiogenic cytokine. *J. Immunol.* **2006**, *176*, 12–15. [CrossRef]
61. van Beijnum, J.R.; Nowak-Sliwinska, P.; van den Boezem, E.; Hautvast, P.; Buurman, W.A.; Griffioen, A.W. Tumor angiogenesis is enforced by autocrine regulation of high-mobility group box 1. *Oncogene* **2013**, *32*, 363–374. [CrossRef]
62. Wu, C.Z.; Zheng, J.J.; Bai, Y.H.; Xia, P.; Zhang, H.C.; Guo, Y. HMGB1/RAGE axis mediates the apoptosis, invasion, autophagy, and angiogenesis of the renal cell carcinoma. *OncoTargets Ther.* **2018**, *11*, 4501–4510. [CrossRef] [PubMed]
63. Lin, Q.; Yang, X.P.; Fang, D.; Ren, X.; Zhou, H.; Fang, J.; Liu, X.; Zhou, S.; Wen, F.; Yao, X.; et al. High-mobility group box-1 mediates toll-like receptor 4-dependent angiogenesis. *Arterioscler. Thromb. Vasc. Biol.* **2011**, *31*, 1024–1032. [CrossRef] [PubMed]
64. Jiang, W.; Jiang, P.; Yang, R.; Liu, D.F. Functional role of SIRT1-induced HMGB1 expression and acetylation in migration, invasion and angiogenesis of ovarian cancer. *Eur. Rev. Med. Pharmacol. Sci.* **2018**, *22*, 4431–4439. [CrossRef] [PubMed]
65. Park, S.Y.; Lee, S.W.; Kim, H.Y.; Lee, W.S.; Hong, K.W.; Kim, C.D. HMGB1 induces angiogenesis in rheumatoid arthritis via HIF-1α activation. *Eur. J. Immunol.* **2015**, *45*, 1216–1227. [CrossRef]
66. Mohammad, G.; Siddiquei, M.M.; Othman, A.; Al-Shabrawey, M.; Abu El-Asrar, A.M. High-mobility group box-1 protein activates inflammatory signaling pathway components and disrupts retinal vascular-barrier in the diabetic retina. *Exp. Eye Res.* **2013**, *107*, 101–109. [CrossRef]
67. Kim, J.; Kim, C.S.; Sohn, E.; Kim, J.S. Cytoplasmic translocation of high-mobility group box-1 protein is induced by diabetes and high glucose in retinal pericytes. *Mol. Med. Rep.* **2016**, *14*, 3655–3661. [CrossRef]
68. Mohammad, G.; Jomar, D.; Siddiquei, M.M.; Alam, K.; Abu El-Asrar, A.M. High-Mobility Group Box-1 Protein Mediates the Regulation of Signal Transducer and Activator of Transcription-3 in the Diabetic Retina and in Human Retinal Müller Cells. *Ophthalmic Res.* **2017**, *57*, 150–160. [CrossRef]

69. Mohammad, G.; Alam, K.; Nawaz, M.I.; Siddiquei, M.M.; Mousa, A.; Abu El-Asrar, A.M. Mutual enhancement between high-mobility group box-1 and NADPH oxidase-derived reactive oxygen species mediates diabetes-induced upregulation of retinal apoptotic markers. *J. Physiol. Biochem.* **2015**, *71*, 359–372. [CrossRef]
70. Ran, R.J.; Zheng, X.Y.; Du, L.P.; Zhang, X.D.; Chen, X.L.; Zhu, S.Y. Upregulated inflammatory associated factors and blood-retinal barrier changes in the retina of type 2 diabetes mellitus model. *Int. J. Ophthalmol.* **2016**, *9*, 1591–1597. [CrossRef]
71. Zhou, M.; Luo, J.; Zhang, H. Role of Sirtuin 1 in the pathogenesis of ocular disease (Review). *Int. J. Mol. Med.* **2018**, *42*, 13–20. [CrossRef]
72. Mohammad, G.; Abdelaziz, G.M.; Siddiquei, M.M.; Ahmad, A.; De Hertogh, G.; Abu El-Asrar, A.M. Cross-Talk between Sirtuin 1 and the Proinflammatory Mediator High-Mobility Group Box-1 in the Regulation of Blood-Retinal Barrier Breakdown in Diabetic Retinopathy. *Curr. Eye Res.* **2019**, *44*, 1133–1143. [CrossRef]
73. Liu, L.; Patel, P.; Steinle, J.J. PKA regulates HMGB1 through activation of IGFBP-3 and SIRT1 in human retinal endothelial cells cultured in high glucose. *Inflamm. Res.* **2018**, *67*, 1013–1019. [CrossRef]
74. Chen, X.L.; Zhang, X.D.; Li, Y.Y.; Chen, X.M.; Tang, D.R.; Ran, R.J. Involvement of HMGB1 mediated signalling pathway in diabetic retinopathy: Evidence from type 2 diabetic rats and ARPE-19 cells under diabetic condition. *Br. J. Ophthalmol.* **2013**, *97*, 1598–1603. [CrossRef]
75. Jiang, S.; Chen, X. Expression of High-Mobility Group Box 1 Protein (HMGB1) and Toll-Like Receptor 9 (TLR9) in Retinas of Diabetic Rats. *Med. Sci. Monit.* **2017**, *23*, 3115–3122. [CrossRef]
76. Zhao, H.; Zhang, J.; Yu, J. HMGB-1 as a Potential Target for the Treatment of Diabetic Retinopathy. *Med. Sci. Monit.* **2015**, *21*, 3062–3067. [CrossRef]
77. Yu, Y.; Yang, L.; Lv, J.; Huang, X.; Yi, J.; Pei, C.; Shao, Y. The role of high mobility group box 1 (HMGB-1) in the diabetic retinopathy inflammation and apoptosis. *Int. J. Clin. Exp. Pathol.* **2015**, *8*, 6807–6813.
78. Gong, Y.; Jin, X.; Wang, Q.S.; Wei, S.H.; Hou, B.K.; Li, H.Y.; Zhang, M.N.; Li, Z.H. The involvement of high mobility group 1 cytokine and phospholipases A2 in diabetic retinopathy. *Lipids Health Dis.* **2014**, *13*, 156. [CrossRef]
79. van Beijnum, J.R.; Buurman, W.A.; Griffioen, A.W. Convergence and amplification of toll-like receptor (TLR) and receptor for advanced glycation end products (RAGE) signaling pathways via high mobility group B1 (HMGB1). *Angiogenesis.* **2008**, *11*, 91–99. [CrossRef]
80. Santos, A.R.; Dvoriantchikova, G.; Li, Y.; Mohammad, G.; Abu El-Asrar, A.M.; Wen, R.; Ivanov, D. Cellular mechanisms of high mobility group 1 (HMGB-1) protein action in the diabetic retinopathy. *PLoS ONE* **2014**, *9*, e87574. [CrossRef]
81. Lee, J.J.; Hsiao, C.C.; Yang, I.H.; Chou, M.H.; Wu, C.L.; Wei, Y.C.; Chen, C.H.; Chuang, J.H. High-mobility group box 1 protein is implicated in advanced glycation end products-induced vascular endothelial growth factor A production in the rat retinal ganglion cell line RGC-5. *Mol. Vis.* **2012**, *18*, 838–850.
82. Fu, D.; Tian, X. Effect of high mobility group box 1 on the human retinal pigment epithelial cell in high-glucose condition. *Int. J. Clin. Exp. Med.* **2015**, *8*, 17796–17803.
83. Jiang, N.; Chen, X. Protective effect of high mobility group box-1 silence on diabetic retinopathy: An in vivo study. *Int. J. Clin. Exp. Pathol.* **2017**, *10*, 8148–8160.
84. Liang, W.J.; Yang, H.W.; Liu, H.N.; Qian, W.; Chen, X.L. HMGB1 upregulates NF-kB by inhibiting IKB-α and associates with diabetic retinopathy. *Life Sci.* **2020**, *241*, 117146. [CrossRef]
85. Abu El-Asrar, A.M.; Alam, K.; Garcia-Ramirez, M.; Ahmad, A.; Siddiquei, M.M.; Mohammad, G.; Mousa, A.; De Hertogh, G.; Opdenakker, G.; Simó, R. Association of HMGB1 with oxidative stress markers and regulators in PDR. *Mol. Vis.* **2017**, *23*, 853–871.
86. El-Asrar, A.M.; Missotten, L.; Geboes, K. Expression of high-mobility groups box-1/receptor for advanced glycation end products/osteopontin/early growth response-1 pathway in proliferative vitreoretinal epiretinal membranes. *Mol. Vis.* **2011**, *17*, 508–518.
87. Abu El-Asrar, A.M.; Imtiaz Nawaz, M.; Kangave, D.; Siddiquei, M.M.; Geboes, K. Osteopontin and other regulators of angiogenesis and fibrogenesis in the vitreous from patients with proliferative vitreoretinal disorders. *Mediat. Inflamm.* **2012**, *2012*, 493043. [CrossRef]
88. El-Asrar, A.M.; Nawaz, M.I.; Kangave, D.; Geboes, K.; Ola, M.S.; Ahmad, S.; Al-Shabrawey, M. High-mobility group box-1 and biomarkers of inflammation in the vitreous from patients with proliferative diabetic retinopathy. *Mol. Vis.* **2011**, *17*, 1829–1838.

89. Shen, Y.; Cao, H.; Chen, F.; Suo, Y.; Wang, N.; Xu, X. A cross-sectional study of vitreous and serum high mobility group box-1 levels in proliferative diabetic retinopathy. *Acta Ophthalmol.* **2020**, *98*, e212–e216. [CrossRef]
90. Abu El-Asrar, A.M.; Nawaz, M.I.; Siddiquei, M.M.; Al-Kharashi, A.S.; Kangave, D.; Mohammad, G. High-mobility group box-1 induces decreased brain-derived neurotrophic factor-mediated neuroprotection in the diabetic retina. *Mediat. Inflamm.* **2013**, *2013*, 863036. [CrossRef]
91. Abu El-Asrar, A.M.; Nawaz, M.I.; Kangave, D.; Abouammoh, M.; Mohammad, G. High-mobility group box-1 and endothelial cell angiogenic markers in the vitreous from patients with proliferative diabetic retinopathy. *Mediat. Inflamm.* **2012**, *2012*, 697489. [CrossRef]
92. Abu El-Asrar, A.M.; Siddiquei, M.M.; Nawaz, M.I.; Geboes, K.; Mohammad, G. The proinflammatory cytokine high-mobility group box-1 mediates retinal neuropathy induced by diabetes. *Mediat. Inflamm.* **2014**, *2014*, 746415. [CrossRef] [PubMed]
93. Abu El-Asrar, A.M.; Mohammad, G.; Nawaz, M.I.; Siddiquei, M.M. High-Mobility Group Box-1 Modulates the Expression of Inflammatory and Angiogenic Signaling Pathways in Diabetic Retina. *Curr. Eye Res.* **2015**, *40*, 1141–1152. [CrossRef] [PubMed]
94. Chang, Y.C.; Lin, C.W.; Hsieh, M.C.; Wu, H.J.; Wu, W.S.; Wu, W.C.; Kao, Y.H. High mobility group B1 up-regulates angiogenic and fibrogenic factors in human retinal pigment epithelial ARPE-19 cells. *Cell Signal.* **2017**, *40*, 248–257. [CrossRef] [PubMed]
95. Surai, P.F.; Kochish, I.I.; Fisinin, V.I.; Kidd, M.T. Antioxidant Defence Systems and Oxidative Stress in Poultry Biology: An Update. *Antioxidants* **2019**, *8*, 235. [CrossRef] [PubMed]
96. Hayashi, H. Molecular biology of secondary metabolism: Case study for *Glycyrrhiza* plants. In *Recent advances in plant biotechnology*; Kirakosyan, A., Kaufman, P.B., Eds.; Springer: New York, NY, USA, 2009; pp. 89–103.
97. Mollica, L.; De Marchis, F.; Spitaleri, A.; Dallacosta, C.; Pennacchini, D.; Zamai, M.; Agresti, A.; Trisciuoglio, L.; Musco, G.; Bianchi, M.E. Glycyrrhizin Binds to High-Mobility Group Box 1 Protein and Inhibits Its Cytokine Activities. *Chem. Biol.* **2007**, *14*, 431–441. [CrossRef]
98. Shirazi, Z.; Aalami, A.; Tohidfar, M.; Sohani, M.M. Metabolic Engineering of Glycyrrhizin Pathway by Over-Expression of Beta-amyrin 11-Oxidase in Transgenic Roots of Glycyrrhiza glabra. *Mol. Biotechnol.* **2018**, *60*, 412–419. [CrossRef]
99. Liu, L.; Jiang, Y.; Steinle, J.J. Glycyrrhizin Protects the Diabetic Retina against Permeability, Neuronal, and Vascular Damage through Anti-Inflammatory Mechanisms. *J. Clin. Med.* **2019**, *8*, 957. [CrossRef]
100. Liu, L.; Jiang, Y.; Steinle, J.J. Inhibition of HMGB1 protects the retina from ischemia-reperfusion, as well as reduces insulin resistance proteins. *PLoS ONE* **2017**, *12*, e0178236. [CrossRef]
101. Liu, L.; Jiang, Y.; Steinle, J.J. Epac1 and Glycyrrhizin Both Inhibit HMGB1 Levels to Reduce Diabetes-Induced Neuronal and Vascular Damage in the Mouse Retina. *J. Clin. Med.* **2019**, *8*, 772. [CrossRef]
102. Fukui, M.; Kitagawa, Y.; Nakamura, N.; Yoshikawa, T. Glycyrrhizin and serum testosterone concentrations in male patients with type 2 diabetes. *Diabetes Care* **2003**, *26*, 2962. [CrossRef]
103. Selvam, C.; Mutisya, D.; Prakash, S.; Ranganna, K.; Thilagavathi, R. Therapeutic potential of chemically modified siRNA: Recent trends. *Chem. Biol. Drug Des.* **2017**, *90*, 665–678. [CrossRef]
104. Bumcrot, D.; Manoharan, M.; Koteliansky, V.; Sah, D.W. RNAi therapeutics: A potential new class of pharmaceutical drugs. *Nat. Chem. Biol.* **2006**, *2*, 711–719. [CrossRef]
105. Jiang, S.; Chen, X. HMGB1 siRNA can reduce damage to retinal cells induced by high glucose in vitro and in vivo. *Drug Des. Dev. Ther.* **2017**, *11*, 783–795. [CrossRef]
106. Bralley, E.E.; Greenspan, P.; Hargrove, J.L.; Wicker, L.; Hartle, D.K. Topical anti-inflammatory activity of Polygonum cuspidatum extract in the TPA model of mouse ear inflammation. *J. Inflamm. (Lond.)* **2008**, *5*, 1. [CrossRef]
107. Peng, W.; Qin, R.; Li, X.; Zhou, H. Botany, phytochemistry, pharmacology, and potential application of Polygonum cuspidatum Sieb.et Zucc.: A review. *J. Ethnopharmacol.* **2013**, *148*, 729–745. [CrossRef]
108. Han, J.H.; Koh, W.; Lee, H.J.; Lee, H.J.; Lee, E.O.; Lee, S.J.; Khil, J.H.; Kim, J.T.; Jeong, S.J.; Kim, S.H. Analgesic and anti-inflammatory effects of ethyl acetate fraction of Polygonum cuspidatum in experimental animals. *Immunopharmacol. Immunotoxicol.* **2012**, *34*, 191–195. [CrossRef]
109. Sohn, E.; Kim, J.; Kim, C.S.; Lee, Y.M.; Kim, J.S. Extract of polygonum cuspidatum attenuates diabetic retinopathy by inhibiting the high-mobility group box-1 (HMGB1) signaling pathway in streptozotocin-induced diabetic rats. *Nutrients* **2016**, *8*, 140. [CrossRef]

110. Zheng, Y.Q.; Wei, W.; Zhu, L.; Liu, J.X. Effects and mechanisms of paeoniflorin, a bioactive glucoside from paeony root, on adjuvant arthritis in rats. *Inflamm. Res.* **2007**, *56*, 182–188. [CrossRef]
111. Jiang, F.; Zhao, Y.; Wang, J.; Wei, S.; Wei, Z.; Li, R.; Zhu, Y.; Sun, Z.; Xiao, X. Comparative pharmacokinetic study of paeoniflorin and albiflorin after oral administration of Radix Paeoniae Rubra in normal rats and the acute cholestasis hepatitis rats. *Fitoterapia* **2012**, *83*, 415–421. [CrossRef]
112. Iwahara, N.; Hisahara, S.; Kawamata, J.; Matsumura, A.; Yokokawa, K.; Saito, T.; Fujikura, M.; Manabe, T.; Suzuki, H.; Matsushita, T. Role of suppressor of cytokine signaling 3 (SOCS3) in altering activated microglia phenotype in APPswe/PS1dE9 mice. *J. Alzheimer's Dis. JAD* **2016**, *55*, 1235–1247. [CrossRef]
113. Zhu, S.H.; Liu, B.Q.; Hao, M.J.; Fan, Y.X.; Qian, C.; Teng, P.; Zhou, X.W.; Hu, L.; Liu, W.T.; Yuan, Z.L.; et al. Paeoniflorin Suppressed High Glucose-Induced Retinal Microglia MMP-9 Expression and Inflammatory Response via Inhibition of TLR4/NF-κB Pathway Through Upregulation of SOCS3 in Diabetic Retinopathy. *Inflammation* **2017**, *40*, 1475–1486. [CrossRef] [PubMed]
114. Yan, C.; Ward, P.A.; Wang, X.; Gao, H. Myeloid depletion of SOCS3 enhances LPS-induced acute lung injury through CCAAT/enhancer binding protein δ pathway. *FASEB J.* **2013**, *27*, 2967–2976. [CrossRef] [PubMed]
115. Vlachojannis, J.E.; Cameron, M.; Chrubasik, S. A systematic review on the effectiveness of willow bark for musculoskeletal pain. *Phytother. Res.* **2009**, *23*, 897–900. [CrossRef] [PubMed]
116. Kong, C.S.; Kim, K.H.; Choi, J.S.; Kim, J.E.; Park, C.; Jeong, J.W. Salicin, an extract from white willow bark, inhibits angiogenesis by blocking the ROS-ERK pathways. *Phytother. Res.* **2014**, *28*, 1246–1251. [CrossRef]
117. Ishikado, A.; Sono, Y.; Matsumoto, M.; Robida-Stubbs, S.; Okuno, A.; Goto, M.; King, G.L.; Keith Blackwell, T.; Makino, T. Willow bark extract increases antioxidant enzymes and reduces oxidative stress through activation of Nrf2 in vascular endothelial cells and Caenorhabditis elegans. *Free Radic. Biol. Med.* **2013**, *65*, 1506–1515. [CrossRef]
118. Song, Y.; Tian, X.; Wang, X.; Feng, H. Vascular protection of salicin on IL-1β-induced endothelial inflammatory response and damages in retinal endothelial cells. *Artif. Cells Nanomed. Biotechnol.* **2019**, *47*, 1995–2002. [CrossRef]
119. Fink, M.P. Ethyl pyruvate: A novel anti-inflammatory agent. *J. Intern. Med.* **2007**, *261*, 349–362. [CrossRef]
120. Lee, Y.M.; Kim, J.; Jo, K.; Shin, S.D.; Kim, C.S.; Sohn, E.J.; Kim, S.G.; Kim, J.S. Ethyl pyruvate inhibits retinal pathogenic neovascularization by downregulating HMGB1 expression. *J. Diabetes Res.* **2013**, *2013*, 245271. [CrossRef]
121. Maurer, M.; Bader, M.; Bas, M.; Bossi, F.; Cicardi, M.; Cugno, M.; Howarth, P.; Kaplan, A.; Kojda, G.; Leeb-Lundberg, F.; et al. New topics in bradykinin research. *Allergy* **2011**, *66*, 1397–1406. [CrossRef]
122. Zhu, Y.; Li, X.Y.; Wang, J.; Zhu, Y.G. Bradykinin alleviates DR retinal endothelial injury by regulating HMGB-1/NF-κB pathway. *Eur. Rev. Med. Pharmacol. Sci.* **2019**, *23*, 5535–5541. [CrossRef]
123. Zhao, L.; Patel, S.H.; Pei, J.; Zhang, K. Antagonizing Wnt pathway in diabetic retinopathy. *Diabetes* **2013**, *62*, 3993–3995. [CrossRef] [PubMed]
124. Chao, J.; Bledsoe, G.; Chao, L. Protective Role of Kallistatin in Vascular and Organ Injury. *Hypertension* **2016**, *68*, 533–541. [CrossRef]
125. Ma, J.X.; King, L.P.; Yang, Z.; Crouch, R.K.; Chao, L.; Chao, J. Kallistatin in human ocular tissues: Reduced levels in vitreous fluids from patients with diabetic retinopathy. *Curr. Eye Res.* **1996**, *15*, 1117–1123. [CrossRef] [PubMed]
126. Xing, Q.; Zhang, G.; Kang, L.; Wu, J.; Chen, H.; Liu, G.; Zhu, R.; Guan, H.; Lu, P. The Suppression of Kallistatin on High-Glucose-Induced Proliferation of Retinal Endothelial Cells in Diabetic Retinopathy. *Ophthalmic Res.* **2017**, *57*, 141–149. [CrossRef] [PubMed]
127. Zhang, Q.; Guy, K.; Pagadala, J.; Jiang, Y.; Walker, R.J.; Liu, L.; Soderland, C.; Kern, T.S.; Ferry, R., Jr.; He, H.; et al. Compound 49b prevents diabetes-induced apoptosis through increased IGFBP-3 levels. *Investig. Ophthalmol. Vis. Sci.* **2012**, *53*, 3004–3013. [CrossRef] [PubMed]
128. Jiang, Y.; Pagadala, J.; Miller, D.; Steinle, J.J. Reduced insulin receptor signaling in retinal Müller cells cultured in high glucose. *Mol. Vis.* **2013**, *19*, 804–811.
129. Berger, E.A.; Carion, T.W.; Jiang, Y.; Liu, L.; Chahine, A.; Walker, R.J.; Steinle, J.J. β-Adrenergic receptor agonist, compound 49b, inhibits TLR4 signaling pathway in diabetic retina. *Immunol. Cell Biol.* **2016**, *94*, 656–661. [CrossRef]

130. Nebbioso, M.; Alisi, L.; Giovannetti, F.; Armentano, M.; Lambiase, A. Eye drop emulsion containing 0.1% cyclosporin (1 mg/mL) for the treatment of severe vernal keratoconjunctivitis: An evidence-based review and place in therapy. *Clin. Ophthalmol.* **2019**, *13*, 1147–1155. [CrossRef]
131. Wang, P.; Chen, F.; Zhang, X. Cyclosporine-a attenuates retinal inflammation by inhibiting HMGB-1 formation in rats with type 2 diabetes mellitus. *BMC Pharmacol. Toxicol.* **2020**, *21*, 9. [CrossRef]
132. Carmo, A.; Cunha-Vaz, J.G.; Carvalho, A.P.; Lopes, M.C. Effect of cyclosporin-A on the blood-retinal barrier permeability in streptozotocin-induced diabetes. *Mediat. Inflamm.* **2000**, *9*, 243–248. [CrossRef]

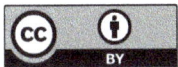 © 2020 by the authors. Licensee MDPI, Basel, Switzerland. This article is an open access article distributed under the terms and conditions of the Creative Commons Attribution (CC BY) license (http://creativecommons.org/licenses/by/4.0/).

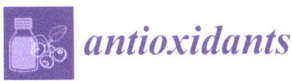

Review

Importance of the Use of Oxidative Stress Biomarkers and Inflammatory Profile in Aqueous and Vitreous Humor in Diabetic Retinopathy

Ana Karen López-Contreras [1], María Guadalupe Martínez-Ruiz [1], Cecilia Olvera-Montaño [1], Ricardo Raúl Robles-Rivera [1], Diana Esperanza Arévalo-Simental [1,2], José Alberto Castellanos-González [1,3], Abel Hernández-Chávez [1], Selene Guadalupe Huerta-Olvera [4], Ernesto German Cardona-Muñoz [1] and Adolfo Daniel Rodríguez-Carrizalez [1,*]

1. Department of Physiology, Health Sciences University Center, Institute of Clinical and Experimental Therapeutics, University of Guadalajara, Guadalajara, Jalisco 44340, Mexico; Karen.LopezC@alumno.udg.mx (A.K.L.-C.); maria.mruiz@alumnos.udg.mx (M.G.M.-R.); cecilia.Olvera@alumno.udg.mx (C.O.-M.); raul.roblesr@alumnos.udg.mx (R.R.R.-R.); darevalo@hcg.gob.mx (D.E.A.-S.); jose.castellanos2223@alumnos.udg.mx (J.A.C.-G.); abel.hchavez@academicos.udg.mx (A.H.-C.); cardona@cucs.udg.mx (E.G.C.-M.)
2. Department of Ophthalmology, Hospital Civil de Guadalajara "Fray Antonio Alcalde", Guadalajara, Jalisco 44280, Mexico
3. Department of Ophthalmology, Specialties Hospital of the National Occidental Medical Center, Mexican Institute of Social Security, Guadalajara, Jalisco 44329, Mexico
4. Medical and Life Sciences Department, La Ciénega University Center, University of Guadalajara, Ocotlán, Jalisco 47810, Mexico; selene.huerta@academicos.udg.mx
* Correspondence: adolfo.rodriguez@academicos.udg.mx

Received: 25 July 2020; Accepted: 10 September 2020; Published: 20 September 2020

Abstract: Diabetic retinopathy is one of the leading causes of visual impairment and morbidity worldwide, being the number one cause of blindness in people between 27 and 75 years old. It is estimated that ~191 million people will be diagnosed with this microvascular complication by 2030. Its pathogenesis is due to alterations in the retinal microvasculature as a result of a high concentration of glucose in the blood for a long time which generates numerous molecular changes like oxidative stress. Therefore, this narrative review aims to approach various biomarkers associated with the development of diabetic retinopathy. Focusing on the molecules showing promise as detection tools, among them we consider markers of oxidative stress (TAC, LPO, MDA, 4-HNE, SOD, GPx, and catalase), inflammation (IL-6, IL-1ß, IL-8, IL-10, IL-17A, TNF-α, and MMPs), apoptosis (NF-kB, *cyt-c*, and caspases), and recently those that have to do with epigenetic modifications, their measurement in different biological matrices obtained from the eye, including importance, obtaining process, handling, and storage of these matrices in order to have the ability to detect the disease in its early stages.

Keywords: diabetic retinopathy; oxidative stress; antioxidants; biomarkers of diabetic retinopathy; metabolic memory; tear film; aqueous humor; vitreous humor

1. Introduction

The retina is a transparent tissue of the eye which has an intricate arrangement of neurons and also requires a highly complex circulation to meet metabolic requirements and the proper functioning of neurotransmission, phototransduction, and complex interaction of metabolites, vasoactive agents, and growth factors [1,2]. The central retinal artery passes through the optic nerve to ensure blood flow, and gas and nutrient exchange, while the central retinal vein is involved in the elimination of waste products [3]. The retinal vasculature is of great importance and within its physiological functions; the most important is to maintain the internal blood–retinal barrier (iBRB), which prevents nonspecific penetration of macromolecules into the retinal neuropile. The outer blood–retinal barrier (oBRB), formed between the tight junctions of retinal pigment cells, maintains ionic concentrations in the avascular region of the retina and the interstitial space for neurotransmission [3]. Retinal vascular dysfunction occurs shortly after the onset of diabetes and is characterized by impaired microvasculature and transport across the blood–retinal barrier playing an important role in the onset and progression of vascular lesions in diabetic retinopathy (DR) [2,4]. There is currently a wide range of treatments available for diabetes mellitus (DM) which has dramatically increased the lifespan of diabetic patients, but in turn gives time for clinically significant microvascular complications to develop [5]. Currently, there is a wide variety of effective treatments for DR, diagnosing the disease in its early stages helps prevent progression to blindness [5,6].

In this narrative review, we aim to approach various biomarkers associated with the development of diabetic retinopathy. In particular, our objective is to focus on the importance of molecules that are promising as detection tools and their measurement in different biological matrices obtained from the eye, in order to achieve an early disease detection or, ideally, even before the actual start of the DR. Articles in English were included that showed relevance both in preclinical and clinical stages of the DR. We take into account the articles that contribute to the discussion of the use of biomarkers of different nature to identify and estimate the stage of the disease in which patients with DR are, in addition to the use of different biological matrices obtained directly from the eyeball such as the tear, aqueous humor, and vitreous humor.

2. Diabetic Retinopathy

Among the 468 million people with diabetes mellitus worldwide, approximately 90 million suffer from some form of DR [7]. It is the number one cause of blindness in people between the ages of 27 and 75. The prevalence of DR is approximately 25% and 90% at 5 and 20 years, respectively, from its diagnosis. Furthermore, it is estimated that ~191 million people will be diagnosed with this microvascular complication by 2030 [8,9], and the number of DR patients whose vision is threatened will increase from 37.3 to 56.3 million. This disturbing prospect makes the DR a significant global public health and economic problem [10].

Chronic hyperglycemia is the main risk factor affecting DR, as part of its pathophysiology it has been shown to induce vascular endothelial dysfunction in the retina [11]. When this state persist, activation of other pathways occurs in addition to glycolysis (such as polyol, hexosamine, and advanced glycation), which are known to induce apoptosis and pericyte degeneration, eventually damaging the retina [12].

DR is classified into nonproliferative diabetic retinopathy (NPDR) and proliferative diabetic retinopathy (PDR) stages according to the presence of visible ophthalmological changes and the manifestation of retinal neovascularization [13,14]. NPDR is usually asymptomatic except when associated with macular edema; however, cases with uncontrolled DM or where retinopathy's progression is not monitored tend to progress to PDR, which is generally linked to complications that could lead to impaired visual acuity [15]. The first clinical sign of DR is the presence of microaneurysms in the retina during the mild version of the disease. In moderate diabetic retinopathy, exudates, hemorrhages, and minimal intraretinal microvascular abnormalities appear and may increase their proportion in severe stages [8]. Retinal detachment, neovascularization, along with fibrovascular tissue proliferation are features of PDR where newly formed vessels are leaky, fragile, misdirected, and the contraction of the aging vitreous cause them to rupture or if a greater force is created, it can lead to tractional retinal detachment resulting in acute or gradual loss of vision [2,9].

3. Role of Oxidants and Antioxidants in the Eye with Diabetic Retinopathy

The eye is an organ exposed to multiple exogenous factors, which are potentially precipitants of injury, including visible light, ultraviolet light, environmental toxins, and ionizing radiation, as well as the endogenous stress induced by the mitochondria within the eye tissues during the physiological functions of the eye [16]. This endogenous and exogenous stress produces an imbalance between oxidants and antioxidants, generating unstable reactive oxygen species (ROS) characterized by one or two unpaired electrons within their outer orbit [17]. ROS generation is normally correlated with cellular metabolic rate. The ocular surface produces lipids, aqueous, and mucin, all together form the tear film, which serves to protect and maintain the health of the ocular surface when it spreads over the eyelids [18]. The aqueous layer is produced by the tear and accessory glands. Mucins are secreted by corneal epithelial cells and conjunctival goblet cells. The lipids are secreted by the Meibomian glands located in the eyelids [18]. The ocular surface is further compromised in those patients with more severe and longer duration of diabetes disease, including those with higher A1c values, or retinopathy [19,20]. That is why the eyeball, as well as being exposed to attacks by ROS, is also provided with different antioxidants in its different segments, especially in the tear film, aqueous humor and vitreous humor.

3.1. Oxidative Stress and the Damage It Causes to the Eye

Oxidative stress (OS) is known as the interruption in free radical production homeostasis during various vital processes, such as the electron transport chain reaction and the sweeping of the oxidant products, or defense mechanisms designed to neutralize these harmful molecules. This imbalance is closely related to the pathophysiology of DR [21]. The addition of an electron to the dioxygen molecule creates the superoxide anion radical, which is generated mainly during the mitochondrial respiration process. Subsequently, the dismutation of this free radical by superoxide dismutase enzymes forms hydrogen peroxide (H_2O_2) [22]; decomposition of this molecule by various transition metals through the Fenton reaction can generate a high reactive hydroxyl radical [23,24]. Moreover, the reaction of the superoxide or hydroxyl radical with polyunsaturated fatty acids can generate the peroxyl radical (Figure 1). The human eye is constantly subject to OS, due to frequent exposure to light, in addition to high metabolic activity and oxygen tension. Solar ultraviolet radiation (UVR) turns out to be the main inducer in the external environment for ROS formation in the eye [24]. Other mechanisms like increased vascular endothelial growth factor (VEGF) production, alteration of the extracellular matrix architecture, genetic factors, and redox signaling are also present along with angiogenesis, collateral vessel formation, and increased permeability in PDR [25–27]. Stress induced by oxygen-derived free radicals such as hydroxyl radical, superoxide anion, and hydrogen peroxide can be harmful to cells [28], due to its ability to diffuse across hydrophobic membranes and their participation in the production of more reactive species, being H_2O_2 the most extensively studied oxygen metabolite [29].

In the anterior segment of the eye, H_2O_2 is present in the uvea and in the aqueous humor of mammals at concentrations between 30 and 70 µM [30]. H_2O_2 is a product of many antioxidant reactions of ascorbate such as those with oxygen and superoxide. High concentrations of this oxidant have been shown to be toxic to the lens [29,31]. Elevated levels up to seven times the normal range of H_2O_2 have been demonstrated in the aqueous humor and the lens of some human patients with cataracts [32]. H_2O_2 injected into the anterior chamber of the eye caused significant morphological changes in the iris and ciliary body and decreased intraocular pressure (IOP) [29].

In the posterior segment, H_2O_2 has been associated with tissue damage in the retina due to light and oxygen [33]. One of the main causes of DR is the development of glycosylated proteins, which generate free radicals, resulting in oxidative tissue damage and subsequent glutathione (GSH) depletion [34]. Glycosylated proteins can even combine with lipids and be further damaged by free radicals, forming advanced glycated end products (AGE), which can then deposit in blood vessels of the retina and promote neovascularization [35]. Diabetics with retinopathy have higher levels of oxidative damage markers in subretinal fluid when compared to diabetics without retinopathy and healthy controls [36]. The retina responds to OS with reactive gliosis: the activation of astrocytes, microglial, and macroglial cells. Microglial cells are resident retinal macrophages that confer neuroprotection against ROS damage and other injuries. OS promotes the degradation of sialic acid residues in membrane proteins, leaving photoreceptors and other cells with a damaged glycocalyx, this leads to greater phagocytosis by microglial cells, and increases neuronal cells death, worsening the pathology [37,38].

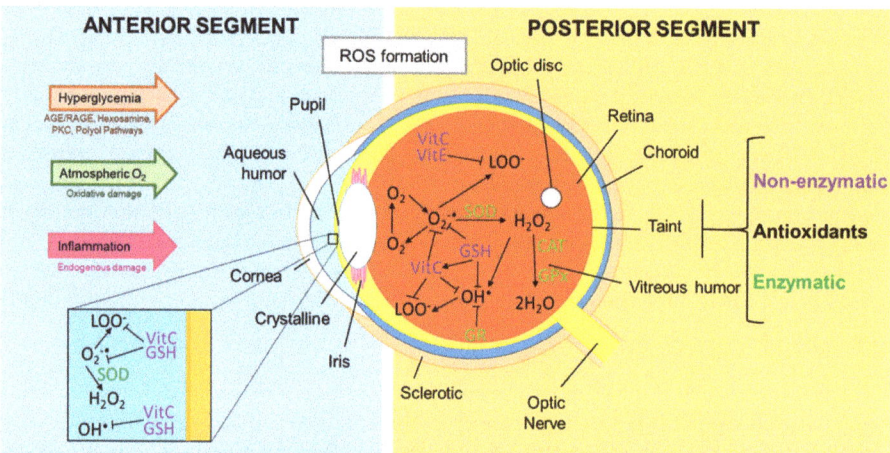

Figure 1. Reactive oxygen species and antioxidants in the eye. In the eye, chronic hyperglycemic state, atmospheric O2, and inflammation processes alter different metabolic pathways which stimulates the formation of reactive oxygen species (ROS) in the anterior and posterior segment, starting with oxygen (O2) to which the addition of one electron forms the superoxide anion radical (O2-•), the dismutation of this molecule by superoxide dismutases (SOD) forms hydrogen peroxide (H2O2), and the breakdown of this molecule can generate hydroxyl radical (OH•) which is highly reactive. In addition the reaction of O2- • or OH• radical with polyunsaturated fatty acids generates the peroxyl radical (LOO•). The formation of this radicals can be countered by enzymatic and non-enzymatic antioxidants like vitamin C, vitamin E, glutathione (GSH), glutathione peroxidase (GPx), superoxide dismutase (SOD), catalase (CAT), and glutathione reductase (GR), among others. (Modified from ref. [24]).

Free radicals have also been reported to cause lipid peroxidation and a decrease in potassium-evoked dopamine release in vitro. OS induced by H_2O_2 has shown to enhance basal release of [3H] d-aspartate but decreased potassium (K+)—evoked release of this amino acid [39]. In one study, H_2O_2 caused a decrease in concentrations of glutamate and glycine in the retina. While low concentrations of H_2O_2 also produced decrease in glycine concentration in the vitreous humor, but had no significant action on glutamate levels [40]. The catalase 3-AT inhibitor caused reduction in both the retina and vitreous humor of the glutamate and glycine concentrations, indicating an important role of endogenously produced peroxides in the regulation of retinal amino acid neurotransmission. The observed inhibitory action of H_2O_2 on glutamate concentrations in ex vivo experiments emulate the effects observed in in vitro assays [40]. Nitric oxide synthase—the enzyme that catalyzes the formation of nitric oxide (NO)—is located in retinal neurons and the pigment epithelium. NO can participate in reactions with superoxide radicals to form the more potent and long-lived oxidant, peroxynitrite, from which there is evidence that can inhibit the absorption of glutamate in the rat's brain [41]. H_2O_2 interacts with the COX pathway that leads to the formation of prostanoids both in vitro and in vivo as well as simulating the biosynthesis of PGE2 and PGI$_2$ and the production of thromboxane B2. Isoprostanes are compounds derived from the free radical catalyzed peroxidation of arachidonic acid independent of COX. Then products such as PGE$_2$ and 8-iso-PGF$_{2\alpha}$, regulate H_2O_2 and its inhibitory action on glutaminergic transmission in the isolated bovine retina [42]. It can be concluded that in the posterior segment H_2O_2 has the ability to alter the availability of amino acids in bovine eyes [29].

3.2. Antioxidants Present in the Tear Film, Aqueous Humor, and Vitreous Humor

The eye is packed with a variety of antioxidants, which mitigates the damaging effects of ROS. An antioxidant is frequently defined as the substance that, when present in low concentration compared to that of an oxidizable substrate, significantly delays or inhibits the oxidation of the substrate [43]. Overproduction or inadequate elimination of ROS beyond the ability to counteract the antioxidant system can cause OS and overload the eye tissues [44]. Tear film and aqueous humor are important components of defense mechanisms on the ocular surface.

The tear film covers the anterior surface of the cornea and is the first line of defense against external aggressions [24]; it contains both non-enzymatic and enzymatic antioxidants. In human tears, ascorbic acid (665 µM) and uric acid (328 µM) represent ~50% of the total antioxidant activity, with ascorbic acid being the most abundant followed by uric acid; some other small molecules found are GSH (107 µM), L-cysteine (48 µM), and L-tyrosine (45 µM). The only antioxidant enzyme reported in the tear film is superoxide dismutase (SOD), which has an activity at 1–32 U/mg protein [24,45].

Aqueous humor is a clear, slightly alkaline liquid that occupies the space between the cornea and the lens, formed and secreted by the ciliary bodies. It plays a crucial role in the nutrition and protection of the corneal endothelium and in the anterior epithelial lining of the lens. Another of its functions is to eliminate metabolic waste and biochemical products generated by the cornea and the lens. ROS can be continuously generated in the aqueous humor in the form of hydrogen peroxide, superoxide anion, singlet oxygen, and peroxyl radicals [46]. The antioxidants found in the aqueous humor are almost the same as in the tear film, among the non-enzymatic antioxidants there is ascorbic acid (530 µM), L-tyrosine (78 µM), uric acid (43 µM), L-cysteine (14.3 µM), and glutathione (5.5 µM) [45]. Ascorbic acid has three different protective mechanisms in the aqueous humor: quenching or blocking the fluorescence of biomolecules, control of the biotransformation generated by the same fluorescence, and the direct absorption of UVR. The amino acid L-tyrosine is electrochemically active and removes hydroxyl radicals and singlet oxygen species. Uric acid (UA), a water-soluble molecule with high reactivity towards singlet oxygen and hydroxyl radicals, serves as a powerful scavenger of ROS [24,47]. In summary, the tear film and aqueous humor are packed with low-molecular weight, water-soluble antioxidants, which support the cornea's defense mechanisms against OS [24].

The vitreous humor is the structure that fills the space within the posterior segment of the eye; it is surrounded by the surface of the posterior lens and by the internal limiting membrane (ILM) of the retina. The vitreous body has a total volume of approximately 4 mL, mainly composed of water (98–99%), collagen fibers, glycosaminoglycans, non-collagen proteins, and small amounts of trace elements [48]. The nature of the vitreous gel is attributed to the interaction between its two main components: collagen and hyaluronan (HA) [44]. The concentration of HA within the vitreous gel varies between 0.02 and 1 mg/cm3 and plays a synergistic role with collagen and other proteoglycans for the regulation of vitreous stiffness [44,49]. The vitreous cortex is a lamellar structure attached to the ILM of the retina posterior to the peripheral vitreous base by an extracellular matrix "adhesive" consisting of laminin, opticin, fibronectin, chondroitin sulfate, and heparan sulfate. It can be said that the vitreous is acellular since it only presents a monolayer of mononuclear phagocytes, hyalocytes, located within the posterior vitreous cortex [50]. Among its functions, the vitreous contributes to the clarity of the intraocular media, the maintenance of IOP, and the regulation of intraocular oxygen tension [51]. In addition, the vitreous body provides protection by acting as a shock absorber, due to the collagen fibers that reduce the compressive forces of HA when the globe is exposed to external pressure [52].

The vitreous accumulates a high amount of water-soluble antioxidants, which could protect the eye from OS. These antioxidants can also be classified into enzymatic and non-enzymatic antioxidants [29]. Non-enzymatic antioxidants have the ability to quickly inactivate radicals and oxidants. Considering the source of non-enzymatic vitreous antioxidants, these can be classified into nutrient non-enzymatic and metabolic antioxidants [53]. Nutrient non-enzymatic antioxidants include those obtained exogenously through food and supplements, such as vitamin C, vitamin B2, and trace metals like zinc and selenium. Metabolic antioxidants are endogenous antioxidants produced by the body itself, such as GSH, metal-chelating proteins like transferrin, and uric acid [44,54].

Vitamin C, also known as ascorbic acid, is a water-soluble molecule present in most tissues in its anionic state but cannot be synthesized by humans: they can only obtain it exogenously. The vitreous gel receives its vitamin C supply from the plasma through active transport from the ciliary body. The ascorbic acid found inside the vitreous body reaches concentrations of approximately 2 mmol/L; this is 33 times more than the plasma concentration. As an antioxidant, ascorbic acid is oxidized to convert superoxide anions and lipid hydroperoxidases into stable forms, thereby preventing lipid peroxidation [55]. Vitamin B2 (riboflavin) has been detected in the human vitreous (0.8 µg/100 mL) and animal (8.0 µg/L). Riboflavin protects against lipid peroxidation and plays an essential role in the glutathione redox cycle [56]. Zinc is the most abundant trace element within the eye that exerts antioxidant effects by protecting sulfhydryl groups from oxidation; its concentration is close to 1.95 µMol/L. Zinc works as a scavenger of free oxygen radicals like hydroxyl as it acts as a stimulus for metallothionein synthesis, it also protects tissues from various forms of oxidative damage, including lipid peroxidation and glycoxidation [57,58]. Selenium is an essential trace element, it has an average concentration of 0.1035 µMol/L. Selenium works indirectly as an antioxidant being incorporated into antioxidant enzymes, such as selenoenzymes [59].

The GSH peptide has cysteine and a thiol antioxidant in its constitution, and is found in an average concentration of 0.26 mmol/L [60]. As an antioxidant, glutathione can directly remove selected oxygen radicals and indirectly aid in the recycling of vitamins C and E [61], it also functions as a cofactor for glutathione peroxidase (GPx) activity allowing the reduction of lipid hydroperoxides [62]. Transferrin (molecular weight ~80 kDa), is found in an average concentration in the vitreous of 0.0878 g/L [44]. As an antioxidant, transferrin is an iron chelator that keeps ionic iron sequestered at physiological pH, and thus minimizes the participation of iron in radical iron-dependent reactions; its activity helps reduce the toxicity of intravitreal iron during vitreous hemorrhage [63]. Uric acid is a breakdown product of purine nucleotides and works as an antioxidant at normal concentrations. However, in the presence of oxidative stress, there is an upregulation of UA concentrations and a change related to redox balance, causing UA to become oxidative [64].

The enzymatic antioxidants detected in the vitreous are GPx, SOD, and catalase. From the glutathione peroxidase family, extracellular GPx3 and phospholipid GPx4 are found within the vitreous body [65]. As a homotetrameric protein, GPx3 catalyzes the reduction of organic hydroperoxides and H_2O_2 until alcohol and water are obtained by using GSH as an electron donor. GPx4 is a monomeric protein capable of directly reducing phospholipid and cholesterol hydroperoxides [66]. SOD is a metalloprotein enzyme that is responsible for catalyzing superoxide radicals into hydrogen peroxide and molecular oxygen. SOD is made up of three isoforms: cytosolic SOD (SOD1), mitochondrial SOD (SOD2), and extracellular SOD (SOD3). SOD1 and SOD3 contain copper and zinc (Cu/Zn-SOD), while SOD2 contains manganese (Mn-SOD) [44,67]. In the vitreous base and cortex we find the concentrated SOD3 isoenzyme where it interacts with proteoglycans and regulates the response to OS in the vitreous preventing local oxidative damage [67]. Catalase is a tetrahedral hemoprotein that also protects tissues from the toxic effects of peroxide by converting peroxides to water and oxygen. The vitreous body in humans has an average concentration of 58 µL O_2 per mg of soluble catalase protein. It has been detected in the vitreous of patients with PDR; this suggests that catalase may be a potential target for the treatment of acute ischemic diseases of the retina [68]. Besides, along with GPx are found in other ocular tissues, including the iris and the ciliary body [30]. Fluorometric and postmortem toxicological analysis studies have shown that the passage of molecules from the systemic circulation to the vitreous through the blood–aqueous and blood–retina barriers is mediated by diffusion, hydrostatic and osmotic pressure gradients, convection, and active transport [69,70].

Repeated long-term administration of these agents may be necessary to achieve sufficient therapeutic doses of exogenous nutrients within the vitreous [71].

4. Ocular Matrices: Tears, Aqueous Humor, and Vitreous Humor

There are many different microenvironments in the body; each organ and tissue can have its own microenvironment, including blood and cells. For example, a given biomarker can be present at multiple sites, and its relationship to the state of retinopathy can vary according to the site where it is measured [72]. The eye is a complex sensory organ that has the ability to receive light and convert it into electrical impulses, which are transmitted to the brain through the optic nerve, resulting in visual perception. In the case of animal models with ocular disorders, the variety of ocular matrices that can be collected and analyzed for biomarker measurement is wide, but the implementation of this biomarker measurement in the clinic together with the type of ocular matrix to be sampled is a key consideration. In humans, the most easily obtained eye matrices are tears and tissues of the ocular surface, such as the cornea and conjunctiva, they provide exact information regarding disorders in the anterior segment. Aqueous humor (AH) and vitreous are the most suitable matrices for evaluating relevant biomarkers for posterior segment disorders, such as DR. They are difficult to access matrices, requiring an invasive procedure performed in the clinic to facilitate specimen collection, leading to significant ocular complications [73]. Evaluation of ocular biomarkers provides valuable information regarding disease progression and this makes it a critical component of the discovery and development of ophthalmic drugs.

4.1. Tears

The tear film is composed by three layers: mucin, aqueous, and lipid that provides functional, nutritional, and protective characteristics for the ocular surface. These layers interact with the meibomian gland, lacrimal gland, conjunctiva, and cornea, which facilitate and regulate the normal production, distribution, and elimination of tears. The tear film creates a refractive surface on the cornea and protects it from environmental damage, each layer contents glycoproteins, amino acids, electrolytes, enzymes and proteins like lipocalin, lysozymes, lactoferrin, and albumin, as well phosphatidylcholine and phosphatidylethanolamine. Particular immunological components include sIgA e IgG, cytokines mainly Tumor necrosis factor-α (TNF-α), IL-α, IL-1ß, IL-6, matrix metalloproteinases (MMP), and chemokines, which are immunological mediators in the ocular surface diseases (Figure 2). Although, they are expressed in other diseases, for example, in autoimmune diseases, diabetic retinopathy, dry eye syndrome, ocular allergies, neurological disorders like Parkinson's disease, and Multiple Sclerosis [74]. Obtaining the tear film requires minimally invasive procedures, making it an accessible matrix that needs to be further studied and used as a starting point for the study of a variety of eye diseases. The determination of a wide variety of cytokines, enzymes and metabolic residues in tears could be useful for the establishment of therapeutics targets, contributing to the improvement of treatments and facilitating their diagnosis.

The number of components in tear samples varies according to the technique used for their collection. Due to the small volume of tear sample (5–10 µL), two techniques are commonly used for their collection:

1. Direct or aspiration: the collection is through microcapillary tubes (MCT) or micropipettes, the tip of the tube is placed in the cul-de-sac for 5 min, in non-stimulated tears (NST), until it forms a lake of tear, then for capillarity tears are absorbed and the sample (5.5–6.5 µL) is transferred immediately into a sterile tube with storage solution or buffer assay to produce a dilution 1:10 and storage at −80 °C. The main advantage is the amount of proteins and biomarkers obtained directly of ocular surface. A disadvantage is the loss of proteins may occur due to incomplete pouring into microvials [75,76].
2. Indirect methods: These methods collect the samples of tears through absorbing papers like cellulose sponges or Schirmer test strips (STS), both are invasive techniques. The cellulose sponges

are used frequently to analyze inflammatory markers like interleukins and MMP-9 and they are measured by enzyme-linked immunosorbent assay (ELISA) or Luminex technology using tears that were collected with Merocel, Pro-ophta, or Weck-Cel sponges. However, comparative studies with simultaneous measurements of cytokines have shown that Merocel is useful for clinical assess for cytokines/chemokines levels but have the limitation with measures of IL-7 and IL-4 due to protein stability problems with the extraction buffer [75–77]. In the case of STS, it may also be used for cytokine analysis assays. For collection of tears, the strip is placed on the inferior fornix of the eye and the patient should close their eyes for 5 min. After completed the time, the patient should open their eyes for remove carefully the strip and then it is collocated into a sterile 1.5 mL tube. Immediately transfer the tube to the laboratory to process later in a bead based multiplex assay or store at −80 °C. With this method the sample contains higher amounts of cellular proteins, lipids, and mucous compared with MCT and the analysis with multiplex provide high sensitivity for analyzing cytokines and other proteins [78].

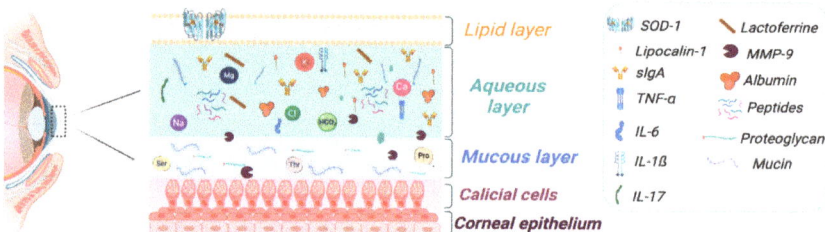

Figure 2. Main components in tear film. The wide variety of components in each layer of the tear film provides function, nutrition, and protection to the ocular surface. However, it is susceptible to change their composition due to oxidative stress and inflammatory processes that involve the eye structures, which makes it an easy access ocular matrix to identify these changes measuring levels of components as biomarkers. SOD1: superoxide dismutase-1, Ser: serine, Thr: Threonine, Pro: Proline, IL: Interleukin, sIgA: surface Immunoglobuline A, MMP-9: matrix metalloproteinase-9, TNF-α: Tumor necrosis factor-α. Image created with BioRender.com.

4.2. Aqueous Humor

AH is primarily composed of water (99.9%) and small amounts of carbohydrates, vitamins, proteins, and other nutrients, as well as growth factors and cytokines. It is responsible for maintaining eye pressure among other things for the support of ocular health. It is important to know that AH is drain from the eye through one of two passive pathways: the traditional trabecular meshwork (TM) pathway and the unconventional one, which is the uveoscleral pathway [79,80].

The samples of AH are collected by aqueous route through a paracenthesis in patients undergoing cataract surgery, trabeculectomy, phacoemulsification, or post-mortem eyes. Collection volumes are small and range from 100 to 150 µL [81,82]. After aqueous humor samples are obtained they are usually stored undiluted directly at −80 °C; they can be aliquoted according to the volume obtained and no more than one freeze–thaw cycle is recommended prior to analysis [83]. Potentially valuable information can be obtained from the analysis of these samples, however, there are potential risks associated with their collection. The methods are highly invasive and can create a risk of additional damage to the cornea and lens [73]. Post-mortem eye samples will have different profiles than those collected from living patients due to the accumulation of metabolic waste and other uncontrolled post-mortem processes. This is why samples collected from living patients are considered more useful.

4.3. Vitreous Humor

The vitreous is located in the posterior segment between the lens and the retina. As stated earlier, it is mainly composed of water and a mesh of fine collagen fibrils embedded with dissolved hyaluronan molecules, inorganic salts and lipids [84]. In addition, the vitreous contains other proteins such as albumin, globulins, clotting proteins, and complement factors that have accumulated from blood filtration or the spread of surrounding tissue and vasculature [85]. The anatomical position of this matrix in contact and close with the retina makes it an ideal compartment for taking samples that reflect biochemical and pathophysiological changes when there are states of retinal or vitreoretinal disease, including PDR [73,86].

Vitreous samples in vivo are generally collected through vitreous taps from vitrectomy patients [87]. Samples obtained from vitreous humor (900–920 uL) are generally stored undiluted at −80 °C as well as aqueous humor, it is recommended to separate them in aliquots to avoid freeze–thaw cycles. For its analysis, the samples can be centrifuged to eliminate cellular components and debris [88]. Given the invasiveness of vitreous sampling, recently has been evaluated the possibility of collecting vitreous reflux after intravitreal injections, being the appropriate time and without the need to enter the operating room, however, the possible risks should be better assessed [89]. In a study by Srividya and colleagues, they used Schirmer's tear strips to collect vitreous reflux from patients with diabetic macular edema (DME) and PDR, where they compared their total protein concentration with undiluted vitrectomy specimens. The results showed similar total protein concentrations between the vitreous reflux and the vitrectomy samples ($P < 0.05$) [89]. The most common method of analysis for biomarkers in this samples are enzyme-linked immunosorbent assays (ELISAs) and enzyme-colorimetric assays. Recently, multiplex bead array assays are now commonly used to maximize the usefulness of the vitreous sample, like in AH because they have the advantage that they can measure multiple analytes simultaneously in small volumes [90]. Proteomic and genomic analysis techniques are also used to analyze biomarkers of different nature in vitreous samples.

5. Measurement of Biomarkers

A biomarker provide a powerful and dynamic approach to improve our understanding of the mechanisms underlying eye disease, supporting information for diagnosis, disease control, or to predict clinical response to treatment [73]. Biomarkers can help to understand DR and contribute to the development of new treatments or new clinical strategies to prevent vision loss [91]. The FDA-NIH Joint Leadership Council updated the BEST Resource (Biomarkers, Endpoints, and Other Tools), modify the original definition of biomarker to "a defined characteristic that is measured as an indicator of normal biological processes, pathogenic processes, or responses to an exposure or intervention, including therapeutic interventions" [92]. New biomarkers are generally considered of interest, as they are associated to predict the disease or its response to treatments, however they are not proven, nor are they widely accepted or used in clinical practice as a decision-making tool [91]. The development of new biomarkers is a complex process that requires high refinement, and depends on the etiological disclosure that is presented. On the other hand, in clinical practice individual biomarkers but also a set or panel of biomarkers can be used, these can include biomarkers of different types, such as exposure, effect, and susceptibility biomarkers. Multiplex immunoassays are ideal for analyzing small volumes of samples, such as tears and now also in AH where they have been shown to be effective in measuring cytokine levels. With Next Generation Sequencing Techniques (NGS), small-sample miRNome analysis can be performed that avoids some of the limitations of hybridization-based detection methods [93]. Genetic matrix analysis is an additional powerful technique for comparing gene expression profiles in AH [94].

5.1. Oxidative Stress: ROS and Relevance in DR

The ocular surface is always subjected to intense exposure to light and solar ultraviolet radiation, also high metabolic activity increases the production of ROS and OS. This is a common adaptation secondary to inflammation and diabetes that produce more mediators to ROS in ocular surface as xanthine oxidase. It is hypothesized that the increase in antioxidant markers may reflect a local, compensatory response in the eye against OS [73]. Therefore, adequate levels of antioxidant enzymes responsible for free radical scavenging are essential for oxidation and reduction (redox) homeostasis [95]. Nezzar et al. analyzed the expression of glutathione peroxidase (GPx1–GPx8), catalase and SOD1 in human tissues of meibomian glands and conjunctiva and they found that both tissues express GPx2, GPx4, and GPx7 to control peroxide concentration in the lipid layer to protects the ocular surface from OS damage. Moreover, SOD1 and catalase were found expressed in conjunctiva and meibomian gland this might suggest their role in recycling ROS and their interaction with inflammation caused by OS [96]. In addition, products such as GPx, SOD and malondialdehyde (MDA) have been observed at irregular levels in the AH of patients with PDR. SOD is a key antioxidant enzyme involved in the metabolism of oxygen free radicals and prevents the formation of other ROS [97].

GPXs are a family of selenium-dependent isoenzymes that catalyze the reduction of H_2O_2 or organic hydroperoxides in water and alcohols through oxidation of GSH to GSSG. Its activity can be measured using cumene hydroperoxide and GSH as substrates in a coupled reaction with glutathione reductase (GR) [98,99]. GPx messenger RNA express mainly in the ocular ciliary epithelium suggests that in AH glutathione peroxidase originates from these cells [100], its activity in the AH of glaucoma patients has been reported to be three times higher than in cataract patients, the mean value of GPx in AH of glaucoma patients was 18.4 ± 2.5 U/mL, and the mean value of the cataract group was 6.1 ± 0.6 U/mL ($p < 0.001$) [101] (see Table 1). Some antioxidant mechanisms, such as glutathione-related enzymes, are likely to work in normal and vitreous lenses to keep proteins in a reduced state. Unstable pro-oxidant molecules in the vitreous can play a role in cataract pathogenesis along with retinal disease. They can spread damage to lens membranes and vitreous proteins [102,103]. The study by Altomare et al. said specific activity of the GPx could not be detected in the vitreous humor; it is probably due to the high dilution of the vitreous humor used for the extraction procedure [103].

Table 1. Biomarker levels in tear, aqueous, and vitreous humor. Levels of the markers of oxidative stress, inflammation, and apoptosis measured in tear, aqueous, and vitreous humor in different ocular conditions, in addition to PDR, differentiating the different methodologies used. PDR: proliferative diabetic retinopathy, DED: dry eye disease, TAC: total antioxidant capacity, LPO: lipoperoxides, MDA: malondialdehyde, GSH: glutathione, GPx: glutathione peroxidase, SOD: superoxide dismutase, 8-OHdG: 8-hidroxi-2-deoxiguanosine, 8-IPGF: 8-isoprostaglandins, NO: nitric oxide, IL-6: interleukin-6, IL-8: interleukin-8, IL-10: interleukin-10, TNF-α: Tumour necrosis factor alpha, VEGF: vascular endothelial growth factor, EGF: epidermal grow factor, MMP-9: metalloproteinase-9, FN-kβ: Nuclear factor kβ, T1DM: type 1 diabetes mellitus, T2DM: type 2 diabetes mellitus.

Profile	Biomarker	Matrix	Pathology	Levels	Method	References
Oxidative Stress	TAC	Aqueous	PDR	0.55 ± 0.28 μmol Trolox/g *	Radical absorbance capacity assay	[104]
		Vitreous	PDR	0.19 ± 0.10 μmol Trolox/g *	Radical absorbance capacity assay	[104]
	LPO	Vitreous	PDR	Male: 145.8 ± 6.3 μM * Female: 135.6 ± 10.9 μM *	Colorimetric assay	[105]
	MDA	Tears	DR	95 μM	Capillary electrophoresis	[106]
		Aqueous humor	Cataract	0.1 ± 0.1 μmol/L *	TBARS method	[107]
		Vitreous	PDR	Male: 101.3 ± 7.6 nmol/mL * Female: 87.6 ± 18.4 nmol/mL *	Colorimetric assay	[105]
	GSH	Tears	DR	107 μM	Chromatography electrochemical	[24]
	GPx	Aqueous	Glaucoma	18.4 ± 2.5 U/mL *	-	[101]
		Aqueous	Cataract	6.1 ± 0.6 U/mL *	-	[101]
	SOD	Tears	DR	1–32 U/mg	Spectrophotometry direct	[45,108]
		Vitreous	PDR	Male: 30.5 ± 2.5 U/mL * Female: 28.5 ± 3.8 U/mL *	Colorimetric Enzyme assay	[105]
	8-OHdG	Aqueous	Cataract	311.6 ± 127.7 μg/mL *	ELISA	[109]
		Aqueous	Myopic	212.5 ± 103.2 μg/mL *	ELISA	[109]
	8-IPGF	Aqueous	Exfoliation syndrome	2429 ± 2940 pg/mL *	Immunoassay	[110]
		Aqueous	Cataract	529.1 ± 226.8 pg/mL *	Immunoassay	[110]
		Aqueous	Diabetic cataract	624 ± 95.7 pg/mL *	ELISA	[111]
	ON	Aqueous humor	PDR	19.43 ± 8.75 μM *	Colorimetric assay	[95]
		Vitreous humor	PDR T1DM	0.524 ± 0.27 μM *	spectrophotometric Griess reaction	[112]
		Vitreous humor	PDR T2DM	0.383 ± 0.17 μM *	spectrophotometric Griess reaction	[112]
	L-tyrosine	Tears	DR	45 μM	Chromatography electrochemical	[24]
	L-cysteine	Tears	DR	48 μM	Chromatography electrochemical	[24]
	Ascorbic acid	Tears	DR	665 μM	Chromatography electrochemical	[24]
	Uric acid	Tears	DR	328 μM	Chromatography electrochemical	[24]
Inflammatory	IL-1β	Tears	DR	16.7 ± 3.2 pg/mL *	Multiplex assay Bio-Plex system	[113]
	IL-6	Tears	DR	63.3 ± 12.3 pg/mL *	Multiplex assay Bio-Plex system	[113]
		Tears	DED	26.25 ± 5.20 pg/mL *	Multiplex bead assay	[114]
		Aqueous humor	DR	40.64 ± 16.52 pg/mL *	Multiplex bead immunoassay	[115]
		Aqueous humor	PDR	37.19 pg/mL (3.992–4577.38) **	Immunology Multiplex Assay	[83]
		Vitreous fluid	PDR progression	347.2 pg/mL (26.2–758.6) **	ELISA	[116]
		Vitreous fluid	DR	42.29 ± 10.94 pg/mL *	ELISA	[117]
		Vitreous	DR	64.2 ± 10.4 pg/mL *	Immunoassay	[118]
	IL-8	Aqueous humor	DR	42.20 ± 33.03 pg/mL *	Multiplex bead immunoassay	[115]
		Aqueous humor	PDR	25.28 pg/mL (13.21–184.62) **	Immunology Multiplex Assay	[83]
		Aqueous humor	PDR	76.55 ± 10.88 pg/mL *	ELISA	[119]
		Vitreous humor	PDR	63.55 ± 10.74 pg/mL *	ELISA	[119]
	IL-10	Aqueous humor	DR	0.24 ± 0.16 pg/mL *	Multiplex bead immunoassay	[115]
		Aqueous humor	Fuchs' uveitis	11.70 ± 6.60 pg/mL *	ELISA	[120]
		Aqueous humor	Behcet's uveitis	7.23 ± 1.73 pg/mL *	ELISA	[120]
		Vitreous humor	PDR	224.789 ± 43.801 pg/mL *	ELISA	[121]
		Vitreous	DR	4.43 ± 0.4 pg/mL *	Immunoassay	[118]
	IL-17A	Tears	DED	454.67 ± 37.70 pg/mL *	Multiplex bead analysis	[114]
	TNF-α	Tears	NPDR	1.2–5.5 pg/mL	ELISA	[122]
		Tears	PDR	9.2–21.7 pg/mL	ELISA	[122]
		Aqueous humor	DR	4.04 ± 1.83 pg/mL *	Multiplex bead immunoassay	[115]
		Aqueous humor	PDR	84.35 ± 30.82 pg/mL *	CBA technique	[123]
		Vitreous fluid	DR	155.8 ± 82.0 pg/mL *	ELISA	[124]
	IFN-γ	Tears	DR	1957.50 ± 166.1 pg/mL *	Multiplex assay Bio-Plex system	[113]
	VEGF-A	Aqueous humor	DR	357.02 ± 84.25 pg/mL *	Multiplex bead immunoassay	[115]
	VEGF	Tears	DR	270.7 ± 40.2 pg/mL *	Multiplex assay Bio-Plex system	[113]
		Aqueous humor	PDR	211.62 pg/mL (48.10–1990.98) **	Immunology Multiplex Assay	[83]
		Vitreous fluid	PDR progression	1789.2 pg/mL (198.5–3436.8) **	ELISA	[116]
		Vitreous	DR	731.20 ± 222.72 pg/mL *	ELISA	[117]
		Vitreous	DR	1491.0 ± 183.1 pg/mL *	ELISA	[125]
Apoptosis	EGF	Tears	DED	1318.9 ± 6 835.0 pg/mL *	Milliplex bead assay	[126]
	MMP-9	Tears	DED	40 ng/mL	Immunoplex	[74,127]
		Aqueous	PDR	160.3 ± 39.5 AU/mL *	Zymographic analysis	[128]
		Vitreous	Macular hole	113.9 ± 229.7 AU/mL *	Zymographic analysis	[129]
	Cytochrome-C	Tears/Cell culture	DED	-	Cell culture	[130]

* Data are expressed as the mean ± SD. ** Median values and 5th and 95th percentile values in pg/mL.

SODs are a family of enzymes that catalyze the dismutation of superoxide into oxygen and H_2O_2 [99,131]. The fluid in the anterior chamber has very low SOD activity, so there are no apparent differences between diabetic patients and controls. However, it should be noted that the humor of the anterior chamber has a high content of ascorbate, which contributes significantly to protection against superoxide [132]. Significantly lower SOD levels in the vitreous have been found in diabetic patients with PDR than in non-diabetic controls examined post mortem [132]. There is a flow of fluid from the vitreous to the choriocapillary that holds the retina together, this is where SOD can contribute to protection against superoxide radicals in the extracellular space of the retina [132].

Determination of total antioxidant capacity (TAC) is a method for rapid quantification of antioxidant efficacy in disease prevention [133,134], defined as the "cumulative action of all antioxidants present in plasma and body fluids, providing an integrated parameter rather than the simple sum of measurable antioxidant values" [135]. Reduced capacity has been observed in the AH of patients with PDR [104] and there is a close correlation between OS and morphological changes in the TM [136], in patients with PDR suggests that the involvement of the anterior chamber may be caused in part by redox state imbalances [104]. Actually, the antioxidants of each system can exert their activity with different mechanisms and different efficiency; therefore, the assessment of TAC could be much more important than the concentration of antioxidants individually [104]. Izuta et al. reported that the TAC scan of the vitreous actually increases in patients with PDR [137].

Oxidation of DNA components by ROS and reactive nitrogen species (RNS) is the main source of DNA damage leading to various types of DNA modification, including chain breakage, nucleotide oxidation, base loss, and adduct formation [138]. The radicals can react with all the purine and pyrimidine bases, as well as with the deoxyribose skeleton, generating several products, one of them 8-hidroxi-2-deoxiguanosine (8-OHdG) [139]. It has been estimated that several thousand 8-OHdG lesions can form daily in a mammalian cell, this represents 5% of all oxidative lesions, which is why it is one of the most widely used DNA oxidation biomarkers to measure OS [140]. Their levels in aqueous humor increases and the total antioxidant status decreases in the serum and aqueous humor of glaucoma patients [141]. High myopia is a degenerative disease [142]. Therefore, 8-OHdG was found at lower levels in it compared to the control group; their levels are positively correlated with central corneal thickness (CCT) and negatively correlated with long axial length (AXL). Myopic patients presented 212.5 ± 103.2 µg/mL versus 311.6 ± 127.7 µg/mL in the control group with cataract patients [109] (see Table 1).

In diabetic patients with PDR, lipid peroxidation is a very pronounced process in humoral parts of the body, which is why it is responsible for the OS induced in diabetic patients [143]. Polyunsaturated fatty acid (PUFA) molecules are present in cell membranes and are prone to oxidation due to the presence of susceptible carbon double bonds [144,145]. The eye, in general, but particularly the macula, is susceptible to OS due to its high metabolic activity and the large amount of PUFA in the photoreceptor membranes [145]. The determination of the final product of lipid oxidation is widely used as a marker of OS. MDA together with 4-hydroxy-2-nonenal (4-HNE) represent the most investigated final product of lipid oxidation. 4-HNE is a stable and biologically very active molecule whose presence is not restricted to the site of its origin, since it can diffuse through the membrane barrier [146]. The elevated blood levels of MDA in patients with diabetes reflect similar increases in the level of AH, which points to the involvement of OS and lipid peroxidation in the progression of DR to the proliferative form [95]. Cell-free vitreous is the target of 4-HNE, although aging has been reported to increase specific conjugates in retinal proteins [147]. After laser treatment, this biomarker accumulates in this relatively separate compartment giving rise to conjugated humor proteins and deterioration of the antioxidant activity by the lipoperoxidation product will make the vitreous more vulnerable to pro-oxidative effect [148]. Besides, it could interfere with the expression of different collagen subtypes effecting a change in the expression profile of the collagen subclasses, having consequences for the functional integrity of the vitreous as seen in the aged eye [149]. On the other hand, the results on the changes of MDA in the vitreous of diabetic patients with PDR obtained by Brzović-Šarić et al. agree with what has been reported, which showed an increase in vitreous MDA in patients with PDR. So in general, direct lipid peroxidation (LPO) method is more sensitive and provides a better picture of the status than MDA [105]. A significant correlation has been shown between the increase in LPO in the vitreous and an increase in the expression of VEGF; therefore, it seems that the determination of LPO in serum could be a good predictor of the onset of OS in the vitreous [105,150]. Because the retina is rich in PUFAs and there is an increase in glucose oxidation and oxygen absorption, it is susceptible to an increase in OS. The structural and functional changes observed in it may be due to lipid peroxidation of the vascular endothelium [151]. Isoprostanes (F2-IsoPs) are stable products, whose formation increases with exposure to OS, they have gained acceptance as a reliable marker of oxidative damage in both in vivo and in vitro animal models and their use is becoming more frequent [32], as a chemically stable prostaglandin-like isomers generated by the reaction of PUFAs in membrane phospholipids. They are formed in lipid membranes and then released freely by the action of phospholipase. An important fact is that they are not affected by lipid content in the diet and, therefore, its measurement in biological fluids can provide an estimate of endogenous production [152].

NO is one of the most abundant free radicals in the human body, which can also react with other ROS, this causes cellular dysfunction and apoptosis [153]. It is synthesized by endothelial cells and is an important vasoactive agent that affects blood flow along with other vascular functions [154]. In the eye, neuronal nitric oxide synthase is believed to be responsible for producing NO in photoreceptors and bipolar cells, and as far as endothelial nitric oxide synthase is concerned, it is present in vascular endothelial cells [155]. However, inducible nitric oxide synthase found in Muller's cells and in the retinal pigment epithelium could be involved in phagocytosis of the external segment of the photoreceptor, in addition to infectious, inflammatory, and ischemic processes, and in the pathogenesis of DR [156]. In a Kulaksızoglu's study, the NO levels found by the measurement of nitrite and nitrate in the aqueous humor were significantly higher in patients with PDR than in controls without diabetes [95]. Another study noted that improved NO production in the eyes of people with diabetes is consistent with reports of it as a mediator of physiological and pathological processes in the retina [157]. NO is a highly important intercellular signaling molecule that plays a role in vasodilatory responses. In addition, it is involved in basal conditions and after retinal ischemia in the control of retinal blood flow [158]. The use of aqueous humor as a biological sample is proposed to assess the course of different eye disorders showing an increase in pro-oxidative molecules and reduction in antioxidants [159,160]. In the study by Yilmaz et al. nitrite levels in vitreous humor of patients with PDR were higher than those of the control group (patients undergoing vitrectomy for idiopathic macular hole). However, among patients with PDR, there were no significant differences between the levels corresponding to type I and type II diabetes ($P = 0.56$). On the other hand, patients with type I diabetes had a mean concentration of 0.524 ± 0.27 µM in vitreous, while those with type II diabetes had a mean of 0.383 ± 0.17 µM [112] (see Table 1). Other possibility is that overproduction of NO can cause damage to the retina by disrupting the rod outer segment membrane phagocytosis by retinal pigment epithelium (RPE) cells. Then, an accumulation of ROS occurs between the photoreceptors and the RPE cells, resulting in the degeneration of the photoreceptors [161].

5.2. Inflammation: Cytokines and Relevance in DR

DM patients with advanced diabetic retinopathy have more dry eye issues associated with neurotrophic keratopathy which could cause severe vision loss due to cornea ulcer or neurotrophic ulcer, this could lead an increased expression of proinflammatory cytokines, like inducible protein-10 (IP-10) and monocyte chemoattractant protein-1 (MCP-1), and decreased levels of antiangiogenic cytokines which demonstrate that an inflammatory reaction occurs in the ocular surface of diabetic patients [162]. The alterations in the ocular surface have been associated to inflammatory processes and microvascular damage that involves mediators like Th1 and Th17 and IL-1ß, IL-17A, TNF-α, and mainly Epidermal Growth Factor (EGF) found elevated in patients with diabetes mellitus [126].

TNF-α a cytokine strongly correlated with insulin resistance by changing phosphorylation of insulin receptor substrate-1 and interfering with insulin signaling cascade and leading chronic inflammation due to leukostasis induce by VEGF, IL-1α and platelet-activating factor in the retinal vasculature, but also it is a mediator of apoptosis in retinal neurons and endothelial cells. TNF-α in tears was significantly higher in patients with PDR (13.5 pg/mL) compared with NPDR (2.8 pg/mL) [122]. In a recent cross-sectional study in Asian patients with DR, there was evaluated the differences in Total Protein Concentrations (TPC) and TNF-α in tears correlated with the three stages of NPDR (mild, moderate and severe), they found a decreased in TPC in moderate and severe NPDR compared with higher concentrations of TNF-α in the same stages, but in mild NPDR and patients without retinopathy the concentrations were similar. In this study, there was also higher levels of TNF-α correlated with higher levels of HbA1c which are explained by AGEs that activate proinflammatory pathways and promotes angiogenesis and microvascular changes in the retina [163]. TNF-α is one of the cytokines that induces disruption of the BRB by loosening the tight junctions between individual retinal endothelial cells and also between cells of the RPE, causing BRB breakdown. It promotes the irreversible adhesion of leukocytes to the endothelium and increases the production of ROS [164]. It also plays an important role in neovascularization and vasomotor reactions [165]. Actually, increased levels of TNF-α have been found in the vitreous body of patients with T2DM and PDR compared with a control group [166]. There is a study where patients with PDR were divided into subgroups based on disease progression and regression, the vitreous levels of VEGF and IL-6 were significantly higher in the eyes of patients in the progression group with 1789.2 pg/mL (198.5–3436.8) and 347.2 pg/mL (26.2–758.6), respectively (see Table 2), than they were in eyes with PDR regression [116].

Table 2. miRNA's found in human eye fluids of patients. A comparison of some of the most commonly found miRNAs in vitreous or aqueous humor from patients with and without proliferative diabetic retinopathy. PDR: proliferative diabetic retinopathy, NDM: non-diabetic, PVD: proliferative vitreoretinal disease, MH: macular hole without any other condition, DME: diabetic macular edema.

MiRNA	Role	Matrix	Comparison	Result	Author(s)
miR-200b	Angiogenesis promotion [167]	Vitreous humor	PDR vs. NDM	Higher	Gomaa A, 2017 [168]
miR-21	Fibrosis and inflammation promotion [169]	Vitreous humor	PVD vs. MH	Higher	Usui-Ouchi A, 2016 [170]
miR-15a	Angiogenesis inhibition [171]	Vitreous humor	PDR vs. MH	Higher	Hirota K, 2015 [172]
	Pro-inflammatory signaling inhibition [173]	Aqueous humor +	DME +		+ Cho Heeyoon, 2020 [174]
miR-320	Apoptosis regulation and angiogenesis repression [175]	Vitreous humor	PVD vs. MH	Higher	Usui-Ouchi A, 2016 [170]
miR-320a miR 320b	Angiogenesis repression [176]	Vitreous humor	PDR vs. MH	Higher	Hirota K, 2015 [172]
miR-184	Apoptosis promotion [177]	Aqueous humor	PDR vs. Cataract	Higher	Chen S, 2019 [178]
miR-93 miR-93-5p	Proliferation and angiogenesis promotion [179]	Vitreous humor Aqueous humor	PDR vs. NDM PDR vs. Cataract	Higher	Hirota K, 2015 [172] Chen S, 2019 [178]
miR-29a	Angiogenesis inhibition [180]	Vitreous humor Aqueous humor +	PDR vs. MH Cataract +	Higher	Hirota K 2015 [172] + Wecker T, 2016 [93]
miR-16 miR-16-5p	Tumor suppression [181]	Vitreous humor Aqueous humor +	PVD vs. MH Cataract +	Higher	Usui-Ouchi A, 2016 [170] Wecker T, 2016 [93]
miR-23a	Senescence promotion [182]	Vitreous humor	PDR vs. MH	Higher	Hirota K, 2015 [172]
miR-126	HMGB1 and VCAM-1 regulation [173]	Aqueous humor	PDR vs. Cataract	Lower	Chen S, 2019 [178]
Let-7e	Proliferation inhibition [183]	Vitreous humor	PVD vs. MH	Lower	Usui-Ouchi A, 2016 [170]
miR-204	Apoptosis promotion [184]	Vitreous humor	PVD vs. macular hole	Lower	Usui-Ouchi A, 2016 [170]

+ Biomarker found but not compared to another matrix or group.

In the inflammatory pathway, IL-6 has a role with induction of multiple process like synthesis and release of acute phase reactants and matrix metalloproteinase 9 (MMP-9), decreased tear production and apoptosis, induced differentiation of Th17, and the release of other proinflammatory cytokines like IL-1ß, the increased levels in this cytokine are particularly associated with increased metaplasia and keratinization of the ocular surface. Additionally, the secretion of interferon gamma (IFN-γ) plays a multiple role with adaptive and innate response on the ocular surfaces inducing cell loss in the conjunctival goblet cells that reduces mucin production and apoptosis on lacrimal acini, associating high levels of this cytokine with severity of the tear film dysfunction [73,113,185]. Furthermore, decrease in the concentrations of proteins lysozyme, lactoferrin and albumin is more frequent in patients with PDR than NPDR [186], that could be associated with changes on ocular surface like tear film dysfunction, progressive loss of corneal epithelia and degeneration of nerve fibers [187], increasing the risk of corneal ulcerations and deteriorate their visual quality. In other studies have been analyze tear samples in different stages of diabetic retinopathy and found a decreased in the content of tears proteins in the onset of DR as well, tear film dysfunction due to malfunctioning in the tear formation or more diluted tears. Lactotransferrin (LTF) and Immunoglobulin λ are increased in PDR together with another tear proteins expressed with frequency in PDR like lipocalin 1 (LCN1), lysozyme C (LYZ), lipophilin A, lacritin (LACRT) lipidic carriers for retinoids required for tear production, their increase are specifically associated as predictors for DR progression, some are linked to inflammation secondary to neovascularization, bleeding or macular edema [188]. Interestingly, IL-6 levels were positively correlated with the DR stage (PDR: 47.68 vs. NPDR: 29.68 pg/mL; $p < 0.001$) [115]. Elevated levels of IL-6 have been reported to participate as a proinflammatory and angiogenic factor in PDR and DM, is also involved in crossing both the blood–brain barrier and the blood–retinal barrier [189,190], and their levels in DR patients increased significantly compared to those in a non-diabetic control group. IL-6 levels were significantly correlated with PDR and it can act as one of the main drivers to generate a change in the cytokine profile in the aqueous humor of DR patients [115,191].

AH analysis provides useful information to understand the pathogenesis and responses to treatment of various eye conditions. The analysis of AH of DR patients has allow to identify some of the mediators (cytokines, chemokines, among other factors) involved in the pathogenesis of DR. Like IL-8, the concentration of VEGF is found to be increased in AH of diabetic patients [192]. Most studies have worked on aqueous humor cytokines in patients with PDR. However, the dynamic changes between the levels of cytokines in the different states of severity of DR must be analyzed in greater detail. Chen et al. found that IL-6 had positive correlations with IL-8, IP-10, leukemia inhibitory factor (LIF) and hepatocyte growth factor (HGF) in the DR group, while it presented negative correlations with IL-9, IL-21, IL-23, IL-27, and IL-31.

IL-8 is an important chemoattractant that regulates chronic leukocytic inflammation in the vascular walls and ultimately leads to capillary occlusion and retinal ischemia [193], its levels have been reported in the AH of DR patients with 42.20 ± 33.03 pg/mL (mean ± SD) [115]. IL-8 expression can be hypoxia-induced and mediated by nuclear factor kappa B (NF-kB). IL-8 can induce angiogenesis in vitro and in vivo, and its elevated levels have been found in aqueous and vitreous of patients with ocular vascular disease, including DR [194]. Other studies have reported that elevated levels of vitreous IL-8 are associated with increasing levels of retinal ischemia and an increased degree of gliotic obliteration of large vessels in patients with PDR (see Table 2) [119,193]. Sun et al. found that the level of IL-8 in aqueous humor was significantly higher than that in the vitreous in PDR patients [119].

IL-10 is an anti-inflammatory cytokine and antiangiogenic mediator produced by monocytes and macrophages its antitumor effects have been associated with its ability to prevent angiogenesis associated with tumor growth [195]. In Mao C study, the median IL-10 concentration was higher in the vitreous of the PDR patients (224.789 pg/mL) than in the control group (160.143 pg/mL) and it was statistically significantly, which was different from Hernández C study [121,196]. A predominance of macrophages (50%) has been determined in the vitreous samples of patients with PDR by cytological examination, this could explain the greater production of IL-10 resistant to other proinflammatory cytokines due to the increase in macrophages [125]. It suppresses the expression of the receptor for proinflammatory cytokines such as IL-1 and tumor necrosis factor α (TNF-α) and inhibits the activation of its receptors by reducing the synthesis of these cytokines it limits inflammation. Its antiangiogenic effect has recently been shown to be associated with the downregulation of VEGF expression [197]. Dong et al. found that IL-10 levels in the AH decreased with increasing severity of DR.

TNF-α is one of the main inflammatory response cytokines with chemotactic action on monocytes and neutrophils that activates them as macrophages, improving their cytotoxicity, while being one of the mediators of this cytotoxicity [198], with levels in aqueous humor of 4.04 ± 1.83 pg/mL (mean ± SD) in DR patients [115]. VEGF, also known as vascular permeability factor (VPF or vasculotropin), considered today the main factor controlling angiogenesis and vascular permeability and causes much of the pathogenesis of PDR and diabetic macular edema [199]. It is produced by endothelial cells, macrophages, CD4 lymphocytes, plasma cells, among others [200,201]. One study showed that the VEGF level was significantly elevated in diabetic subjects compared to the non-diabetic control group. However, there was no correlation between VEGF and DR severity ($p = 0.357$) [115].

The vitreous cavity contains different types of unique cells, such as retinal cells, RPE, choroid, and retinal vessels. Although the AH and the vitreous fluid do not flow with each other, some proteins can be exchanged between these two compartments. IL-6, IL-8, VEGF, and TNF-α have been observed to be elevated in serum and vitreous fluid from patients with DR [202]. Murugeswari et al. found that the levels of IL-6, IL-8, MCP-1, and VEGF present in the vitreous humor were significantly higher in PDR patients than in patients with macular hole [203]. In another study, a comprehensive analysis of mediators in the vitreous fluids of patients with PDR and in patients with other eye diseases was performed and elevated levels of VEGF, MCP-1, IL-8 and IL-6 were found compared to the control group [204]. IL-6 normally participates in acute phase reactions such as hematopoiesis, IL-2 induction, and differentiation of keratinocytes and B and T lymphocytes. In vitro studies suggest that NO may be acting as the intermediate molecule in IL-6-induced VEGF synthesis. Precisely, the synthesis of IL-6 can be induced in vitro by hypoxia and tissue hyperglycemia [205].

Interleukin 17 (IL-17) plays an important role in a wide variety of immunological diseases, but on the ocular surface it promotes neutrophil infiltration in tissues that induce synthesis and secretion of matrix metalloproteinases and ROS that generate disruption in the corneal epithelium, loss of epithelial functionality and induction of apoptosis. This contributes to the induction of neovascularization with stimulation of proangiogenic factor and modulation of cytoskeleton, which was examined in the vitreous and plasma of patients with DR, with levels significantly increased in PDR [114,206,207].

5.3. Apoptosis

Apoptosis is the most studied type of cell death in diabetic retinopathy its characteristics are well defined and it is easily detected with techniques such as TUNEL (Terminal dUTP Nick End Labeling). Despite this, there are types of cell death that are difficult to detect due to the lack of defined markers and available techniques [208]. The hyperosmolar state has a relevant change in various tissues, but in tear film and cornea increases desquamation, loss of intercellular connections, disruption of cell membranes and decreases cytoplasmic density, it was found that proinflammatory stimulus in the corneal epithelium increases the expression of cytokines like IL-1ß, TNF-α, IL-8, MMP-9 activating the MAPK signaling pathway then the expression of proapoptotic markers (Fas, Fas ligand, APO2, CD40 and CD40 ligand) and cytochrome-c, this mediates an apoptotic pathway reported in vitro with an hyperosmotic state (≥450 mOsm) which converge on proteolytic activation of caspase-3 capable of cleaving various cellular proteinases to finally cause apoptotic death [130]. An increase in pericyte apoptosis in retinal tissue of diabetic patients compared to non-diabetic patients has been demonstrated with the use of TUNEL staining [208,209].

Lipocalin is a tear endonuclease which plays a role in the catalytic activity of DNA and its effect in the concentration of NaCl, Mg^{2+}, Ca^{2+} and variation in pH facilitates lipocalin its role in prevention of viral infections and anti-inflammatory activity by regelation of tear viscosity, capture and release of lipids, inactivating endonucleases and pathogens binding sites on the ocular surface [210,211]. In diabetic patients with neurotrophic keratopathy, have been found increasing levels of AGE's products in cornea which activates a signal pathway mediated by NK-kB, generating an increase on oxidative stress, and anormal accumulation of MMP-9, this is correlated with ocular surface inflammation and induce a cycle of damage and apoptosis [212,213]. Cathepsins are a group of proteases key players in extracellular space, they have collagenase and elastase activity and participate in extracellular matrix (ECM) remodeling, but also are signaling molecules. Cathepsin C and B are present in tears, but its role in the ocular surface is not well explained. Cathepsin S is involved in initiating inflammatory responses by effecting degradation of lysosomal protein and ECM which is essential for homeostasis and cellular differentiation [127].

Matrix metalloproteinases (MMPs) are a family of calcium-activated zinc-containing enzymes that are involved in turnover and remodeling of the ECM and collectively are capable of breaking down most of their protein components, including collagens, laminin, fibronectin, elastin and other components. MMPs can also degrade a number of non-ECM proteins, including growth factors, chemokines, cytokines, and some surface receptors [214]. Metalloproteinases are involved in a number of both physiological and pathological processes, the enzymes may participate in pathological processes such as neovascularization [128]. MMP-2 and MMP-9 can degrade pigment epithelial derived factor (PEDF), which is the main antiangiogenic protein of the eye, specifically it is a 50 kDa glycoprotein highly expressed in the retinal pigment epithelium [215]. We know that one of the first characteristics of DR is the rupture of the blood–retina barrier. This results in vascular permeability in the retina and the development of retinal edema. These types of findings suggest that elevated MMP expression in AH may facilitate an increase in vascular permeability [216]. MMP-9 belongs to the group of type IV collagenases which plays an important role in new vessel formation and were previously found to be upregulated by VEGF [217]. Increased levels of pro-MMP-9 and activated MMP-9 have previously been found in the vitreous of patients with PDR associated with vitreous hemorrhage [218]. MMPs can also act in the early stages of DR, in the breakdown of the BRB and in the destruction of the tight junctions of endothelial cells [216]. Among the different MMPs examined in the vitreous samples, only the levels of MMP-2 and MMP-9 levels are significantly increased in the PDR eyes. In another study both metalloproteinases are present in the vitreous samples from PDR patients, being MMP-9 the only one elevated in PDR patients [128]. Noda et al. discovered that the vitreous proliferative membranes in diabetic retinopathy, in addition to having elevated levels of MMP-9, contain high levels of MMP-2. Furthermore, elevated levels of MMP-9 have been previously reported in the vitreous humor and fibrovascular membranes of patients with PDR [219].

The release of cytochrome c (*cyt c*) from the mitochondria is a fundamental step for the beginning of the apoptotic process [220]. *Cyt c* is a small globular protein that contains iron porphyrin cofactor (heme c) that covalently binds to the unique polypeptide chain. Its main function is its participation in the electron transport chain of the inner mitochondrial membrane (IMM). *Cyt c* is reversibly reduced and oxidized as an electron is transferred from ubiquinol-cytochrome c reductase (complex III) to *cyt c* oxidase (complex IV) in the mitochondrial respiratory chain [221]. Premature death of retinal cells occurs prior to the development of other lesions characteristic of retinopathy, suggesting that it may play a critical role in the development of DR [222]. The rate of apoptosis of vascular and nonvascular retinal cells in diabetes is low, but statistically higher than normal, which is consistent with the slow development of DR [223]. *Cyt c* has the ability to perform a variety of functions depending on the site and conditions of the cell where it is located; These properties have allowed it to be identified as an "extremely multifunctional" protein (EMF) [224]. So the structural and biological properties of the complex (ferric) *Cyt c-CL* (cytochrome c—cardiolipin), promotes the transformation of proteins into a peroxidase in the early stages of cellular apoptosis [225]. Besides, *cyt c* in mammalian cells can activate caspases, a family of cysteine proteases that have within their functions that of cleaving crucial substrates to induce cell dismantling [225].

Caspase-3 activation is a slower process compared to increased OS in diabetes, or from another point of view, its activation may be occurring as a consequence of increased OS [226]. Caspases involved in the activation of proinflammatory cytokines and the initiation and execution of apoptosis [223]. Because apoptosis of retinal capillary cells probably contributes to capillary "dropout" and retinal ischemia in DR, there is an interest in caspases that may be involved in initiating and executing this apoptotic process [223]. Caspase-3 is the executioner caspase that plays a central role in the proteolytic cascade during apoptosis its immunoreactivity occurred in ganglion cells in diabetic retinas, following their apoptotic death induced by ischemia, excitotoxicity, axotomy, and chronic ocular hypertension, their inhibition reduces apoptotic cell death induced in retinal cells [227]. Nuclear factor-kβ (NF-kβ) is an important polyphenic nuclear factor which participates in apoptosis and cellular neovascularization, it can be activated by a variety of signals such as IL-1β, TNF-α, and OS. Several studies have shown that is closely related to inflammation, the appearance of tumors, cellular apoptosis, among other pathological processes. However, the main pathological changes in the DR include retinal cell apoptosis and neovascularization. This highlights that NF-kβ plays a role in DR [228,229]. In another scenario when cells are stimulated by hypoxia, hyperglycemia, and some inflammatory cytokines, the NF-kβ-specific inhibitor protein (IkB-α) is phosphorylated and degraded just to be released and activated, entering the nucleus to regulate gene transcription [229].

The BRB function of endothelial cells is supported by surrounding cells, such as Müller cells, pericytes, and astrocytes. As the blood–retinal barrier depends to a large extent on this microenvironment where the function of a specific type of cell depends on the support of other types of cells, any cellular injury or cellular loss will have great effects on the proper function of the retinal barrier and, in fact, any retinal function [230,231]. The NF-kβ present in the subretinal membranes and micro vessels is activated in response to increased ROS and AGE, which in turn further activate the apoptosis process. The activated NF-kβ is then further bound to nuclear DNA and thereby overexpresses different genes that lead to free radical production and further cell death [232]. Activated NF-kβ also increases the expression of cytokines IL-1b, IL-6, and IL-8 and the proapoptotic molecule caspase-3 in vitreous fluid and serum, leading to inflammation-mediated cellular apoptosis [233]. Together, the activation of NF-kβ, TNF-α, and interleukins improve MMP-9 transcription leading to DNA alkylation and the development of DR [234].

6. Metabolic Memory of Oxidative Stress in Diabetic Retinopathy

Several studies maintain that epigenetic modification is a significant factor in the development of DR. The duration of hyperglycemia decides if better subsequent glycemic control would be effective in the DR, which implies that the sustained state of hyperglycemia produces a metabolic memory phenomenon and be attributed to epigenetics, which may be the reason for inter-individual differences in drug response and variation in the progression of diabetes complications [235–237].

There have been several epigenetic modifications studied in DR: methylation directly to DNA molecule, which can repress transcription of certain genes; chromatin remodeling and modifications to the DNA condensing proteins, histones, which can also activate or suppress DNA on its own; and non-coding RNA that post-transcriptionally regulates gene expression. Although there are more epigenetics modifications known involved in DM or cancer, these alterations are the most studied in DR functioning as potential prognostic, therapeutic, or diagnostic biomarkers.

6.1. DNA Methylation

The most primitive epigenetic modification is DNA methylation and, according to various studies, it has a correlation with the progression of DR. In DNA methylation the methyl group is transferred from S-adenosylmethionine (SAM) to DNA molecules, this reaction is catalyzed by DNA methyltransferases. It was found that patients with DR have shown a significantly higher level of DNA methylation compared to those without DR, indicating that increased DNA methylation is a relevant component in the development of DR [237]. Another study revealed that methylation and activation of the matrix metalloproteinase 9 (MMP-9) gene associated with DR has an important role in accelerating apoptosis of retinal vascular endothelium [238]. This indicates that DNA methylation in DR is a highly dynamic process, which involves various epigenetic changes targeting extracellular matrix, manganese superoxide dismutase (MnSOD) also cross-linking with OS, and mitochondrial homeostasis causing mitochondrial dysfunction with subsequent capillary damage [238–241].

ROS generated from mitochondrial oxidative phosphorylation is the most representative source of OS in endothelial cells, which cause peroxidation of PUFAs, protein damage and consequently mitochondrial DNA (mtDNA) damage [239,242,243]. Methylation of mtDNA has recently been associated with the development of diseases and as a potential biomarker. Iacobazzi divided mtDNA methylation into global mtDNA methylation biomarkers, such as 5-methylcytosine (5mc) derived from the incorporation of a methyl group at position 5 of cytosine, and 5-hydroxymethylcytosine (5hmc), produced from 5mc through a hydroxymethylation reaction catalyzed by ten-eleven-translocation, which are related to aging and neurodegenerative disorders; and specific methylation biomarkers such as ND6 gene, which is suppressed under OS conditions by increased DNA methyltransferase (DNMT) [244]. As a general methylation biomarker, 5hmc can be seen at rac family small GTPase 1, which leads to increased binding of NF-kB linking this epigenetic modification with inflammation in DR [245]. In the retina, there is a more specific area where methylation is occurring called *D-loop* where transcription and replication of mtDNA is controlled [243,246] which has been used as a biomarker in a clinical study that showed significantly higher methylation rates in the serum of patients with PDR than patients without DR, these had higher methylation rates than non-diabetic patients [247] functioning as a novel diagnostic tool. Another potential biomarker related with DNA methylation in DR is homocysteine, of which high levels have been associated with increased risk of developing DR in diabetic patients, and with higher global DNA methylation probably linking it to altered metabolic memory phenomenon [248,249]. Interestingly, high homocysteine levels have been associated with increased inflammatory cytokines and activation of NF-kB [250].

Several therapeutic approaches have been assessed targeting mitochondrial dysfunction despite the low specificity of DNMT, synthetic DNA methylation inhibitors such as hydralazine and procainamide are being evaluated in clinical trials, or polyphenols like resveratrol have shown to directly inhibit DNMTs as well as being a powerful antioxidant which ultimately lead to epigenetic changes with altered gene expression [251–254].

6.2. Modification of Histones

Other relevant epigenetic alteration is the modification of histones, which has also been a key contributor to the pathophysiology of the DR. Histones are proteins in the nucleus related to DNA and play a role in regulation of gene expression and can be post-translational modified by methylation, acetylation, ubiquitination and phosphorylation regulating chromatin structure, and these histones can have an active cross-talk with other histone modifications [235,255]. Relevant examples of these epigenetic changes are histone acetyltransferase (HAT) and histone deacetylases are involved in regulating gene expression in the complications of diabetes [256]. For example, H3 acetylated histone expression was decreased in induced diabetic models. Furthermore, it was discovered that these changes were irreversible once the blood glucose of these rats was restored to a normal level, indicating that the development of DR is associated with the modification of histones and that it would also be participating in the phenomenon of metabolic memory [241,257]. When there is a high-glucose environment in the retina, histone acetylation is increased due to a decreased activity of histone deacetylase (HDAC) inducing an increased expression of pro-inflammatory cytokines in Müller cells [256].

During DR, an alteration of mitochondrial homeostasis and dynamics occurs, where a vicious circle is created between the alteration of mitochondrial enzymes that induce the formation of superoxide, which in turn alters the physiology of the organelles. Furthermore, dysfunction of the repair pathways generates even more mitochondrial damage [239]. However, regulation of the mtDNA replication/repair machinery has the ability to prevent mitochondrial dysfunction and the development of DR to some extent [239,258]. Decreased mitochondrial SOD2 and inhibition of Nrf2 (nuclear factor-(erythroid-derived 2-)like 2), a transcription factor affecting antioxidants, have been observed. What happens is that during the state of OS, Nrf2 translocate to the nucleus where it binds to the antioxidant response element (ARE). On the other hand, Keap1, an inhibitor of Nrf2, binds it in the cytosol and leads it to proteomic degradation through cullin-3-dependent degradation [2,252,259]. Moreover, in vitro studies have shown metabolic memory phenomenon through exposure of retinal capillary cells to high glucose concentrations, inducing epigenetic modification of SOD2; the gene that encodes for MnSOD, by decreasing methylation of H3K4 at Sod2 promoter predisposing to worsening of the oxidative stress damage cycle [255,260]. There have been different therapeutic approaches regarding histone acetylation/deacetylation in diabetic nephropathy; histone deacetylase inhibitors like Vorinostat may have a protecting effect by decreasing OS, agents like sodium butyrate inhibited HDAC activity and thus elevated the expression of Nrf2, both protecting against renal injury [256]. These therapeutic approaches have yet to be assessed in DR, but HDAC inhibition may have ameliorative effects in diabetic microvascular complications.

A study of the effects of diabetes on nuclear–mitochondrial communication in the retina revealed that the mitochondrial biogenesis of the retina is weakened in diabetes and is under the control of superoxide radicals. Therefore, this makes us think that the regulation of biogenesis by pharmaceutical or molecular means could provide a way to prevent the development/progression of DR [261]. Examples of these are approaches with intravitreal adeno associated viral MnSOD which showed to reduce retinal capillary basement membrane thickness, inhibit apoptosis of these capillaries, by effectively overexpressing MnSOD, suggesting an ameliorative effect on the metabolic memory phenomenon [254,262]. Moreover, different approaches have been made with different polyphenols, the most promising one is resveratrol that is associated with decreased phosphorylation of 5'-adenosine monophosphate activated protein kinase (AMPK) that regulates histone deacetylase Sirtuin 1 (Sirt1) which may ultimately suppress NF-kB activation [252].

6.3. Chromatin Remodeling

Chromatin remodeling is the conjunction of various structural and/or molecular changes that ultimately modify DNA functions as expression, replication and recombination of genes. Therefore, without having genomic alterations the production of proteins will be affected and may be inherited to offspring [258].

Histone modifiers (acetylation, deacetylation, methylation, and demethylation enzymes), histone chaperons and ATP-dependent chromatin remodelers are responsible for chromatin restructuring [263]. Four families of chromatin remodelers have been described: SWI/SNF, NO80, CHD and ISWI. This very last is associated to the Base Excision Repair (BER) and the Nucleotide Excision Repair (NER) mechanisms to help repair DNA after an oxidative insult [264]. Chromatin remodeling by its remodeler family SWI/SNF contributes to the response against stress and senescence, at the same time mitochondrial dysfunction induces chromatin remodeling responses [265]. The thioredoxing-interacting protein (TXNIP) is a protein known to have an important impact over OS, inflammation and apoptosis in the pancreas and the retina [266], in recent years it has been considered that these modifications lead to chromatin remodeling in retinal cells. During hyperglycemia some molecules such as Angiotensin II, transforming growth factor-β (TGF-β) and AGEs are overexpressed leading to enhanced activation of their receptors causing augmented production or intracellular factors that end up modifying chromatin structure [267].

The DNA binding proteins HMGBs (high mobility group B) can mediate nucleosome remodeling. Such proteins lower their affinity to DNA and their function when oxidized [268]. OS promotes alterations in chromatin by histone acetylation and increased activation of NF-kB resulting in major inflammatory genes expression [269]. Second messengers are also able to modify chromatin structure via chromatin-binding proteins. PI5P (phosphoinositide phosphatidylinositol-5-phosphate) is an example, its production augments in OS environment, it binds to ING2 (inhibitor of growth family member 2) to repress pro-proliferative genes and promote apoptosis [270,271].

6.4. Non-Coding RNA

Non-Coding RNAs are RNAs that are not translated into proteins, and instead they play a role as gene expression modulators. There are two types of non-coding RNAs classified by their length, small RNAs formed by 20–30 nucleotides and LncRNAs (long non-coding RNAs) having up to 200 nucleotides [272]. Small non-coding RNAs (20–30 nucleotides) are categorized as microRNAs (miRNAs), short interfering RNAs (siRNAs), and piwi-interacting RNAs (piRNAs). The first two are more similar between each other as they both have double-stranded precursors, while piRNAs appear to derive from single-stranded precursors [273].

MiRNAs have a regulatory function on endogenous genes, and siRNAs protect the genome from invasive nucleic acids [273]. Both molecules work primarily by silencing genes recognized by a specific sequence in the miRNA or siRNA chain. Normally, miRNAs inhibit the expression of their target genes promoting its mRNAs degradation or inhibition of its translation [274], but this programmed action may be modified in response to external threats (viruses, transposons) or changes within the cell. Then, siRNAs will co-opt the invader into their own mechanism and prevent it from its expression; on the other hand, miRNAs may be diluted or exchanged by different miRNAs or even new miRNAs will be expressed to silence genes that will have the effect of counteracting the previous silencing [273,275]. Most lncRNAs are transcribed by RNA polymerase II and spliced into various isoforms which act as epigenetic regulators. They can regulate DNA polymerase activity, around 20% of lncRNAs recruit chromatin remodeling complexes to repress transcription of target genes [276,277].

Through the years non-coding RNAs have been related to many degenerative illnesses, including Alzheimer, cancer and diabetes [272,274,277]. As mentioned before, when cells encounter environmental modifications, such as hyperglycemia, they promote altered expression of miRNAs. The downregulation of certain miRNAs (miR-126 and miR-200b) and the upregulation of others (miR-18a, miR-20b, miR31 an mir-155) are now related to augmented VEGF production [278], miR-146 is a miRNA that functions as a negative feedback to NF-kB activation induced by IL-1β in retinal endothelial cells and it is also upregulated after 3 months following the onset of diabetes [278].

Some miRNas such as miR27b respond to stress by reducing the expression of pro-antioxidant proteins as Nrf2 resulting in a pro-oxidant environment [279]. mR27b also has a pro-angiogenic effect targeting Notch ligand D114, Sprouty -2, PPARgamma and Semaphorin 6A [280]. Another miRNA; miR-211 is upregulated in diabetes causing impaired expression of sirtuin-1 [281], a protein that protects mitochondria from damage [282]. In the past years over 47 miRNAs have been found differential between patients with diabetes and patients with DR, five of them, including miR-21 implicated in angiogenic processes, have been considered as biomarkers for early detection of such microvascular complication [283,284].

miRNAs associate with groups of proteins known as Argonaute proteins to silence the target gene. Argonaute proteins are usually found scattered in the cytoplasm, in oxidative stress conditions they tend to gather around stress granules, an action mediated by miRNAs [285]. On the other hand, argonaute2 is enhanced by hypoxia which leads to an inhibited maturation of miRNAs that respond to stress as defense mechanisms [286]. Previously mentioned miRNAs have been found in serum, some of them and others are found in vitreous humor and aqueous humor in PDR as seen in Table 2. miR-126 has recently been considered as a potential serum biomarker for PDR nonetheless, other studies have shown that the concentration of miRNAs in eye matrices with PDR differs even two times fold from those in serum [287].

H-19, a lncRNA that prevents glucose-induced endothelial mesenchymal transition in the retina, is downregulated in hyperglycemic conditions leading to activation of endothelial transition via TFGF-beta [288]. A recent study has found that lncRNA AK077216 is downregulated in subjects with DR independently from glycemic conditions, this lncRNA is able to inhibit ARPE-19 cells apoptosis via inhibition of miR-383 proapototic function [289]. The proliferation promoting lncRNA BANCR has also been found overexpressed in patients with DR which may play a role as a potential therapeutic target [290,291]. According to Awata and cols. there is an association between susceptibility to DR and lncRNA RP1-90L14 [91].

Studies have shown that these alterations occur early in hyperglycemic states in retinal and endothelial cells [292], furthermore; they are maintained even after returning to normoglycemia [293–295]. Since non-coding RNA, specially miRNAs have a regulatory function, relatively prompt response to alterations in the body and, more importantly, such responses are maintained for a period of time after glycemic control they represent a potential therapeutic target in DR to delay its progression. Nevertheless more studies are needed so far.

7. Conclusions

In the review article, we summarize the studies and take information that contributed to elucidating the most widely used biomarkers that produce more information about the different stages of diabetic retinopathy. Currently, there is still no definitive marker for the detection of early stages of DR or even one that can be detected before retinopathy develops. The reviewed studies have suggested a large number of potential markers, however, it must be taken into account that the multifactorial etiology of DR further complicates the detection strategy, so instead of a single definitive marker, the use of a panel or set of markers representing each affected aspect in DR. For this, it is necessary to choose a biological matrix that meets characteristics such as accessibility, suitability and representativeness of the disease state. At the ocular level, there are very few biomarkers whose measurement has FDA approval. Most of the biomarkers are exploratory in nature; however, they are very useful for solving issues during drug development. Tears, aqueous humor, and vitreous are among the fluid ocular matrices most frequently used for human biomarker evaluation. The use of these matrices has posed difficulties, including non-standardized collection processes and little available sample volume. For this reason, it is of great importance to continue working on studies that provide more information to establish optimized processing and analysis methods in order to make the most of the information obtained from the measurement of biomarkers in them. Large-scale prospective multicenter studies are necessary to be able to accurately determine the veracity and reliability of various biomarkers in the early stages of DR. Therefore, the OS associated with chronic hyperglycemia plays a central role in the stimulation and alteration of the molecular and biochemical signaling pathways along with cellular damage involved in the DR, the evidence suggests that metabolic defects that alter epigenetic substrates they will also affect epigenetic chromatin modifications. The epigenetic alterations that were discussed play a critical role in the pathogenesis of DR, further analysis and comparison of the results that have been obtained so far is necessary to also consolidate the path towards the discovery of new treatments and therapeutic strategies.

Author Contributions: First, second and thirth chapter preparation, A.K.L.-C. & A.D.R.-C.; fourth and fifth chapter preparation, A.K.L.-C., M.G.M.-R. & S.G.H.-O.; sixth chapter preparation, C.O.-M. & R.R.R.-R.; Figures, A.K.L.-C. & M.G.M.-R.; Tables, A.K.L.-C., M.G.M.-R. & C.O.-M.; Investigation, A.K.L.-C., M.G.M.-R., C.O.-M. & R.R.R.-R.; Original Draft Preparation, A.K.L.-C., M.G.M.-R., C.O.-M., R.R.R.-R. & A.D.R.-C.; Supervision, D.E.A.-S., J.A.C.-G., A.H.-C. & S.G.H.-O.; Project administration, E.G.C.-M. & A.D.R.-C.; Writing-review and editing, All authors. All authors have read and agreed to the published version of the manuscript.

Funding: This research received no external funding.

Conflicts of Interest: The authors declare no conflict of interest.

References

1. Campochiaro, P.A. Molecular pathogenesis of retinal and choroidal vascular diseases. *Prog. Retin. Eye Res.* **2015**, *49*, 67–81. [CrossRef] [PubMed]
2. Mahajan, N.; Arora, P.; Sandhir, R.A.-O. Perturbed Biochemical Pathways and Associated Oxidative Stress Lead to Vascular Dysfunctions in Diabetic Retinopathy. *Oxid. Med. Cell. Longev.* **2019**. [CrossRef] [PubMed]
3. Cunha-Vaz, J.; Bernardes, R.; Lobo, C. Blood-retinal barrier. *Eur. J. Ophthalmol.* **2011**, *21*, S3–S9. [CrossRef]
4. Alder, V.A.; Su, E.N.; Yu, D.Y.; Cringle, S.; Yu, D.-Y. Overview of studies on metabolic and vascular regulatory changes in early diabetic retinopathy. *Aust. N. Z. J. Ophthalmol.* **1998**, *26*, 141–148. [CrossRef] [PubMed]
5. Pusparajah, P.; Lee, L.-H.; Kadir, K.A. Molecular Markers of Diabetic Retinopathy: Potential Screening Tool of the Future? *Front. Physiol.* **2016**, *7*, 200. [CrossRef] [PubMed]
6. Aiello, L.P.; Cahill, M.T.; Wong, J.S. Systemic considerations in the management of diabetic retinopathy. *Am. J. Ophthalmol.* **2001**, *132*, 760–776. [CrossRef]
7. Yau, J.W.; Rogers, S.L.; Kawasaki, R.; Lamoureux, E.L.; Kowalski, J.W.; Bek, T.; Chen, S.-J.; Dekker, J.M.; Fletcher, A.; Grauslund, J.; et al. Global prevalence and major risk factors of diabetic retinopathy. *Diabetes Care* **2012**, *35*, 556–564. [CrossRef]

8. Cecilia, O.-M.; Alberto, C.-G.J.; José, N.-P.; Germán, C.-M.E.; Karen, L.-C.A.; Miguel, R.-P.L.; Raúl, R.-R.R.; Daniel, R.-C.A. Oxidative Stress as the Main Target in Diabetic Retinopathy Pathophysiology. *J. Diabetes Res.* **2019**, *2019*, 8562408. [CrossRef]
9. Zheng, Y.; He, M.; Congdon, N. The worldwide epidemic of diabetic retinopathy. *Indian J. Ophthalmol.* **2012**, *60*, 428–431. [CrossRef]
10. Avidor, D.; Loewenstein, A.; Waisbourd, M.; Nutman, A. Cost-effectiveness of diabetic retinopathy screening programs using telemedicine: A systematic review. *Cost Eff. Resour. Alloc.* **2020**, *18*, 16. [CrossRef]
11. Whitehead, M.; Wickremasinghe, S.; Osborne, A.; Wijngaarden, P.; Martin, K.R. Diabetic retinopathy: A complex pathophysiology requiring novel therapeutic strategies. *Expert Opin. Biol. Ther.* **2018**, *18*, 1257–1270. [CrossRef]
12. Robles-Rivera, R.R.; Castellanos-González, J.A.; Olvera-Montaño, C.; Flores-Martin, R.A.; López-Contreras, A.K.; Arevalo-Simental, D.E.; Cardona-Muñoz, E.G.; Roman-Pintos, L.M.; Rodríguez-Carrizalez, A.D. Adjuvant Therapies in Diabetic Retinopathy as an Early Approach to Delay Its Progression: The Importance of Oxidative Stress and Inflammation. *Oxid. Med. Cell. Longev.* **2020**, *2020*, 3096470. [CrossRef] [PubMed]
13. Santiago, A.R.; Boia, R.; Aires, I.D.; Ambrósio, A.F.; Fernandes, R. Sweet Stress: Coping With Vascular Dysfunction in Diabetic Retinopathy. *Front. Physiol.* **2018**, *13*, 820. [CrossRef] [PubMed]
14. Flaxman, S.R.; Bourne, R.R.A.; Resnikoff, S.; Ackland, P.; Braithwaite, T.; Cicinelli, M.V.; Das, A.; Jonas, J.B.; Keeffe, J.; Kempen, J.H.; et al. Global causes of blindness and distance vision impairment 1990–2020: A systematic review and meta-analysis. *Lancet Glob. Health* **2017**, *5*, 1221–1234. [CrossRef]
15. van der Giet, M.; Henkel, C.; Schuchardt, M.; Tolle, M. Anti-VEGF Drugs in Eye Diseases: Local Therapy with Potential Systemic Effects. *Curr. Pharm. Des.* **2015**, *21*, 3548–3556. [CrossRef] [PubMed]
16. Saccà, S.C.; Roszkowska, A.M.; Izzotti, A. Environmental light and endogenous antioxidants as the main determinants of non-cancer ocular diseases. *Mutat. Res. Rev. Mutat. Res.* **2013**, *752*, 153–171. [CrossRef] [PubMed]
17. Riley, P.A. Free Radicals in Biology: Oxidative Stress and the Effects of Ionizing Radiation. *Int. J. Radiat. Biol.* **1994**, *65*, 27–33. [CrossRef]
18. Richdale, K.; Chao, C.; Hamilton, M. Eye care providers' emerging roles in early detection of diabetes and management of diabetic changes to the ocular surface: A review. *BMJ Open Diabetes Res. Care* **2020**, *8*, e001094. [CrossRef]
19. DeMill, D.L.; Hussain, M.; Pop-Busui, R.; Shtein, R.M. Ocular surface disease in patients with diabetic peripheral neuropathy. *Br. J. Ophthalmol.* **2016**, *100*, 924. [CrossRef]
20. Yoon, K.C.; Im, S.K.; Seo, M.S. Changes of Tear Film and Ocular Surface in Diabetes Mellitus. *Korean J. Ophthalmol.* **2004**, *18*, 168–174. [CrossRef]
21. Behl, T.; Kaur, I.; Kotwani, A. Implication of oxidative stress in progression of diabetic retinopathy. *Surv. Ophthalmol.* **2016**, *61*, 187–196. [CrossRef] [PubMed]
22. Johnson, F.; Giulivi, C. Superoxide dismutases and their impact upon human health. *Mol. Asp. Med.* **2005**, *26*, 340–352. [CrossRef] [PubMed]
23. Leonard, S.S.; Harris, G.K.; Shi, X. Metal-induced oxidative stress and signal transduction. *Free Radic. Biol. Med.* **2004**, *37*, 1921–1942. [CrossRef] [PubMed]
24. Chen, Y.; Mehta, G.; Vasiliou, V. Antioxidant defenses in the ocular surface. *Ocul. Surf.* **2009**, *7*, 176–185. [CrossRef]
25. Hardy, P.; Beauchamp, M.; Sennlaub, F.; Gobeil, F.J.; Tremblay, L.; Mwaikambo, B.; Lachapelle, P.; Chemtob, S. New insights into the retinal circulation: Inflammatory lipid mediators in ischemic retinopathy. *Prostaglandins Leukot. Essent. Fat. Acids* **2005**, *72*, 301–325. [CrossRef]
26. Bishop, P.N. The role of extracellular matrix in retinal vascular development and preretinal neovascularization. *Exp. Eye Res.* **2015**, *133*, 30–36. [CrossRef]
27. Géhl, Z.; Bakondi, E.; Resch, M.D.; Hegedűs, C.; Kovács, K.; Lakatos, P.; Szabó, A.; Nagy, Z.; Virág, L. Diabetes-induced oxidative stress in the vitreous humor. *Redox Biol.* **2016**, *9*, 100–103. [CrossRef]
28. Blokhina, O.; Virolainen, E.; Fagerstedt, K.V. Antioxidants, oxidative damage and oxygen deprivation stress: A review. *Ann. Bot.* **2003**, *91*, 179–194. [CrossRef]
29. Ohia, S.E.; Opere, C.A.; LeDay, A.M. Pharmacological consequences of oxidative stress in ocular tissues. *Mutat. Res. Fundam. Mol. Mech. Mutagenes.* **2005**, *579*, 22–36. [CrossRef]

30. Rose, R.C.; Richer, S.P.; Bode, A.M. Ocular Oxidants and Antioxidant Protection. *Proc. Soc. Exp. Biol. Med.* **1998**, *217*, 397–407. [CrossRef]
31. Shang, F.; Lu, M.; Dudek, E.; Reddan, J.; Taylor, A. Vitamin C and vitamin E restore the resistance of GSH-depleted lens cells to H_2O_2. *Free Radic. Biol. Med.* **2003**, *34*, 521–530. [CrossRef]
32. Shichi, H. Cataract formation and prevention. *Expert Opin. Investig. Drugs* **2004**, *13*, 691–701. [CrossRef] [PubMed]
33. Beatty, S.; Koh, H.-H.; Phil, M.; Henson, D.; Boulton, M. The Role of Oxidative Stress in the Pathogenesis of Age-Related Macular Degeneration. *Surv. Ophthalmol.* **2000**, *45*, 115–134. [CrossRef]
34. Kowluru, R.; Kern, T.S.; Engerman, R.L. Abnormalities of retinal metabolism in diabetes or galactosemia II. Comparison of γ-glutamyl transpeptidase in retina and cerebral cortex, and effects of antioxidant therapy. *Curr. Eye Res.* **1994**, *13*, 891–896. [CrossRef] [PubMed]
35. Lu, M.; Kuroki, M.; Amano, S.; Tolentino, M.; Keough, K.; Kim, I.; Bucala, R.; Adamis, A.P. Advanced glycation end products increase retinal vascular endothelial growth factor expression. *J. Clin. Investig.* **1998**, *101*, 1219–1224. [CrossRef]
36. van Reyk, D.M.; Gillies, M.C.; Davies, M.J. The retina: Oxidative stress and diabetes. *Redox Rep.* **2003**, *8*, 187–192. [CrossRef] [PubMed]
37. Domènech, E.; Marfany, G. The Relevance of Oxidative Stress in the Pathogenesis and Therapy of Retinal Dystrophies. *Antioxidants* **2020**, *9*, 347. [CrossRef]
38. Rashid, K.; Akhtar-Schaefer, I.; Langmann, T. Microglia in Retinal Degeneration. *Front. Immunol.* **2019**, *10*, 1975. [CrossRef]
39. Maan-Yuh Lin, A.; Yang, C.-H.; Chai, C.-Y. Striatal Dopamine Dynamics Are Altered Following an Intranigral Infusion of Iron in Adult Rats. *Free Radic. Biol. Med.* **1998**, *24*, 988–993. [CrossRef]
40. LeDay, A.M.; Ganguly, S.; Kulkarni, K.; Dash, A.; Opere, C.; Ohia, S. Effect of hydrogen peroxide on amino acid concentrations in bovine retina and vitreous humor, ex vivo. *Methods Find Exp. Clin. Pharmacol.* **2003**, *25*, 695–701. [CrossRef]
41. Sharpe, M.A.; Robb, S.J.; Clark, J.B. Nitric oxide and Fenton/Haber–Weiss chemistry: Nitric oxide is a potent antioxidant at physiological concentrations. *J. Neurochem.* **2003**, *87*, 386–394. [CrossRef] [PubMed]
42. LeDay, A.M.; Kulkarni, K.H.; Opere, C.A.; Ohia, S.E. Arachidonic acid metabolites and peroxide-induced inhibition of [3H]D-aspartate release from bovine isolated retinae. *Curr. Eye Res.* **2004**, *28*, 367–372. [CrossRef] [PubMed]
43. Halliwell, B.; Gutteridge, J.M.C. The definition and measurement of antioxidants in biological systems. *Free Radic. Biol. Med.* **1995**, *18*, 125–126. [CrossRef]
44. Ankamah, E.; Sebag, J.; Ng, E.; Nolan, J. Vitreous Antioxidants, Degeneration, and Vitreo-Retinopathy: Exploring the Links. *Antioxidants* **2019**, *9*, 7. [CrossRef]
45. Behndig, A.; Svensson, B.; Marklund, S.L.; Karlsson, K. Superoxide dismutase isoenzymes in the human eye. *Investig. Ophthalmol. Vis. Sci.* **1998**, *39*, 471–475.
46. Richer, S.P.; Rose, R.C. Water soluble antioxidants in mammalian aqueous humor: Interaction with UV B and hydrogen peroxide. *Vis. Res.* **1998**, *38*, 2881–2888. [CrossRef]
47. Horwath-Winter, J.; Kirchengast, S.; Meinitzer, A.; Wachswender, C.; Faschinger, C.; Schmut, O. Determination of uric acid concentrations in human tear fluid, aqueous humour and serum. *Acta Ophthalmol.* **2009**, *87*, 188–192. [CrossRef]
48. Milston, R.; Madigan, M.C.; Sebag, J. Vitreous floaters: Etiology, diagnostics, and management. *Surv. Ophthalmol.* **2016**, *61*, 211–227. [CrossRef]
49. Filas, B.A.; Zhang, Q.; Okamoto, R.J.; Shui, Y.-B.; Beebe, D.C. Enzymatic degradation identifies components responsible for the structural properties of the vitreous body. *Investig. Ophthalmol. Vis. Sci.* **2014**, *55*, 55–63. [CrossRef]
50. Kita, T.; Sakamoto, T.; Ishibashi, T. II.D. Hyalocytes: Essential Vitreous Cells in Vitreoretinal Health and Disease. In *Vitreous: In Health and Disease*; Sebag, J., Ed.; Springer: New York, NY, USA, 2014; pp. 151–164.
51. Shui, Y.-B.; Holekamp, N.M.; Kramer, B.C.; Crowley, J.R.; Wilkins, M.A.; Chu, F.; Malone, P.E.; Mangers, S.J.; Hou, J.H.; Siegfried, C.J.; et al. The gel state of the vitreous and ascorbate-dependent oxygen consumption: Relationship to the etiology of nuclear cataracts. *Arch. Ophthalmol.* **2009**, *127*, 475–482. [CrossRef]
52. Sa, A.; Elawadi, A.I. Liquefaction of the Vitreous Humor floaters is a Risk Factor for Lens Opacity and Retinal Dysfunction. *J. Am. Sci.* **2011**, *7*, 927–936.

53. Mirończuk-Chodakowska, I.; Witkowska, A.M.; Zujko, M.E. Endogenous non-enzymatic antioxidants in the human body. *Adv. Med Sci.* **2018**, *63*, 68–78. [CrossRef] [PubMed]
54. Pham-Huy, L.A.; He, H.; Pham-Huy, C. Free radicals, antioxidants in disease and health. *Int. J. Biomed. Sci. IJBS* **2008**, *4*, 89–96.
55. Park, S.W.; Ghim, W.; Oh, S.; Kim, Y.; Park, U.C.; Kang, J.; Yu, H.G. Association of vitreous vitamin C depletion with diabetic macular ischemia in proliferative diabetic retinopathy. *PLoS ONE* **2019**, *14*, e0218433. [CrossRef] [PubMed]
56. Ashoori, M.; Saedisomeolia, A. Riboflavin (vitamin B2) and oxidative stress: A review. *Br. J. Nutr.* **2014**, *111*, 1985–1991. [CrossRef] [PubMed]
57. Konerirajapuram, N.; Coral, K.; Punitham, R.; Sharma, T.; Kasinathan, N.; Sivaramakrishnan, R. Trace Elements Iron, Copper and Zinc in Vitreous of Patients with Various Vitreoretinal Diseases. *Indian J. Ophthalmol.* **2004**, *52*, 145–148.
58. Sato, M.; Kondoh, M. Recent Studies on Metallothionein: Protection Against Toxicity of Heavy Metals and Oxygen Free Radicals. *Tohoku J. Exp. Med.* **2002**, *196*, 9–22. [CrossRef]
59. Tinggi, U. Selenium: Its role as antioxidant in human health. *Environ. Health Prev. Med.* **2008**, *13*, 102–108. [CrossRef]
60. Golbidi, S.; Laher, I. Antioxidant therapy in human endocrine disorders. *Med. Sci. Monit.* **2010**, *16*, RA9–RA24.
61. Golbidi, S.; Badran, M.; Laher, I. Antioxidant and anti-inflammatory effects of exercise in diabetic patients. *Exp. Diabetes Res.* **2012**, *2012*, 941868. [CrossRef]
62. Sunitha, K.; Suresh, P.; Santhosh, M.S.; Hemshekhar, M.; Thushara, R.; Marathe, G.K.; Thirunavukkarasu, C.; Kemparaju, K.; Kumar, M.S.; Girish, K. Inhibition of hyaluronidase by N-acetyl cysteine and glutathione: Role of thiol group in hyaluronan protection. *Int. J. Biol. Macromol.* **2013**, *55*, 39–46. [CrossRef] [PubMed]
63. Wong, R.W.; Richa, D.C.; Hahn, P.; Green, W.R.; Dunaief, J.L. Iron toxicity as a potential factor in AMD. *Retina* **2007**, *7*, 997–1003. [CrossRef] [PubMed]
64. Krizova, L.; Kalousova, M.; Kubena, A.; Benakova, H.; Zima, T.; Kovarik, Z.; Kalvoda, J.; Kalvodova, B. Increased Uric Acid and Glucose Concentrations in Vitreous and Serum of Patients with Diabetic Macular Oedema. *Ophthalmic Res.* **2011**, *46*, 73–79. [CrossRef]
65. González de Vega, R.; Fernández-Sánchez, M.L.; González-Iglesias, H.; Prados, M.C.; Sanz-Medel, A. Quantitative selenium speciation by HPLC-ICP-MS(IDA) and simultaneous activity measurements in human vitreous humor. *Anal. Bioanal. Chem.* **2015**, *407*, 2405–2413. [CrossRef]
66. Herbette, S.; Roeckel-Drevet, P.; Drevet, J.R. Seleno-independent glutathione peroxidases. *FEBS J.* **2007**, *274*, 2163–2180. [CrossRef]
67. Wert, K.J.; Vélez, G.; Cross, M.R.; Wagner, B.A.; Teoh-Fitzgerald, M.L.; Buettner, G.R.; McAnany, J.J.; Olivier, A.; Tsang, S.H.; Harper, M.M.; et al. Extracellular superoxide dismutase (SOD3) regulates oxidative stress at the vitreoretinal interface. *Free Radic. Biol. Med.* **2018**, *124*, 408–419. [CrossRef]
68. Yamane, K.; Minamoto, A.; Yamashita, H.; Takamura, H.; Miyamoto-Myoken, Y.; Yoshizato, K.; Nabetani, T.; Tsugita, A.; Mishima, H.K. Proteome Analysis of Human Vitreous Proteins. *Mol. Cell. Proteom.* **2003**, *2*, 1177. [CrossRef]
69. Murthy, K.R.; Goel, R.; Subbannayya, Y.; Jacob, H.K.C.; Murthy, P.R.; Manda, S.S.; Patil, A.H.; Sharma, R.; Sahasrabuddhe, N.A.; Parashar, A.; et al. Proteomic analysis of human vitreous humor. *Clin. Proteom.* **2014**, *11*, 29. [CrossRef]
70. Łukasik, M.; Szutowski, M.; Sołtyszewski, I.; Cieślak, P.A.; Małkowska, A. Postmortem Vitreous Humor Analysis for Xenobiotics and their Metabolites. *Law Forensic Sci.* **2018**, *15*, 1–8.
71. Yadav, D.; Varma, L.T.; Yadav, K. Drug Delivery to Posterior Segment of the Eye: Conventional Delivery Strategies, Their Barriers, and Restrictions. In *Drug Delivery for the Retina and Posterior Segment Disease*; Springer: Cham, Switzerland, 2018; pp. 51–67. [CrossRef]
72. Li, S.; Fu, X.-A.; Zhou, X.-F.; Chen, Y.-Y.; Chen, W.-Q. Angiogenesis-related cytokines in serum of proliferative diabetic retinopathy patients before and after vitrectomy. *Int. J. Ophthalmol.* **2012**, *5*, 726–730. [CrossRef]
73. Tamhane, M.; Cabrera-Ghayouri, S.; Abelian, G.; Viswanath, V. Review of Biomarkers in Ocular Matrices: Challenges and Opportunities. *Pharm. Res.* **2019**, *36*, 40. [CrossRef] [PubMed]
74. Fong, P.Y.; Shih, K.C.; Lam, P.Y.; Chan, T.C.Y.; Jhanji, V.; Tong, L. Role of tear film biomarkers in the diagnosis and management of dry eye disease. *Taiwan J. Ophthalmol.* **2019**, *9*, 150–159. [CrossRef] [PubMed]

75. Rentka, A.; Koroskenyi, K.; Hársfalvi, J.; Szekanecz, Z.; Szucs, G.; Szodoray, P.; Kemeny-Beke, A. Evaluation of commonly used tear sampling methods and their relevance in subsequent biochemical analysis. *Ann. Clin. Biochem.* **2017**, *54*, 521–529. [CrossRef] [PubMed]
76. Di Zazzo, A.; Micera, A.; De Piano, M.; Cortes, M.; Bonini, S. Tears and ocular surface disorders: Usefulness of biomarkers. *J. Cell. Physiol.* **2019**, *234*, 9982–9993. [CrossRef]
77. Inic-Kanada, A.; Nussbaumer, A.; Montanaro, J.; Belij, S.; Schlacher, S.; Stein, E.; Bintner, N.; Merio, M.; Zlabinger, G.J.; Barisani-Asenbauer, T. Comparison of ophthalmic sponges and extraction buffers for quantifying cytokine profiles in tears using Luminex technology. *Mol. Vis.* **2012**, *18*, 2717–2725.
78. Balne, P.K.; Au, V.B.; Tong, L.; Ghosh, A.; Agrawal, M.; Connolly, J. Bead Based Multiplex Assay for Analysis of Tear Cytokine Profiles. *J. Vis. Exp.* **2017**. [CrossRef]
79. Johnson, M.; McLaren, J.W.; Overby, D.R. Unconventional aqueous humor outflow: A review. *Exp. Eye Res.* **2017**, *158*, 94–111. [CrossRef]
80. Chowdhury, U.R.; Madden, B.J.; Charlesworth, M.C.; Fautsch, M.P. Proteome analysis of human aqueous humor. *Investig. Ophthalmol. Vis. Sci.* **2010**, *51*, 4921–4931. [CrossRef]
81. Murthy, K.R.; Rajagopalan, P.; Pinto, S.M.; Advani, J.; Murthy, P.R.; Goel, R.; Subbannayya, Y.; Balakrishnan, L.; Dash, M.; Anil, A.K.; et al. Proteomics of Human Aqueous Humor. *Omics J. Integr. Biol.* **2015**, *19*, 283–293. [CrossRef]
82. Goel, M.; Picciani, R.G.; Lee, R.K.; Bhattacharya, S.K. Aqueous humor dynamics: A review. *Open Ophthalmol. J.* **2010**, *4*, 52–59. [CrossRef]
83. Rusnak, S.; Vrzalová, J.; Sobotova, M.; Hecová, L.; Ricarova, R.; Topolcan, O. The Measurement of Intraocular Biomarkers in Various Stages of Proliferative Diabetic Retinopathy Using Multiplex xMAP Technology. *J. Ophthalmol.* **2015**, *2015*, 424783. [CrossRef] [PubMed]
84. Scott, J.E. The chemical morphology of the vitreous. *Eye* **1992**, *6*, 553–555. [CrossRef] [PubMed]
85. Ulrich, J.N.; Spannagl, M.; Kampik, A.; Gandorfer, A. Components of the fibrinolytic system in the vitreous body in patients with vitreoretinal disorders. *Clin. Exp. Ophthalmol.* **2008**, *36*, 431–436. [CrossRef] [PubMed]
86. Wu, C.W.; Sauter, J.L.; Johnson, P.K.; Chen, C.-D.; Olsen, T.W. Identification and localization of major soluble vitreous proteins in human ocular tissue. *Am. J. Ophthalmol.* **2004**, *137*, 655–661. [CrossRef] [PubMed]
87. Ghodasra, D.H.; Fante, R.; Gardner, T.W.; Langue, M.; Niziol, L.M.; Besirli, C.; Cohen, S.R.; Dedania, V.S.; Demirci, H.; Jain, N.; et al. Safety and Feasibility of Quantitative Multiplexed Cytokine Analysis From Office-Based Vitreous Aspiration. *Investig. Ophthalmol. Vis. Sci.* **2016**, *57*, 3017–3023. [CrossRef]
88. Bergandi, L.; Skorokhod, O.A.; La Grotta, R.; Schwarzer, E.; Nuzzi, R. Oxidative Stress, Lipid Peroxidation, and Loss of Hyaluronic Acid in the Human Vitreous Affected by Synchysis Scintillans. *J. Ophthalmol.* **2019**, *2019*, 7231015. [CrossRef]
89. Srividya, G.; Jain, M.; Mahalakshmi, K.; Gayathri, S.; Raman, R.; Angayarkanni, N. A novel and less invasive technique to assess cytokine profile of vitreous in patients of diabetic macular oedema. *Eye* **2018**, *32*, 820–829. [CrossRef]
90. García-Ramírez, M.; Canals, F.; Hernandez, C.; Colomé, N.; Ferrer, C.; Carrasco, E.; García-Arumí, J.; Simó, R. Proteomic analysis of human vitreous fluid by fluorescence-based difference gel electrophoresis (DIGE): A new strategy for identifying potential candidates in the pathogenesis of proliferative diabetic retinopathy. *Diabetología* **2007**, *50*, 1294–1303. [CrossRef]
91. Jenkins, A.J.; Joglekar, M.V.; Hardikar, A.A.; Keech, A.C.; O'Neal, D.N.; Januszewski, A.S. Biomarkers in Diabetic Retinopathy. *Rev. Diabet. Stud.* **2015**, *12*, 159–195. [CrossRef]
92. FDANIH Biomarker Working Group. *BEST (Biomarkers, EndpointS, and other Tools) Resource*; Food and Drug Administration: Silver Spring, MD, USA, 2018; p. 61.
93. Wecker, T.; Hoffmeier, K.; Plötner, A.; Grüning, B.; Horres, R.; Backofen, R.; Reinhard, T.; Schlunck, G. MicroRNA Profiling in Aqueous Humor of Individual Human Eyes by Next-Generation Sequencing. *Investig. Ophthalmol. Vis. Sci.* **2016**, *57*, 1706–1713. [CrossRef]
94. Tanaka, Y.; Tsuda, S.; Kunikata, H.; Sato, J.; Kokubun, T.; Yasuda, M.; Nishiguchi, K.M.; Inada, T.; Nakazawa, T. Profiles of Extracellular miRNAs in the Aqueous Humor of Glaucoma Patients Assessed with a Microarray System. *Sci. Rep.* **2014**, *4*, 5089. [CrossRef] [PubMed]
95. Kulaksızoglu, S.; Karalezli, A. Aqueous Humour and Serum Levels of Nitric Oxide, Malondialdehyde and Total Antioxidant Status in Patients with Type 2 Diabetes with Proliferative Diabetic Retinopathy and Nondiabetic Senile Cataracts. *Can. J. Diabetes* **2016**, *40*, 115–119. [CrossRef] [PubMed]

96. Nezzar, H.; Chiambaretta, F.; Marceau, G.; Blanchon, L.; Faye, B.; Dechelotte, P.; Rigal, D.; Sapin, V. Molecular and metabolic retinoid pathways in the human ocular surface. *Mol. Vis.* **2007**, *13*, 1641–1650. [PubMed]
97. Goyal, A.; Srivastava, A.; Sihota, R.; Kaur, J. Evaluation of Oxidative Stress Markers in Aqueous Humor of Primary Open Angle Glaucoma and Primary Angle Closure Glaucoma Patients. *Curr. Eye Res.* **2014**, *39*, 823–829. [CrossRef] [PubMed]
98. Flohé, L.; Günzler, W.A. Assays of glutathione peroxidase. *Methods Enzymol.* **1984**, *105*, 114–120. [CrossRef]
99. Marrocco, I.; Altieri, F.; Peluso, I. Measurement and Clinical Significance of Biomarkers of Oxidative Stress in Humans. *Oxid. Med. Cell. Longev.* **2017**, *2017*, 6501046. [CrossRef]
100. Huang, W.; Koralewska-Makár, A.; Bauer, B.; Åkesson, B. Extracellular glutathione peroxidase and ascorbic acid in aqueous humor and serum of patients operated on for cataract. *Clin. Chim. Acta* **1997**, *261*, 117–130. [CrossRef]
101. Ferreira, S.M.; Lerner, S.F.; Brunzini, R.; Evelson, P.; Llesuy, S. Oxidative stress markers in aqueous humor of glaucoma patients. *Am. J. Ophthalmol.* **2004**, *137*, 62–69. [CrossRef]
102. Stadtman, E.R.; Oliver, C.N. Metal-catalyzed oxidation of proteins. Physiological consequences. *J. Biol. Chem.* **1991**, *266*, 2005–2008.
103. Altomare, E.; Grattagliano, I.; Vendemaile, G.; Micelli-Ferrari, T.; Signorile, A.; Cardia, L. Oxidative protein damage in human diabetic eye: Evidence of a retinal participation. *Eur. J. Clin. Investig.* **1997**, *27*, 141–147. [CrossRef]
104. Mancino, R.; Di Pierro, N.; Varesi, C.; Cerulli, A.; Feraco, A.; Cedrone, C.; Pinazo-Duran, M.D.; Coletta, M.; Nucci, C. Lipid peroxidation and total antioxidant capacity in vitreous, aqueous humor, and blood samples from patients with diabetic retinopathy. *Mol. Vis.* **2011**, *17*, 1298–1304.
105. Brzović-Šarić, V.; Landeka, I.; Šarić, B.; Barberić, M.; Andrijašević, L.; Cerovski, B.; Oršolić, N.; Đikić, D. Levels of selected oxidative stress markers in the vitreous and serum of diabetic retinopathy patients. *Mol. Vis.* **2015**, *21*, 649–664. [PubMed]
106. Georgakopoulos, C.D.; Lamari, F.N.; Karathanasopoulou, I.N.; Gartaganis, V.S.; Pharmakakis, N.M.; Karamanos, N. Tear analysis of ascorbic acid, uric acid and malondialdehyde with capillary electrophoresis. *Biomed. Chromatogr.* **2010**, *24*, 852–857. [CrossRef] [PubMed]
107. Hernández-Martínez, F.J.; Piñas-García, P.; Lleó-Pérez, A.; Zanon-Moreno, V.C.; Bendala-Tufanisco, E.; García-Medina, J.; Vinuesa-Silva, I.; Pinazo-Durán, M.D. Biomarkers of lipid peroxidation in the aqueous humor of primary open-angle glaucoma patients. *Arch. Soc. Esp. Oftalmol.* **2016**, *91*, 357–362. [CrossRef]
108. Behndig, A.; Karlsson, K.; Johansson, B.O.; Brännström, T.; Marklund, S.L. Superoxide dismutase isoenzymes in the normal and diseased human cornea. *Investig. Ophthalmol. Vis. Sci.* **2001**, *42*, 2293–2296.
109. Kim, E.B.; Kim, H.K.; Hyon, J.Y.; Wee, W.R.; Shin, Y.J. Oxidative Stress Levels in Aqueous Humor from High Myopic Patients. *Korean J. Ophthalmol.* **2016**, *30*, 172–179. [CrossRef] [PubMed]
110. Koliakos, G.G.; Konstas, A.G.P.; Schlötzer-Schrehardt, U.; Hollo, G.; Katsimbris, I.E.; Georgiadis, N.; Ritch, R. 8-Isoprostaglandin F2a and ascorbic acid concentration in the aqueous humour of patients with exfoliation syndrome. *Br. J. Ophthalmol.* **2003**, *87*, 353–356. [CrossRef]
111. Rahim, A. 8-Isoprostaglandin F2a Levels in Aqueous Humor of Senile and Diabetic Cataract Patients. *Iosr J. Dent. Med Sci.* **2012**, *2*, 40–42. [CrossRef]
112. Yilmaz, G.; Esser, P.; Kociek, N.; Aydin, P.; Heimann, K. Elevated vitreous nitric oxide levels in patients with proliferative diabetic retinopathy. *Am. J. Ophthalmol.* **2000**, *130*, 87–90. [CrossRef]
113. Liu, J.; Shi, B.; He, S.; Yao, X.; Willcox, M.D.; Zhao, Z. Changes to tear cytokines of type 2 diabetic patients with or without retinopathy. *Mol. Vis.* **2010**, *16*, 2931–2938. [PubMed]
114. Liu, R.; Gao, C.; Chen, H.; Li, Y.; Jin, Y.; Qi, H. Analysis of Th17-associated cytokines and clinical correlations in patients with dry eye disease. *PLoS ONE* **2017**, *12*, e0173301. [CrossRef]
115. Chen, H.; Zhang, X.; Liao, N.; Wen, F. Assessment of biomarkers using multiplex assays in aqueous humor of patients with diabetic retinopathy. *BMC Ophthalmol.* **2017**, *17*, 176. [CrossRef]
116. Funatsu, H.; Yamashita, H.; Mimura, T.; Noma, H.; Nakamura, S.; Hori, S. Risk evaluation of outcome of vitreous surgery based on vitreous levels of cytokines. *Eye* **2007**, *21*, 377–382. [CrossRef]
117. Tsai, T.; Kuehn, S.; Tsiampalis, N.; Vu, M.-K.; Kakkassery, V.; Stute, G.; Dick, H.B.; Joachim, S.C. Anti-inflammatory cytokine and angiogenic factors levels in vitreous samples of diabetic retinopathy patients. *PLoS ONE* **2018**, *13*, e0194603. [CrossRef]

118. Chernykh, V.; Smirnov, E.; Varvarinsky, Y.; Chernykh, D.; Obukhova, O.; Trunov, A. IL-4, IL-6, IL-10, IL-17A and vascular endothelial growth factor in the vitreous of patients with proliferative diabetic retinopathy. *Adv. Biosci. Biotechnol.* **2015**, *5*, 184–187. [CrossRef]
119. Sun, C.; Zhang, H.; Jiang, J.; Li, Y.; Nie, C.; Gu, J.; Luo, L.; Wang, Z. Angiogenic and inflammatory biomarker levels in aqueous humor and vitreous of neovascular glaucoma and proliferative diabetic retinopathy. *Int. Ophthalmol.* **2020**, *40*, 467–475. [CrossRef]
120. Simsek, M.; Ozdal, P.C.; Akbiyik, F.; Citirik, M.; Berker, N.; Erol, Y.O.; Yilmazbas, P. Aqueous humor IL-8, IL-10, and VEGF levels in Fuchs' uveitis syndrome and Behçet's uveitis. *Int. Ophthalmol.* **2019**, *39*, 2629–2636. [CrossRef]
121. Mao, C.; Yan, H. Roles of elevated intravitreal IL-1β and IL-10 levels in proliferative diabetic retinopathy. *Indian J. Ophthalmol.* **2014**, *62*, 699–701. [CrossRef]
122. Costagliola, C.; Romano, V.; De Tollis, M.; Aceto, F.; Dell'Omo, R.; Romano, M.; Pedicino, C.; Semeraro, F. TNF-alpha levels in tears: A novel biomarker to assess the degree of diabetic retinopathy. *Mediat. Inflamm.* **2013**, *2013*, 629529. [CrossRef]
123. Wu, H.; Hwang, D.-K.; Song, X.; Tao, Y. Association between Aqueous Cytokines and Diabetic Retinopathy Stage. *J. Ophthalmol.* **2017**, *2017*, 9402198. [CrossRef]
124. Boss, J.D.; Singh, P.K.; Pandya, H.K.; Tosi, J.; Kim, C.; Tewari, A.; Juzych, M.S.; Abrams, G.W.; Kumar, A. Assessment of Neurotrophins and Inflammatory Mediators in Vitreous of Patients With Diabetic Retinopathy. *Investig. Ophthalmol. Vis. Sci.* **2017**, *58*, 5594–5603. [CrossRef]
125. Canataroglu, H.; Varinli, I.; Ozcan, A.; Canataroglu, A.; Doran, F.; Varinli, S. Interleukin (IL)-6, Interleukin (IL)-8 Levels and Cellular Composition of the Vitreous Humor in Proliferative Diabetic Retinopathy, Proliferative Vitreoretinopathy, and Traumatic Proliferative Vitreoretinopathy. *Ocul. Immunol. Inflamm.* **2005**, *13*, 375–381. [CrossRef]
126. Liu, R.; Ma, B.; Gao, Y.; Ma, B.; Liu, Y.; Qi, H. Tear Inflammatory Cytokines Analysis and Clinical Correlations in Diabetes and Nondiabetes With Dry Eye. *Am. J. Ophthalmol.* **2019**, *200*, 10–15. [CrossRef]
127. Fu, R.; Klinngam, W.; Heur, M.; Edman, M.C.; Hamm-Alvarez, S.F. Tear Proteases and Protease Inhibitors: Potential Biomarkers and Disease Drivers in Ocular Surface Disease. *Eye Contact Lenses* **2020**, *46* (Suppl. 2), S70–S83. [CrossRef]
128. Kłysik, A.; Naduk-Kik, J.; Hrabec, Z.; Gos, R.; Hrabec, E. Intraocular matrix metalloproteinase 2 and 9 in patients with diabetes mellitus with and without diabetic retinopathy. *Arch. Med Sci. AMS* **2010**, *6*, 375–381. [CrossRef]
129. Tuuminen, R.; Loukovaara, S. High intravitreal TGF-β1 and MMP-9 levels in eyes with retinal vein occlusion. *Eye* **2014**, *28*, 1095–1099. [CrossRef]
130. Luo, L.; Li, D.Q.; Pflugfelder, S.C. Hyperosmolarity-induced apoptosis in human corneal epithelial cells is mediated by cytochrome c and MAPK pathways. *Cornea* **2007**, *26*, 452–460. [CrossRef]
131. Peskin, A.V.; Winterbourn, C.C. Assay of superoxide dismutase activity in a plate assay using WST-1. *Free Radic. Biol. Med.* **2017**, *103*, 188–191. [CrossRef]
132. Kernell, A.; Lundh, B.L.; Marklund, S.L.; Skoog, K.O.; Björkstén, B. Superoxide dismutase in the anterior chamber and the vitreous of diabetic patients. *Investig. Ophthalmol. Vis. Sci.* **1992**, *33*, 3131–3135.
133. Sies, H. Total Antioxidant Capacity: Appraisal of a Concept. *J. Nutr.* **2007**, *137*, 1493–1495. [CrossRef]
134. Huang, D.; Ou, B.; Prior, R.L. The Chemistry behind Antioxidant Capacity Assays. *J. Agric. Food Chem.* **2005**, *53*, 1841–1856. [CrossRef]
135. Ghiselli, A.; Serafini, M.; Natella, F.; Scaccini, C. Total antioxidant capacity as a tool to assess redox status: Critical view and experimental data. *Free Radic. Biol. Med.* **2000**, *29*, 1106–1114. [CrossRef]
136. Saccà, S.C.; Pascotto, A.; Camicione, P.; Capris, P.; Izzotti, A. Oxidative DNA Damage in the Human Trabecular Meshwork: Clinical Correlation in Patients With Primary Open-Angle Glaucoma. *Arch. Ophthalmol.* **2005**, *123*, 458–463. [CrossRef]
137. Izuta, H.; Matsunaga, N.; Shimazawa, M.; Sugiyama, T.; Ikeda, T.; Hara, H. Proliferative diabetic retinopathy and relations among antioxidant activity, oxidative stress, and VEGF in the vitreous body. *Mol. Vis.* **2010**, *16*, 130–136.
138. Dizdaroglu, M.; Jaruga, P.; Birincioglu, M.; Rodriguez, H. Free radical-induced damage to DNA: Mechanisms and measurement. *Free Radic. Biol. Med.* **2002**, *32*, 1102–1115. [CrossRef]

139. Cadet, J.; Douki, T.; Gasparutto, D.; Ravanat, J.L. Oxidative damage to DNA: Formation, measurement and biochemical features. *Mutat. Res. Fundam. Mol. Mech. Mutagenesis* **2003**, *531*, 5–23. [CrossRef]
140. Cadet, J.; Wagner, J.R. Oxidatively generated base damage to cellular DNA by hydroxyl radical and one-electron oxidants: Similarities and differences. *Arch. Biochem. Biophys.* **2014**, *557*, 47–54. [CrossRef]
141. Thiagarajan, R.; Manikandan, R. Antioxidants and cataract. *Free Radic. Res.* **2013**, *47*, 337–345. [CrossRef]
142. Jia, Y.; Hu, D.-N.; Zhu, D.; Zhang, L.; Gu, P.; Fan, X.; Zhou, J.-B. MMP-2, MMP-3, TIMP-1, TIMP-2, and TIMP-3 Protein Levels in Human Aqueous Humor: Relationship With Axial Length. *Investig. Ophthalmol. Vis. Sci.* **2014**, *55*, 3922–3928. [CrossRef]
143. Saxena, S.; Srivastava, P.; Khanna, V.K. Elevated lipid peroxides induced angiogenesis in proliferative diabetic retinopathy. *J. Ocul. Biol. Dis. Inform.* **2010**, *3*, 85–87. [CrossRef]
144. Kersten, E.; Paun, C.C.; Schellevis, R.L.; Hoyng, C.B.; Delcourt, C.; Lengyel, I.; Peto, T.; Ueffing, M.; Klaver, C.C.W.; Dammeier, S.; et al. Systemic and ocular fluid compounds as potential biomarkers in age-related macular degeneration. *Surv. Ophthalmol.* **2018**, *63*, 9–39. [CrossRef] [PubMed]
145. Cai, J.; Nelson, K.C.; Wu, M.; Sternberg, P.; Jones, D.P. Oxidative damage and protection of the RPE. *Prog. Retin. Eye Res.* **2000**, *19*, 205–221. [CrossRef]
146. Bergandi, L.; Skorokhod, O.A.; Franzone, F.; La Grotta, R.; Schwarzer, E.; Nuzzi, R. Induction of oxidative stress in human aqueous and vitreous humors by Nd:YAG laser posterior capsulotomy. *Int. J. Ophthalmol.* **2018**, *11*, 1145–1151. [CrossRef]
147. Ethen, C.M.; Reilly, C.; Feng, X.; Olsen, T.W.; Ferrington, D.A. Age-Related Macular Degeneration and Retinal Protein Modification by 4-Hydroxy-2-nonenal. *Investig. Ophthalmol. Vis. Sci.* **2007**, *48*, 3469–3479. [CrossRef]
148. Cipak, A.; Mrakovcic, L.; Ciz, M.; Lojek, A.; Mihaylova, B.; Goshev, I.; Jaganjac, M.; Cindric, M.; Sitic, S.; Margaritoni, M.; et al. Growth suppression of human breast carcinoma stem cells by lipid peroxidation product 4-hydroxy-2-nonenal and hydroxyl radicalmodified collagen. *Acta Biochim. Pol.* **2010**, *57*, 165–171. [CrossRef]
149. Bishop, P.N.; Holmes, D.F.; Kadler, K.E.; McLeod, D.; Bos, K.J. Age-Related Changes on the Surface of Vitreous Collagen Fibrils. *Investig. Ophthalmol. Vis. Sci.* **2004**, *45*, 1041–1046. [CrossRef]
150. Kamegawa, M.; Nakanishi-Ueda, T.; Iwai, S.; Ueda, T.; Kosuge, S.; Ogura, H.; Sasuga, K.; Inagaki, M.; Watanabe, M.; Oguchi, K.; et al. Effect of Lipid-Hydroperoxide-Induced Oxidative Stress on Vitamin E, Ascorbate and Glutathione in the Rabbit Retina. *Ophthalmic Res.* **2007**, *39*, 49–54. [CrossRef]
151. Madsen-Bouterse, S.A.; Kowluru, R.A. Oxidative stress and diabetic retinopathy: Pathophysiological mechanisms and treatment perspectives. *Rev. Endocr. Metab. Disord.* **2008**, *9*, 315–327. [CrossRef]
152. Smith, K.A.; Shepherd, J.; Wakil, A.; Kilpatrick, E.S. A comparison of methods for the measurement of 8-isoPGF2α: A marker of oxidative stress. *Ann. Clin. Biochem.* **2011**, *48*, 147–154. [CrossRef]
153. Evereklioglu, C.; Er, H.; Doganay, S.; Cekmen, M.; Turkoz, Y.; Otlu, B.; Ozerol, E. Nitric oxide and lipid peroxidation are increased and associated with decreased antioxidant enzyme activities in patients with age-related macular degeneration. *Doc. Ophthalmol.* **2003**, *106*, 129–136. [CrossRef]
154. Bhutto, I.A.; Baba, T.; Merges, C.; McLeod, D.S.; Lutty, G.A. Low nitric oxide synthases (NOSs) in eyes with age-related macular degeneration (AMD). *Exp. Eye Res.* **2010**, *90*, 155–167. [CrossRef] [PubMed]
155. Chakravarthy, U.; Stitt, A.W.; McNally, J.; Bailie, J.R.; Hoey, E.M.; Duprex, P.; Duprex, W.P. Nitric oxide synthase activity and expression in retinal capillary endothelial cells and pericytes. *Curr. Eye Res.* **1995**, *14*, 285–294. [CrossRef] [PubMed]
156. Becquet, F.; Courtois, Y.; Goureau, O. Nitric oxide in the eye: Multifaceted roles and diverse outcomes. *Surv. Ophthalmol.* **1997**, *42*, 71–82. [CrossRef]
157. Hattenbach, L.-O.; Allers, A.; Klais, C.; Koch, F.; Hecker, M. L-Arginine–Nitric Oxide Pathway–Related Metabolites in the Aqueous Humor of Diabetic Patients. *Investig. Ophthalmol. Vis. Sci.* **2000**, *41*, 213–217.
158. Wiederholt, M.; Sturm, A.; Lepple-Wienhues, A. Relaxation of trabecular meshwork and ciliary muscle by release of nitric oxide. *Investig. Ophthalmol. Vis. Sci.* **1994**, *35*, 2515–2520.
159. Bhattacharya, S.K.; Lee, R.K.; Grus, F.H. Molecular biomarkers in glaucoma. *Investig. Ophthalmol. Vis. Sci.* **2013**, *54*, 121–131. [CrossRef] [PubMed]
160. Pinazo-Durán, M.D.; Gallego-Pinazo, R.; García-Medina, J.J.; Zanon-Moreno, V.C.; Nucci, C.; Dolz-Marco, R.; Martinez-Castillo, S.; Galbis-Estrada, C.; Marco-Ramírez, C.; López-Gálvez, M.I.; et al. Oxidative stress and its downstream signaling in aging eyes. *Clin. Interv. Aging* **2014**, *9*, 637–652. [CrossRef]

161. Diederen, R.M.; La Heij, E.C.; Deutz, N.; Kessels, A.G.H.; Van Eijk, H.M.H.; Hendrikse, F. Increased nitric oxide (NO) pathway metabolites in the vitreous fluid of patients with rhegmatogenous retinal detachment or diabetic traction retinal detachment. *Graefe Arch. Clin. Exp. Ophthalmol.* **2006**, *244*, 683–688. [CrossRef] [PubMed]
162. und Hohenstein-Blaul NV, T.; Funke, S.; Grus, F.H. Tears as a source of biomarkers for ocular and systemic diseases. *Exp. Eye Res.* **2013**, *117*, 126–137. [CrossRef] [PubMed]
163. Amil-Bangsa, N.H.; Mohd-Ali, B.; Ishak, B.; Abdul-Aziz, C.N.N.; Ngah, N.F.; Hashim, H.; Ghazali, A.R. Total Protein Concentration and Tumor Necrosis Factor α in Tears of Nonproliferative Diabetic Retinopathy. *Optom. Vis. Sci.* **2019**, *96*, 934–939. [CrossRef]
164. Aveleira, C.A.; Lin, C.-M.; Abcouwer, S.F.; Ambrósio, A.F.; Antonetti, D.A. TNF-α signals through PKCζ/NF-κB to alter the tight junction complex and increase retinal endothelial cell permeability. *Diabetes* **2010**, *59*, 2872–2882. [CrossRef] [PubMed]
165. Arita, R.; Nakao, S.; Kita, T.; Kawahara, S.; Asato, R.; Yoshida, S.; Enaida, H.; Hafezi-Moghadam, A.; Ishibashi, T. A Key Role for ROCK in TNF-α–Mediated Diabetic Microvascular Damage. *Investig. Ophthalmol. Vis. Sci.* **2013**, *54*, 2373–2383. [CrossRef] [PubMed]
166. Adamiec-Mroczek, J.; Oficjalska-Młyńczak, J. Assessment of selected adhesion molecule and proinflammatory cytokine levels in the vitreous body of patients with type 2 diabetes—Role of the inflammatory-immune process in the pathogenesis of proliferative diabetic retinopathy. *Graefe Arch. Clin. Exp. Ophthalmol. Albrecht Graefes Arch. Klin. Exp. Ophthalmol.* **2008**, *246*, 1665–1670. [CrossRef] [PubMed]
167. McArthur, K.; Feng, B.; Wu, Y.; Chen, S.; Chakrabarti, S. MicroRNA-200b regulates vascular endothelial growth factor-mediated alterations in diabetic retinopathy. *Diabetes* **2011**, *60*, 1314–1323. [CrossRef] [PubMed]
168. Gomaa, A.R.; Elsayed, E.T.; Moftah, R.F. MicroRNA-200b Expression in the Vitreous Humor of Patients with Proliferative Diabetic Retinopathy. *Ophthalmic Res.* **2017**, *58*, 168–175. [CrossRef] [PubMed]
169. Chen, Q.; Qiu, F.; Zhou, K.; Matlock, H.G.; Takahashi, Y.; Rajala, R.V.; Yang, Y.; Moran, E.; Ma, J.-X. Pathogenic Role of microRNA-21 in Diabetic Retinopathy Through Downregulation of PPARα. *Diabetes* **2017**, *66*, 1671–1682. [CrossRef]
170. Usui-Ouchi, A.; Ouchi, Y.; Kiyokawa, M.; Sakuma, T.; Ito, R.; Ebihara, N. Upregulation of Mir-21 Levels in the Vitreous Humor Is Associated with Development of Proliferative Vitreoretinal Disease. *PLoS ONE* **2016**, *11*, e0158043. [CrossRef]
171. Besnier, M.; Shantikumar, S.; Anwar, M.; Dixit, P.; Chamorro-Jorganes, A.; Sweaad, W.; Sala-Newby, G.; Madeddu, P.; Thomas, A.C.; Howard, L.; et al. miR-15a/-16 Inhibit Angiogenesis by Targeting the Tie2 Coding Sequence: Therapeutic Potential of a miR-15a/16 Decoy System in Limb Ischemia. *Molecular therapy. Nucleic Acids* **2019**, *17*, 49–62. [CrossRef]
172. Hirota, K.; Keino, H.; Inoue, M.; Ishida, H.; Hirakata, A. Comparisons of microRNA expression profiles in vitreous humor between eyes with macular hole and eyes with proliferative diabetic retinopathy. *Graefe Arch. Clin. Exp. Ophthalmol.* **2015**, *253*, 335–342. [CrossRef]
173. Ye, E.-A.; Steinle, J.J. Regulatory role of microRNA on inflammatory responses of diabetic retinopathy. *Neural Regen. Res.* **2017**, *12*, 580–581. [CrossRef]
174. Cho, H.; Hwang, M.; Hong, E.H.; Yu, H.; Park, H.; Koh, S.; Shin, Y.U. Micro-RNAs in the aqueous humour of patients with diabetic macular oedema. *Clin. Exp. Ophthalmol.* **2020**, *48*, 624–635. [CrossRef] [PubMed]
175. Feng, B.; Chakrabarti, S. miR-320 Regulates Glucose-Induced Gene Expression in Diabetes. *Isrn Endocrinol.* **2012**, *2012*, 549875. [CrossRef] [PubMed]
176. Zampetaki, A.; Willeit, P.; Burr, S.; Yin, X.; Langley, S.R.; Kiechl, S.; Klein, R.; Rossing, P.; Chaturvedi, N.; Mayr, M. Angiogenic microRNAs Linked to Incidence and Progression of Diabetic Retinopathy in Type 1. *Diabetes* **2016**, *65*, 216–227. [CrossRef] [PubMed]
177. Zhang, Y.; Zhou, J.; Li, M.-Q.; Xu, J.; Zhang, J.-P.; Jin, L.-P. MicroRNA-184 promotes apoptosis of trophoblast cells via targeting WIG1 and induces early spontaneous abortion. *Cell Death Dis.* **2019**, *10*, 223. [CrossRef]
178. Chen, S.; Yuan, M.; Liu, Y.; Zhao, X.; Lian, P.; Chen, Y.; Liu, B.; Lu, L. Landscape of microRNA in the aqueous humour of proliferative diabetic retinopathy as assessed by next-generation sequencing. *Clin. Exp. Ophthalmol.* **2019**, *47*, 925–936. [CrossRef]
179. Fang, L.; Deng, Z.; Shatseva, T.; Yang, J.; Peng, C.; Du, W.W.; Yee, A.J.; Ang, L.C.; He, C.; Shan, S.W.; et al. MicroRNA miR-93 promotes tumor growth and angiogenesis by targeting integrin-β8. *Oncogene* **2011**, *30*, 806–821. [CrossRef]

180. Zhang, L.-Q.; Cui, H.; Wang, L.; Fang, X.; Su, S. Role of microRNA-29a in the development of diabetic retinopathy by targeting AGT gene in a rat model. *Exp. Mol. Pathol.* **2017**, *102*, 296–302. [CrossRef]
181. Qu, Y.; Liu, H.; Lv, X.; Liu, Y.; Wang, X.; Zhang, M.; Zhang, X.; Li, Y.; Lou, Q.; Li, S.; et al. MicroRNA-16-5p overexpression suppresses proliferation and invasion as well as triggers apoptosis by targeting VEGFA expression in breast carcinoma. *Oncotarget* **2017**, *8*, 72400–72410. [CrossRef]
182. Luo, Z.; Feng, X.; Wang, H.; Xu, W.; Zhao, Y.; Ma, W.; Jiang, S.; Liu, D.; Huang, J.; Songyang, Z. Mir-23a induces telomere dysfunction and cellular senescence by inhibiting TRF2 expression. *Aging Cell* **2015**, *14*, 391–399. [CrossRef]
183. Su, J.L.; Chen, P.S.; Johansson, G.; Kuo, M.L. Function and regulation of let-7 family microRNAs. *Microrna* **2012**, *1*, 34–39. [CrossRef]
184. Li, T.; Pan, H.; Li, R. The dual regulatory role of miR-204 in cancer. *Tumour Biol. J. Int. Soc. Oncodev. Biol. Med.* **2016**, *37*, 11667. [CrossRef]
185. Jackson, D.C.; Zeng, W.; Wong, C.Y.; Mifsud, E.J.; Williamson, N.A.; Ang, C.-S.; Vingrys, A.J.; Downie, L.E. Tear Interferon-Gamma as a Biomarker for Evaporative Dry Eye Disease. *Investig. Ophthalmol. Vis. Sci.* **2016**, *57*, 4824–4830. [CrossRef] [PubMed]
186. Yu, L.; Chen, X.; Qin, G.; Xie, H.; Lv, P. Tear film function in type 2 diabetic patients with retinopathy. *Ophthalmologica* **2008**, *222*, 284–291. [CrossRef]
187. Gao, Y.; Zhang, Y.; Ru, Y.-S.; Wang, X.-W.; Yang, J.-Z.; Li, C.-H.; Wang, H.-X.; Li, X.-R.; Li, B. Ocular surface changes in type II diabetic patients with proliferative diabetic retinopathy. *Int. J. Ophthalmol.* **2015**, *8*, 358–364. [CrossRef] [PubMed]
188. Csősz, É.; Boross, P.; Csutak, A.; Berta, A.; Toth, F.; Poliska, S.; Török, Z.; Tőzsér, J. Quantitative analysis of proteins in the tear fluid of patients with diabetic retinopathy. *J. Proteom.* **2012**, *75*, 2196–2204. [CrossRef] [PubMed]
189. Banks, W.A.; Kastin, A.J.; Gutierrez, E.G. Penetration of interleukin-6 across the murine blood-brain barrier. *Neurosci. Lett.* **1994**, *179*, 53–56. [CrossRef]
190. Moriarty, A.; Spalton, D.; Moriarty, B.; Shilling, J.; Ffytche, T.; Bulsara, M. Studies of the Blood-Aqueous Barrier in Diabetes Mellitus. *Am. J. Ophthalmol.* **1994**, *117*, 768–771. [CrossRef]
191. Holzinger, C.; Weissinger, E.; Zuckermann, A.; Imhof, M.; Kink, F.; Schöllhammer, A.; Kopp, C.; Wolner, E. Effects of interleukin-1, -2, -4, -6, interferon-gamma and granulocyte/macrophage colony stimulating factor on human vascular endothelial cells. *Immunol. Lett.* **1993**, *35*, 109–117. [CrossRef]
192. Sharma, R.K.; Rogojina, A.T.; Chalam, K.V. Multiplex immunoassay analysis of biomarkers in clinically accessible quantities of human aqueous humor. *Mol. Vis.* **2009**, *15*, 60–69.
193. Globočnik Petrovič, M.; Korošec, P.; Košnik, M.; Hawlina, M. Vitreous Levels of Interleukin-8 in Patients With Proliferative Diabetic Retinopathy. *Am. J. Ophthalmol.* **2007**, *143*, 175–176. [CrossRef]
194. Chono, I.; Miyazaki, D.; Miyake, H.; Komatsu, N.; Ehara, F.; Nagase, D.; Kawamoto, Y.; Shimizu, Y.; Ideta, R.; Inoue, Y. High interleukin-8 level in aqueous humor is associated with poor prognosis in eyes with open angle glaucoma and neovascular glaucoma. *Sci. Rep.* **2018**, *8*, 14533. [CrossRef] [PubMed]
195. Paine, S.K.; Sen, A.; Choudhuri, S.; Mondal, L.K.; Chowdhury, I.H.; Basu, A.; Mukherjee, A.; Bhattacharya, B. Association of tumor necrosis factor α, interleukin 6, and interleukin 10 promoter polymorphism with proliferative diabetic retinopathy in type 2 diabetic subjects. *Retina* **2012**, *32*. [CrossRef] [PubMed]
196. Hernández, C.; Segura, R.M.; Fonollosa, A.; Carrasco, E.; Francisco, G.; Simo, R. Interleukin-8, monocyte chemoattractant protein-1 and IL-10 in the vitreous fluid of patients with proliferative diabetic retinopathy. *Diabet. Med.* **2005**, *22*, 719–722. [CrossRef] [PubMed]
197. Rubio-Perez, J.M.; Morillas-Ruiz, J.M. A review: Inflammatory process in Alzheimer's disease, role of cytokines. *Sci. World J.* **2012**, *2012*, 756357. [CrossRef]
198. Bigda, J.; Beletsky, I.; Brakebusch, C.; Varfolomeev, Y.; Engelmann, H.; Holtmann, H.; Wallach, D. Dual role of the p75 tumor necrosis factor (TNF) receptor in TNF cytotoxicity. *J. Exp. Med.* **1994**, *180*, 445–460. [CrossRef]
199. Ozturk, B.T.; Bozkurt, B.; Kerimoglu, H.; Okka, M.; Kamis, U.; Gunduz, K. Effect of serum cytokines and VEGF levels on diabetic retinopathy and macular thickness. *Mol. Vis.* **2009**, *15*, 1906–1914.
200. Zorena, K.; Raczyńska, D.; Raczyńska, K. Biomarkers in Diabetic Retinopathy and the Therapeutic Implications. *Mediat. Inflamm.* **2013**, *2013*, 193604. [CrossRef]
201. Ferrara, N.; Gerber, H.-P.; LeCouter, J. The biology of VEGF and its receptors. *Nat. Med.* **2003**, *9*, 669–676. [CrossRef]

202. Vignali, D.A.A. Multiplexed particle-based flow cytometric assays. *J. Immunol. Methods* **2000**, *243*, 243–255. [CrossRef]
203. Murugeswari, P.; Shukla, D.; Rajendran, A.; Kim, R.; Namperumalsamy, P.; Muthukkaruppan, V. Proinflammatory cytokines and angiogenic and anti-angiogenic factors in vitreous of patients with proliferative diabetic retinopathy and eales' disease. *RETINA* **2008**, *28*. [CrossRef]
204. Yoshimura, T.; Sonoda, K.-H.; Sugahara, M.; Mochizuki, Y.; Enaida, H.; Oshima, Y.; Ueno, A.; Hata, Y.; Yoshida, H.; Ishibashi, T. Comprehensive Analysis of Inflammatory Immune Mediators in Vitreoretinal Diseases. *PLoS ONE* **2009**, *4*, e8158. [CrossRef] [PubMed]
205. Mocan, M.C.; Kadayifcilar, S.; Eldem, B. Elevated intravitreal interleukin-6 levels in patients with proliferative diabetic retinopathy. *Can. J. Ophthalmol.* **2006**, *41*, 747–752. [CrossRef] [PubMed]
206. Garbutcheon-Singh, K.B.; Carnt, N.; Pattamatta, U.; Samarawickrama, C.; White, A.; Calder, V. A Review of the Cytokine IL-17 in Ocular Surface and Corneal Disease. *Curr. Eye Res.* **2019**, *44*, 1–10. [CrossRef] [PubMed]
207. Li, Y.; Zhou, Y. Interleukin-17: The Role for Pathological Angiogenesis in Ocular Neovascular Diseases. *Tohoku J. Exp. Med.* **2019**, *247*, 87–98. [CrossRef]
208. Feenstra, D.J.; Yego, E.C.; Mohr, S. Modes of Retinal Cell Death in Diabetic Retinopathy. *J. Clin. Exp. Ophthalmol.* **2013**, *4*, 298. [CrossRef]
209. Devi, T.S.; Hosoya, K.-I.; Terasaki, T.; Singh, L.P. Critical role of TXNIP in oxidative stress, DNA damage and retinal pericyte apoptosis under high glucose: Implications for diabetic retinopathy. *Exp. Cell Res.* **2013**, *319*, 1001–1012. [CrossRef]
210. Dartt, D.A. Tear lipocalin: Structure and function. *Ocul. Surf.* **2011**, *9*, 126–138. [CrossRef]
211. Yusifov, T.N.; Abduragimov, A.R.; Narsinh, K.; Gasymov, O.K.; Glasgow, B.J. Tear lipocalin is the major endonuclease in tears. *Mol. Vis.* **2008**, *14*, 180–188.
212. Zhao, H.; He, Y.; Ren, Y.-R.; Chen, B.-H. Corneal alteration and pathogenesis in diabetes mellitus. *Int. J. Ophthalmol.* **2019**, *12*, 1939–1950. [CrossRef]
213. Kim, J.; Kim, C.-S.; Sohn, E.; Jeong, I.-H.; Kim, H.; Kim, J.S. Involvement of advanced glycation end products, oxidative stress and nuclear factor-kappaB in the development of diabetic keratopathy. *Graefe Arch. Clin. Exp. Ophthalmol.* **2011**, *4*, 529–536. [CrossRef]
214. Hrabec, E.; Naduk, J.; Strek, M.; Hrabec, Z. Type IV collagenases (MMP-2 and MMP-9) and their substrates–intracellular proteins, hormones, cytokines, chemokines and their receptors. *Postepy Biochem.* **2007**, *53*, 37–45. [PubMed]
215. Notari, L.; Miller, A.; Martínez, A.; Amaral, J.; Ju, M.; Robinson, G.; Smith, L.E.H.; Becerra, S.P. Pigment Epithelium–Derived Factor Is a Substrate for Matrix Metalloproteinase Type 2 and Type 9: Implications for Downregulation in Hypoxia. *Investig. Ophthalmol. Vis. Sci.* **2005**, *46*, 2736–2747. [CrossRef]
216. Giebel, S.J.; Menicucci, G.; McGuire, P.G.; Das, A. Matrix metalloproteinases in early diabetic retinopathy and their role in alteration of the blood–retinal barrier. *Lab. Investig.* **2005**, *85*, 597–607. [CrossRef] [PubMed]
217. Zucker, S.; Mirza, H.; Conner, C.E.; Lorenz, A.F.; Drews, M.D.; Bahou, W.F.; Jesty, J. Vascular endothelial groth factor induces tissue factor and matrix metalloproteinase production in endothelial cells: Conversion of prothrombin to thrombin results in progelatininase a activation and cell proliferation. *Int. J. Cancer* **1998**, *75*, 780–786. [CrossRef]
218. Descamps, F.J.; Martens, E.; Kangave, D.; Struyf, S.; Geboes, K.; Van Damme, J.; Opdenakker, G.; Abu El-Asrar, A.M. The activated form of gelatinase B/matrix metalloproteinase-9 is associated with diabetic vitreous hemorrhage. *Exp. Eye Res.* **2006**, *83*, 401–407. [CrossRef]
219. Noda, K.; Ishida, S.; Inoue, M.; Obata, K.-I.; Oguchi, Y.; Okada, Y.; Ikeda, E. Production and Activation of Matrix Metalloproteinase-2 in Proliferative Diabetic Retinopathy. *Investig. Ophthalmol. Vis. Sci.* **2003**, *44*, 2163–2170. [CrossRef]
220. Ow, Y.-L.P.; Green, D.R.; Hao, Z.; Mak, T.W. Cytochrome c: Functions beyond respiration. *Nat. Rev. Mol. Cell Biol.* **2008**, *9*, 532–542. [CrossRef]
221. Chertkova, R.V.; Brazhe, N.A.; Bryantseva, T.V.; Nekrasov, A.N.; Dolgikh, D.A.; Yusipovich, A.; Sosnovtseva, O.V.; Maksimov, G.V.; Rubin, A.B.; Kirpichnikov, M.P. New insight into the mechanism of mitochondrial cytochrome c function. *PLoS ONE* **2017**, *12*, e0178280. [CrossRef]
222. Mizutani, M.; Kern, T.S.; Lorenzi, M. Accelerated death of retinal microvascular cells in human and experimental diabetic retinopathy. *J. Clin. Investig.* **1996**, *97*, 2883–2890. [CrossRef]

223. Mohr, S.; Xi, X.; Tang, J.; Kern, T.S. Caspase Activation in Retinas of Diabetic and Galactosemic Mice and Diabetic Patients. *Diabetes* **2002**, *51*, 1172. [CrossRef]
224. Chapple, C.E.; Robisson, B.; Spinelli, L.; Guien, C.; Becker, E.; Brun, C. Extreme multifunctional proteins identified from a human protein interaction network. *Nat. Commun.* **2015**, *6*, 7412. [CrossRef]
225. Santucci, R.; Sinibaldi, F.; Cozza, P.; Polticelli, F.; Fiorucci, L. Cytochrome c: An extreme multifunctional protein with a key role in cell fate. *Int. J. Biol. Macromol.* **2019**, *136*, 1237–1246. [CrossRef] [PubMed]
226. Kowluru, R.A.; Tang, J.; Kern, T.S. Abnormalities of Retinal Metabolism in Diabetes and Experimental Galactosemia. *Diabetes* **2001**, *50*, 1938. [CrossRef] [PubMed]
227. McKinnon, S.J.; Lehman, D.M.; Kerrigan-Baumrind, L.A.; Merges, C.A.; Pease, M.E.; Kerrigan, D.F.; Ransom, N.L.; Tahzib, N.G.; A Reitsamer, H.; Levkovitch-Verbin, H.; et al. Caspase Activation and Amyloid Precursor Protein Cleavage in Rat Ocular Hypertension. *Investig. Ophthalmol. Vis. Sci.* **2002**, *43*, 1077–1087.
228. Tang, J.; Kern, T.S. Inflammation in diabetic retinopathy. *Prog. Retin. Eye Res.* **2011**, *30*, 343–358. [CrossRef]
229. Jiang, N.; Chen, X.-L.; Yang, H.-W.; Ma, Y.-R. Effects of nuclear factor κB expression on retinal neovascularization and apoptosis in a diabetic retinopathy rat model. *Int. J. Ophthalmol.* **2015**, *8*, 448–452. [CrossRef]
230. Hammes, H.-P.; Lin, J.; Renner, O.; Shani, M.; Lundqvist, A.; Betsholtz, C.; Brownlee, M.; Deutsch, U. Pericytes and the Pathogenesis of Diabetic Retinopathy. *Diabetes* **2002**, *51*, 3107. [CrossRef]
231. Busik, J.V.; Mohr, S.; Grant, M.B. Hyperglycemia-induced reactive oxygen species toxicity to endothelial cells is dependent on paracrine mediators. *Diabetes* **2008**, *57*, 1952–1965. [CrossRef]
232. Kowluru, R.A.; Koppolu, P.; Chakrabarti, S.; Chen, S. Diabetes-induced Activation of Nuclear Transcriptional Factor in the Retina, and its Inhibition by Antioxidants. *Free Radic. Res.* **2003**, *37*, 1169–1180. [CrossRef]
233. Yuuki, T.; Kanda, T.; Kimura, Y.; Kotajima, N.; Tamura, J.; Kobayashi, I.; Kishi, S. Inflammatory cytokines in vitreous fluid and serum of patients with diabetic vitreoretinopathy. *J. Diabetes Complicat.* **2001**, *15*, 257–259. [CrossRef]
234. Kowluru, R.A.; Shan, Y.; Mishra, M. Dynamic DNA methylation of matrix metalloproteinase-9 in the development of diabetic retinopathy. *Lab. Investig. J. Technol. Methods Pathol.* **2016**, *96*, 1040–1049. [CrossRef]
235. Coco, C.; Sgarra, L.; Potenza, M.A.; Nacci, C.; Ms, B.P.; Barbano, R.; Parrella, P.; Montagnani, M. Can Epigenetics of Endothelial Dysfunction Represent the Key to Precision Medicine in Type 2 Diabetes Mellitus? *Int. J. Mol. Sci.* **2019**, *20*, 2949. [CrossRef] [PubMed]
236. Kanda, A.; Noda, K.; Saito, W.; Ishida, S. Vitreous renin activity correlates with vascular endothelial growth factor in proliferative diabetic retinopathy. *Br. J. Ophthalmol.* **2013**, *97*, 666–668. [CrossRef] [PubMed]
237. Maghbooli, Z.; Hossein-Nezhad, A.; Larijani, B.; Amini, M.; Keshtkar, A. Global DNA methylation as a possible biomarker for diabetic retinopathy. *Diabetes Metab. Res. Rev.* **2015**, *31*, 183–189. [CrossRef] [PubMed]
238. Zhong, Q.; Kowluru, R.A. Regulation of matrix metalloproteinase-9 by epigenetic modifications and the development of diabetic retinopathy. *Diabetes Care* **2013**, *62*, 2559–2568. [CrossRef] [PubMed]
239. Tewari, S.; Zhong, Q.; Santos, J.M.; Kowluru, A. Mitochondria DNA replication and DNA methylation in the metabolic memory associated with continued progression of diabetic retinopathy. *Investig. Ophthalmol. Vis. Sci.* **2012**, *53*, 4881–4888. [CrossRef]
240. Mishra, M.; Kowluru, R.A. The Role of DNA Methylation in the Metabolic Memory Phenomenon Associated With the Continued Progression of Diabetic Retinopathy. *Investig. Ophthalmol. Vis. Sci.* **2016**, *57*, 5748–5757. [CrossRef]
241. Shafabakhsh, R.; Aghadavod, E.; Ghayour-Mobarhan, M.; Ferns, G.; Asemi, Z. Role of histone modification and DNA methylation in signaling pathways involved in diabetic retinopathy. *J. Cell. Physiol.* **2019**, *234*, 7839–7846. [CrossRef]
242. Mishra, M.; Kowluru, R.A. DNA Methylation—A Potential Source of Mitochondria DNA Base Mismatch in the Development of Diabetic Retinopathy. *Mol. Neurobiol.* **2019**, *56*, 88–101. [CrossRef]
243. Mohammed, S.A.; Ambrosini, S.; Lüscher, T.; Paneni, F.; Costantino, S. Epigenetic Control of Mitochondrial Function in the Vasculature. *Front. Cardiovasc. Med.* **2020**, *7*, 28. [CrossRef]
244. Iacobazzi, V.; Castegna, A.; Infantino, V.; Andria, G. Mitochondrial DNA methylation as a next-generation biomarker and diagnostic tool. *Mol. Genet. Metab.* **2013**, *110*, 25–34. [CrossRef]
245. Lanza, M.; Benincasa, G.; Costa, D.; Napoli, C. Clinical Role of Epigenetics and Network Analysis in Eye Diseases: A Translational Science Review. *J. Ophthalmol.* **2019**, *2019*, 2424956. [CrossRef] [PubMed]

246. Duraisamy, A.J.; Mishra, M.; Kowluru, A.; Kowluru, A. Epigenetics and Regulation of Oxidative Stress in Diabetic Retinopathy. *Investig. Ophthalmol. Vis. Sci.* **2018**, *59*, 4831–4840. [CrossRef] [PubMed]
247. Duraisamy, A.J.; Radhakrishnan, R.; Seyoum, B.; Abrams, G.W.; Kowluru, A. Epigenetic Modifications in Peripheral Blood as Potential Noninvasive Biomarker of Diabetic Retinopathy. *Transl. Vis. Sci. Technol.* **2019**, *8*, 43. [CrossRef] [PubMed]
248. Xu, C.; Wu, Y.; Liu, G.; Liu, X.; Wang, F.; Yu, J. Relationship between homocysteine level and diabetic retinopathy: A systematic review and meta-analysis. *Diagn. Pathol.* **2014**, *9*, 167. [CrossRef] [PubMed]
249. Tawfik, A.; Mohamed, R.; Elsherbiny, N.M.; DeAngelis, M.M.; Bartoli, M.; Al-Shabrawey, M. Homocysteine: A Potential Biomarker for Diabetic Retinopathy. *J. Clin. Med.* **2019**, *8*, 121. [CrossRef] [PubMed]
250. Elsherbiny, N.M.; Sharma, I.; Kira, D.; Alhusban, S.; Samra, Y.A.; Jadeja, R.; Martin, P.; Al-Shabrawey, M.; Tawfik, A. Homocysteine Induces Inflammation in Retina and Brain. *Biomolecules* **2020**, *10*, 393. [CrossRef]
251. Kowluru, R.A.; Mishra, M. Therapeutic targets for altering mitochondrial dysfunction associated with diabetic retinopathy. *Expert Opin. Ther. Targets* **2018**, *22*, 233–245. [CrossRef]
252. Rodríguez, M.L.; Pérez, S.; Mena-Mollá, S.; Desco, M.C.; Ortega, Á.L. Oxidative Stress and Microvascular Alterations in Diabetic Retinopathy: Future Therapies. *Oxid. Med. Cell. Longev.* **2019**, *2019*, 4940825. [CrossRef]
253. Sinclair, S.H.; Schwartz, S.S. Diabetic Retinopathy-An Underdiagnosed and Undertreated Inflammatory, Neuro-Vascular Complication of Diabetes. *Front. Endocrinol.* **2019**, *10*, 843. [CrossRef]
254. Zhang, L.W.; Zhao, H.; Chen, B.H. Reactive oxygen species mediates a metabolic memory of high glucose stress signaling in bovine retinal pericytes. *Int. J. Ophthalmol.* **2019**, *12*, 1067–1074. [CrossRef]
255. Kowluru, R.A. Mitochondrial Stability in Diabetic Retinopathy: Lessons Learned From Epigenetics. *Diabetes* **2019**, *68*, 241–247. [CrossRef] [PubMed]
256. Khullar, M.; Cheema, B.S.; Raut, S.K. Emerging Evidence of Epigenetic Modifications in Vascular Complication of Diabetes. *Front. Endocrinol.* **2017**, *8*, 237. [CrossRef] [PubMed]
257. Zhang, X.; Bao, S.; Lai, D.; Rapkins, R.W.; Gillies, M.C. Intravitreal triamcinolone acetonide inhibits breakdown of the blood-retinal barrier through differential regulation of VEGF-A and its receptors in early diabetic rat retinas. *Diabetes* **2008**, *57*, 1026–1033. [CrossRef] [PubMed]
258. Zhang, X.; Zhao, L.; Hambly, B.D.; Bao, S.; Wang, K. Diabetic retinopathy: Reversibility of epigenetic modifications and new therapeutic targets. *Cell Biosci.* **2017**, *15*, 42. [CrossRef]
259. Kaspar, J.W.; Niture, S.K.; Jaiswal, A.K. Nrf2:INrf2 (Keap1) signaling in oxidative stress. *Free Radic. Biol. Med.* **2009**, *47*, 1304–1309. [CrossRef]
260. Zhong, Q.; Kowluru, R.A. Epigenetic modification of Sod2 in the development of diabetic retinopathy and in the metabolic memory: Role of histone methylation. *Investig. Ophthalmol. Vis. Sci.* **2013**, *54*, 244–250. [CrossRef]
261. Santos, J.M.; Tewari, S.; Goldberg, A.F.X.; Kowluru, A. Mitochondrial biogenesis and the development of diabetic retinopathy. *Free Radic Biol Med.* **2011**, *51*, 1849–1860. [CrossRef]
262. Zhang, L.W.; Xia, H.; Han, Q.; Chen, B. Effects of antioxidant gene therapy on the development of diabetic retinopathy and the metabolic memory phenomenon. *Graefe Arch. Clin. Exp. Ophthalmol.* **2015**, *253*, 249–259. [CrossRef]
263. Sundar, I.K.; Yao, H.; Rahman, I. Oxidative stress and chromatin remodeling in chronic obstructive pulmonary disease and smoking-related diseases. *Antioxid. Redox Signal.* **2013**, *18*, 1956–1971. [CrossRef]
264. Aydin, Ö.Z.; Vermeulen, W.; Lans, H. ISWI chromatin remodeling complexes in the DNA damage response. *Cell Cycle* **2014**, *13*, 3016–3025. [CrossRef]
265. Matilainen, O.; Sleiman, M.S.B.; Quirós, P.M.; Garcia, S.M.D.A.; Auwerx, J. The chromatin remodeling factor ISW-1 integrates organismal responses against nuclear and mitochondrial stress. *Nat. Commun.* **2017**, *8*, 1818. [CrossRef] [PubMed]
266. Perrone, L.; Devi, T.S.; Hosoya, K.-I.; Terasaki, T.; Singh, L.P. Inhibition of TXNIP expression in vivo blocks early pathologies of diabetic retinopathy. *Cell Death Dis.* **2010**, *1*, e65. [CrossRef] [PubMed]
267. Reddy, M.A.; Zhang, E.; Natarajan, R. Epigenetic mechanisms in diabetic complications and metabolic memory. *Diabetologia* **2015**, *58*, 443–455. [CrossRef]
268. Kreuz, S.; Fischle, W. Oxidative stress signaling to chromatin in health and disease. *Epigenomics* **2016**, *8*, 843–862. [CrossRef]

269. Moodie, F.M.; Marwick, J.A.; Anderson, C.S.; Szulakowski, P.; Biswas, S.K.; Bauter, M.R.; Kilty, I.; Rahman, I. Oxidative stress and cigarette smoke alter chromatin remodeling but differentially regulate NF-kappaB activation and proinflammatory cytokine release in alveolar epithelial cells. *FASEB J.* **2004**, *18*, 1897–1899. [CrossRef]
270. Gozani, O.; Karuman, P.; Jones, D.R.; Ivanov, D.; Cha, J.; Lugovskoy, A.A.; Baird, C.L.; Zhu, H.; Field, S.J.; Lessnick, S.L.; et al. The PHD finger of the chromatin-associated protein ING2 functions as a nuclear phosphoinositide receptor. *Cell* **2003**, *114*, 99–111. [CrossRef]
271. Bua, D.J.; Martin, G.M.; Binda, O.; Gozani, O. Nuclear phosphatidylinositol-5-phosphate regulates ING2 stability at discrete chromatin targets in response to DNA damage. *Sci. Rep.* **2013**, *3*, 2137. [CrossRef]
272. Saeidi, L.; Ghaedi, H.; Sadatamini, M.; Vahabpour, R.; Rahimipour, A.; Shanaki, M.; Mansoori, Z.; Kazerouni, F. Long non-coding RNA LY86-AS1 and HCG27_201 expression in type 2 diabetes mellitus. *Mol. Biol. Rep.* **2018**, *45*, 2601–2608. [CrossRef]
273. Carthew, R.W.; Sontheimer, E.J. Origins and Mechanisms of miRNAs and siRNAs. *Cell* **2009**, *136*, 642–655. [CrossRef]
274. Xue, M.; Zhuo, Y.; Shan, B. MicroRNAs, Long Noncoding RNAs, and Their Functions in Human Disease. *Methods Mol. Biol.* **2017**, *1617*, 1–25. [CrossRef]
275. Ha, T.-Y. MicroRNAs in Human Diseases: From Cancer to Cardiovascular Disease. *Immune Netw.* **2011**, *11*, 135–154. [CrossRef]
276. Khalil, A.M.; Guttman, M.; Huarte, M.; Garber, M.; Raj, A.; Morales, D.R.; Thomas, K.; Presser, A.; Bernstein, B.E.; Van Oudenaarden, A.; et al. Many human large intergenic noncoding RNAs associate with chromatin-modifying complexes and affect gene expression. *Proc. Natl. Acad. Sci. USA* **2009**, *106*, 11667–11672. [CrossRef]
277. Panchapakesan, U.; Pollock, C. Long non-coding RNAs-towards precision medicine in diabetic kidney disease? *Clin. Sci.* **2016**, *130*, 1599–1602. [CrossRef]
278. Kovacs, B.; Lumayag, S.; Cowan, C.; Xu, S. MicroRNAs in early diabetic retinopathy in streptozotocin-induced diabetic rats. *Investig. Ophthalmol. Vis. Sci.* **2011**, *52*, 4402–4409. [CrossRef]
279. Xu, W.; Li, F.; Liu, Z.; Xu, Z.; Sun, B.; Cao, J.; Liu, Y. MicroRNA-27b inhibition promotes Nrf2/ARE pathway activation and alleviates intracerebral hemorrhage-induced brain injury. *Oncotarget* **2017**, *8*, 70669–70684. [CrossRef]
280. Veliceasa, D.; Biyashev, D.; Qin, G.; Misener, S.; Mackie, A.R.; Kishore, R.; Volpert, O.V. Therapeutic manipulation of angiogenesis with miR-27b. *Vasc. Cell* **2015**, *7*, 6. [CrossRef]
281. Liu, H.N.; Cao, N.; Li, X.; Qian, W.; Chen, X.-L. Serum microRNA-211 as a biomarker for diabetic retinopathy via modulating Sirtuin 1. *Biochem. Biophys. Res. Commun.* **2018**, *505*, 1236–1243. [CrossRef]
282. Mishra, M.; Duraisamy, A.J.; Kowluru, R.A. Sirt1: A Guardian of the Development of Diabetic Retinopathy. *Diabetes* **2018**, *67*, 745–754. [CrossRef]
283. Liang, Z.; Gao, K.P.; Wang, Y.X.; Liu, Z.C.; Tian, L.; Yang, X.Z.; Ding, J.; Wu, W.T.; Yang, W.H.; Li, Y.L.; et al. RNA sequencing identified specific circulating miRNA biomarkers for early detection of diabetes retinopathy. *Am. J. Physiol. Endocrinol. Metab.* **2018**, *315*, 374–385. [CrossRef]
284. Desmettre, T. Epigenetics in age-related macular degeneration (AMD)—French translation of the article. *J. Fr. Ophtalmol.* **2018**, *41*, 981–990. [CrossRef]
285. Leung, A.K.; Calabrese, J.M.; Sharp, P.A. Quantitative analysis of Argonaute protein reveals microRNA-dependent localization to stress granules. *Proc. Natl. Acad. Sci. USA* **2006**, *103*, 18125–18130. [CrossRef]
286. Shen, J.; Xia, W.; Khotskaya, Y.B.; Huo, L.; Nakanishi, K.; Lim, S.-O.; Du, Y.; Wang, Y.; Chang, W.-C.; Chen, C.-H.; et al. EGFR modulates microRNA maturation in response to hypoxia through phosphorylation of AGO2. *Nature* **2013**, *497*, 383–387. [CrossRef]
287. Qin, L.L.; An, M.-X.; Liu, Y.-L.; Xu, H.-C.; Lu, Z.-Q. MicroRNA-126: A promising novel biomarker in peripheral blood for diabetic retinopathy. *Int. J. Ophthalmol.* **2017**, *10*, 530–534. [CrossRef]
288. Thomas, A.A.; Biswas, S.; Feng, B.; Chen, S.; Gonder, J.; Chakrabarti, S. lncRNA H19 prevents endothelial-mesenchymal transition in diabetic retinopathy. *Diabetologia* **2019**, *62*, 517–530. [CrossRef]
289. Zhang, X.; Shi, E.; Yang, L.; Fu, W.; Hu, F.; Zhou, X. LncRNA AK077216 is downregulated in diabetic retinopathy and inhibited the apoptosis of retinal pigment epithelial cells by downregulating miR-383. *Endocr. J.* **2019**, *66*, 1011–1016. [CrossRef]

290. Yin, L.; Sun, Z.; Ren, Q.; Su, X.; Zhang, D. Long Non-Coding RNA BANCR Is Overexpressed in Patients with Diabetic Retinopathy and Promotes Apoptosis of Retinal Pigment Epithelial Cells. *Med. Sci. Monit.* **2019**, *25*, 2845–2851. [CrossRef]
291. Zhang, X.; Zou, X.; Li, Y.; Wang, Y. Downregulation of lncRNA BANCR participates in the development of retinopathy among diabetic patients. *Exp. Ther. Med.* **2019**, *17*, 4132–4138. [CrossRef]
292. Perrone, L.; Matrone, C.; Singh, L.P. Epigenetic modifications and potential new treatment targets in diabetic retinopathy. *J. Ophthalmol.* **2014**, *2014*, 789120. [CrossRef]
293. El-Osta, A. Redox mediating epigenetic changes confer metabolic memories. *Circ. Res.* **2012**, 262–264. [CrossRef]
294. Santos, J.M.; Kowluru, R.A. Role of mitochondria biogenesis in the metabolic memory associated with the continued progression of diabetic retinopathy and its regulation by lipoic acid. *Investig. Ophthalmol. Vis. Sci.* **2011**, *52*, 8791–8798. [CrossRef]
295. Kowluru, R.A. Diabetic retinopathy, metabolic memory and epigenetic modifications. *Vis. Res.* **2017**, *139*, 30–38. [CrossRef] [PubMed]

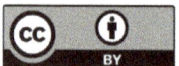

© 2020 by the authors. Licensee MDPI, Basel, Switzerland. This article is an open access article distributed under the terms and conditions of the Creative Commons Attribution (CC BY) license (http://creativecommons.org/licenses/by/4.0/).

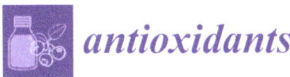

Review

Extracellular Vesicles and MicroRNA: Putative Role in Diagnosis and Treatment of Diabetic Retinopathy

Beatriz Martins [1,2,†], Madania Amorim [1,2,†], Flávio Reis [1,2], António Francisco Ambrósio [1,2,3] and Rosa Fernandes [1,2,3,*]

1. Coimbra Institute for Clinical and Biomedical Research (iCBR), Faculty of Medicine, University of Coimbra, 3000-548 Coimbra, Portugal; mrro_54@hotmail.com (B.M.); madaniyah.gaffur@gmail.com (M.A.); freis@fmed.uc.pt (F.R.); afambrosio@fmed.uc.pt (A.F.A.)
2. Center for Innovative Biomedicine and Biotechnology, University of Coimbra, 3000-548 Coimbra, Portugal
3. Association for Innovation and Biomedical Research on Light and Image (AIBILI), 3000-548 Coimbra, Portugal
* Correspondence: rcfernandes@fmed.uc.pt; Tel.: +351-239480072
† These authors contributed equally to this work.

Received: 30 June 2020; Accepted: 2 August 2020; Published: 4 August 2020

Abstract: Diabetic retinopathy (DR) is a complex, progressive, and heterogenous retinal degenerative disease associated with diabetes duration. It is characterized by glial, neural, and microvascular dysfunction, being the blood-retinal barrier (BRB) breakdown a hallmark of the early stages. In advanced stages, there is formation of new blood vessels, which are fragile and prone to leaking. This disease, if left untreated, may result in severe vision loss and eventually legal blindness. Although there are some available treatment options for DR, most of them are targeted to the advanced stages of the disease, have some adverse effects, and many patients do not adequately respond to the treatment, which demands further research. Oxidative stress and low-grade inflammation are closely associated processes that play a critical role in the development of DR. Retinal cells communicate with each other or with another one, using cell junctions, adhesion contacts, and secreted soluble factors that can act in neighboring or long-distance cells. Another mechanism of cell communication is via secreted extracellular vesicles (EVs), through exchange of material. Here, we review the current knowledge on deregulation of cell-to-cell communication through EVs, discussing the changes in miRNA expression profiling in body fluids and their role in the development of DR. Thereafter, current and promising therapeutic agents for preventing the progression of DR will be discussed.

Keywords: diabetic retinopathy (DR); inflammation; oxidative stress; angiogenesis; extracellular vesicles; miRNA; biomarkers; antioxidants

1. Introduction

Diabetes mellitus (DM) is one of the most common metabolic disorders that has become both a major public health threat and an economic burden for society. According to estimates from the International Diabetes Federation (IDF) in 2019, 463 million adults (one in eleven between 20–79 years) were living with diabetes and this number is expected to increase to around 700 million by 2045 [1]. Diabetes is a systemic disease that can affect almost any part of the body, including the eye, especially the retinal tissue, causing a microvascular complication known as diabetic retinopathy (DR). Diabetic retinopathy is a leading cause of visual impairment among working-age adults worldwide [2], affecting more than 149 million individuals [3]. The global prevalence of this disease has increased to epidemic proportions [4], and is responsible for 50,000 new cases of retinal neovascularization and diabetic macular edema worldwide every year [5]. This means that it affects around one-third of the diabetic population, with approximately one-tenth of these patients having vision-threatening retinopathy [6,7]. Although DR is not a mortal illness, it leads to emotional distress and reduces daily life functionality, thus significantly impacting the quality of life in patients with advanced stages of the disease. In addition to the visual impairment, it is associated with significant economic consequences for public health systems [7].

During the first two decades after the onset of diabetes, almost all type 1 diabetes (T1D) cases develop DR and about two thirds of patients with type 2 diabetes (T2D) also have some form of the disease [8]. DR is a silent complication that in its early stages causes no symptoms. However, chronic hyperglycemia can produce noticeable retina damage over time, involving blood and other fluids leakage out of retinal capillaries, which may result in cloudy or blurred vision. Therefore, if left untreated DR may result in severe visual impairment or even blindness. Although over the past several decades significant advances have been made and a variety of treatments for DR are currently available, none of them are yet curative. In the early stages of the disease, a tight blood glucose control and regular monitoring can help prevent its progression to more advanced stages. In advanced stages, the main treatments of DR include intraocular injections of anti-VEGF antibodies, laser treatments, and vitrectomy [7,9]. Although the results are encouraging and these treatments can halt the progression of DR or even temporarily improve the vision loss, they are associated with two major concerns/limitations: Can produce several adverse effects and are ineffective in some of the patients (non-responders). A better understanding of the exact cellular and molecular mechanisms underlying DR and the discovery of reliable early biomarkers will decisively contribute to the identification of putative targets for the development of new and more effective options than existing treatments offer.

Extracellular vesicles (EVs) are a heterogenous population of membranous vesicles that can be released into the extracellular milieu by the majority of the cells of the body [10]. They can be classified into three categories (microvesicles, exosomes, and apoptotic bodies) based on their size and mode of biogenesis. It is now known that tissue homeostasis strongly depends on an effective cell-to-cell communication mediated by EVs. These vesicles released from the parent cells are extracellular carriers of both proteins, RNA, and miRNA, which are capable of inducing a wide range of effects on recipient cells [11]. In fact, many miRNAs were described to play critical roles in the regulation of several cellular processes, including cell cycle, proliferation, and apoptosis [12], contributing therefore to the maintenance of the retinal tissue homeostasis. Hence, it is expected that miRNA expression dysregulation also affects those processes, directly contributing to pathological conditions, such as DR. Importantly, changes in the miRNA expression profile may reflect the pathological state, highlighting the putative use of miRNAs as biomarkers to predict DR progression [13].

Herein, we describe and discuss how inflammation and oxidative stress contribute to retinal endothelial cells dysfunction in DR, highlighting the deregulation of cell-to-cell communication mediated by extracellular vesicles. Moreover, we will summarize the most recent studies about the role of miRNAs in the pathogenesis of DR and the potential beneficial effects of therapeutic agents with anti-inflammatory and antioxidant properties.

2. Pathophysiologic Changes and Clinical Definition of DR

Diabetic retinopathy is a progressive disease, whose major risk factor is the duration of diabetes. It develops through a series of stages of increasing degrees of severity [14] and affects the microvascular circulation of the retina, compromising the integrity and function of retinal tissue. Endothelial cells, the building blocks of the microvasculature, are particularly sensitive to sustained hyperglycemia-induced damage [15,16]. The retina is not only a network of blood vessels, rather it is a multilayered neuronal (photoreceptors, and horizontal, bipolar, amacrine and ganglion cells) and glial (astrocytes, Müller cells, and microglia) cells that covers approximately 95% of the tissue, with blood vessels (endothelial cells and pericytes) comprising only a small portion (<5%) [17]. In healthy conditions, a synergistic interaction between retinal neurons, glial cells, and blood vessels contributes to the autoregulation of vascular flow and metabolic activity. Indeed, retinal blood vessels provide nutrients to the neural tissue, and neuroglial cells are essential players in transmission of visual information, being therefore crucial to the maintenance of the retinal homeostasis [18]. Thus, the intimate relationship between neuroglial and vascular networks is only possible by a metabolic synergy and cell-to-cell communication [18]. Although microvascular changes are found in DR and its diagnosis is based on their screening, many studies using electrophysiological tests pointed to changes in the neuroretinal function before the onset of microvascular lesions in the human retina [19–22]. In addition, early thinning on the inner retina can be detected in type 2 diabetes by spectral-domain optical coherence tomography (SD-OCT) scans analysis, even before visible vascular changes are present, which supports the presence of a neurodegenerative process in diabetic patients [23].

During the development and progression of DR several changes take place, which can be grouped into categories, such as physiological, rheological, hormonal, and biochemical, etc. [24]. It is well established that hyperglycemia contributes both to DR and other microvascular complications of diabetes, but it is not the single factor. There are several biochemical pathways that are involved in the onset and progression of DR. Moreover, no specific mechanism can be regarded as the main responsiblility for DR, rather a complex relationship between several pathways and factors may be important to the disease process. Functional and/or morphological changes are found in various retinal cell types, including endothelial cells, pericytes, microglial cells, ganglion cells, Müller cells, astrocytes, and microglia, in the diabetic retina, before clinical symptoms and diagnosis are attained (Figure 1) [25]. The development of the disease is believed to be due to a dysregulation of the neuroglial vascular unit. Nevertheless, this whole scenario is dynamic at different stages of the natural history of DR and varies from individual to individual [24,26]. In the first stage (preclinical retinopathy) there are significant biochemical and histological changes in the retinal vessels [27], which include increased permeability of the blood-retinal barrier (BRB), loss of perivascular cells, vascular basement membrane thickening with subsequent capillary occlusion, and neuronal and glial abnormalities. This is followed by a stage of morphostructural and pathophysiological changes, in which the progressive dysfunction of endothelial cells plays a crucial role, leading to worsening of previous changes and culminating in neovascularization (Figure 1) [28]. These changes are ophthalmoscopically visible and based on them, according to the multicenter Early Treatment DR Study (ETDRS), the DR may be classified as non-proliferative DR (NPDR) and proliferative DR (PDR) [29].

The presence of a few microaneurysms characterizes the mild NPDR while their presence associated with intraretinal hemorrhages or venous beading characterizes the moderated NPRD [30]. Progressively, retinopathy can be characterized by deposits of lipids in the retina (hard retinal exudates), small infarctions located in the retinal nerve fiber layer (cotton patches), collateral dilated capillary channels in areas of retinal ischemia (intraretinal microvascular abnormalities), and irregular dilation of retinal veins associated with significant retinal ischemia (venous beading). Then, the disease may further advance to a stage characterized by the development of new blood vessels (PDR) in the retina in response to oxygen deprivation through upregulation of angiogenic factors and, in some cases, development of fibrous tissue at the optic disc or near venules in the retina [31]. Advanced PDR is commonly associated with preretinal and vitreous hemorrhage as a result of the bleeding of new retinal blood vessels, and a traction on the macula due to fibrovascular tissue, which will then lead to a significant vision loss [24,32]. Notwithstanding, it is important to highlight an additional category of DR, which is characterized by leakage of the retinal vessels and thickening of the retina thus leading to what is called diabetic macular edema (DME). DME can be developed in all of the stages of retinopathy, although being more prevalent in the late stages of the disease, being the most common cause of vision loss in diabetic individuals [24,30,33].

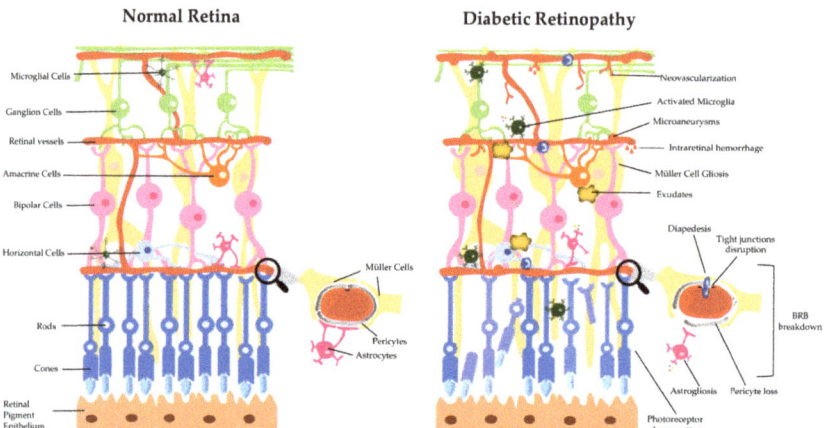

Figure 1. Schematic drawing of a cross-section of a healthy retina and a retina with diabetic retinopathy. The retina is a multilayered tissue composed by neuronal (photoreceptors, and horizontal, bipolar, amacrine and ganglion cells) and glial (astrocytes, Müller cells, and microglia) cells, that closely embed with three capillary plexuses. The blood-retinal barrier (BRB), that regulates the exchange of fluids between blood and retinal tissue, plays an important role in the maintenance of the retinal homeostasis. However, in diabetic retinopathy (DR) several retinal abnormalities appear, including microvascular changes (microaneurysms, intra-retinal hemorrhages, and neovascularization), the appearance of exudates, ganglion cell and photoreceptor degeneration, and glial dysfunction (astrogliosis, Müller cell gliosis, and activation of microglia). The reactivity of glial cells promotes the secretion of inflammatory cytokines, leukocyte adhesion, and diapedesis. These alterations lead to the breakdown of the BRB, characterized by pericyte loss and tight junctions' disruption.

3. The Role of Oxidative Stress and Inflammation in DR

The pathogenesis of DR is very complex and several mechanisms, such as hypoxia, oxidative stress, and inflammation are involved in the disease development and progression [30,34,35]. The retina is one of the most metabolically active tissues in the body, making it extremely sensitive to changes in oxygen levels [7]. In addition to the high content of polyunsaturated fatty acids (PUFAs), this tissue needs to produce energy (ATP) by consuming large amounts of glucose and oxygen, through the mitochondrial electron transport chain in the inner mitochondrial membrane. During this process, the electron transport chain can leak electrons directly onto molecular oxygen, generating free radicals/reactive oxygen species (ROS) [36]. Mitochondria are an important endogenous source of ROS in the retina. Although ROS play an important role in the immune response, excessive intracellular levels of ROS may damage cellular lipids, proteins, and nucleic acids. When ROS production exceeds cellular antioxidant capacity, ROS can thus contribute in a large scale to oxidative stress due to the limited mitochondrial reserve capacity, being particularly vulnerable to small changes in energy homeostasis [37]. Therefore, ROS can cause oxidative stress, damaging mitochondria [2], which results in a reduced efficiency of ATP production [36]. In the context of hyperglycemia, it has been shown that there is a dysregulation of mitochondrial biogenesis, leading to bioenergetics deficits [38]. Moreover, mitochondrial functional changes were detected in the retinas of diabetic rodents, before clinical manifestations of DR (pericyte loss and capillary degeneration) are present. Altogether, these data suggest that oxidative stress and mitochondrial dysfunction may play an important role in the onset and progression of DR.

The contribution of mitochondria to diabetes-induced oxidative stress is well established and, according to Brownlee [39], in his "unifying theory" of hyperglycemia-induced endothelial cell damage, ROS overproduction is the common upstream event that can stimulate the biochemical pathways which have a pathogenic role in DR: 1) The polyol (sorbitol) pathway, which can deplete the cytosolic nicotinamide adenine dinucleotide phosphate (NADPH), necessary to maintain glutathione (GSH), the main intracellular antioxidant, in its reduced state [24]; 2) the formation of advanced glycation end products (AGEs) intracellularly, which can induce cross-linking of proteins to promote vascular stiffness and enhance oxidative stress; 3) activation of different isoforms of protein kinase C (PKC) can induce changes in endothelial cell monolayer permeability (PKCα), cell proliferation (PKCβ) and increased ROS production, activation of the NF-kB, and platelet-derived growth factor (PDGF) survival signaling pathway (PKCδ) [40,41]; and 4) the hexosamine pathway, which decreases NADPH-dependent GSH production, is implicated in the apoptosis of endothelial cells and the limited proliferation of pericytes, as well as retinal neuronal apoptosis [42–44].

When intracellular antioxidant enzymes fail to remove efficiently ROS that are produced by retinal cells, excessive ROS can be accumulated within the cell cytoplasm, mitochondria, and nucleus. In the nucleus, ROS can cause DNA strand breaks [45,46].

Chronic hyperglycemia can trigger Müller cells and astrocytes reactivity, activating the transcription nuclear factor NF-κB [18]. Once activated, NF-κB is translocated into the nucleus, where it binds to nuclear DNA and promotes the expression of pro-inflammatory cytokines, such as interleukin (IL)-1β, IL-6, IL-8, interferon gamma (IFN-γ), and tumor necrosis factor-alpha (TNF-α). On the other hand, activation of the PI3K/Akt/mTOR signaling pathway mediates the secretion of inflammatory cytokines by ROS induced-hyperglycemia itself. Moreover, it has been proposed that Müller cells can directly initiate retinal inflammation in diabetes through stimulation of cluster of differentiation 40 (CD40) and indirectly signal to microglia to elicit inflammation [47].

Chronic hyperglycemia-induced vascular dysfunction is mediated through increased levels of intercellular adhesion molecule 1 (ICAM-1) in endothelial cells, that results in leukocyte adhesion to the endothelium, change of BRB permeability, and thrombus formation [48]. Increased levels of other inflammatory mediators have been also found in the vitreous of diabetic patients with retinopathy, such as the monocyte chemotactic protein 1(MCP-1), that is an important chemotactic factor for monocytes, and vascular endothelial growth factor (VEGF), an important mediator of angiogenesis and effector of permeability [49]. Cyclooxygenase-2 (COX-2) is another inflammatory agent that is increased in diabetic retinas and is released by activated inflammatory cells and glial cells, and may play an important role in the degeneration of retinal capillaries [50]. Under inflammation conditions, this enzyme increases the synthesis of prostaglandins, which stabilizes hypoxia-induced factor-1 (HIF-1), leading to VEGF expression and NF-kB activation. In parallel, mitochondrial ROS and oxidized mtDNA, when released into the cytosol, are recognized as damaged associated molecular patterns (DAMPs) by cytosolic pattern recognition receptors (PRRs), including toll-like receptors, namely TLR4 and TLR9. This recognition triggers cell death by different pathways: A NLR family pyrin domain containing 3 (NLRP3) inflammasome is formed, which leads to activation of caspase-1 and secretion of IL-1β and IL-18, leading to pyroptosis, a highly inflammatory form of programmed cell death [2,30,36]. Other types of cell death can occur, such as apoptosis and autophagy-dependent cell death. Apoptosis can be triggered by matrix metalloproteinases 2 and 9 (MMP-2 and MMP-9) that compromise the mitochondrial membrane potential [51,52]. Autophagy can lead to cell death by modulation of mTOR/AMPK, activating caspase 3 [53].

In summary, oxidative stress and low-grade inflammation associated with chronic hyperglycemia are considered to play a key role in the onset and progression of DR, being difficult to pinpoint exactly which of the mechanisms/pathways are most important in the pathogenesis of DR, rather the coexistence between them contribute to BRB breakdown and neovascularization [30]. Therefore, hyperglycemia leads to a series of successive triggered events, leading to neural, glial, and microvascular dysfunction, that culminate in DR [54].

4. Crosstalk between Endothelial Cells and Other Retinal Cells through Extracellular Vesicles (EVs)

Intercellular communication is an essential component in all multicellular organisms, ensuring the exchange of information between cells in response to normal homeostatic processes or to possible pathological threats. One of the most important components involved in both short- and long-distance communication are the EVs, a heterogenous group of cell-derived membrane vesicles limited by a lipid bilayer that are secreted from almost all cell types and contain proteins, lipids, and nucleic acids, such as mRNAs and miRNAs [11,55]. Depending on their size and biogenesis pathway, EVs can be classified into exosomes, microvesicles, or apoptotic bodies. Exosomes are nano-sized vesicles of endocytic origin, with a diameter between 30–150 nm. This subtype of vesicles is originated through the inward budding of a multivesicular body (MVB) membrane that fuses with the cell membrane releasing the intraluminal vesicles (ILVs) to the extracellular space which generate the exosomes [56]. Microvesicles, also known as ectosomes or microparticles, are cell membrane-derived vesicles with a size range between 100–1000 nm. These vesicles are formed through the direct outward budding of the plasma membrane after vertical trafficking of a specific molecular cargo and consequent release of the microvesicles [57]. Apoptotic bodies are the largest subtype of EVs, with a wide range of sizes between 50–5000 nm, that are released also by outward budding of the cell membrane, exclusively during apoptotic cell death (Figure 2) [58].

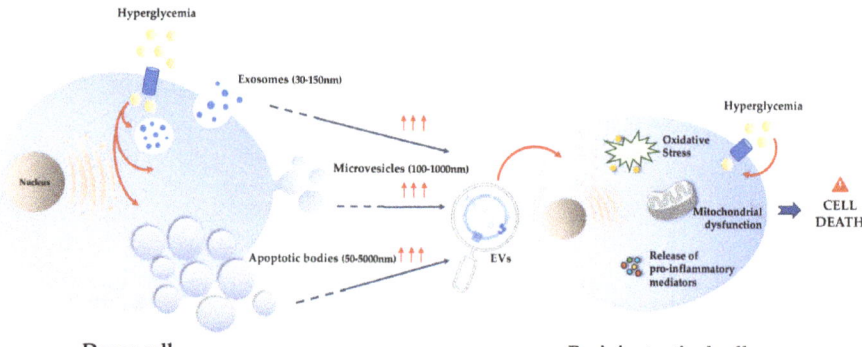

Figure 2. Extracellular vesicles (EVs) and their role in the pathogenesis of diabetic retinopathy (DR). EVs can be classified into three different types depending on their size and biogenesis—exosomes, microvesicles, and apoptotic bodies. Hyperglycemia leads to the increase of EVs released from donor cells. These EVs, derived from other retinal cells or from circulation, can interact with recipient/target retinal cells contributing, along with chronic hyperglycemia, to oxidative stress and release of pro-inflammatory mediators. These mechanisms may contribute to mitochondrial dysfunction leading to retinal cell death.

All types of EVs normally reflect the phenotype of their parental cells, since different cells secrete different EVs with specific cargo molecules depending on their function. This suggests that EVs molecular profile can be used to detect not only their origin but also somehow the molecular content of the cell of origin. This feature makes these vesicles very interesting candidates as biomarkers and therapeutic drug delivery systems for a variety of chronic diseases, including cancer and degenerative diseases, such as DR [59]. A recent study characterized the EVs released by adult neural retina in culture and this allowed to determine the cellular origin of different types of EVs through the analysis of their molecular cargo (RNA and proteins) [60]. The authors were able to detect EVs derived from photoreceptors which contain proteins such as rhodopsin, the photo-responsive receptor of rod cells, and cadherin related family member 1 (Cdhr1), an adhesion protein that is normally present in the outer and inner segments of photoreceptors. They have also detected the presence of neuronal-specific nuclear protein (NeuN) in the isolated EVs, a marker for amacrine and retinal ganglion cells. Additionally, through their molecular content, they were able to conclude that the retinal-derived EVs are mainly related with processes such as phototransduction, synapse structure, RNA processing, and transcription regulation [60]. Furthermore, other studies have also demonstrated that EVs from distinct retinal cells, such as astrocytes and retinal pigment epithelial (RPE) cells present different protein profiles, which suffer alterations during pathophysiological processes [61,62]. Therefore, besides intercellular communication being essential to the maintenance of retinal function, a small alteration in this balance can lead to the appearance of several retinal diseases. Although EVs biology in the visual system is not extensively investigated, some studies have already described that EVs are closely involved in the progression of several retinal diseases, such as age-related macular degeneration (AMD) and glaucoma [63,64].

It is known that diabetes and its macro- and microvascular complications are associated to increased levels of EVs with distinct molecular profiles [65], presenting for instance procoagulant, proinflammatory, and proangiogenic properties [66]. We can speculate that in the diabetic eye, and in particular in the retina, a single alteration in the number of EVs is able to disturb the normal visual homeostasis (Figure 2). In fact, EVs biological effects in the eye were described to be concentration-dependent at their target site [67]. Concerning DR, the chronic low-grade inflammation and oxidative stress, which play an important role in diabetes progression, are closely related with the dysfunction of metabolic pathways in retinal endothelial cells. Early diabetes-related endothelial dysfunction can lead to a deregulation of intercellular communication between retinal endothelial cells, leukocytes, and neuroglial cells, which results in increased BRB permeability [30]. This deregulation of intercellular communication between retinal cells is closely related to the release of EVs with different profiles. For example, a report involving diabetic patients showed the presence of increased levels of photoreceptor-derived and microglial-derived microvesicles in the vitreous of patients with proliferative DR. Additionally, this study also demonstrated that these EVs were able to stimulate endothelial cell proliferation and neovascularization both in vitro and in vivo, confirming their different molecular cargo in the context of hyperglycemia [68]. Regarding DR progression, the intercellular communication between retinal endothelial cells and pericytes is critical for the vascular damage present in the eye of diabetic patients [14]. A recent study has highlighted the role of exosomes containing a specific circular RNA (circRNA) in the progression of DR. In that study, the authors demonstrated that circRNA cPWW2P2A, which is upregulated in pericytes during the disease, is transferred through exosomes to endothelial cells contributing to retinal vascular dysfunction [69]. In the same context, another study has demonstrated that under diabetic-like conditions, mesenchymal stem cells-derived EVs were able to cause pericyte detachment and endothelial cell proliferation, which may be mediated by MMP-2, with consequent BRB disruption [70]. In this study, the authors have also addressed the involvement of EVs-derived MMPs in the progression of DR. In fact, several MMPs, such as MMP-2, MMP-9, and MMP-14 have been described as being increased in the vitreous fluid and in the retina of both patients with DR and animal models of DR, contributing to vessel destabilization and consequent BRB breakdown [71].

Other important mediators involved in DR onset and progression appear to be closely related with EVs-mediated communication. In fact, TNF-α, C-reactive protein and thrombin, commonly increased in the eye of diabetic patients, can stimulate the formation of endothelial microvesicles in vitro [72–74]. As a consequence, the increased release of endothelial EVs can stimulate the production of ROS in the target cells, which may contribute to retinal vascular damage in the context of DR progression [75]. Nonetheless, in the early stages of the disease, EVs can also exhibit protective effects, preventing the rapid progression of the retinal damage. For example, in vitro and in vivo studies have demonstrated that EVs derived from microglial cells were able to inhibit hypoxia-induced photoreceptor apoptosis, thus preventing neovascularization and alleviating visual injury [76].

All these studies highlighted the importance of a tight regulated intercellular communication between retinal cells and the role of retinal-derived EVs in the progression of retinal disorders, namely DR.

5. Contribution of Plasma EVs to Microvascular Damage in DR

With diabetes being a chronic systemic disorder, circulating EVs have an important role in the progression of several complications associated with this disease. Increased levels of cytokines (namely TNF-α), angiogenic factors, RANTES (regulated on activation, normal T-cell expressed and secreted), and angiotensin-2 have been detected in the plasma EVs of diabetic patients, highlighting their role in diabetes progression [77]. Although some EVs can pass the BRB [59], they can also act pathologically in the BRB. During the development of DR, increased vascular permeability can also facilitate the accumulation of these circulating EVs in the eye, which may be crucial to the development of the most progressive forms of the disease. In this sense, several studies have been reporting the role of plasma EVs on the activation of inflammatory and oxidative mechanisms involved in the microvascular damage in DR (Figure 2) [78].

It is known that the complement activation, due to proinflammatory changes and impairment of complement regulatory proteins, has a main role in the vascular damage and DR progression [79,80]. A recent study from Huang et al. has proven the involvement of plasma EVs on complement activation in the retina, using a diabetic animal model [81]. Increased levels of plasma exosomes were associated with increased levels of IgG, which was present in the membrane of the vesicles, resulting in the activation of the classic complement pathway. Additionally, the lack of IgG-laden exosomes resulted in a decrease of complement activation and consequent reduction of retinal vascular damage, proving the involvement of the circulating EVs in the microvascular damage through complement activation [81]. In the same way, a more recent study from the same group has demonstrated that, using the same animal model and primary cultures of human retinal endothelial cells (hRECs), this mechanism, by which plasma EVs can lead to retinal vascular damage, occurs due to the deposition of membrane attack complex (MAC) and cytosolic damage [82]. In fact, increased levels of MAC on the eyes of diabetic patients have been already described, when compared to the eyes of non-diabetic patients [83]. In the end, the IgG-laden plasma exosomes may contribute to the microvascular damage in the context of DR activating the classic complement pathway which leads to MAC deposition and consequent endothelial damage.

Concerning plasma EVs, both platelet- and monocyte-derived microvesicles have been receiving a lot of attention in this field, since two studies from Ogata et al. have described increased levels of both types of EVs in diabetic patients with DR. These vesicles appear to be closely related with DR progression as their levels were increased in advanced stages of DR [84,85]. Specifically, platelet-derived vesicles appear to mediate hyperglycemia-induced retinal endothelial damage through the release of CXCL10 which is going to activate the TLR4 pathway. These platelet-derived EVs also induce the production of ROS and inhibit the activity of superoxide dismutase (SOD) which, in addition to TLR4 activation, leads to decreased levels of tight junction proteins, such as ZO-1 and occludin, and retinal endothelial injury, including BRB breakdown [86].

Other studies have correlated changes in plasma EVs molecular profile with DR progression. For example, a recent study has reported a correlation of RANTES and CCR5-positive microvesicles, both proangiogenic factors, with the progression of NPDR [87]. Furthermore, high glucose conditions are able to increase NADPH oxidase activity on endothelium-derived microparticles, which are also increased in diabetic patients, leading to increased levels of ROS and inflammatory mediators and consequent impaired endothelial function [88]. These circulating EVs may also contribute to early endothelial dysfunction by decreasing nitric oxide (NO) and prostacyclin activity, increasing macrophage and leukocyte infiltration [71]. Thus, EVs appear to be closely related with the endothelial dysfunction and microvascular damage in DR.

Some studies have described a procoagulant property of these EVs in the context of DR [89], suggesting that plasma EVs may play a role in the coagulation cascade during the progression of the disease. Moreover, Su et al. described that increased levels of phosphatidylserine (PS)-positive microvesicles in patients with non-proliferative and proliferative DR are related with an increased procoagulant activity, which may explain the role of EVs on microvascular complications in patients with DR [90].

Together, these studies highlight the role of plasma EVs in DR progression, which appear to be a great promise not only to use them as biomarkers but also as therapeutic targets for the treatment of DR in the future.

6. miRNA in DR: Role in Oxidative Stress and Inflammatory Signaling Pathways

MicroRNA (miRNA) are a class of evolutionarily conserved single-stranded RNA molecules. These are non-coding small molecules (19–25 nucleotides long) that are involved in the regulation of gene expression. In this way, they can affect nearly all aspects of cell physiology, such as cell growth, differentiation, metabolism, and apoptosis [12,91–93]. Dysregulation of miRNA expression has been extensively recognized to be linked to the development of many diseases, including DR [94–96]. In fact, several reports have found an association of miRNA with the risk to develop DR [97–99]. Changes in circulating/extracellular miRNA expression levels in biological fluids, such as plasma, serum, vitreous, and aqueous humor in diabetic patients with retinopathy have been reported (Figure 3) [100–103]. An important and challenging question is whether these biofluid miRNAs execute protective/deleterious effects in the retina or simply serve as (read-outs) biosignatures that can aid in diagnosing and monitoring DR.

Extracellular miRNA in biological fluids can be found associated with proteins or enwrapped with vesicles [104]. In the former, miRNAs can be coupled with proteins, such as Argonaute (AGO) [105–107], nucleophosmin 1 (NPM1) [108], and high-density lipoproteins (HDLs) [109,110], and be released into the extracellular milieu; the binding to proteins protect miRNA from degradation by RNases, increasing their stability in body fluids. In the latter, miRNA can be incorporated in three broad secretory vesicles, based upon their mode of biogenesis: Exosomes, shedding microvesicles, and apoptotic bodies [111], and then released to the extracellular environment.

Multiple studies focusing in the identification of circulating miRNA from biofluids that differentiate between diabetic patients with retinopathy and diabetic patients without retinopathy or healthy controls have been published in the last years. Some of these studies have shown remarkable predictive value for detecting DR. Wang et al., in a cohort study with a small sample size, found five miRNAs (miR-4448, miR-338-3p, miR-485-5p and miR-9-5p, and miR-190a-5p) differentially expressed in serum samples in DR and non-DR groups [112]. The first four miRNAs were downregulated and the remaining (miR-190a-5p) was upregulated in T2D patients with retinopathy. The five miRNAs regulate 55 target genes, with a substantial overlapping with sirtuins, which are known to play a significant role by influencing various pathological processes such as inflammation, oxidative stress, and angiogenesis [113].

In another study, the expression of two miRNA, miR-20b and miR-17-3p, using also a relatively small sample size, has been investigated [114]. MiR-20b and miR-17-3p belong to the miR-17 family and target the 3′ UTRs of genes encoding HIF-1α and VEGF-A. Therefore, they may play a role in angiogenesis in DR. While a significant decrease in serum miR-20b was found in diabetic patients compared to healthy subjects, a decrease in serum miR-20b and miR-17-3p was found in NPDR and PDR groups when compared with healthy subjects. A combined analysis of these noncoding RNAs with two regulators of retinal endothelial dysfunction, Homebox antisense intergenic RNA (HOTAIR) and metastasis-associated lung adenocarcinoma transcript 1 (MALAT1), was able to discriminate diabetic patients without retinopathy from healthy controls and NPDR and PDR from diabetic patients without retinopathy, suggesting that miR-20b and miR-17-3p may be used as noninvasive biomarkers for screening of DR and the early diagnosis of PDR [115].

A study conducted by Qing et al. validated three miRNAs (elevated levels of plasma miR-21, miR-181c, and miR-1179) in predicting PDR [98]. A rise in plasma miR-21 levels in patients with T2D and PDR has also been found in another study [102]. From a mechanistic point of view, miR-21 seems to be involved in tumor-induced angiogenesis through targeting PTEN, leading to the activation of AKT and ERK1/2 signaling pathways, and thereby enhancing HIF-1α and VEGF expression [116]. Moreover, it has been also described to protect endothelial cells against high glucose-induced cytotoxicity [117]. Therefore, miR-21 may be associated with angiogenesis in a diabetic microenvironment. Concerning miR-181c, its levels are elevated in high glucose conditions, but they are inhibited in endothelial cells exposed to hypoxia, suggesting that it plays a key role in the regulation of angiogenesis in ischemia and in diabetes [118].

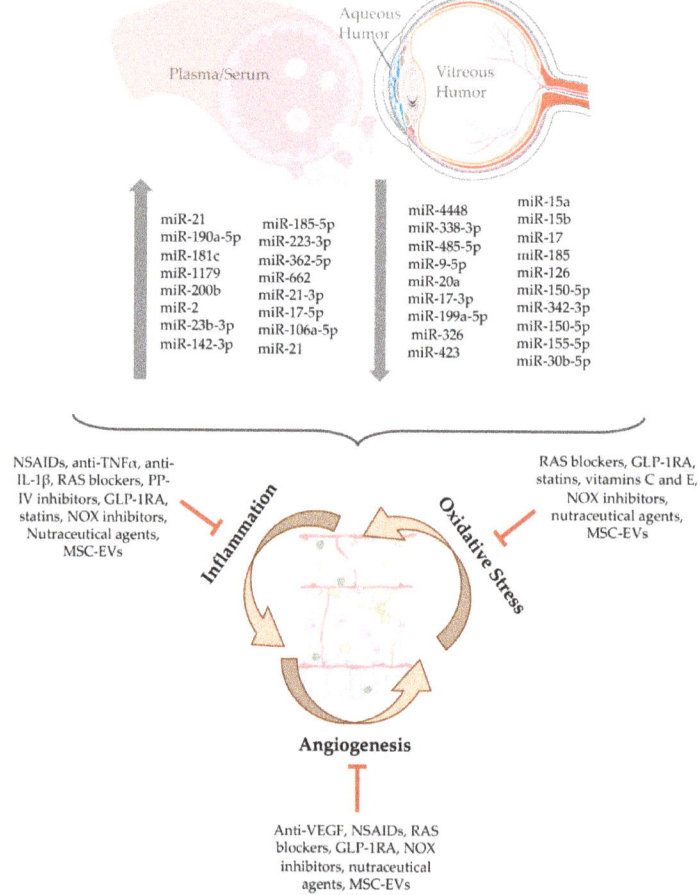

Figure 3. Alterations of miRNAs profile in DR and possible therapeutic interventions. The progression of DR is associated with the deregulation of miRNA expression, which leads to the increase (↑) or decrease (↓) of some miRNA involved in oxidative stress, inflammatory, and angiogenic processes. However, some therapeutic and nutraceutical strategies targeting inflammatory pathways, oxidative stress, and neovascularization, can be useful in preventing or arresting DR progression.

The information available regarding the expression profiles of the miRNAs in the vitreous of eyes with DR is scarce, mainly because healthy individuals cannot be used as controls due to ethical considerations. For example, Gomaa et al. reported increased VEGF and miR-200b expression levels in the vitreous of diabetic patients with PDR compared to age- and sex-matched nondiabetic individuals (nondiabetic patients indicated for pars plana vitrectomy due to idiopathic macular holes). In addition to being present in the vitreous, miR-200b has been described in neuronal, glial, and vascular elements in the retina [119]. MiR-200b expression was previously reported in the diabetic retina of experimental animal models of diabetes, but there was no consensus among the results of these studies [119–121]. Murray et al. found an upregulation of miR-200b in the retina of Akita mouse at nine months of age [120]. In agreement, Kovas et al. also reported increased expression levels of this miRNA both in the retina and retinal endothelial cells from diabetic rats after three months upon diabetes induction with streptozotocin (STZ) [121]. However, McArthur et al. reported decreased miR-200b expression levels in the retinas of STZ-induced diabetic rats after one month of diabetes [119]. As VEGF is one of the direct targets of miR200b, the rise of VEGF expression in DR may be attributable to the downregulation of miR-200b. In addition to the direct inhibitory effect of miR-200b on VEGF expression in response to diabetes, it may also mediate such effect indirectly via p300, a histone acetylation and transcription coactivator in malignancies, affecting in this way the gene expression of multiple vasoactive genes [122]. A recent cohort study using vitreous samples from PDR patients has revealed that miR-20a-5p, miR-23b-3p, miR-142-3p, miR-185-5p, miR-223-3p, miR-362-5p, and miR-662 expression levels were significantly higher compared to controls (vitreous from non-diabetic patients with macular holes), whereas miR-199a-5p and miR-326 were significantly lower [123]. Interestingly, all six overexpressed miRNAs have been previously described as potentially targeting proteins that are increased in the vitreous during PDR, such as VEGF-A, angiopoietin 2, PDGF-B, and connective tissue growth factor (CTGF). These authors claimed that the observed increase in miRNA expression can play a role in the regulation of angiogenesis and wound healing processes in the context of PDR, and the interplay between miRNA and their targets may result in a variety of gene expression profiles [123].

Several other studies tried to give insight into the mechanistic pathways possibly affected in DR by analyzing altered serum miRNA levels. Recently, Tamir et al. have performed a study involving 47 T2D patients (10 without retinopathy, 22 with NPDR, and 15 with PDR) and 22 healthy subjects, to study the potential involvement of 16 candidate miRNAs that were previously described in the literature to be altered in the plasma/serum of diabetic patients (miR423, miR-486-3p, miR-320a-3p, miR-320b, miR-200b-3p, miR-221-3p, miR-146a-5p, miR-183-5p, miR-122-5p, miR126-5p, miR-30d, miR-93-5p, miR-21, miR-27b-3p, let7f-5p, and miR-16-2-3p) [99,119,124–139]. They detected decreased miR-423 levels in T2D with PDR compared to healthy controls. Moreover, the authors found a correlation between lowered miR-423 in diabetic patients and VEGF, and an inverse correlation between NO and eNOS expression, suggesting a crosstalk between miR-423 and VEGF signaling, affecting the eNOS function. A recent report has found that five miRNAs—miR-15a, miR-15b, miR-17, miR20a, and miR-185—are downregulated in the aqueous humor of NPDR patients with DME, which is a leading cause of legal blindness in patients with T2D. Most of the downregulated miRNAs were related to inflammation, oxidative stress, and angiogenesis. MiR-15a has been associated with a dual anti-inflammatory and anti-angiogenic action. It has been reported that human retinal endothelial cells cultured in high glucose conditions decrease the expression levels of miR-15a [140]. Moreover, this downregulation in vascular cells is associated to increased leukostasis in the retina (an indication of retinal inflammation), together with activation of pro-inflammatory signaling of IL-1β, TNF-α, and NF-κB [140]. It has been suggested that miR-15a inhibits angiogenesis by binding to VEGF-A or Tie2 angiopoietin receptor [141,142]. Reduced levels of TNF-α and suppressor of cytokine signaling 3 (SOCS3) induced by miR-15b have been reported to inhibit insulin resistance in retinal endothelial cells [143]. MiR-17-5p is known to regulate hypoxia-induced NLRP3 inflammasome activation [144], downregulating inflammatory mediators such as IL-1β and TNF-α, and negatively regulates TLR4 expression [145]. MiR-20a has been shown to ameliorate the altered markers of endothelial function and oxidative stress as well as mediators of inflammation in an animal model of diabetes [146]. MiR-185 is decreased in diabetic patients and mice [147]. It is also known that miR-185 inhibits angiogenesis through direct interaction with stromal interaction molecule 1 (STIM1) in human microvascular endothelial cells [148].

Lu et al. detected decreased miR-126 serum content in diabetic patients with NPDR compared to healthy controls [149]. Moreover, it has been demonstrated that insulin receptor substrate 1 (IRS-1) is a target gene of miR-126 in endothelial cells and retinal pericytes in an animal model of DR. Furthermore, the interaction between them downregulates the expression of PI3K/Akt pathway proteins and negatively influences the viability and invasion of endothelial cells and retinal pericytes isolated from a mice model of DR [150]. The PI3K/Akt pathway is crucial for a long-term upregulation of VEGF, which is an angiogenic factor involved in the pathogenesis of DR. Therefore, miR-126 and its target gene IRS-1 may be promising molecular targets for the prevention and treatment of DR. Although it has been claimed that miR-126 can be used as a biomarker for early diagnosis of PDR, no single biomarker is enough to give a clear predictive sign of DR, being necessary a combination of molecular biomarkers, as well as anatomical and functional biomarkers, to increase the specificity and diagnosis accuracy.

Although there are many reports showing differences in circulating miRNAs in diabetic patients with retinopathy, the information regarding the importance of miRNA shuttled by EVs in the onset and progression of DR is scarce. In a recent study, using plasma from T1D subjects with PDR, the miRNA profiling patterns in the circulating EVs were different compared with healthy controls [151]. From 11 miRNA differentially expressed in DR patients in comparison with healthy controls, four were found to be upregulated, namely miR-21-3p, miR-17-5p, miR-106a-5p, and miR-21. These miRNAs were previously correlated to angiogenesis, inflammation, diabetes, and response to ischemia [152–156]. Three downregulated miRNA (miR-150-5p, miR-342-3p, miR-155-5p) were described as anti-angiogenic and also found to be decreased in T1D or T2D patients [155,157–159]. Furthermore, Mazzeo et al. [151] have shown that EVs isolated from the plasma of diabetic patients with retinopathy were able to induce pericyte detachment, increased permeability of pericyte/endothelial cell bilayers, and capillary-like tubular structures formation, which are some of the early features of DR. More recently, the same authors have investigated the role of miR-150-5p, miR-21-3p, and miR-30b-5p in the regulation of microvessels homeostasis and angiogenesis. They found the involvement of those miRNAs in abnormal angiogenesis and hypoxia-induced retinal injury characteristic of the diabetic eye [160]. Altogether, these data suggest that miRNA shuttled in EVs appears to be involved in the onset of DR, and miR-150-5p, miR-21-3p, and miR-30b-5p extracted from circulating EVs were identified as putative prognostic biomarkers for DR.

7. Therapeutic and Nutraceutical Agents with Anti-Inflammatory and Antioxidant Properties against DR

In clinical terms, the management of DR has been focused on intensive control of glycemia, as well as blood pressure and lipidemia, together with therapeutic interventions, such as photocoagulation with argon laser and immunotherapy through the intravitreal injection of anti-VEGF drugs [161]. DR progression and loss of sight can be prevented or delayed, but the existing retinal blood vessels damage and lost neuronal cell functions are typically irreversible, which is a major concern because those treatments are particularly directed to late-stage DR. In addition, there are relevant limitations associated with the discomfort caused to patients, the poor effectiveness in some individuals, the possibility of long-term side effects, as well as the economic cost [161]. Thus, it is crucial to develop novel and more efficient strategies to treat or retard progression of DR in early stages. In this regard, therapeutic and nutraceutical strategies targeting inflammation and oxidative stress have received renewed attention in recent years (Figure 3) [7,162,163]. In a small cohort, anti-VEGF therapy has been associated with a lower expression of miR-23b-3p in PDR as compared to untreated PDR patients, which suggests the involvement of a regulatory mechanism [123]. However, in this study it was not investigated whether differences exist between responders and non-responders to anti-VEGF therapy.

Corticosteroids have the ability to reduce inflammation by genomic and non-genomic mechanisms [162,164]. Regarding the genomic, corticosteroid-binding globulin (CBG) protein transports corticosteroid molecules through the serum and allows the entry into the cytoplasm after crossing the cell membrane, where it binds to a glucocorticoid receptor thus admitting penetration into the cell nucleus. By interfering with a diversity of genes modulated by specific miRNAs, corticosteroids can influence the production of hundreds of proteins involved in inflammation and cell metabolism, which in the eye can contribute to anti-inflammatory properties and preservation of BRB. In addition, corticosteroids act directly by extracellular mechanisms linked with reduction of permeability and induction of vasoconstriction of the blood vessels as well as related with alleviation of cellular swelling and stimulation of adenosine production on Müller cells [162,164]. Furthermore, corticosteroids can stabilize blood–ocular barrier functions namely due to protection of tight junction integrity, which contributes to reduce serum leakage and the expression of extracellular MMP [165].

Currently, corticosteroids are viewed as a second-line therapy for DR patients that are poorly responsive to anti-VEGF therapy in cases of DME [166]. Triamcinolone acetonide, fluocinolone acetonide, and dexamethasone sodium phosphate have been successfully used as an intravitreal steroid treatment to reduce the frequency of anti-VEGF intravitreal injections, which is particularly useful in patients with contraindications for anti-VEGF therapy, such as those with coronary diseases [166]. Mounting evidence show that glucocorticoids exert anti-inflammatory activities by reducing the expression of adhesion molecules related to leukostasis (such as ICAM-1 and E-selectin), decreasing the release of other pro-inflammatory mediators (namely IL-6, NF-kB, TNF-α, and IFN-γ, etc.) and inhibiting the inflammatory cells (leucocytes, monocytes, macrophages) infiltration [167,168]. In vitro studies have shown that dexamethasone is able to reduce the secretion of exosomes containing pro-inflammatory miRNA-155 in RAW264.7 macrophages treated with lipopolysaccharide (LPS) [169]. Furthermore, glucocorticoids have been also associated with an angiostatic effect due to the inhibition of a variety of proangiogenesis mediators, namely VEGF, BFGF, and TGF-b [170,171]. Complementarily, in vitro and in vivo preclinical evidences have demonstrated that corticosteroids can also modulate vascular permeability by attenuating VEGF and SDF-1 pathways in different cell types and conditions [162], as well as exert neuroprotective effects on the retina [172].

Gathering evidences support a role for COX-2 in retinal inflammation, which opens up the possibility of using non-steroidal anti-inflammatory drugs (NSAIDs) in DR [50,173,174]. In diabetic animals, aspirin was able to prevent capillary cell apoptosis and vessel degeneration [50,175,176]. Regarding human data, the Dipyridamole Aspirin Microangiopathy of Diabetes (DAMAD) study reported beneficial effects of higher doses of aspirin (990 mg) in patients with early DR, in contrast to the poor results obtained in the advanced DR patients enrolled in the Early Treatment DR Study (ETDRS), using 650 mg of aspirin [177]. More recently, a prospective study showed beneficial effects of sulindac against DR development and progression [178]. Preclinical studies with specific COX-2 inhibitors have shown beneficial effects translated in reduced vascular leakage, capillary cell apoptosis, and vessel degeneration [179,180]. While the clinical use when administered systemically is discouraged due to increased risk of heart attack and stroke [164], the topical administration of a COX-2 inhibitor in preclinical studies was found to reduce DR symptoms similarly to systemic administration [174,179,180]. Topical use of NSAIDs in the eyes is overall of limited efficacy due to the reduced bioavailability and effect in the retina for the majority of these drugs, including bromfenac, nepafenac, and ketorolac [174]. To the best of our knowledge, no information is available in the literature concerning comparison of miRNA expression profiles in fluid samples between PDR patients treated with corticosteroids or NSAIDS and untreated PDR patients.

There are other therapeutic strategies under evaluation using inhibitors of proinflammatory molecules, such as the cytokines TNF-α and IL-1β, etc. Anti-TNF-α therapy has been mainly evaluated in preclinical studies and in a few cases of DME or PDR. A clinical study in a small number of patients with refractory DME were unable to present amelioration when treated with intravenous (IV) etanercept, a recombinant fusion protein having anti-TNF-α properties [181]. Intravenous therapy with infliximab, a monoclonal antibody directed against TNF-α, showed amelioration of visual acuity and reduction of macular thickness in DME patients non-responsive to laser photocoagulation [182]. However, other studies related with non-ophthalmic conditions, in which similar doses of infliximab were used, reported an increase in the incidence of serious adverse events [183,184]. Moreover, infliximab relieves BRB breakdown through the activation of the p38 MAPK pathway in a diabetic rodent model [185]. Regarding anti-IL-1β therapy with canakinumab (a selective IL-1β antibody), patients with proliferative DR presented stabilization (not regression) of retinal neovascularization [186].

Other drugs often used for other clinical conditions have been tested as anti-inflammatory agents against DR. Since the renin–angiotensin system (RAS) is involved in oxidative stress and AGEs formation, thus contributing to retinal inflammation in diabetes, RAS blockers have been evaluated in preclinical and clinical studies. Losartan and candesartan, which are angiotensin II type 1 receptor (AT1R) blockers, and enalapril, an angiotensin-converting enzyme (ACE) inhibitor, were able to promote beneficial effects against DR progression in animal models of diabetes due to the prevention of oxidative stress, inflammation, and vascular damage [187]. Similar benefits were observed in clinical trials [188], except in the DR Candesartan Trials (DIRECT), whose results showed reduced DR incidence but unaffected progression [189,190], recommending further research. MiR-152 has been pointed to be a regulator of the (Pro)renin receptor (PRR), a component of the RAS, in hREC. When hREC are exposed to high glucose conditions, PPR expression is induced via the inhibition of the miR-152, which is able to regulate the expression of VEGF, VEGFR-2, and TGFb1 [191].

Furthermore, dipeptidyl peptidase 4 (DPP-4) inhibitors (also known as gliptins), which are second-line oral anti-diabetic drugs, have been demonstrating anti-inflammatory properties and prevention of BRB breakdown in preclinical models of diabetes [192–194]. Similar benefits were obtained using glucagon-like peptide 1 receptor agonists (GLP1RAs) in experimental models, including protection against hyperglycemia-induced inflammation, oxidative stress, BRB breakdown, angiogenesis, and neurodegeneration, which seems to be at least in part mediated by the AKT pathway [195–197]. A recent report has described that liraglutide, a GLP1RA, has also vasoprotective effects in diabetic rats. Liraglutide was able to inhibit miR-93-5p, miR-181a-5p, and miR-34a-5p expression, and activate miR-26a-5p expression, which then stimulate the PI3K-Akt-Bcl2 activation pathway, thus inhibiting endothelial cell apoptosis [198].

Moreover, some lipid-lowering drugs, such as statins and fenofibrate, have been associated with protection against DR progression, which could be attributed to anti-inflammatory and antioxidant properties [199,200]. The promising results for some of these drugs in preclinical settings recommends further clinical evaluation in the perspective of possible repurposing to treat DR.

In preclinical studies, some vitamins (namely C and E) have been demonstrating antioxidant activity able to improve DR phenotype, particularly decreasing the development of acellular capillaries and the number of pericyte ghosts [201]. However, the clinical efficacy is contradictory. Some studies report beneficial effects whereas others mentioned a lack of a positive impact regardless of the antioxidant capacity [202]. Targeting specific promoters of oxidative stress could eventually be a more promising strategy. Several NAD(P)H-oxidase (NOX) inhibitors, including diphenyleneiodonium and apocynin, have been demonstrating preventive actions against DR progression, which might be due to reduction of ROS and VEGF levels, although NOX-independent effects have been also reported [203]. In preclinical studies, NOX blockers were able to reduce vascular leakage and neovascularization, as well as oxidative stress and inflammation, by mechanisms involving the prevention of NF-kB activation and CCL2 production [204–206]. It is known that in diabetes miRNAs can regulate the expression of ROS generating proteins, such as NOX, and antioxidant proteins, such as sirtuins or superoxide dismutase, influencing therefore the oxidative stress response [207]. However, the information available concerning the effect of NOX inhibitors on oxidative stress in DR is scarce. Further investigation is warranted in order to investigate whether changes of miRNA profiles may have an impact on regulating oxidative stress in the context of DR.

In recent years, much attention has been focused on the possibility that nutraceuticals agents can complement pharmacological therapy to prevent or delay the evolution of DR. Among the main candidates there are several natural molecules, including a variety of polyphenols (such as resveratrol, curcumin, quercetin, pterostilbene, epicatechin, epigallocatechin gallate, etc.) and anthocyanins, sesamin (a lignan isolated from sesame seeds and sesame oil), bromelain (a cysteine protease found in pineapple juice and stems), as well as alpha-lipoic acid (a vitamin-like chemical present in liver, kidney, and some vegetables), and lutein (a carotenoid present in green vegetables), etc. Several recently good reviews highlighted their strong anti-inflammatory and antioxidant properties, as well as their capacity to afford protection against hypoxia and angiogenesis, which have been associated with interference with adhesion, angiogenesis, and inflammation molecules/mediators (such as ICAM-1, VEGF, and TNF-a) and signaling (namely via NF-kB, NRF2-Keap1, and TLRs) [7,33,162,163]. These molecules could be an attractive nutraceutical alternative to the pharmacological approaches, but more clinical research is needed to complement the preclinical evidences. In addition, efficient delivery systems should be developed to overcome the well-known low bioavailability of some of them that still limits their efficacy.

As natural vehicles for the transfer of miRNAs, lipids, and proteins, EVs-based therapies have been recognized as having a number of potential applications for ocular diseases, namely DR. Particularly, stem cell (SC)-derived EVs are the most extensive explored since several studies have highlighted their positive therapeutic effects on immunomodulation and tissue remodeling without negative secondary effects [59]. Especially in the retina, pre-clinical studies have been using mesenchymal stem cells (MSC)-derived EVs to positively modulate injury responses. Intravitreal administration of MSC-derived exosomes are able to reduce retinal ischemia and neovascularization in a murine model of oxygen-induced retinopathy (OIR) [208] and reduce apoptosis and inflammatory responses through the reduction of MCP-1 in the retina of a mouse model of retinal laser injury [209]. In the context of DR, MSC-derived EVs also present protective effects in the retina of STZ-induced diabetic animals, being able to prevent retinal degeneration through the upregulation of miRNA-222 expression [210] and to reduce hyperglycemia-induced retinal inflammation, decreasing the levels of inflammatory markers, namely IL-1β, IL-18, and caspase-1 through miR-126 overexpression [211]. However, not only MSC-derived EVs present protective effects. In fact, Hajrasouliha et al. have shown that exosomes from retinal astrocytes cells were able to prevent retinal vessel leakage and inhibit neovascularization in a laser-induced choroidal neovascularization model [61]. These initial findings encourage further research and the development of novel EVs-based therapies for the treatment of DR.

8. Conclusions and Perspectives

The diagnosis of DR depends mainly on the detection of microvascular changes in the retina. Over the past decades, a significant progress has been made in the management of DR and a number of treatments are able to prevent, delay, or reduce vision loss. However, there is still no cure for DR. To tackle this challenge more effectively, early diagnosis is the most decisive factor.

Oxidative stress and low-grade inflammation play an important role in the pathogenesis of DR, but the exact molecular signaling pathways and key players involved are not completely elucidated yet. Evidence suggests that EVs can deliver their miRNA cargo to other cells, thus playing a role in cell-to-cell communication. As was highlighted in this manuscript, EVs and miRNAs might contribute to DR development through their important roles in inflammation, oxidative stress, and angiogenesis. However, the complete picture of miRNAs repertoire and their regulation in DR is highly complex and there are still many unknowns. As biomarkers, miRNAs do not yet allow to predict who will develop advanced forms of DR or to distinguish the stage of the disease. To take steps forward, some limitations associated with several studies must be overcome, such as small-cohorts, isolation of different subpopulations of vesicles or study groups. A better understanding of the role of EVs and changes in miRNA levels in DR could provide a more detailed characterization of the different stages of the disease. Future research approaches should be carefully charted to strengthen and confirm the current findings. As DR is a heterogenous and molecularly complex disease, miRNA-based therapeutics in combination with other anti-inflammatory and/or antioxidant therapeutic and nutraceutical agents could be an interesting opportunity for future exploration in the context of personalized combination therapy.

Author Contributions: R.F. conceptualized the review; R.F., F.R., B.M., and M.A. wrote the manuscript; B.M. and M.A. designed the figures; R.F., F.R., and A.F.A. reviewed and edited the manuscript. All authors have read and agreed to the published version of the manuscript.

Funding: This work was supported by the European Regional Development Fund (FEDER), through Programa Operacional Factores de Competitividade COMPETE2020 (CENTRO-01-0145-FEDER-000008: BRAINHEALTH 2020; CENTRO-01-0145-FEDER-000012: HealthyAging2020) and by National funds via Portuguese Science and Technology Foundation (FCT): Strategic Projects UID/NEU/04539/2019 (CNC.IBILI), UIDB/04539/2020, UIDP/04539/2020 (CIBB), and PTDC/SAU-NUT/31712/2017, as well as by COMPETE-FEDER funds (POCI-01-0145-FEDER-007440 and POCI-01-0145-FEDER-031712).

Conflicts of Interest: The authors declare no conflict of interest.

References

1. Federation, I.D. *IDF Diabetes Atlas*, 9th ed.; International Diabetes Federation: Brussels, Belgium, 2019.
2. Wang, P.; Chen, F.; Wang, W.; Zhang, X.D. Hydrogen Sulfide Attenuates High Glucose-Induced Human Retinal Pigment Epithelial Cell Inflammation by Inhibiting ROS Formation and NLRP3 Inflammasome Activation. *Mediat. Inflamm.* **2019**, *2019*, 1–13. [CrossRef]
3. Youngblood, H.; Robinson, R.; Sharma, A.; Sharma, S. Proteomic Biomarkers of Retinal Inflammation in Diabetic Retinopathy. *Int. J. Mol. Sci.* **2019**, *20*, 4755. [CrossRef] [PubMed]
4. Biswas, S.; Sarabusky, M.; Chakrabarti, S. Diabetic Retinopathy, lncRNAs, and Inflammation: A Dynamic, Interconnected Network. *J. Clin. Med.* **2019**, *8*, 1033. [CrossRef] [PubMed]
5. Petrie, J.R.; Guzik, T.J.; Touyz, R.M. Diabetes, Hypertension, and Cardiovascular Disease: Clinical Insights and Vascular Mechanisms. *Can. J. Cardiol.* **2018**, *34*, 575–584. [CrossRef] [PubMed]
6. Simo, R.; Stitt, A.W.; Gardner, T.W. Neurodegeneration in diabetic retinopathy: Does it really matter? *Diabetologia* **2018**, *61*, 1902–1912. [CrossRef] [PubMed]
7. Rodriguez, M.L.; Perez, S.; Mena-Molla, S.; Desco, M.C.; Ortega, A.L. Oxidative Stress and Microvascular Alterations in Diabetic Retinopathy: Future Therapies. *Oxid. Med. Cell Longev.* **2019**, *2019*, 4940825. [CrossRef] [PubMed]
8. Fong, D.S.; Aiello, L.P.; Ferris, F.L., 3rd; Klein, R. Diabetic retinopathy. *Diabetes Care* **2004**, *27*, 2540–2553. [CrossRef]
9. Tarr, J.M.; Kaul, K.; Chopra, M.; Kohner, E.M.; Chibber, R. Pathophysiology of diabetic retinopathy. *ISRN Ophthalmol.* **2013**, *2013*, 343560. [CrossRef]
10. Colombo, M.; Raposo, G.; Thery, C. Biogenesis, secretion, and intercellular interactions of exosomes and other extracellular vesicles. *Annu. Rev. Cell Dev. Biol.* **2014**, *30*, 255–289. [CrossRef]
11. van Niel, G.; D'Angelo, G.; Raposo, G. Shedding light on the cell biology of extracellular vesicles. *Nat. Rev. Mol. Cell Biol.* **2018**, *19*, 213–228. [CrossRef]
12. O'Brien, J.; Hayder, H.; Zayed, Y.; Peng, C. Overview of MicroRNA Biogenesis, Mechanisms of Actions, and Circulation. *Front. Endocrinol. (Lausanne)* **2018**, *9*, 402. [CrossRef] [PubMed]
13. Li, X.; Yu, Z.W.; Wang, Y.; Fu, Y.H.; Gao, X.Y. MicroRNAs: Potential Targets in Diabetic Retinopathy. *Horm. Metab. Res.* **2020**, *52*, 142–148. [CrossRef]
14. Wong, T.Y.; Cheung, C.M.; Larsen, M.; Sharma, S.; Simo, R. Diabetic retinopathy. *Nat. Rev. Dis. Primers* **2016**, *2*, 16012. [CrossRef] [PubMed]
15. Liao, P.L.; Lin, C.H.; Li, C.H.; Tsai, C.H.; Ho, J.D.; Chiou, G.C.; Kang, J.J.; Cheng, Y.W. Anti-inflammatory properties of shikonin contribute to improved early-stage diabetic retinopathy. *Sci. Rep.* **2017**, *7*, 44985. [CrossRef] [PubMed]
16. Wu, M.Y.; Yiang, G.T.; Lai, T.T.; Li, C.J. The Oxidative Stress and Mitochondrial Dysfunction during the Pathogenesis of Diabetic Retinopathy. *Oxid. Med. Cell Longev.* **2018**, *2018*, 3420187. [CrossRef]
17. Gardner, T.W.; Abcouwer, S.F.; Barber, A.J.; Jackson, G.R. An integrated approach to diabetic retinopathy research. *Arch. Ophthalmol.* **2011**, *129*, 230–235. [CrossRef]
18. de Hoz, R.; Rojas, B.; Ramirez, A.I.; Salazar, J.J.; Gallego, B.I.; Trivino, A.; Ramirez, J.M. Retinal Macroglial Responses in Health and Disease. *Biomed. Res. Int.* **2016**, *2016*, 2954721. [CrossRef]
19. Bresnick, G.H. Diabetic retinopathy viewed as a neurosensory disorder. *Arch. Ophthalmol.* **1986**, *104*, 989–990. [CrossRef]

20. Ghirlanda, G.; Di Leo, M.A.; Caputo, S.; Cercone, S.; Greco, A.V. From functional to microvascular abnormalities in early diabetic retinopathy. *Diabetes Metab. Rev.* **1997**, *13*, 15–35. [CrossRef]
21. Greenstein, V.C.; Shapiro, A.; Zaidi, Q.; Hood, D.C. Psychophysical evidence for post-receptoral sensitivity loss in diabetics. *Investig. Ophthalmol. Vis. Sci.* **1992**, *33*, 2781–2790.
22. Antonetti, D.A.; Barber, A.J.; Bronson, S.K.; Freeman, W.M.; Gardner, T.W.; Jefferson, L.S.; Kester, M.; Kimball, S.R.; Krady, J.K.; LaNoue, K.F.; et al. Diabetic retinopathy: Seeing beyond glucose-induced microvascular disease. *Diabetes* **2006**, *55*, 2401–2411. [CrossRef] [PubMed]
23. Chhablani, J.; Sharma, A.; Goud, A.; Peguda, H.K.; Rao, H.L.; Begum, V.U.; Barteselli, G. Neurodegeneration in Type 2 Diabetes: Evidence From Spectral-Domain Optical Coherence Tomography. *Investig. Ophthalmol. Vis. Sci.* **2015**, *56*, 6333–6338. [CrossRef] [PubMed]
24. Barrett, E.J.; Liu, Z.; Khamaisi, M.; King, G.L.; Klein, R.; Klein, B.E.K.; Hughes, T.M.; Craft, S.; Freedman, B.I.; Bowden, D.W.; et al. Diabetic Microvascular Disease: An Endocrine Society Scientific Statement. *J. Clin. Endocrinol. Metab.* **2017**, *102*, 4343–4410. [CrossRef] [PubMed]
25. Al-Shabrawey, M.; Zhang, W.; McDonald, D. Diabetic retinopathy: Mechanism, diagnosis, prevention, and treatment. *Biomed. Res. Int.* **2015**, *2015*, 854593. [CrossRef]
26. Rubsam, A.; Parikh, S.; Fort, P.E. Role of Inflammation in Diabetic Retinopathy. *Int. J. Mol. Sci.* **2018**, *19*, 942. [CrossRef]
27. Othman, R.; Vaucher, E.; Couture, R. Bradykinin Type 1 Receptor—Inducible Nitric Oxide Synthase: A New Axis Implicated in Diabetic Retinopathy. *Front. Pharmacol.* **2019**, *10*, 300. [CrossRef]
28. Sorrentino, F.S.; Matteini, S.; Bonifazzi, C.; Sebastiani, A.; Parmeggiani, F. Diabetic retinopathy and endothelin system: Microangiopathy versus endothelial dysfunction. *Eye (Lond.)* **2018**, *32*, 1157–1163. [CrossRef]
29. Early Treatment Diabetic Retinopathy Study Research Group. Early photocoagulation for diabetic retinopathy. ETDRS report number 9. *Ophthalmology* **1991**, *98*, 766–785. [CrossRef]
30. Santiago, A.R.; Boia, R.; Aires, I.D.; Ambrosio, A.F.; Fernandes, R. Sweet Stress: Coping With Vascular Dysfunction in Diabetic Retinopathy. *Front. Physiol.* **2018**, *9*, 820. [CrossRef]
31. Abu El-Asrar, A.M.; Ahmad, A.; Siddiquei, M.M.; De Zutter, A.; Allegaert, E.; Gikandi, P.W.; De Hertogh, G.; Van Damme, J.; Opdenakker, G.; Struyf, S. The Proinflammatory and Proangiogenic Macrophage Migration Inhibitory Factor Is a Potential Regulator in Proliferative Diabetic Retinopathy. *Front. Immunol.* **2019**, *10*, 2752. [CrossRef]
32. Aouiss, A.; Anka Idrissi, D.; Kabine, M.; Zaid, Y. Update of inflammatory proliferative retinopathy: Ischemia, hypoxia and angiogenesis. *Curr. Res. Transl. Med.* **2019**, *67*, 62–71. [CrossRef]
33. Wang, W.; Lo, A.C.Y. Diabetic Retinopathy: Pathophysiology and Treatments. *Int. J. Mol. Sci.* **2018**, *19*, 1816. [CrossRef]
34. Al-Kharashi, A.S. Role of oxidative stress, inflammation, hypoxia and angiogenesis in the development of diabetic retinopathy. *Saudi J. Ophthalmol.* **2018**, *32*, 318–323. [CrossRef] [PubMed]
35. Brownlee, M. Biochemistry and molecular cell biology of diabetic complications. *Nature* **2001**, *414*, 813–820. [CrossRef] [PubMed]
36. Yumnamcha, T.; Devi, T.S.; Singh, L.P. Auranofin Mediates Mitochondrial Dysregulation and Inflammatory Cell Death in Human Retinal Pigment Epithelial Cells: Implications of Retinal Neurodegenerative Diseases. *Front. Neurosci.* **2019**, *13*, 1065. [CrossRef] [PubMed]
37. Kooragayala, K.; Gotoh, N.; Cogliati, T.; Nellissery, J.; Kaden, T.R.; French, S.; Balaban, R.; Li, W.; Covian, R.; Swaroop, A. Quantification of Oxygen Consumption in Retina Ex Vivo Demonstrates Limited Reserve Capacity of Photoreceptor Mitochondria. *Investig. Ophthalmol. Vis. Sci.* **2015**, *56*, 8428–8436. [CrossRef]
38. Hombrebueno, J.R.; Cairns, L.; Dutton, L.R.; Lyons, T.J.; Brazil, D.P.; Moynagh, P.; Curtis, T.M.; Xu, H. Uncoupled turnover disrupts mitochondrial quality control in diabetic retinopathy. *JCI Insight* **2019**, *4*, e129760. [CrossRef]
39. Brownlee, M. The pathobiology of diabetic complications: A unifying mechanism. *Diabetes* **2005**, *54*, 1615–1625. [CrossRef]
40. Berezin, A. Neutrophil extracellular traps: The core player in vascular complications of diabetes mellitus. *Diabetes Metab. Syndr.* **2019**, *13*, 3017–3023. [CrossRef]
41. Geraldes, P.; King, G.L. Activation of protein kinase C isoforms and its impact on diabetic complications. *Circ. Res.* **2010**, *106*, 1319–1331. [CrossRef]

42. Nakamura, M.; Barber, A.J.; Antonetti, D.A.; LaNoue, K.F.; Robinson, K.A.; Buse, M.G.; Gardner, T.W. Excessive hexosamines block the neuroprotective effect of insulin and induce apoptosis in retinal neurons. *J. Biol. Chem.* **2001**, *276*, 43748–43755. [CrossRef] [PubMed]
43. Kowluru, R.A.; Mishra, M. Oxidative stress, mitochondrial damage and diabetic retinopathy. *Biochim. Biophys. Acta* **2015**, *1852*, 2474–2483. [CrossRef] [PubMed]
44. Du, X.; Matsumura, T.; Edelstein, D.; Rossetti, L.; Zsengeller, Z.; Szabo, C.; Brownlee, M. Inhibition of GAPDH activity by poly(ADP-ribose) polymerase activates three major pathways of hyperglycemic damage in endothelial cells. *J. Clin. Investig.* **2003**, *112*, 1049–1057. [CrossRef] [PubMed]
45. Giacco, F.; Brownlee, M. Oxidative stress and diabetic complications. *Circ. Res.* **2010**, *107*, 1058–1070. [CrossRef]
46. Adhya, P.; Sharma, S.S. Redox TRPs in diabetes and diabetic complications: Mechanisms and pharmacological modulation. *Pharmacol. Res.* **2019**, *146*, 104271. [CrossRef]
47. Abcouwer, S.F. Muller Cell-Microglia Cross Talk Drives Neuroinflammation in Diabetic Retinopathy. *Diabetes* **2017**, *66*, 261–263. [CrossRef]
48. Rangasamy, S.; McGuire, P.G.; Franco Nitta, C.; Monickaraj, F.; Oruganti, S.R.; Das, A. Chemokine mediated monocyte trafficking into the retina: Role of inflammation in alteration of the blood-retinal barrier in diabetic retinopathy. *PLoS ONE* **2014**, *9*, e108508. [CrossRef]
49. Semeraro, F.; Cancarini, A.; dell'Omo, R.; Rezzola, S.; Romano, M.R.; Costagliola, C. Diabetic Retinopathy: Vascular and Inflammatory Disease. *J. Diabetes Res.* **2015**, *2015*, 582060. [CrossRef]
50. Zheng, L.; Howell, S.J.; Hatala, D.A.; Huang, K.; Kern, T.S. Salicylate-based anti-inflammatory drugs inhibit the early lesion of diabetic retinopathy. *Diabetes* **2007**, *56*, 337–345. [CrossRef]
51. Kowluru, R.A.; Zhong, Q.; Santos, J.M. Matrix metalloproteinases in diabetic retinopathy: Potential role of MMP-9. *Expert Opin. Investig. Drugs* **2012**, *21*, 797–805. [CrossRef] [PubMed]
52. Mohammad, G.; Kowluru, R.A. Novel role of mitochondrial matrix metalloproteinase-2 in the development of diabetic retinopathy. *Investig. Ophthalmol. Vis. Sci.* **2011**, *52*, 3832–3841. [CrossRef]
53. Rosa, M.D.; Distefano, G.; Gagliano, C.; Rusciano, D.; Malaguarnera, L. Autophagy in Diabetic Retinopathy. *Curr. Neuropharmacol.* **2016**, *14*, 810–825. [CrossRef] [PubMed]
54. Picconi, F.; Parravano, M.; Ylli, D.; Pasqualetti, P.; Coluzzi, S.; Giordani, I.; Malandrucco, I.; Lauro, D.; Scarinci, F.; Giorno, P.; et al. Retinal neurodegeneration in patients with type 1 diabetes mellitus: The role of glycemic variability. *Acta Diabetol.* **2017**, *54*, 489–497. [CrossRef] [PubMed]
55. Pitt, J.M.; Kroemer, G.; Zitvogel, L. Extracellular vesicles: Masters of intercellular communication and potential clinical interventions. *J. Clin. Investig.* **2016**, *126*, 1139–1143. [CrossRef] [PubMed]
56. Mathieu, M.; Martin-Jaular, L.; Lavieu, G.; Thery, C. Specificities of secretion and uptake of exosomes and other extracellular vesicles for cell-to-cell communication. *Nat. Cell Biol.* **2019**, *21*, 9–17. [CrossRef]
57. Tricarico, C.; Clancy, J.; D'Souza-Schorey, C. Biology and biogenesis of shed microvesicles. *Small GTPases* **2017**, *8*, 220–232. [CrossRef]
58. Hauser, P.; Wang, S.; Didenko, V.V. Apoptotic Bodies: Selective Detection in Extracellular Vesicles. *Methods Mol. Biol.* **2017**, *1554*, 193–200.
59. van der Merwe, Y.; Steketee, M.B. Extracellular Vesicles: Biomarkers, Therapeutics, and Vehicles in the Visual System. *Curr. Ophthalmol. Rep.* **2017**, *5*, 276–282. [CrossRef]
60. Mighty, J.; Zhou, J.; Benito-Martin, A.; Sauma, S.; Hanna, S.; Onwumere, O.; Shi, C.; Muntzel, M.; Sauane, M.; Young, M.; et al. Analysis of Adult Neural Retina Extracellular Vesicle Release, RNA Transport and Proteomic Cargo. *Investig. Ophthalmol. Vis. Sci.* **2020**, *61*, 30. [CrossRef]
61. Hajrasouliha, A.R.; Jiang, G.; Lu, Q.; Lu, H.; Kaplan, H.J.; Zhang, H.G.; Shao, H. Exosomes from retinal astrocytes contain antiangiogenic components that inhibit laser-induced choroidal neovascularization. *J. Biol. Chem.* **2013**, *288*, 28058–28067. [CrossRef]
62. Klingeborn, M.; Dismuke, W.M.; Skiba, N.P.; Kelly, U.; Stamer, W.D.; Bowes Rickman, C. Directional Exosome Proteomes Reflect Polarity-Specific Functions in Retinal Pigmented Epithelium Monolayers. *Sci. Rep.* **2018**, *8*, 17327. [CrossRef] [PubMed]
63. Kang, G.Y.; Bang, J.Y.; Choi, A.J.; Yoon, J.; Lee, W.C.; Choi, S.; Yoon, S.; Kim, H.C.; Baek, J.H.; Park, H.S.; et al. Exosomal proteins in the aqueous humor as novel biomarkers in patients with neovascular age-related macular degeneration. *J. Proteome Res.* **2014**, *13*, 581–595. [CrossRef] [PubMed]

64. Lerner, N.; Avissar, S.; Beit-Yannai, E. Extracellular vesicles mediate signaling between the aqueous humor producing and draining cells in the ocular system. *PLoS ONE* **2017**, *12*, e0171153. [CrossRef] [PubMed]
65. Garcia-Contreras, M.; Brooks, R.W.; Boccuzzi, L.; Robbins, P.D.; Ricordi, C. Exosomes as biomarkers and therapeutic tools for type 1 diabetes mellitus. *Eur. Rev. Med. Pharmacol. Sci.* **2017**, *21*, 2940–2956.
66. Zhou, F.; Huang, L.; Qu, S.L.; Chao, R.; Yang, C.; Jiang, Z.S.; Zhang, C. The emerging roles of extracellular vesicles in diabetes and diabetic complications. *Clin. Chim. Acta* **2019**, *497*, 130–136. [CrossRef]
67. Tabak, S.; Schreiber-Avissar, S.; Beit-Yannai, E. Extracellular vesicles have variable dose-dependent effects on cultured draining cells in the eye. *J. Cell Mol. Med.* **2018**, *22*, 1992–2000. [CrossRef]
68. Chahed, S.; Leroyer, A.S.; Benzerroug, M.; Gaucher, D.; Georgescu, A.; Picaud, S.; Silvestre, J.S.; Gaudric, A.; Tedgui, A.; Massin, P.; et al. Increased vitreous shedding of microparticles in proliferative diabetic retinopathy stimulates endothelial proliferation. *Diabetes* **2010**, *59*, 694–701. [CrossRef]
69. Liu, C.; Ge, H.M.; Liu, B.H.; Dong, R.; Shan, K.; Chen, X.; Yao, M.D.; Li, X.M.; Yao, J.; Zhou, R.M.; et al. Targeting pericyte-endothelial cell crosstalk by circular RNA-cPWWP2A inhibition aggravates diabetes-induced microvascular dysfunction. *Proc. Natl. Acad. Sci. USA* **2019**, *116*, 7455–7464. [CrossRef]
70. Beltramo, E.; Lopatina, T.; Berrone, E.; Mazzeo, A.; Iavello, A.; Camussi, G.; Porta, M. Extracellular vesicles derived from mesenchymal stem cells induce features of diabetic retinopathy in vitro. *Acta Diabetol.* **2014**, *51*, 1055–1064. [CrossRef]
71. Zhang, W.; Chen, S.; Liu, M.L. Pathogenic roles of microvesicles in diabetic retinopathy. *Acta Pharmacol. Sin.* **2018**, *39*, 1–11. [CrossRef]
72. Vitkova, V.; Zivny, J.; Janota, J. Endothelial cell-derived microvesicles: Potential mediators and biomarkers of pathologic processes. *Biomark. Med.* **2018**, *12*, 161–175. [CrossRef] [PubMed]
73. Bastiaans, J.; van Meurs, J.C.; Mulder, V.C.; Nagtzaam, N.M.; Smits-te Nijenhuis, M.; Dufour-van den Goorbergh, D.C.; van Hagen, P.M.; Hooijkaas, H.; Dik, W.A. The role of thrombin in proliferative vitreoretinopathy. *Investig. Ophthalmol. Vis. Sci.* **2014**, *55*, 4659–4666. [CrossRef]
74. Huang, H.; Gandhi, J.K.; Zhong, X.; Wei, Y.; Gong, J.; Duh, E.J.; Vinores, S.A. TNFalpha is required for late BRB breakdown in diabetic retinopathy, and its inhibition prevents leukostasis and protects vessels and neurons from apoptosis. *Investig. Ophthalmol. Vis. Sci.* **2011**, *52*, 1336–1344. [CrossRef] [PubMed]
75. Burger, D.; Montezano, A.C.; Nishigaki, N.; He, Y.; Carter, A.; Touyz, R.M. Endothelial Microparticle Formation by Angiotensin II Is Mediated via Ang II Receptor Type I/NADPH Oxidase/Rho Kinase Pathways Targeted to Lipid Rafts. *Arterioscler. Thromb. Vasc. Biol.* **2011**, *31*, 1898–1907. [CrossRef]
76. Xu, W.; Wu, Y.; Hu, Z.; Sun, L.; Dou, G.; Zhang, Z.; Wang, H.; Guo, C.; Wang, Y. Exosomes from Microglia Attenuate Photoreceptor Injury and Neovascularization in an Animal Model of Retinopathy of Prematurity. *Mol. Ther. Nucleic Acids* **2019**, *16*, 778–790. [CrossRef]
77. Tokarz, A.; Szuscik, I.; Kusnierz-Cabala, B.; Kapusta, M.; Konkolewska, M.; Zurakowski, A.; Georgescu, A.; Stepien, E. Extracellular vesicles participate in the transport of cytokines and angiogenic factors in diabetic patients with ocular complications. *Folia Med. Cracov.* **2015**, *55*, 35–48.
78. Tsimerman, G.; Roguin, A.; Bachar, A.; Melamed, E.; Brenner, B.; Aharon, A. Involvement of microparticles in diabetic vascular complications. *Thromb. Haemost.* **2011**, *106*, 310–321. [CrossRef] [PubMed]
79. Xu, H.; Chen, M. Targeting the complement system for the management of retinal inflammatory and degenerative diseases. *Eur. J. Pharmacol.* **2016**, *787*, 94–104. [CrossRef] [PubMed]
80. Chrzanowska, M.; Modrzejewska, A.; Modrzejewska, M. New insight into the role of the complement in the most common types of retinopathy-current literature review. *Int. J. Ophthalmol.* **2018**, *11*, 1856–1864.
81. Huang, C.; Fisher, K.P.; Hammer, S.S.; Navitskaya, S.; Blanchard, G.J.; Busik, J.V. Plasma Exosomes Contribute to Microvascular Damage in Diabetic Retinopathy by Activating the Classical Complement Pathway. *Diabetes* **2018**, *67*, 1639–1649. [CrossRef]
82. Huang, C.; Fisher, K.P.; Hammer, S.S.; Busik, J.V. Extracellular Vesicle-Induced Classical Complement Activation Leads to Retinal Endothelial Cell Damage via MAC Deposition. *Int. J. Mol. Sci.* **2020**, *21*, 1693. [CrossRef] [PubMed]
83. Gerl, V.B.; Bohl, J.; Pitz, S.; Stoffelns, B.; Pfeiffer, N.; Bhakdi, S. Extensive deposits of complement C3d and C5b-9 in the choriocapillaris of eyes of patients with diabetic retinopathy. *Investig. Ophthalmol. Vis. Sci.* **2002**, *43*, 1104–1108.

84. Ogata, N.; Nomura, S.; Shouzu, A.; Imaizumi, M.; Arichi, M.; Matsumura, M. Elevation of monocyte-derived microparticles in patients with diabetic retinopathy. *Diabetes Res. Clin. Pract.* **2006**, *73*, 241–248. [CrossRef] [PubMed]
85. Ogata, N.; Imaizumi, M.; Nomura, S.; Shozu, A.; Arichi, M.; Matsuoka, M.; Matsumura, M. Increased levels of platelet-derived microparticles in patients with diabetic retinopathy. *Diabetes Res. Clin. Pract.* **2005**, *68*, 193–201. [CrossRef] [PubMed]
86. Zhang, W.; Dong, X.; Wang, T.; Kong, Y. Exosomes derived from platelet-rich plasma mediate hyperglycemia-induced retinal endothelial injury via targeting the TLR4 signaling pathway. *Exp. Eye Res.* **2019**, *189*, 107813. [CrossRef] [PubMed]
87. Tokarz, A.; Konkolewska, M.; Kusnierz-Cabala, B.; Maziarz, B.; Hanarz, P.; Zurakowski, A.; Szuscik, I.; Stepien, E.L. Retinopathy severity correlates with RANTES concentrations and CCR 5-positive microvesicles in diabetes. *Folia Med. Cracov.* **2019**, *59*, 95–112.
88. Jansen, F.; Yang, X.; Franklin, B.S.; Hoelscher, M.; Schmitz, T.; Bedorf, J.; Nickenig, G.; Werner, N. High glucose condition increases NADPH oxidase activity in endothelial microparticles that promote vascular inflammation. *Cardiovasc. Res.* **2013**, *98*, 94–106. [CrossRef]
89. Razmara, M.; Hjemdahl, P.; Ostenson, C.G.; Li, N. Platelet hyperprocoagulant activity in Type 2 diabetes mellitus: Attenuation by glycoprotein IIb/IIIa inhibition. *J. Thromb. Haemost.* **2008**, *6*, 2186–2192. [CrossRef]
90. Su, Y.; Chen, J.; Dong, Z.; Zhang, Y.; Ma, R.; Kou, J.; Wang, F.; Shi, J. Procoagulant Activity of Blood and Endothelial Cells via Phosphatidylserine Exposure and Microparticle Delivery in Patients with Diabetic Retinopathy. *Cell Physiol. Biochem.* **2018**, *45*, 2411–2420. [CrossRef]
91. Hausser, J.; Zavolan, M. Identification and consequences of miRNA-target interactions–beyond repression of gene expression. *Nat. Rev. Genet.* **2014**, *15*, 599–612. [CrossRef]
92. Jonas, S.; Izaurralde, E. Towards a molecular understanding of microRNA-mediated gene silencing. *Nat. Rev. Genet.* **2015**, *16*, 421–433. [CrossRef]
93. Bushati, N.; Cohen, S.M. microRNA functions. *Annu. Rev. Cell Dev. Biol.* **2007**, *23*, 175–205. [CrossRef] [PubMed]
94. Tufekci, K.U.; Oner, M.G.; Meuwissen, R.L.; Genc, S. The role of microRNAs in human diseases. *Methods Mol. Biol.* **2014**, *1107*, 33–50. [PubMed]
95. Konovalova, J.; Gerasymchuk, D.; Parkkinen, I.; Chmielarz, P.; Domanskyi, A. Interplay between MicroRNAs and Oxidative Stress in Neurodegenerative Diseases. *Int. J. Mol. Sci.* **2019**, *20*, 6055. [CrossRef] [PubMed]
96. Shafabakhsh, R.; Aghadavod, E.; Mobini, M.; Heidari-Soureshjani, R.; Asemi, Z. Association between microRNAs expression and signaling pathways of inflammatory markers in diabetic retinopathy. *J. Cell Physiol.* **2019**, *234*, 7781–7787. [CrossRef]
97. Garcia de la Torre, N.; Fernandez-Durango, R.; Gomez, R.; Fuentes, M.; Roldan-Pallares, M.; Donate, J.; Barabash, A.; Alonso, B.; Runkle, I.; Duran, A.; et al. Expression of Angiogenic MicroRNAs in Endothelial Progenitor Cells From Type 1 Diabetic Patients With and Without Diabetic Retinopathy. *Investig. Ophthalmol. Vis. Sci.* **2015**, *56*, 4090–4098. [CrossRef]
98. Qing, S.; Yuan, S.; Yun, C.; Hui, H.; Mao, P.; Wen, F.; Ding, Y.; Liu, Q. Serum miRNA biomarkers serve as a fingerprint for proliferative diabetic retinopathy. *Cell Physiol. Biochem.* **2014**, *34*, 1733–1740. [CrossRef]
99. Zampetaki, A.; Willeit, P.; Burr, S.; Yin, X.; Langley, S.R.; Kiechl, S.; Klein, R.; Rossing, P.; Chaturvedi, N.; Mayr, M. Angiogenic microRNAs Linked to Incidence and Progression of Diabetic Retinopathy in Type 1 Diabetes. *Diabetes* **2016**, *65*, 216–227. [CrossRef]
100. Chen, S.; Yuan, M.; Liu, Y.; Zhao, X.; Lian, P.; Chen, Y.; Liu, B.; Lu, L. Landscape of microRNA in the aqueous humour of proliferative diabetic retinopathy as assessed by next-generation sequencing. *Clin. Exp. Ophthalmol.* **2019**, *47*, 925–936. [CrossRef]
101. Martinez, B.; Peplow, P.V. MicroRNAs as biomarkers of diabetic retinopathy and disease progression. *Neural Regen. Res.* **2019**, *14*, 1858–1869.
102. Jiang, Q.; Lyu, X.M.; Yuan, Y.; Wang, L. Plasma miR-21 expression: An indicator for the severity of Type 2 diabetes with diabetic retinopathy. *Biosci. Rep.* **2017**, *37*. [CrossRef]
103. Zhou, H.; Peng, C.; Huang, D.S.; Liu, L.; Guan, P. microRNA Expression Profiling Based on Microarray Approach in Human Diabetic Retinopathy: A Systematic Review and Meta-Analysis. *DNA Cell Biol.* **2020**, *39*, 441–450. [CrossRef]

104. Iftikhar, H.; Carney, G.E. Evidence and potential in vivo functions for biofluid miRNAs: From expression profiling to functional testing: Potential roles of extracellular miRNAs as indicators of physiological change and as agents of intercellular information exchange. *Bioessays* **2016**, *38*, 367–378. [CrossRef]
105. Arroyo, J.D.; Chevillet, J.R.; Kroh, E.M.; Ruf, I.K.; Pritchard, C.C.; Gibson, D.F.; Mitchell, P.S.; Bennett, C.F.; Pogosova-Agadjanyan, E.L.; Stirewalt, D.L.; et al. Argonaute2 complexes carry a population of circulating microRNAs independent of vesicles in human plasma. *Proc. Natl. Acad. Sci. USA* **2011**, *108*, 5003–5008. [CrossRef]
106. Turchinovich, A.; Weiz, L.; Langheinz, A.; Burwinkel, B. Characterization of extracellular circulating microRNA. *Nucleic Acids Res.* **2011**, *39*, 7223–7233. [CrossRef]
107. Ferreira, R.; Santos, T.; Amar, A.; Gong, A.; Chen, T.C.; Tahara, S.M.; Giannotta, S.L.; Hofman, F.M. Argonaute-2 promotes miR-18a entry in human brain endothelial cells. *J. Am. Heart Assoc.* **2014**, *3*, e000968. [CrossRef]
108. Wang, K.; Zhang, S.; Weber, J.; Baxter, D.; Galas, D.J. Export of microRNAs and microRNA-protective protein by mammalian cells. *Nucleic Acids Res.* **2010**, *38*, 7248–7259. [CrossRef]
109. Vickers, K.C.; Palmisano, B.T.; Shoucri, B.M.; Shamburek, R.D.; Remaley, A.T. MicroRNAs are transported in plasma and delivered to recipient cells by high-density lipoproteins. *Nat. Cell Biol.* **2011**, *13*, 423–433. [CrossRef]
110. Sedgeman, L.R.; Beysen, C.; Ramirez Solano, M.A.; Michell, D.L.; Sheng, Q.; Zhao, S.; Turner, S.; Linton, M.F.; Vickers, K.C. Beta cell secretion of miR-375 to HDL is inversely associated with insulin secretion. *Sci. Rep.* **2019**, *9*, 3803. [CrossRef]
111. Kalra, H.; Simpson, R.J.; Ji, H.; Aikawa, E.; Altevogt, P.; Askenase, P.; Bond, V.C.; Borras, F.E.; Breakefield, X.; Budnik, V.; et al. Vesiclepedia: A compendium for extracellular vesicles with continuous community annotation. *PLoS Biol.* **2012**, *10*, e1001450. [CrossRef]
112. Li, Z.; Dong, Y.; He, C.; Pan, X.; Liu, D.; Yang, J.; Sun, L.; Chen, P.; Wang, Q. RNA-Seq Revealed Novel Non-proliferative Retinopathy Specific Circulating MiRNAs in T2DM Patients. *Front. Genet.* **2019**, *10*, 531. [CrossRef]
113. Zhou, M.; Luo, J.; Zhang, H. Role of Sirtuin 1 in the pathogenesis of ocular disease (Review). *Int. J. Mol. Med.* **2018**, *42*, 13–20. [CrossRef]
114. Betel, D.; Wilson, M.; Gabow, A.; Marks, D.S.; Sander, C. The microRNA.org resource: Targets and expression. *Nucleic Acids Res.* **2008**, *36*, 149–153. [CrossRef]
115. Shaker, O.G.; Abdelaleem, O.O.; Mahmoud, R.H.; Abdelghaffar, N.K.; Ahmed, T.I.; Said, O.M.; Zaki, O.M. Diagnostic and prognostic role of serum miR-20b, miR-17-3p, HOTAIR, and MALAT1 in diabetic retinopathy. *IUBMB Life* **2019**, *71*, 310–320. [CrossRef]
116. Liu, L.Z.; Li, C.; Chen, Q.; Jing, Y.; Carpenter, R.; Jiang, Y.; Kung, H.F.; Lai, L.; Jiang, B.H. MiR-21 induced angiogenesis through AKT and ERK activation and HIF-1alpha expression. *PLoS ONE* **2011**, *6*, e19139.
117. Zeng, J.; Xiong, Y.; Li, G.; Liu, M.; He, T.; Tang, Y.; Chen, Y.; Cai, L.; Jiang, R.; Tao, J. MiR-21 is overexpressed in response to high glucose and protects endothelial cells from apoptosis. *Exp. Clin. Endocrinol. Diabetes* **2013**, *121*, 425–430. [CrossRef]
118. Solly, E.; Hourigan, S.T.; Mulangala, J.; Psaltis, P.J.; Di Bartolo, B.; NG, M.; Nicholas, S.; Bursill, C.; Tan, J.T.M. Inhibition of miR-181c Rescues Diabetes-Impaired Angiogenesis. *Diabetes* **2019**, *68* (Suppl. 1). [CrossRef]
119. McArthur, K.; Feng, B.; Wu, Y.; Chen, S.; Chakrabarti, S. MicroRNA-200b regulates vascular endothelial growth factor-mediated alterations in diabetic retinopathy. *Diabetes* **2011**, *60*, 1314–1323. [CrossRef]
120. Murray, A.R.; Chen, Q.; Takahashi, Y.; Zhou, K.K.; Park, K.; Ma, J.X. MicroRNA-200b downregulates oxidation resistance 1 (Oxr1) expression in the retina of type 1 diabetes model. *Investig. Ophthalmol. Vis. Sci.* **2013**, *54*, 1689–1697. [CrossRef]
121. Kovacs, B.; Lumayag, S.; Cowan, C.; Xu, S. MicroRNAs in early diabetic retinopathy in streptozotocin-induced diabetic rats. *Investig. Ophthalmol. Vis. Sci.* **2011**, *52*, 4402–4409. [CrossRef]
122. Chen, S.; Feng, B.; George, B.; Chakrabarti, R.; Chen, M.; Chakrabarti, S. Transcriptional coactivator p300 regulates glucose-induced gene expression in endothelial cells. *Am. J. Physiol. Endocrinol. Metab.* **2010**, *298*, 127–137. [CrossRef]
123. Friedrich, J.; Steel, D.H.W.; Schlingemann, R.O.; Koss, M.J.; Hammes, H.P.; Krenning, G.; Klaassen, I. microRNA Expression Profile in the Vitreous of Proliferative Diabetic Retinopathy Patients and Differences from Patients Treated with Anti-VEGF Therapy. *Transl. Vis. Sci. Technol.* **2020**, *9*, 16. [CrossRef]

124. Pezzolesi, M.G.; Satake, E.; McDonnell, K.P.; Major, M.; Smiles, A.M.; Krolewski, A.S. Circulating TGF-beta1-Regulated miRNAs and the Risk of Rapid Progression to ESRD in Type 1 Diabetes. *Diabetes* **2015**, *64*, 3285–3293. [CrossRef] [PubMed]
125. Jones, A.; Danielson, K.M.; Benton, M.C.; Ziegler, O.; Shah, R.; Stubbs, R.S.; Das, S.; Macartney-Coxson, D. miRNA Signatures of Insulin Resistance in Obesity. *Obesity (Silver Spring)* **2017**, *25*, 1734–1744. [CrossRef] [PubMed]
126. Meerson, A.; Najjar, A.; Saad, E.; Sbeit, W.; Barhoum, M.; Assy, N. Sex Differences in Plasma MicroRNA Biomarkers of Early and Complicated Diabetes Mellitus in Israeli Arab and Jewish Patients. *Noncoding RNA* **2019**, *5*, 32. [CrossRef]
127. Zampetaki, A.; Kiechl, S.; Drozdov, I.; Willeit, P.; Mayr, U.; Prokopi, M.; Mayr, A.; Weger, S.; Oberhollenzer, F.; Bonora, E.; et al. Plasma microRNA profiling reveals loss of endothelial miR-126 and other microRNAs in type 2 diabetes. *Circ. Res.* **2010**, *107*, 810–817. [CrossRef] [PubMed]
128. Jimenez-Lucena, R.; Rangel-Zuniga, O.A.; Alcala-Diaz, J.F.; Lopez-Moreno, J.; Roncero-Ramos, I.; Molina-Abril, H.; Yubero-Serrano, E.M.; Caballero-Villarraso, J.; Delgado-Lista, J.; Castano, J.P.; et al. Circulating miRNAs as Predictive Biomarkers of Type 2 Diabetes Mellitus Development in Coronary Heart Disease Patients from the CORDIOPREV Study. *Mol. Ther. Nucleic Acids* **2018**, *12*, 146–157. [CrossRef]
129. Seyhan, A.A.; Nunez Lopez, Y.O.; Xie, H.; Yi, F.; Mathews, C.; Pasarica, M.; Pratley, R.E. Pancreas-enriched miRNAs are altered in the circulation of subjects with diabetes: A pilot cross-sectional study. *Sci. Rep.* **2016**, *6*, 31479. [CrossRef]
130. de Candia, P.; Spinetti, G.; Specchia, C.; Sangalli, E.; La Sala, L.; Uccellatore, A.; Lupini, S.; Genovese, S.; Matarese, G.; Ceriello, A. A unique plasma microRNA profile defines type 2 diabetes progression. *PLoS ONE* **2017**, *12*, e0188980. [CrossRef]
131. Hirota, K.; Keino, H.; Inoue, M.; Ishida, H.; Hirakata, A. Comparisons of microRNA expression profiles in vitreous humor between eyes with macular hole and eyes with proliferative diabetic retinopathy. *Graefes Arch. Clin. Exp. Ophthalmol.* **2015**, *253*, 335–342. [CrossRef]
132. Blum, A.; Yehuda, H.; Geron, N.; Meerson, A. Elevated Levels of miR-122 in Serum May Contribute to Improved Endothelial Function and Lower Oncologic Risk Following Bariatric Surgery. *Isr. Med. Assoc. J.* **2017**, *19*, 620–624.
133. Pastukh, N.; Meerson, A.; Kalish, D.; Jabaly, H.; Blum, A. Serum miR-122 levels correlate with diabetic retinopathy. *Clin. Exp. Med.* **2019**, *19*, 255–260. [CrossRef]
134. Wang, X.; Sundquist, J.; Zoller, B.; Memon, A.A.; Palmer, K.; Sundquist, K.; Bennet, L. Determination of 14 circulating microRNAs in Swedes and Iraqis with and without diabetes mellitus type 2. *PLoS ONE* **2014**, *9*, e86792. [CrossRef]
135. Kong, L.; Zhu, J.; Han, W.; Jiang, X.; Xu, M.; Zhao, Y.; Dong, Q.; Pang, Z.; Guan, Q.; Gao, L.; et al. Significance of serum microRNAs in pre-diabetes and newly diagnosed type 2 diabetes: A clinical study. *Acta Diabetol.* **2011**, *48*, 61–69. [CrossRef]
136. Flowers, E.; Kanaya, A.M.; Fukuoka, Y.; Allen, I.E.; Cooper, B.; Aouizerat, B.E. Preliminary evidence supports circulating microRNAs as prognostic biomarkers for type 2 diabetes. *Obes. Sci. Pract.* **2017**, *3*, 446–452. [CrossRef]
137. Carreras-Badosa, G.; Bonmati, A.; Ortega, F.J.; Mercader, J.M.; Guindo-Martinez, M.; Torrents, D.; Prats-Puig, A.; Martinez-Calcerrada, J.M.; Platero-Gutierrez, E.; De Zegher, F.; et al. Altered Circulating miRNA Expression Profile in Pregestational and Gestational Obesity. *J. Clin. Endocrinol. Metab.* **2015**, *100*, E1446–E1456. [CrossRef]
138. Farr, R.J.; Januszewski, A.S.; Joglekar, M.V.; Liang, H.; McAulley, A.K.; Hewitt, A.W.; Thomas, H.E.; Loudovaris, T.; Kay, T.W.; Jenkins, A.; et al. A comparative analysis of high-throughput platforms for validation of a circulating microRNA signature in diabetic retinopathy. *Sci. Rep.* **2015**, *5*, 10375. [CrossRef]
139. Blum, A.; Meerson, A.; Rohana, H.; Jabaly, H.; Nahul, N.; Celesh, D.; Romanenko, O.; Tamir, S. MicroRNA-423 may regulate diabetic vasculopathy. *Clin. Exp. Med.* **2019**, *19*, 469–477. [CrossRef]
140. Ye, E.A.; Liu, L.; Jiang, Y.; Jan, J.; Gaddipati, S.; Suvas, S.; Steinle, J.J. miR-15a/16 reduces retinal leukostasis through decreased pro-inflammatory signaling. *J. Neuroinflammation* **2016**, *13*, 305. [CrossRef]

141. Besnier, M.; Shantikumar, S.; Anwar, M.; Dixit, P.; Chamorro-Jorganes, A.; Sweaad, W.; Sala-Newby, G.; Madeddu, P.; Thomas, A.C.; Howard, L.; et al. miR-15a/-16 Inhibit Angiogenesis by Targeting the Tie2 Coding Sequence: Therapeutic Potential of a miR-15a/16 Decoy System in Limb Ischemia. *Mol. Ther. Nucleic Acids* **2019**, *17*, 49–62. [CrossRef]
142. Wang, Q.; Navitskaya, S.; Chakravarthy, H.; Huang, C.; Kady, N.; Lydic, T.A.; Chen, Y.E.; Yin, K.J.; Powell, F.L.; Martin, P.M.; et al. Dual Anti-Inflammatory and Anti-Angiogenic Action of miR-15a in Diabetic Retinopathy. *EBioMedicine* **2016**, *11*, 138–150. [CrossRef] [PubMed]
143. Ye, E.A.; Steinle, J.J. miR-15b/16 protects primary human retinal microvascular endothelial cells against hyperglycemia-induced increases in tumor necrosis factor alpha and suppressor of cytokine signaling 3. *J. Neuroinflammation* **2015**, *12*, 44. [CrossRef] [PubMed]
144. Chen, D.; Dixon, B.J.; Doycheva, D.M.; Li, B.; Zhang, Y.; Hu, Q.; He, Y.; Guo, Z.; Nowrangi, D.; Flores, J.; et al. IRE1alpha inhibition decreased TXNIP/NLRP3 inflammasome activation through miR-17-5p after neonatal hypoxic-ischemic brain injury in rats. *J. Neuroinflammation* **2018**, *15*, 32. [CrossRef] [PubMed]
145. Ji, Z.R.; Xue, W.L.; Zhang, L. Schisandrin B Attenuates Inflammation in LPS-Induced Sepsis Through miR-17-5p Downregulating TLR4. *Inflammation* **2019**, *42*, 731–739. [CrossRef]
146. Li, Y.; Zheng, L.; Li, Y.H.; Wang, Y.L.; Li, L. MiR-20a ameliorates diabetic angiopathy in streptozotocin-induced diabetic rats by regulating intracellular antioxidant enzymes and VEGF. *Eur. Rev. Med. Pharmacol. Sci.* **2020**, *24*, 1948–1955.
147. Bao, L.; Fu, X.; Si, M.; Wang, Y.; Ma, R.; Ren, X.; Lv, H. MicroRNA-185 targets SOCS3 to inhibit beta-cell dysfunction in diabetes. *PLoS ONE* **2015**, *10*, e0116067. [CrossRef]
148. Hou, J.; Liu, L.; Zhu, Q.; Wu, Y.; Tian, B.; Cui, L.; Liu, Y.; Li, X. MicroRNA-185 inhibits angiogenesis in human microvascular endothelial cells through targeting stromal interaction molecule 1. *Cell Biol. Int.* **2016**, *40*, 318–328. [CrossRef]
149. Qin, L.L.; An, M.X.; Liu, Y.L.; Xu, H.C.; Lu, Z.Q. MicroRNA-126: A promising novel biomarker in peripheral blood for diabetic retinopathy. *Int. J. Ophthalmol.* **2017**, *10*, 530–534.
150. Fang, S.; Ma, X.; Guo, S.; Lu, J. MicroRNA-126 inhibits cell viability and invasion in a diabetic retinopathy model via targeting IRS-1. *Oncol. Lett.* **2017**, *14*, 4311–4318. [CrossRef]
151. Mazzeo, A.; Beltramo, E.; Lopatina, T.; Gai, C.; Trento, M.; Porta, M. Molecular and functional characterization of circulating extracellular vesicles from diabetic patients with and without retinopathy and healthy subjects. *Exp. Eye Res.* **2018**, *176*, 69–77. [CrossRef]
152. Ng, P.C.; Chan, K.Y.; Leung, K.T.; Tam, Y.H.; Ma, T.P.; Lam, H.S.; Cheung, H.M.; Lee, K.H.; To, K.F.; Li, K. Comparative MiRNA Expressional Profiles and Molecular Networks in Human Small Bowel Tissues of Necrotizing Enterocolitis and Spontaneous Intestinal Perforation. *PLoS ONE* **2015**, *10*, e0135737. [CrossRef] [PubMed]
153. Snowhite, I.V.; Allende, G.; Sosenko, J.; Pastori, R.L.; Messinger Cayetano, S.; Pugliese, A. Association of serum microRNAs with islet autoimmunity, disease progression and metabolic impairment in relatives at risk of type 1 diabetes. *Diabetologia* **2017**, *60*, 1409–1422. [CrossRef] [PubMed]
154. Otsuka, M.; Zheng, M.; Hayashi, M.; Lee, J.D.; Yoshino, O.; Lin, S.; Han, J. Impaired microRNA processing causes corpus luteum insufficiency and infertility in mice. *J. Clin. Investig.* **2008**, *118*, 1944–1954. [CrossRef] [PubMed]
155. Shen, J.; Yang, X.; Xie, B.; Chen, Y.; Swaim, M.; Hackett, S.F.; Campochiaro, P.A. MicroRNAs regulate ocular neovascularization. *Mol. Ther.* **2008**, *16*, 1208–1216. [CrossRef]
156. Chen, Q.; Qiu, F.; Zhou, K.; Matlock, H.G.; Takahashi, Y.; Rajala, R.V.S.; Yang, Y.; Moran, E.; Ma, J.X. Pathogenic Role of microRNA-21 in Diabetic Retinopathy Through Downregulation of PPARalpha. *Diabetes* **2017**, *66*, 1671–1682. [CrossRef] [PubMed]
157. Fayyad-Kazan, H.; Bitar, N.; Najar, M.; Lewalle, P.; Fayyad-Kazan, M.; Badran, R.; Hamade, E.; Daher, A.; Hussein, N.; ElDirani, R.; et al. Circulating miR-150 and miR-342 in plasma are novel potential biomarkers for acute myeloid leukemia. *J. Transl. Med.* **2013**, *11*, 31. [CrossRef]
158. Li, X.R.; Chu, H.J.; Lv, T.; Wang, L.; Kong, S.F.; Dai, S.Z. miR-342-3p suppresses proliferation, migration and invasion by targeting FOXM1 in human cervical cancer. *FEBS Lett.* **2014**, *588*, 3298–3307. [CrossRef]
159. Estrella, S.; Garcia-Diaz, D.F.; Codner, E.; Camacho-Guillen, P.; Perez-Bravo, F. [Expression of miR-22 and miR-150 in type 1 diabetes mellitus: Possible relationship with autoimmunity and clinical characteristics]. *Med. Clin. (Barc)* **2016**, *147*, 245–247. [CrossRef]

160. Mazzeo, A.; Lopatina, T.; Gai, C.; Trento, M.; Porta, M.; Beltramo, E. Functional analysis of miR-21-3p, miR-30b-5p and miR-150-5p shuttled by extracellular vesicles from diabetic subjects reveals their association with diabetic retinopathy. *Exp. Eye Res.* **2019**, *184*, 56–63. [CrossRef]
161. Mansour, S.E.; Browning, D.J.; Wong, K.; Flynn, H.W., Jr.; Bhavsar, A.R. The Evolving Treatment of Diabetic Retinopathy. *Clin. Ophthalmol.* **2020**, *14*, 653–678. [CrossRef]
162. Semeraro, F.; Morescalchi, F.; Cancarini, A.; Russo, A.; Rezzola, S.; Costagliola, C. Diabetic retinopathy, a vascular and inflammatory disease: Therapeutic implications. *Diabetes Metab.* **2019**, *45*, 517–527. [CrossRef] [PubMed]
163. Rossino, M.G.; Casini, G. Nutraceuticals for the Treatment of Diabetic Retinopathy. *Nutrients* **2019**, *11*, 771. [CrossRef]
164. Stewart, M.W. Corticosteroid use for diabetic macular edema: Old fad or new trend? *Curr. Diab. Rep.* **2012**, *12*, 364–375. [CrossRef] [PubMed]
165. Wang, Y.S.; Friedrichs, U.; Eichler, W.; Hoffmann, S.; Wiedemann, P. Inhibitory effects of triamcinolone acetonide on bFGF-induced migration and tube formation in choroidal microvascular endothelial cells. *Graefes Arch. Clin. Exp. Ophthalmol.* **2002**, *240*, 42–48. [CrossRef] [PubMed]
166. Lattanzio, R.; Cicinelli, M.V.; Bandello, F. Intravitreal Steroids in Diabetic Macular Edema. *Dev. Ophthalmol.* **2017**, *60*, 78–90. [PubMed]
167. Penfold, P.L.; Wen, L.; Madigan, M.C.; King, N.J.; Provis, J.M. Modulation of permeability and adhesion molecule expression by human choroidal endothelial cells. *Investig. Ophthalmol. Vis. Sci.* **2002**, *43*, 3125–3130.
168. Penfold, P.L.; Wen, L.; Madigan, M.C.; Gillies, M.C.; King, N.J.; Provis, J.M. Triamcinolone acetonide modulates permeability and intercellular adhesion molecule-1 (ICAM-1) expression of the ECV304 cell line: Implications for macular degeneration. *Clin. Exp. Immunol.* **2000**, *121*, 458–465. [CrossRef]
169. Chen, Y.; Zhang, M.; Zheng, Y. Glucocorticoids inhibit production of exosomes containing inflammatory microRNA-155 in lipopolysaccharide-induced macrophage inflammatory responses. *Int. J. Clin. Exp. Pathol.* **2018**, *11*, 3391–3397.
170. Edelman, J.L.; Lutz, D.; Castro, M.R. Corticosteroids inhibit VEGF-induced vascular leakage in a rabbit model of blood-retinal and blood-aqueous barrier breakdown. *Exp. Eye Res.* **2005**, *80*, 249–258. [CrossRef]
171. Lassota, N. Clinical and histological aspects of CNV formation: Studies in an animal model. *Acta Ophthalmol.* **2008**, *86*, 1–28. [CrossRef]
172. Bhisitkul, R.B.; Winn, B.J.; Lee, O.T.; Wong, J.; Pereira Dde, S.; Porco, T.C.; He, X.; Hahn, P.; Dunaief, J.L. Neuroprotective effect of intravitreal triamcinolone acetonide against photoreceptor apoptosis in a rabbit model of subretinal hemorrhage. *Investig. Ophthalmol. Vis. Sci.* **2008**, *49*, 4071–4077. [CrossRef] [PubMed]
173. Ayalasomayajula, S.P.; Amrite, A.C.; Kompella, U.B. Inhibition of cyclooxygenase-2, but not cyclooxygenase-1, reduces prostaglandin E2 secretion from diabetic rat retinas. *Eur. J. Pharmacol.* **2004**, *498*, 275–278. [CrossRef] [PubMed]
174. Zhang, W.; Liu, H.; Rojas, M.; Caldwell, R.W.; Caldwell, R.B. Anti-inflammatory therapy for diabetic retinopathy. *Immunotherapy* **2011**, *3*, 609–628. [CrossRef] [PubMed]
175. Sun, W.; Gerhardinger, C.; Dagher, Z.; Hoehn, T.; Lorenzi, M. Aspirin at low-intermediate concentrations protects retinal vessels in experimental diabetic retinopathy through non-platelet-mediated effects. *Diabetes* **2005**, *54*, 3418–3426. [CrossRef] [PubMed]
176. Kern, T.S.; Engerman, R.L. Pharmacological inhibition of diabetic retinopathy: Aminoguanidine and aspirin. *Diabetes* **2001**, *50*, 1636–1642. [CrossRef] [PubMed]
177. Group, T.D.S. Effect of aspirin alone and aspirin plus dipyridamole in early diabetic retinopathy. A multicenter randomized controlled clinical trial. The DAMAD Study Group. *Diabetes* **1989**, *38*, 491–498. [CrossRef]
178. Hattori, Y.; Hashizume, K.; Nakajima, K.; Nishimura, Y.; Naka, M.; Miyanaga, K. The effect of long-term treatment with sulindac on the progression of diabetic retinopathy. *Curr. Med. Res. Opin.* **2007**, *23*, 1913–1917. [CrossRef]
179. Amrite, A.C.; Ayalasomayajula, S.P.; Cheruvu, N.P.; Kompella, U.B. Single periocular injection of celecoxib-PLGA microparticles inhibits diabetes-induced elevations in retinal PGE2, VEGF, and vascular leakage. *Investig. Ophthalmol. Vis. Sci.* **2006**, *47*, 1149–1160. [CrossRef]
180. Kern, T.S.; Miller, C.M.; Du, Y.; Zheng, L.; Mohr, S.; Ball, S.L.; Kim, M.; Jamison, J.A.; Bingaman, D.P. Topical administration of nepafenac inhibits diabetes-induced retinal microvascular disease and underlying abnormalities of retinal metabolism and physiology. *Diabetes* **2007**, *56*, 373–379. [CrossRef]

181. Tsilimbaris, M.K.; Panagiotoglou, T.D.; Charisis, S.K.; Anastasakis, A.; Krikonis, T.S.; Christodoulakis, E. The use of intravitreal etanercept in diabetic macular oedema. *Semin. Ophthalmol.* **2007**, *22*, 75–79. [CrossRef]
182. Markomichelakis, N.N.; Theodossiadis, P.G.; Sfikakis, P.P. Regression of neovascular age-related macular degeneration following infliximab therapy. *Am. J. Ophthalmol.* **2005**, *139*, 537–540. [CrossRef] [PubMed]
183. Suhler, E.B.; Smith, J.R.; Wertheim, M.S.; Lauer, A.K.; Kurz, D.E.; Pickard, T.D.; Rosenbaum, J.T. A prospective trial of infliximab therapy for refractory uveitis: Preliminary safety and efficacy outcomes. *Arch. Ophthalmol.* **2005**, *123*, 903–912. [CrossRef] [PubMed]
184. Klotz, U.; Teml, A.; Schwab, M. Clinical pharmacokinetics and use of infliximab. *Clin. Pharm.* **2007**, *46*, 645–660. [CrossRef] [PubMed]
185. Xie, M.S.; Zheng, Y.Z.; Huang, L.B.; Xu, G.X. Infliximab relieves blood retinal barrier breakdown through the p38 MAPK pathway in a diabetic rat model. *Int. J. Ophthalmol.* **2017**, *10*, 1824–1829. [PubMed]
186. Stahel, M.; Becker, M.; Graf, N.; Michels, S. SYSTEMIC INTERLEUKIN 1beta INHIBITION IN PROLIFERATIVE DIABETIC RETINOPATHY: A Prospective Open-Label Study Using Canakinumab. *Retina* **2016**, *36*, 385–391. [CrossRef]
187. Sjolie, A.K.; Dodson, P.; Hobbs, F.R. Does renin-angiotensin system blockade have a role in preventing diabetic retinopathy? A clinical review. *Int. J. Clin. Pract.* **2011**, *65*, 148–153. [CrossRef]
188. Tamsma, J.T. Renal and retinal effects of enalapril and losartan in type 1 diabetes. *N. Engl. J. Med.* **2009**, *361*, 1410.
189. Chaturvedi, N.; Porta, M.; Klein, R.; Orchard, T.; Fuller, J.; Parving, H.H.; Bilous, R.; Sjolie, A.K.; DIRECT Programme Study Group. Effect of candesartan on prevention (DIRECT-Prevent 1) and progression (DIRECT-Protect 1) of retinopathy in type 1 diabetes: Randomised, placebo-controlled trials. *Lancet* **2008**, *372*, 1394–1402. [CrossRef]
190. Sjolie, A.K.; Klein, R.; Porta, M.; Orchard, T.; Fuller, J.; Parving, H.H.; Bilous, R.; Chaturvedi, N.; DIRECT Programme Study Group. Effect of candesartan on progression and regression of retinopathy in type 2 diabetes (DIRECT-Protect 2): A randomised placebo-controlled trial. *Lancet* **2008**, *372*, 1385–1393. [CrossRef]
191. Haque, R.; Hur, E.H.; Farrell, A.N.; Iuvone, P.M.; Howell, J.C. MicroRNA-152 represses VEGF and TGFbeta1 expressions through post-transcriptional inhibition of (Pro)renin receptor in human retinal endothelial cells. *Mol. Vis.* **2015**, *21*, 224–235.
192. Goncalves, A.; Marques, C.; Leal, E.; Ribeiro, C.F.; Reis, F.; Ambrosio, A.F.; Fernandes, R. Dipeptidyl peptidase-IV inhibition prevents blood-retinal barrier breakdown, inflammation and neuronal cell death in the retina of type 1 diabetic rats. *Biochim. Biophys. Acta* **2014**, *1842*, 1454–1463. [CrossRef] [PubMed]
193. Goncalves, A.; Leal, E.; Paiva, A.; Teixeira Lemos, E.; Teixeira, F.; Ribeiro, C.F.; Reis, F.; Ambrosio, A.F.; Fernandes, R. Protective effects of the dipeptidyl peptidase IV inhibitor sitagliptin in the blood-retinal barrier in a type 2 diabetes animal model. *Diabetes Obes. Metab.* **2012**, *14*, 454–463. [CrossRef] [PubMed]
194. Goncalves, A.; Almeida, L.; Silva, A.P.; Fontes-Ribeiro, C.; Ambrosio, A.F.; Cristovao, A.; Fernandes, R. The dipeptidyl peptidase-4 (DPP-4) inhibitor sitagliptin ameliorates retinal endothelial cell dysfunction triggered by inflammation. *Biomed. Pharmacother.* **2018**, *102*, 833–838. [CrossRef] [PubMed]
195. Zeng, Y.; Yang, K.; Wang, F.; Zhou, L.; Hu, Y.; Tang, M.; Zhang, S.; Jin, S.; Zhang, J.; Wang, J.; et al. The glucagon like peptide 1 analogue, exendin-4, attenuates oxidative stress-induced retinal cell death in early diabetic rats through promoting Sirt1 and Sirt3 expression. *Exp. Eye Res.* **2016**, *151*, 203–211. [CrossRef]
196. Fan, Y.; Liu, K.; Wang, Q.; Ruan, Y.; Ye, W.; Zhang, Y. Exendin-4 alleviates retinal vascular leakage by protecting the blood-retinal barrier and reducing retinal vascular permeability in diabetic Goto-Kakizaki rats. *Exp. Eye Res.* **2014**, *127*, 104–116. [CrossRef]
197. Hernandez, C.; Bogdanov, P.; Corraliza, L.; Garcia-Ramirez, M.; Sola-Adell, C.; Arranz, J.A.; Arroba, A.I.; Valverde, A.M.; Simo, R. Topical Administration of GLP-1 Receptor Agonists Prevents Retinal Neurodegeneration in Experimental Diabetes. *Diabetes* **2016**, *65*, 172–187. [CrossRef]
198. Zhang, Q.; Xiao, X.; Zheng, J.; Li, M. A glucagon-like peptide-1 analog, liraglutide, ameliorates endothelial dysfunction through miRNAs to inhibit apoptosis in rats. *PeerJ* **2019**, *7*, e6567. [CrossRef]
199. Al-Janabi, A.; Lightman, S.; Tomkins-Netzer, O. 'Statins in retinal disease'. *Eye (Lond.)* **2018**, *32*, 981–991. [CrossRef]
200. Yeh, P.T.; Wang, L.C.; Chang, S.W.; Yang, W.S.; Yang, C.M.; Yang, C.H. Effect of Fenofibrate on the Expression of Inflammatory Mediators in a Diabetic Rat Model. *Curr. Eye Res.* **2019**, *44*, 1121–1132. [CrossRef]

201. Kowluru, R.A.; Tang, J.; Kern, T.S. Abnormalities of retinal metabolism in diabetes and experimental galactosemia. VII. Effect of long-term administration of antioxidants on the development of retinopathy. *Diabetes* **2001**, *50*, 1938–1942. [CrossRef]
202. Ali, T.K.; El-Remessy, A.B. Diabetic retinopathy: Current management and experimental therapeutic targets. *Pharmacotherapy* **2009**, *29*, 182–192. [CrossRef] [PubMed]
203. Peng, J.J.; Xiong, S.Q.; Ding, L.X.; Peng, J.; Xia, X.B. Diabetic retinopathy: Focus on NADPH oxidase and its potential as therapeutic target. *Eur. J. Pharmacol.* **2019**, *853*, 381–387. [CrossRef] [PubMed]
204. Al-Shabrawey, M.; Rojas, M.; Sanders, T.; Behzadian, A.; El-Remessy, A.; Bartoli, M.; Parpia, A.K.; Liou, G.; Caldwell, R.B. Role of NADPH oxidase in retinal vascular inflammation. *Investig. Ophthalmol. Vis. Sci.* **2008**, *49*, 3239–3244. [CrossRef]
205. Zhang, W.; Rojas, M.; Lilly, B.; Tsai, N.T.; Lemtalsi, T.; Liou, G.I.; Caldwell, R.W.; Caldwell, R.B. NAD(P)H oxidase-dependent regulation of CCL2 production during retinal inflammation. *Investig. Ophthalmol. Vis. Sci.* **2009**, *50*, 3033–3040. [CrossRef] [PubMed]
206. Kowluru, R.A.; Koppolu, P.; Chakrabarti, S.; Chen, S. Diabetes-induced activation of nuclear transcriptional factor in the retina, and its inhibition by antioxidants. *Free Radic. Res.* **2003**, *37*, 1169–1180. [CrossRef]
207. *Diabetes: Oxidative Stress and Dietary Antioxidants*, 2nd ed.; Preedy, V.R. (Ed.) Elsevier: Amsterdam, The Netherlands, 2020; 454p.
208. Moisseiev, E.; Anderson, J.D.; Oltjen, S.; Goswami, M.; Zawadzki, R.J.; Nolta, J.A.; Park, S.S. Protective Effect of Intravitreal Administration of Exosomes Derived from Mesenchymal Stem Cells on Retinal Ischemia. *Curr. Eye Res.* **2017**, *42*, 1358–1367. [CrossRef]
209. Yu, B.; Shao, H.; Su, C.; Jiang, Y.; Chen, X.; Bai, L.; Zhang, Y.; Li, Q.; Zhang, X.; Li, X. Exosomes derived from MSCs ameliorate retinal laser injury partially by inhibition of MCP-1. *Sci. Rep.* **2016**, *6*, 34562. [CrossRef]
210. Safwat, A.; Sabry, D.; Ragiae, A.; Amer, E.; Mahmoud, R.H.; Shamardan, R.M. Adipose mesenchymal stem cells-derived exosomes attenuate retina degeneration of streptozotocin-induced diabetes in rabbits. *J. Circ. Biomark.* **2018**, *7*. [CrossRef]
211. Zhang, W.; Wang, Y.; Kong, Y. Exosomes Derived from Mesenchymal Stem Cells Modulate miR-126 to Ameliorate Hyperglycemia-Induced Retinal Inflammation Via Targeting HMGB1. *Investig. Ophthalmol. Vis. Sci.* **2019**, *60*, 294–303. [CrossRef]

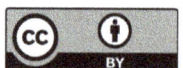

© 2020 by the authors. Licensee MDPI, Basel, Switzerland. This article is an open access article distributed under the terms and conditions of the Creative Commons Attribution (CC BY) license (http://creativecommons.org/licenses/by/4.0/).

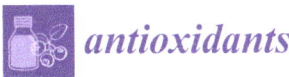

Article

Vitamin D Protects against Oxidative Stress and Inflammation in Human Retinal Cells

Patricia Fernandez-Robredo [1,2,3,†], Jorge González-Zamora [1,†], Sergio Recalde [1,2,3,*], Valentina Bilbao-Malavé [1], Jaione Bezunartea [1], Maria Hernandez [1,2,3,‡] and Alfredo Garcia-Layana [1,2,3,‡]

1. Retinal Pathologies and New Therapies Group, Experimental Ophthalmology Laboratory, Department of Ophthalmology, Clinica Universidad de Navarra, 31008 Pamplona, Spain; pfrobredo@unav.es (P.F.-R.); jgzamora@unav.es (J.G.-Z.); vbilbao@unav.es (V.B.-M.); jbezunartea@unav.es (J.B.); mahersan@unav.es (M.H.); aglayana@unav.es (A.G.-L.)
2. Navarra Institute for Health Research, IdiSNA, 31008 Pamplona, Spain
3. Red Temática de Investigación Cooperativa Sanitaria en Enfermedades Oculares (Oftared), 31008 Pamplona, Spain
* Correspondence: srecalde@unav.es
† These authors contributed equally to this work.
‡ These authors contributed equally to this work.

Received: 31 July 2020; Accepted: 4 September 2020; Published: 8 September 2020

Abstract: Diabetic retinopathy is a vision-threatening microvascular complication of diabetes and is one of the leading causes of blindness. Oxidative stress and inflammation play a major role in its pathogenesis, and new therapies counteracting these contributors could be of great interest. In the current study, we investigated the role of vitamin D against oxidative stress and inflammation in human retinal pigment epithelium (RPE) and human retinal endothelial cell lines. We demonstrate that vitamin D effectively counteracts the oxidative stress induced by hydrogen peroxide (H_2O_2). In addition, the increased levels of proinflammatory proteins such as Interleukin (IL)-6, IL-8, Monocyte chemoattractant protein (MCP)-1, Interferon (IFN)-γ, and tumor necrosis factor (TNF)-α triggered by lipopolysaccharide (LPS) exposure were significantly decreased by vitamin D addition. Interestingly, the increased IL-18 only decreased by vitamin D addition in endothelial cells but not in RPE cells, suggesting a main antiangiogenic role under inflammatory conditions. Moreover, H_2O_2 and LPS induced the alteration and morphological damage of tight junctions in adult retinal pigment epithelium (ARPE-19) cells that were restored under oxidative and inflammatory conditions by the addition of vitamin D to the media. In conclusion, our data suggest that vitamin D could protect the retina by enhancing antioxidant defense and through exhibiting anti-inflammatory properties.

Keywords: vitamin D; oxidative stress; inflammation; diabetic retinopathy

1. Introduction

Diabetic retinopathy (DR) is the main cause of blindness among adults of working age globally [1]. An effective management of diabetes reduces the risk of complications, however, poor control of the condition can result in microvascular complications [2]. Nevertheless, even patients with intensive glycemic control have rate of progression over 7% [3]. The Diabetes Control and Complications Trial (DCCT) found that intensive glycemic control can effectively reduce or slow down the development or progression of DR by 76% in patients with type 1 diabetes, while the U.K. Prospective Diabetes Study (UKPDS) came to a similar conclusion in patients with type 2 diabetes [2,4].

The investigation of the underlying mechanisms of DR is of great importance and may provide potential new alternative treatments. Several studies have shown that diabetes can lead to DR by several mechanisms including the polyol pathway [5], non-enzymatic glycation [6], activation of protein kinase C [7], oxidative stress [8–12], and inflammation [13]. Oxidative stress is considered to be one of the crucial causative factors in the development of DR, in combination with other biochemical imbalances, leading to both structural and functional changes and also promoting an increased loss of capillary cells in the microvasculature of the retina [11,12]. In addition, a significant body of evidence supports the role of proinflammatory cytokines, chemokines, and other inflammatory mediators in the pathogenesis of DR, leading to chronic low-grade inflammation of the retina and eventually to neovascularization [14].

Vitamin D (VITD) is a fat-soluble molecule that is found in two forms: vitamin D_2 and vitamin D_3 [15]. Vitamin D_3 is well recognized as a secosteroid hormone that regulates many cellular signaling activities through its nuclear VITD receptor (VDR) in target cells [15]. Previous studies reported that VITD treatment can protect cells and tissues from oxidative damage [16] and it has also been found to prevent oxidative stress damage in DR in a high-glucose environment [17,18] and in diabetic rats [19]. In addition, some polymorphisms in the VITD receptor gene are associated with increased risk of DR [20–23] and VITD-deficient patients have increased risk of DR [24,25]. VITD also appears to be beneficial in other retinopathies such as age-related macular degeneration (AMD) [26–28]. Therefore, VITD may be suggested as a useful candidate for diabetic patients to reduce the pathological complications of diabetes. However, further research needs to be made to clarify the possible therapeutic potential of VITD in the DR.

In the current study, we investigated the safety of VITD in adult retinal pigment epithelium (ARPE-19) and human retinal endothelial (HREC) cell lines, focusing on its antioxidant and anti-inflammatory effect on cell integrity, oxidative stress, and cytokines release. This study constitutes an in vitro evaluation of the molecular pathways by which VITD might tackle the oxidative stress and inflammation observed in patients suffering from retinal pathologies such as DR.

2. Materials and Methods

2.1. Expression of Genes Related to VITD Metabolism

Total RNA was isolated from cell lines using an ABI PRISM 6100 Nucleic Acid PrepStation (Life Technologies, Carlsbad, CA, USA). Subsequently, the quantity and quality of purified messenger RNA (mRNA) was checked using a NanoDrop spectrophotometer (Nanodrop Technologies, Montchanin, DE, USA) at 260/280. Using the qScript cDNA Supermix Kit (Quanta Biosciences, Inc., Gaithersburg, MD, USA), we reverse-transcribed 1000 ng of each mRNA under the manufactured conditions. The primers of the relevant genes are as follows: cytochrome P450 *(CYP)27A1* (Unigene ID-Hs.516700, 5'-GGCAAGTACCCAGTACGG-3' and 5'-AGCAAATAGCTTCCAAGG-3'), *CYP27B1* (Unigene ID-Hs.524528, 5'-CACCTGACCC ACTTCCTGTT-3' and 5'-TCTGGGACACGAGAATTTCC-3'), *CYP2R1* (Unigene ID-Hs.371427, 5'-AGAGACCCAGAAGTGTTCCAT-3' and 5'-GTCTTTCAGCACAGATGAGGTA-3'), *CYP24A1* (Unigene ID-Hs.89663, 5'-CCCACTAGCCACCTCGTACCAAC-3' and 5'-CGTAGCCCTTCTTT GCGGTAGTC-3'), *VDR* (Unigene ID-Hs.524368, 5'-CGCTCCAATGAGT CCTTCACC-3' and 5'-GCTTCATGCTGCACTCAGGC-3'), *Cubilin* (Unigene ID-Hs.166206, 5'-GCGGCTTCACTGC TTCCTA-3' and 5'-GAGTGATGGTGTGCCCTTGT-3'), *Megalin* (Unigene ID-Hs.657729, 5'-TAAGT CAGTGCCCAACCTTT-3'and 5'-GCGGTTGTTCCTGGAG-3'). A 2720 Thermal Cycler (Life Technologies, Gaithersburg, MD, USA) was used for amplification with the following protocol: 10 min at 95 °C, 40 cycles of 30 s at 95 °C, 1 min 58 °C, and extension of 45 s at 72 °C. Two housekeeping genes, *18S* (Unigene ID-Hs.99999901_s1, and glyceraldehyde 3-phosphate dehydrogenase, *GAPDH* (Unigene ID-Hs.99999905_m1), Life Technologies, Gaithersburg, MD, USA) were used as internal controls, and 18S (5'-GTTGGTGGAGCGATTTGTCT-3' and 5'-GGCCTCACTAAACCATCCAA-3') was selected as the best control.

2.2. Cell Culture

Human retinal pigment epithelial cells, ARPE-19 (CRL-2302, ATCC, Manassas, VA, USA), and human retinal endothelial cells, HREC (p10880, Innoprot, Vizcaya, Spain), were used. ARPE-19 cells (three passages) were grown to confluence (37 °C, 5% CO_2) in Dulbecco's modified Eagle's medium (DMEM; D6429, Sigma-Aldrich, St. Louis, MO, USA) containing 10% fetal bovine serum (FBS; 10270106 Gibco ThermoFisher, Paisley, UK), 1% fungizone (Gibco, Carlsbad, CA, USA), and penicillin–streptomycin (Gibco, Carlsbad, CA, USA). HREC cells were seeded in T75 flasks (353136, Falcon, Corning Life Science, Tewksbury, MA, USA) covered with 1 mg/mL of fibronectin (Innoprot, p8248, Vizcaya, Spain) and grown to confluence in a standard incubator at 37 °C under humidified 5% CO_2 conditions in Endothelial Cell Medium (Innoprot, p60104, Vizcaya, Spain) containing 5% FBS (Innoprot, Vizcaya, Spain), 1% Endothelial Cell Grow Supplement (ECGS, Innoprot, Vizcaya, Spain), and penicillin–streptomycin solution (Innoprot, Vizcaya, Spain).

2.3. Validation of the Cell Lines: Stable Phenotypic Characterization

To verify that ARPE-19 and HREC cells preserved their phenotype, we performed retinoid isomerohydrolase *RPE65* (RPE65) (1:100, 78036, Abcam, Cambridge, MA, USA) and caveolin (1:250, 3238S, Cell Signaling, Danvers, MA, USA) staining by immunofluorescence. Briefly, 100,000 ARPE-19 and 50,000 HREC cells were seeded on a 10 mm dish (Menzel-Glaser, Waltham, MA, USA). Cold methanol was used for cellular fixing. Afterward, cells were washed with 1% phosphate buffer saline (PBS) and then incubated with blocking buffer containing 1% bovine serum albumin (BSA), 0.5% Triton X-100, 0.2% sodium azide, and 1% fetal bovine serum (FBS) for 1 h at 4 °C. Cells were incubated with the primary antibodies, diluted in blocking buffer at 4 °C for 24 h, and washed once more with PBS and then incubated with the secondary fluorescent antibodies goat anti-mouse 488 (1:250, A11029, Life technologies, Gaithersburg, MD, USA) and donkey anti-rabbit 488 (1:250, A21206, Invitrogen, Carlsbad, CA, USA) for RPE65 marker diluted in blocking buffer during 1 h in the dark. Nuclei were labelled with 4′,6-diamidino-2-phenylindole (DAPI; Sigma-Aldrich, St. Louis, MO, USA). The morphology of cells was observed under an inverted phase-contrast microscope (Olympus CKX41, Tokyo, Japan) and photographed by a digital camera, and fluorescent images were obtained using a confocal microscope (LSM800, Zeiss, Oberkochen, Germany).

2.4. Treatments and Experimental Design: Oxidative Stress and Inflammation-Like Conditions

ARPE-19 and HREC cell lines were treated with VITD (1 nM; C9756-1G, Sigma-Aldrich, St. Louis, MO, USA) for 1 h to test its effect on cells. To induce in vitro oxidative stress, we subjected cells to H_2O_2 (1000 µM, Panreac, Barcelona, Spain) for 2 h. To evaluate the protective effect of VITD, we added it (1 nM; Sigma-Aldrich, St. Louis, MO, USA) in concomitance 1 h before the end of the induction time. Lipopolysaccharide (LPS; Sigma-Aldrich, St. Louis, MO, USA) was added for 24 h (20 µg/mL for ARPE-19 and 50 µg/mL for HREC cells) to induce an inflammatory response, and then VITD (1 nM; Sigma-Aldrich, St. Louis, MO, USA) was added to the supernatant for 1 h in concomitance.

2.5. Cell Structure and Integrity: Zonula Occludens (ZO)-1 Immunofluorescence and Western Blot

The effect of VITD on intercellular tight junction status was evaluated by zonula occludens-1 (ZO-1) immunofluorescence. One-hundred thousand ARPE-19 cells per well were seeded on laminin-coated polycarbonate membrane cell culture inserts (Corning Life Science, Tewksbury, MA, USA) and were grown in 1% FBS-DMEM for 4 weeks. Immunofluorescence was then performed using a ZO-1 anti-rabbit Alexa Fluor 594 antibody (1:100, 339194, Invitrogen-Life Technologies, Gaithersburg, MD, USA) diluted in blocking buffer, following the same protocol described above. DAPI (4′,6-diamidino-2-phenylindole; Sigma-Aldrich, St. Louis, MO, USA) was used to stain cell nuclei. Images were obtained with a laser scanning confocal imaging system (LSM800, Zeiss, Oberkochen, Germany). H_2O_2 (1600 µM, Panreac,

Barcelona, Spain) over 6 h was used as a positive control for oxidative stress conditions, and LPS (20 µg/mL; L2880 Sigma-Aldrich, St. Louis, MO, USA) was used for 24 h for inflammatory conditions.

A total of 5 µg of ARPE-19 cell homogenates from three passages were mixed with NuPage (4x, Bio-Rad, Hercules, CA, USA), boiled for 5 min, separated on 7% sodium dodecyl sulfate polyacrylamide gel electrophoresis (SDS-PAGE) gels, and transferred onto a nitrocellulose membrane. After we blocked them with 5% skimmed milk (w/v; Scharlau, Barcelona, Spain), 0.1% Tween-20 (w/v; Sigma-Aldrich, St. Louis, MO, USA) in tris buffer saline (TBS) for 1 h at room temperature (RT), membranes were exposed to the mouse monoclonal ZO-1 antibody (1:1000, #33-9100, Invitrogen, Carlsbad, CA, USA) at RT for 1 h, followed by a horseradish peroxidase-conjugated goat anti-mouse antibody (sc-2005; 1:5000, 1 h, RT Santa Cruz Biotechnology Inc., Santa Cruz, CA, USA). Signal was detected with an enhanced chemoluminescence (ECL) kit (ECL-Select, #RPN2235, GE Healthcare, Fairfield, CT, USA) and images were captured with ImageQuant 400 (GE Healthcare). The relative intensities of the immunoreactive bands were analyzed with ImageQuant TL (GE Healthcare, Fairfield, CT, USA). The loading was verified by Ponceau S red and an anti-β-actin monoclonal antibody (1:10,000, 1 h, RT; Sigma-Aldrich, St. Louis, MO, USA), followed by a goat anti-mouse antibody (sc-2005; 1:10,000, 5% skimmed milk, 1 h, RT; Santa Cruz Biotechnology Inc., Santa Cruz, CA), and signal was detected using ECL-Prime, #RPN2232 (GE Healthcare, Fairfield, CT, USA). Data are presented as absorbance units (AU) ZO-1/β-actin (% vs. saline).

2.6. Assay to Detect Cell Apoptosis

Apoptosis in ARPE-19 and HREC was performed in cultured plates using an in situ cell death detection kit with TMR Red according to the manufacturer's instructions (#12156792910, Roche, West Sussex, UK) and stored at 4 °C until analysis, with the apoptotic cells being labelled with active caspase-3 antibody (1:100, G7481; Promega, Madison, Wisconsin, USA) using the protocol mentioned above and incubated with the secondary fluorescent antibody donkey anti-rabbit 488 (A21206, Invitrogen). Nuclei were labelled with DAPI and images were obtained using a confocal microscope (LSM800, Zeiss, Oberkochen, Germany). H_2O_2 (600 µM, Panreac, Barcelona, Spain) for 2 h was used as positive control for oxidative stress conditions.

2.7. Viability/Toxicity Assay (MTT)

Cell viability/toxicity in ARPE-19 and HREC cell lines was determined by the 3-(4,5-dimethylthiazol-2-yl)-2,5-diphenyltetrazolium bromide (MTT) reduction assay CellTiter 96 AQueous One Solution Cell Proliferation Assay (Promega, Madison, WI, USA), following the manufacturer's instructions. A total of 10,000 ARPE-19 or HREC cells were grown until confluence in DMEM with 10% FBS onto 96-well plates. Then, cells were cultivated for 1 additional week in serum-reduced medium (1% FBS-DMEM), and VITD was added to the culture medium for 24 h at 1, 5, 10, and 50 nM doses.

2.8. Proliferation Assay (Bromodeoxyuridine, BrdU)

To examine the effect of VITD on ARPE-19 and HREC cell proliferation, we seeded 10,000 cells onto 96-well plates. After 24 h, cells were exposed to VITD (1 nM) for 1 h and the Calbiochem BrdU Cell Proliferation Assay (Calbiochem, La Jolla, CA, USA) was performed in accordance with the manufacturer's instructions.

2.9. Measurement of 8-Hydroxidioxiguanosine (8-OHdG) under Oxidative Stress Conditions

Oxidative damage was measured in ARPE-19 and HREC supernatants subjected to oxidative stress conditions, as described above. To evaluate the effect of VITD, we added 1 nM to the media. Supernatants (100 µL) were evaluated by using the Enzyme-Linked ImmunoSorbent Assay (ELISA) kit #ab201734 (Abcam, Cambridge, MA, USA). Data are presented in nanograms per milliliter (ng/mL).

2.10. Multiplex Cytokine Analysis under Inflammatory and Basal Conditions: Interleukin (IL)-1β, IL-6, IL-8, IL-10, IL-12p70, and IL-18; Interferon (IFN)-γ; Monocyte Chemoattractant Protein (MCP)-1; and Tumor Necrosis Factor (TNF)-α

The cytokine analysis for IL-1β, -6, -8, -10, -12p70, and -18; IFN-γ; MCP1; and TNF-α was made using FirePlex Firefly (Abcam, Cambridge, MA, USA) particle multiplex immunoassay for Flow Cytometry and Analysis Workbench, a software for multiplex protein expression assays from Abcam Laboratories. Supernatants were used for this purpose and were measured under inflammatory conditions as abovementioned. All cytokines are expressed in pictograms per milliliter (pg/mL), with the exception of MCP-1 and IL-8, which were expressed in ng/mL.

2.11. Statistical Analysis

All parameters were subjected to analysis of the variance (ANOVA) test followed by the Bonferroni post-hoc for multiple comparisons. A difference $p < 0.05$ was considered statistically significant. GraphPad Prism 6.0 (GraphPad Prism Software Inc., San Diego, CA, USA) was used for statistical analysis.

3. Results

3.1. Confirmation of VITD Receptor Expression in ARPE-19 and HREC Cell Lines

In this study, we demonstrated that ARPE-19 and HREC cell lines expressed the machinery for vitamin D_3 and could produce $1,25(OH)_2D_3$. This is the first time that the expression of Vit D_3-synthesizing components has been reported in HREC cells.

We performed conventional polymerase chain reaction (PCR) experiments in order to determine the expression of the following genes involved in VITD synthesis. ARPE-19 cell line highly expressed the genes cytochrome P450 *(CYP)2R1*, *CYP27B*, and *CYP24A* and showed a low expression of vitamin D receptor *(VDR)*, *CYP27A*, and *cubilin* genes; however, they did not express the *megalin* gene. HREC cell line highly expressed the genes *CYP2R1* and *CYP27B*. HREC showed a lower expression of *VDR*, *CYP27A*, *cubilin*, and *megalin* genes and did not express the *CYP24A* gene (Table 1). Ribosomal 18S was used as an internal PCR control (Figure 1).

Table 1. Summary of the main vitamin D (VITD) synthesizing genes in human retinal pigment epithelial cells (ARPE-19) and human retinal endothelial cells (HREC).

	VDR	CYP2R1	CYP27A	CYP27B	CYP24A	Cubilin	Megalin	18S
ARPE-19	++	+++	++	+++	+++	++	−	+++
HREC	++	+++	++	+++	−	++	++	+++

+++: high expression; ++: medium expression; −: no expression.

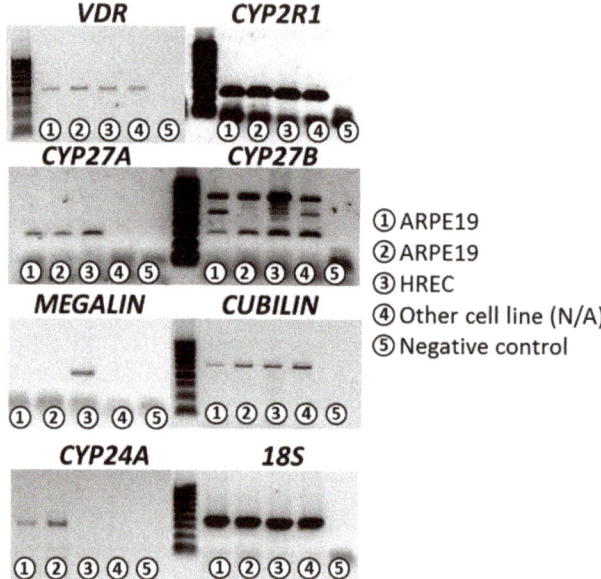

Figure 1. Conventional PCR was carried out using total RNA extracted from ARPE-19 (lines 1 and 2) and HREC cells (line 3). We analyzed the gene expression of *VDR, CYP27B1, CYP24A1, CYP27A1, CYP2R1, cubilin,* and *megalin*. Ribosomal 18S was used as an internal PCR control. Results are representative of at least three independent experiments. Molecular sizes (base pairs [bp]): *18S* (400), *VDR* (421), *CYP27B1* (302), *CYP24A1* (485), *CYP27A1* (292), *CYP2R1* (259), *cubilin* (518), and *megalin* (290).

3.2. Validation of the Cell Lines: Stable Phenotypic Characterization

We performed immunofluorescence for specific ARPE-19 and HREC cell lines' markers. We used RPE65 protein (Abcam 78036) for ARPE-19 cells and caveolin protein (Cell Signalling 3238S) for HREC cells. No changes in the phenotypic characteristics were found, and the cells expressed all the selected markers (Figure 2).

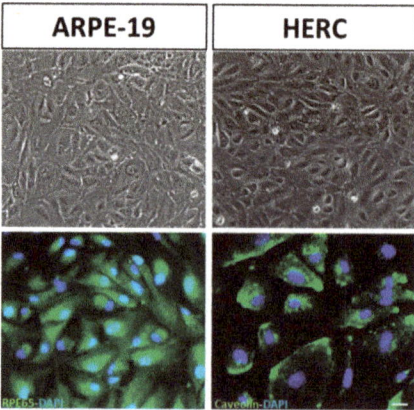

Figure 2. ARPE-19 and HREC cells' phenotyping. Immunofluorescence of RPE65 (green) and caveolin (green) for ARPE-19 and HREC cell lines' labelling, respectively. Upper panel shows cells at bright-field microscopy and down panel shows cells under fluorescence microscopy. Nuclei were labeled with 4′,6-diamidino-2-phenylindole (DAPI) (blue). Scale bar: 20 µm.

3.3. Effect of VITD Addition on Cytoxicity and Proliferation

VITD at 1 nM and for 1 h did not show cytotoxic effects in ARPE-19 cells and HREC cells (Figure 3A,B). Moreover, proliferation was not affected by VITD addition at 1 nM and 1 h of exposure time (Figure 3C,D).

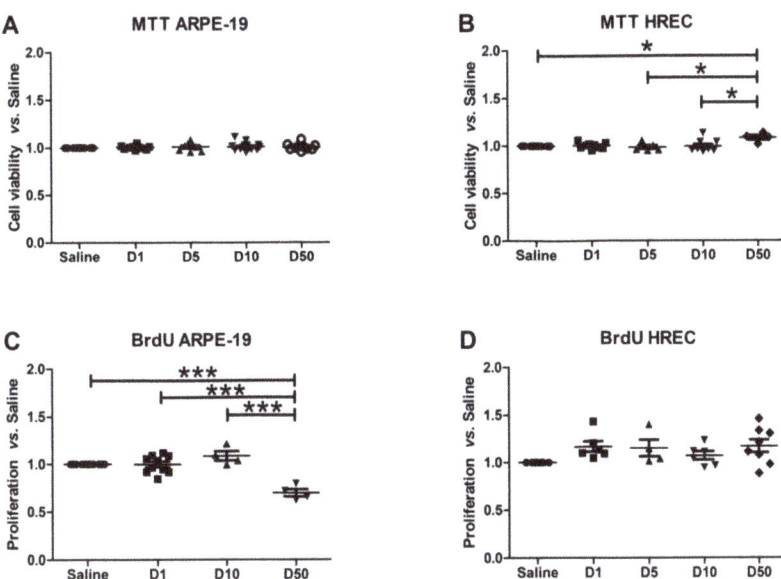

Figure 3. Graphs showing 3-(4,5-dimethylthiazol-2-yl)-2,5-diphenyltetrazolium bromide (MTT) (**A,B**) and Bromodeoxyuridine (BrdU) (**C,D**) results for ARPE-19 (**A,C**) and HREC (**B,D**) cells treated with different VITD concentrations (1, 5, 10, and 50 nM) for 1 h. Any VITD dose showed cytotoxic effects on ARPE-19 cells compared to saline group. HREC showed significant alterations in MTT D50 compared to the rest of the groups (* $p < 0.05$). ARPE-19 proliferation was statistically reduced (*** $p < 0.001$) in the highest dose analyzed (50 nM) compared to saline and to all the remaining doses. HREC cells' proliferation was not affected by any VITD dose.

VITD doses ranged from 1 to 50 nM for both cell types tested. All doses were safe for ARPE-19 cells at any time measured, and the highest dose used significantly reduced proliferation ($p < 0.001$). HREC cells showed an increase in viability, with the highest vitamin D dose ($p < 0.05$) response being in the highest dose at 50 nM. In addition, proliferation was reduced in ARPE-19 cells subjected to a 50 nM VITD dose. To be sure that the effects observed in the subsequent analysis were caused by vitamin D itself and that they were not masked by deleterious effects on cell viability and proliferation, we decided to use 1 nM of VITD, which did not affect proliferation and viability.

3.4. Effect of VITD Addition on Integrity and Apoptosis of Cells

ARPE-19 cells' integrity was conserved after adding VITD at 1 nM. Hydrogen peroxide and LPS induced an increase in tortuosity of the junction contacts in ARPE-19 cells that were stabilized in oxidative and inflammatory conditions by the addition of VITD to the media (Figure 4).

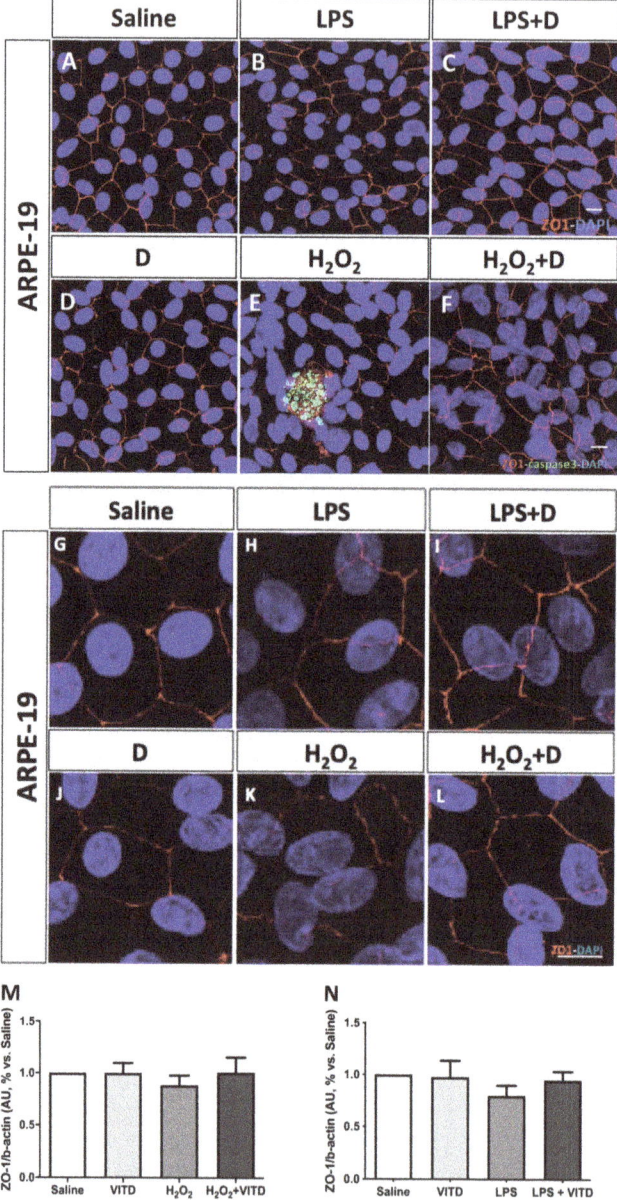

Figure 4. Integrity of ARPE-19 cells evaluated by zonula occludens-1 (ZO-1) (red) and caspase-3 (green) immunofluorescence. VITD (1 nM, 1 h; (**D**)) did not affect ZO-1 structure compared to saline (**A**,**G**). Lipopolysaccharide (LPS) (**B**,**H**) and H_2O_2 (**E**,**K**) addition damaged tight junctions and concomitant incubation with VITD (1 nM, 1 h; (**C**,**I**) and (**F**,**L**)) restored the altered structure. (**G–L**) show the apical junction in higher magnification. Caspase-3 was highly observed in the H_2O_2 group (**E**) compared to saline (**A**) and VITD (**D**). VITD addition showed restoration, and caspase-3 activation was absent (**F**). Nuclei were labeled with DAPI (blue). Scale bar: 20 µm. Densitometry of ZO-1 expression in ARPE-19 cells under oxidative stress (**M**) and inflammatory (**N**) conditions. Although a tendency to reduce the ZO-1 expression was observed, no statistical differences were found. VITD restored values similar to saline group. $n = 3$.

LPS and H_2O_2 addition showed a tendency to reduce ZO-1 expression, although that difference was not significant. Moreover, the supplementation with VITD partly increased the ZO-1 expression, but this result did not reach statistical significance.

Early (caspase-3, Figure 4) and late (TDT- mediated dUTP-biotin nick end-labeling, TUNEL, Figure 5) apoptosis markers revealed that VITD (1 nM) addition did not affect cell death processes. After inflammatory and oxidative induction, ARPE-19 cells and HREC cells showed alterations and an increase labelling for both markers. VITD (1 nM) addition was able to restore those alterations (Figure 5).

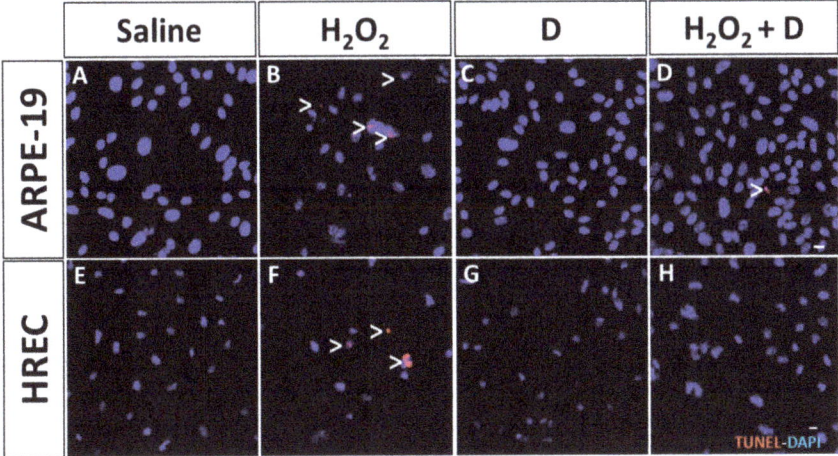

Figure 5. Late apoptosis measured in ARPE-19 (**A–D**) and HREC (**E–H**) cells by TDT- mediated dUTP-biotin nick end-labeling (TUNEL) and analyzed by fluorescence. TUNEL-positive ARPE-19 and HREC cells were observed after H_2O_2 stimulation (2 h; (**B,F**)) compared to saline (**A,E**). VITD (1 nM, 1 h; (**C,G**)) showed similar results to saline groups for both cell types. VITD, in concomitance with H_2O_2 (1 h; (**D,H**)), showed a reduction in altered nuclei, especially in ARPE-19 cells (**D**), and absence of TUNEL labeling. Nuclei were labeled with DAPI (blue). Scale bar: 20 µm.

3.5. Antioxidative and Anti-Inflammatory Properties of VITD Addition

Figure 6 shows that oxidative stress induction by H_2O_2 significantly ($p < 0.001$) increased 8-OHdG in supernatants from ARPE-19 cells. VITD alone did not modify oxidative damage compared to saline. VITD was able to significantly ($p < 0.001$) reduce 8-OHdG production under oxidative-induced conditions.

Figure 7 shows that LPS induction increased IL-8, IFN-γ, IL-1β, MCP-1, TNF-α, IL-10, IL-18, IL-6, and IL-12p70 in ARPE-19 cells. Under inflammatory conditions, VITD was able to significantly ($p < 0.05$) reduce IL-8, IFN-γ, MCP-1, TNF-α, and IL-6.

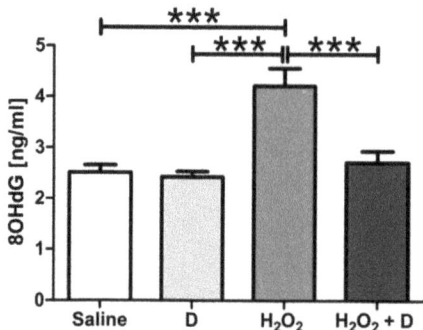

Figure 6. Graph showing 8-OHdG results for ARPE-19 cells measured by ELISA. VITD was able to significantly reduce the 8-OHdG levels elevated by H_2O_2 (*** $p < 0.001$). $n = 3$.

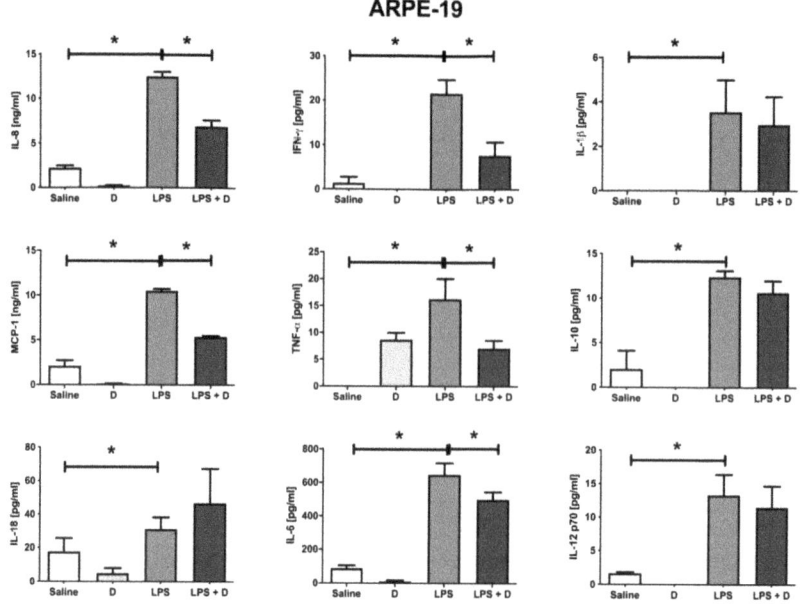

Figure 7. Multiplex inflammatory cytokine array in ARPE-19 cells. All inflammatory cytokine levels were increased by adding LPS (* $p < 0.05$), and Interleukin (IL)-8, Interferon (IFN)-γ, Monocyte chemoattractant protein (MCP)-1, Tumor necrosis factor (TNF)-α, and IL-6 levels were reduced (* $p < 0.05$) with the addition of VITD in concomitance. $n = 3$.

HREC cells subjected to LPS induction showed an increase in IL-8, IFN-γ, IL-1β, MCP-1, IL-10, IL-6, and IL-12p70 cytokines. VITD significantly ($p < 0.05$) decreased IL-8, IFN-γ, IL-1β, MCP-1, TNF-α, IL-6, and IL-12p70 under inflammatory conditions in HREC cells (Figure 8).

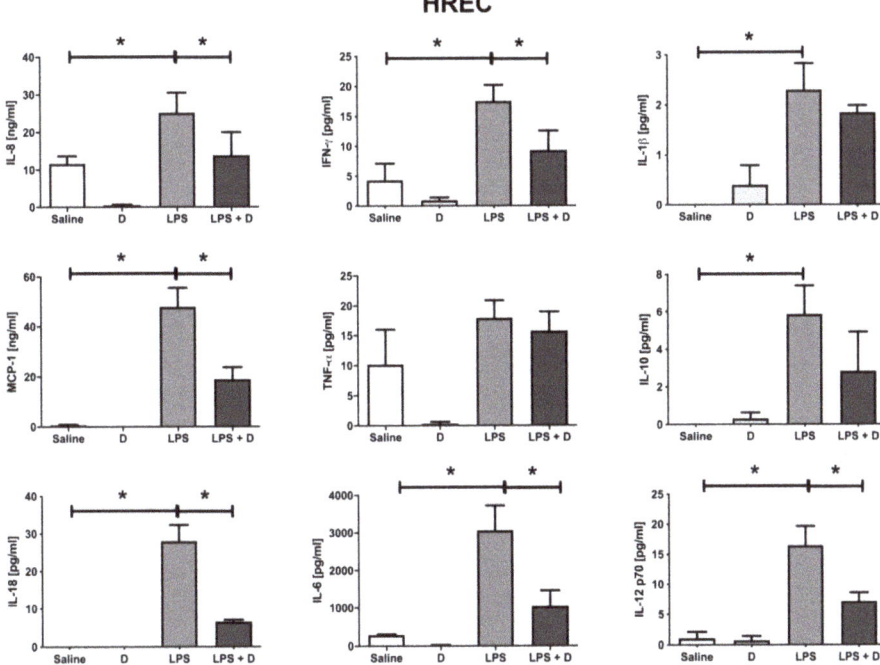

Figure 8. Multiplex inflammatory cytokine array in HREC cells. IL-8, IFN-γ, IL-1β, MCP-1, IL-10, IL-6, and IL-12p70 inflammatory cytokine levels were increased by adding LPS (* $p < 0.05$), and IL-8, IFN-γ, IL-1β, MCP-1, TNF-α, IL-6, and IL-12p70 levels were reduced (* $p < 0.05$) with the addition of VITD in concomitance. $n = 3$.

4. Discussion

The present study shows that damage observed in human retinal pigmented epithelium (RPE) and retinal endothelium cells under oxidative and inflammatory conditions were restored by the addition of VITD to the media. More specifically, induced inflammatory cytokine levels, early and late apoptosis, and oxidative stress markers were reduced back to control levels. This result suggests that VITD could be a useful candidate in modulating the chronic low-grade inflammation and oxidative stress responsible for the complications in retinal pathologies involving RPE and endothelial cells.

It is well established that glycemic control is an effective management to lower the incidence of complications such as DR. However, even an intensive glycemic control is not sufficient to prevent diabetic microvascular pathologies in all patients [4], and hyperglycemia on its own is not sufficient to trigger widespread diabetic microvascular pathologies in all patients [29–31]. Diabetic patients with an initial poor glycemic control have persistent higher incidence of diabetic complications after glucose normalization, a phenomenon described as metabolic memory, suggesting that oxidative stress, non-enzymatic glycation of proteins, epigenetic changes, and chronic inflammation may play a major role in the development and progression of diabetic microvascular complications [32,33] such as diabetic kidney disease [34–36], diabetic polyneuropathy [37,38], and DR [9–11,14]. VITD deficiency is related to a higher risk of DR in type 1 and 2 diabetes mellitus [24,39]. Apart from its role in tissues related to calcium homeostasis [40], high levels of VDR are also present in inflammatory cells such as dendritic cells, macrophages, T-cells, and B-cells, thus supporting the fact that VITD may have a role in inflammatory and immune responses [41].

25-Hydroxylase (encoded by the *CYP27A1* and *CYP2R1* genes), a cytochrome P450 enzyme, catalyzes the formation of vitamin D_3 to 25-hydroxyvitamin D_3 (25(OH)D_3), the main circulating VITD metabolite, and then 25(OH)D_3 is converted to 1,25-dihydroxyvitamin D_3 (1,25[OH]$_2D_3$), the most active form by the enzyme 1 alpha-hydroxylase (encoded by the *CYP27B1* gene). 1,25[OH]$_2D_3$ is inactivated by 24-hydroxylase (encoded by the *CYP24A1* gene) [42]. Megalin and cubilin, endocytic receptors in the cell membrane, allow the internalization of 25(OH)D_3 and 1,25[OH]$_2D_3$ into the cell [43]. We demonstrated that the ARPE-19 cell line highly expressed *CYP2R1*, *CYP27B*, and *CYP24A* genes and showed a low expression of *CYP27A* and *cubilin* genes; however, they did not express the megalin gene. The HREC cell line highly expressed the *CYP2R1* and *CYP27B* genes. HREC showed a lower expression of *VDR*, *CYP27A*, *cubilin*, and *megalin* genes and did not express the *CYP24A* gene. This is the first time that the machinery for VITD internalization and metabolization is reported in HREC cells. A recent study reported that VITD treatment enhanced VDR expression in ARPE-19 cells treated with H_2O_2 [27].

The antioxidant role of vitamin D has been demonstrated in many other micro-environments in the body, especially in the context of diabetes or obesity, including the liver [44], the kidney filtration [45], the heart [46], the hippocampus [47], and the adipose tissue [48], among others. Recently, it has been discovered that vitamin D is not only produced systemically at the renal level, but that extrarenal production is also important. In the eye, there are several tissues in which local production of 1.25(OH)2D3 has been demonstrated, including the sclera, corneal endothelium, ciliary body epithelium, and pigment epithelium, with the corneal endothelium being the eye tissue with the highest conversion rate [49]. We did not find studies focused on the permeability of the retinal blood barrier to VITD; however, it has been demonstrated that the retinal blood barrier has a high permeability to lipophilic substances [50] and also, oral supplemented vitamin D increases the concentration in aqueous humor and tears [49]. To better understand the effect of VITD in the retina, ARPE-19 and HREC cells were subjected to oxidative stress and inflammatory conditions that provoked alterations in tight junctions and also apoptotic signs. Some studies have suggested that VITD can protect against the deleterious effects of reactive oxygen species (ROS), free radicals generated during physiological energy production in the mitochondria [51], therefore improving cell viability in ARPE-19 cells [27] and various tissues [16,52–54]. In line with these observations, we demonstrated that H_2O_2 and LPS induced the alteration and partial loss of tight junction protein organization (i.e., tortuosity and cytosol localization) in ARPE-19 cells and were restored in oxidative and inflammatory conditions by the addition of VITD to the media. However, results observed in protein expression did not show significant differences in the amount of ZO-1. This phenomenon has been also described by other authors, observing that ZO-1 remains localized in junction despite loss of tight junction protein organization by oxidative stress [55], as observed also in our immunofluorescence images. Inflammatory conditions showed a similar behavior on tight junctions, and their expression was not modified but the organization was altered. VITD addition restored morphological alterations observed in immunofluorescence. The increased early and late apoptosis under oxidative stress and inflammatory conditions was also restored by addition of VITD in ARPE-19 and HREC cells, in concordance with other studies after H_2O_2 [27] and after high-glucose-induced oxidative stress and inflammation [17].

A recent study showed that VITD treatment also upregulated the expression of antioxidant genes (*catalase, CAT; superoxide dismutase SOD1* and *SOD2; Glutathione peroxidase GPX2* and *GPX3*) in ARPE-19 cells under similar stress conditions [27]. Accordingly, we found that H_2O_2-treated ARPE-19 cells had significantly increased oxidative stress, and VITD exposure counteracted this 8-OHdG production under oxidative-induced conditions. Other authors showed that increased ROS production and lipid peroxidation downregulated expression of antioxidant genes, and decreased activities of SOD and catalase induced in high glucose-treated ARPE-19 cells was counteracted by VITD exposure [17].

In addition to oxidative stress, the levels of proinflammatory proteins such as MCP-1, IL-1β, IL-6, IL-8, and TNF-α influence the development of DR [56,57], and increased aqueous concentration of those molecules in eyes with severe non-proliferative DR suggests that inflammatory changes precede the development of neovascularization [58,59]. Endothelial damage is also linked to increased leukocyte adhesion that is explained by the overexpression of endothelial adhesion molecules such as Intercellular adhesion molecule (ICAM)-1, Vascular cell adhesion molecule (VCAM)-1, Platelet endothelial cell adhesion molecule (PECAM)-1, and P-selectin [59,60]. Vascular endothelial growth factor (VEGF) also alters adherens and tight junctional proteins between the endothelial cells [61,62], favoring the infiltration of leukocytes into the retina. This complex of inflammatory events leads to blood–retinal barrier breakdown and with it some of the vision threatening complications such as macular edema. Directly or indirectly VITD regulate over 200 genes involved in cellular proliferation, differentiation, apoptosis, angiogenesis, and inflammation [63]. VITD have shown to prevent, slow the progression of, ameliorate inflammation markers of, or decrease the severity of many immune-related disorders such diabetes mellitus [64,65]. In our study, all the inflammatory cytokines investigated were upregulated under inflammatory conditions. TNF-α did not result in a statistically significant elevation after LPS induction in HREC cells, probably due to the dispersion observed in control samples. Herein, we observed that the addition of VITD to the media downregulated levels of IL-6, IL-8, MCP-1, IFN-γ, and TNF-α in retinal epithelial cells, as also shown by other authors in ARPE-19 cells [66,67]. These results suggest that VITD can control the broad inflammatory spectrum studied that is present in non-proliferative DR, indicating a clear anti-inflammatory response. In the case of retinal endothelial cells, similar results were observed, with the exception of TNF-α that were unmodified and IL-18 and IL-12p70 that were also downregulated. Elevated levels of IL1-β and IL18 have been demonstrated in streptozotocin (STZ)-induced diabetic rats [68]. Similarly, serum IL-18 levels have also been reported to be elevated in type 1 diabetic patients, half of which had a form of DR [68]. IL-1β, IL-18, and IL-1α have pro-inflammatory actions, and in the case of IL-18, a role in angiogenesis [69]. The inflammasome is an oligomer protein complex that triggers the secretion of IL-1β and IL-18 into the extracellular space [70]. Interestingly, the inflammasome has been particularly related to the neovascular pathology occurring in proliferative DR (PDR) [71,72]. While the major pro-inflammatory cytokines such as IL-6, TNF-α, and IFN-γ could be detected both in non-PDR and in PDR eyes, inflammasome-related cytokine, IL-18, and caspase-1 were particularly increased in the eyes of PDR patients [72]. In our study, IL-18 levels were effectively reduced by VITD in endothelial cells, but not in RPE cells, suggesting a main antiangiogenic role under inflammatory conditions. Moreover, the primary leukocyte populations found in the retina during disease are microglia and macrophages, and it is well known that the activation of the inflammasome is an important mechanism by which these cells cause damage in retinal degenerations. VITD could help to reduce macrophage recruiting by reducing MCP1 levels.

Analyzing the secretome in ARPE-19 cells, researchers found that adding TNF-α to the media regulated different proteins secreted by the RPE, which play a critical role in extracellular matrix remodeling, complement network, and angiogenesis [73]. Thus, VITD supplementation could contribute to reduce those effects. A mixture of IFN-γ, TNF-α, and IL-1β has been shown to decrease the expression of specific genes that play an important role in processes, such as visual cycle, epithelial morphology, melanogenesis, and phagocytosis, in cultured ARPE-19 cells [74]. Therefore, downregulation of those levels by VITD may potentially contribute to restore the RPE dysfunction implicated in retinal diseases, including DR [75,76]. It has been demonstrated that a higher secretion of IL-10 would be a protective factor against the development of proliferative DR (PDR) when proinflammatory cytokines, such as IL-1β, are elevated, as shown in vitreous of PDR patients [77]. In our study, VITD maintained high IL-10 levels, suggesting a possible contribution to an anti-inflammatory environment that must be investigated deeply. Surprisingly, in contrast to other authors [17], IL-1β was not reduced by VITD addition. The bioactive IL12p70 molecule is primarily produced by monocytes, macrophages, dendritic cells, and B-cells. The main functions of IL-12 include the promotion of IFN-γ production from natural killer in cell-mediated immunity [78]. IL-10 is a major inhibitor of IL-12 production by decreasing Nuclear factor κB (NF-κB) and activator protein 1 (AP-1) activation and the association of IL-12p40 promoter with RNA polymerase [78].

Consistent with the anti-inflammation and anti-oxidation role, our results suggested that VITD effectively downregulated in vitro the production of targeted cytokines in DR-related stimuli, suggesting that VITD could block retinal inflammation and oxidative stress associated with DR. Retinal pathologies such as DR are complex diseases with several and different processes involved. We evaluated the effect of vitamin D as an option to restore or to help with the damage provoked by oxidative stress and inflammation. However, different therapies could target multiple steps of oxidative stress for the prevention of this multifactorial blinding complication of diabetes. Santos et al. revised therapies with vitamins and supplements used to treat diabetic retinopathy, and there are various strategies in order to prevent superoxide accumulation, maintain mitochondrial homeostasis, or protect against DNA damage [79]. Other molecules could also be beneficial, even in combination with vitamin D. Although promising, one of the main limitations of this research is the use of an immortalized cell line in which some transcription alterations are produced. Therefore, the results obtained need to be confirmed in primary cells and in experimental in vivo models of retinopathy. Whether these results can be replicated in in vivo models of DR and clinical trials remains to be elucidated.

5. Conclusions

In summary, VITD could play a role in the protection of the retina and RPE from oxidative stress, inflammation, and apoptosis through the suppression of pro-inflammatory mediators and by enhancing the antioxidant defense capacity. Taking into consideration all the results we have observed, VITD could be a useful candidate in modulating the chronic low-grade inflammation and oxidative stress responsible for the complications in DR. However, further preclinical in vivo tests and DR patient clinical trials are needed to verify the therapeutic potential of VITD.

Author Contributions: Conceptualization, P.F.-R., S.R., M.H. and A.G.-L.; data curation, J.B.; funding acquisition, P.F.-R. and A.G.-L.; investigation, S.R. and J.B.; methodology, S.R. and M.H.; project administration, P.F.-R.; supervision, P.F.-R., S.R. and M.H.; visualization, P.F.-R., J.B. and M.H.; writing—original draft, P.F.-R., J.G.-Z. and V.B.-M.; writing—review and editing, P.F.-R., S.R., V.B.-M., M.H. and A.G.-L. All authors have read and agreed to the published version of the manuscript.

Funding: The present work was partially funded by Thea Laboratoires, Fundación Jesús de Gangoiti Barrera, and partially supported by RETICS (RD16/0008) from ISCIII, Ministerio de Economía y Competitividad, Spain.

Acknowledgments: The authors want to acknowledge Idoia Belza Zuazu and Maite Moreno Orduña for their excellent technical assistance.

Conflicts of Interest: A.G.-L. is a consultant for Bayer, Novartis, Allergan, Thea, and Roche. The rest of the authors declare no conflict of interest. The funders had no role in the design of the study; in the collection, analyses, or interpretation of data; in the writing of the manuscript; or in the decision to publish the results.

References

1. Yau, J.W.Y.; Rogers, S.L.; Kawasaki, R.; Lamoureux, E.L.; Kowalski, J.W.; Bek, T.; Chen, S.-J.; Dekker, J.M.; Fletcher, A.; Grauslund, J.; et al. Global Prevalence and Major Risk Factors of Diabetic Retinopathy. *Diabetes Care* **2012**, *35*, 556–564. [CrossRef] [PubMed]
2. Stratton, I.M. Association of glycaemia with macrovascular and microvascular complications of type 2 diabetes (UKPDS 35): Prospective observational study. *BMJ* **2000**, *321*, 405–412. [CrossRef] [PubMed]
3. The ACCORD Study Group and ACCORD Eye Study Group Effects of Medical Therapies on Retinopathy Progression in Type 2 Diabetes. *N. Engl. J. Med.* **2010**, *363*, 233–244. [CrossRef] [PubMed]
4. The Effect of Intensive Treatment of Diabetes on the Development and Progression of Long-Term Complications in Insulin-Dependent Diabetes Mellitus. *N. Engl. J. Med.* **1993**, *329*, 977–986. [CrossRef] [PubMed]
5. Lorenzi, M. The polyol pathway as a mechanism for diabetic retinopathy: Attractive, elusive, and resilient. *Exp. Diabetes Res.* **2007**, *2007*, 61038. [CrossRef] [PubMed]
6. Stitt, A.W. The role of advanced glycation in the pathogenesis of diabetic retinopathy. *Exp. Mol. Pathol.* **2003**, *75*, 95–108. [CrossRef]

7. Donnelly, R.; Idris, I.; Forrester, J.V. Protein kinase C inhibition and diabetic retinopathy: A shot in the dark at translational research. *Br. J. Ophthalmol.* **2004**, *88*, 145–151. [CrossRef]
8. Madsen-Bouterse, S.A.; Kowluru, R.A. Oxidative stress and diabetic retinopathy: Pathophysiological mechanisms and treatment perspectives. *Rev. Endocr. Metab. Disord.* **2008**, *9*, 315–327. [CrossRef]
9. Calderon, G.D.; Juarez, O.H.; Hernandez, G.E.; Punzo, S.M.; De la Cruz, Z.D. Oxidative stress and diabetic retinopathy: Development and treatment. *Eye* **2017**, *31*, 1122–1130. [CrossRef]
10. Cecilia, O.-M.; José Alberto, C.-G.; José, N.-P.; Ernesto Germán, C.-M.; Ana Karen, L.-C.; Luis Miguel, R.-P.; Ricardo Raúl, R.-R.; Adolfo Daniel, R.-C. Oxidative Stress as the Main Target in Diabetic Retinopathy Pathophysiology. *J. Diabetes Res.* **2019**, *2019*, 1–21. [CrossRef]
11. Li, C.; Miao, X.; Li, F.; Wang, S.; Liu, Q.; Wang, Y.; Sun, J. Oxidative Stress-Related Mechanisms and Antioxidant Therapy in Diabetic Retinopathy. *Oxid. Med. Cell. Longev.* **2017**, *2017*, 1–15. [CrossRef] [PubMed]
12. Yaribeygi, H.; Sathyapalan, T.; Atkin, S.L.; Sahebkar, A. Molecular Mechanisms Linking Oxidative Stress and Diabetes Mellitus. *Oxid. Med. Cell. Longev.* **2020**, *2020*, 8609213. [CrossRef] [PubMed]
13. Mesquida, M.; Drawnel, F.; Fauser, S. The role of inflammation in diabetic eye disease. *Semin. Immunopathol.* **2019**, *41*, 427–445. [CrossRef] [PubMed]
14. Abu El-Asrar, A. Role of inflammation in the pathogenesis of diabetic retinopathy. *Middle East Afr. J. Ophthalmol.* **2012**, *19*, 70. [CrossRef]
15. Bikle, D.D. Vitamin D Metabolism, Mechanism of Action, and Clinical Applications. *Chem. Biol.* **2014**, *21*, 319–329. [CrossRef]
16. Hamden, K.; Carreau, S.; Jamoussi, K.; Miladi, S.; Lajmi, S.; Aloulou, D.; Ayadi, F.; Elfeki, A. 1α,25 Dihydroxyvitamin D3: Therapeutic and Preventive Effects against Oxidative Stress, Hepatic, Pancreatic and Renal Injury in Alloxan-Induced Diabetes in Rats. *J. Nutr. Sci. Vitaminol.* **2009**, *55*, 215–222. [CrossRef]
17. Tohari, A.M.; Almarhoun, M.; Alhasani, R.H.; Biswas, L.; Zhou, X.; Reilly, J.; Zeng, Z.; Shu, X. Protection by vitamin D against high-glucose-induced damage in retinal pigment epithelial cells. *Exp. Cell Res.* **2020**, *392*, 112023. [CrossRef]
18. Lu, L.; Lu, Q.; Chen, W.; Li, J.; Li, C.; Zheng, Z. Vitamin D$_3$ Protects against Diabetic Retinopathy by Inhibiting High-Glucose-Induced Activation of the ROS/TXNIP/NLRP3 Inflammasome Pathway. *J. Diabetes Res.* **2018**, *2018*, 8193523. [CrossRef]
19. Alatawi, F.S.; Faridi, U.A.; Alatawi, M.S. Effect of treatment with vitamin D plus calcium on oxidative stress in streptozotocin-induced diabetic rats. *Saudi Pharm. J.* **2018**, *26*, 1208–1213. [CrossRef]
20. Cyganek, K.; Mirkiewicz-Sieradzka, B.; Malecki, M.T.; Wolkow, P.; Skupien, J.; Bobrek, J.; Czogala, M.; Klupa, T.; Sieradzki, J. Clinical risk factors and the role of VDR gene polymorphisms in diabetic retinopathy in Polish type 2 diabetes patients. *Acta Diabetol.* **2006**, *43*, 114–119. [CrossRef]
21. Zhong, X.; Du, Y.; Lei, Y.; Liu, N.; Guo, Y.; Pan, T. Effects of vitamin D receptor gene polymorphism and clinical characteristics on risk of diabetic retinopathy in Han Chinese type 2 diabetes patients. *Gene* **2015**, *566*, 212–216. [CrossRef] [PubMed]
22. Taverna, M.J.; Sola, A.; Guyot-Argenton, C.; Pacher, N.; Bruzzo, F.; Slama, G.; Reach, G.; Selam, J.-L. Taq I polymorphism of the vitamin D receptor and risk of severe diabetic retinopathy. *Diabetologia* **2002**, *45*, 436–442. [CrossRef] [PubMed]
23. Taverna, M.J.; Selam, J.-L.; Slama, G. Association between a Protein Polymorphism in the Start Codon of the Vitamin D Receptor Gene and Severe Diabetic Retinopathy in C-Peptide-Negative Type 1 Diabetes. *J. Clin. Endocrinol. Metab.* **2005**, *90*, 4803–4808. [CrossRef] [PubMed]
24. Afarid, M.; Ghattavi, N.; Karim Johari, M. Serum Levels of Vitamin D in Diabetic Patients with and without Retinopathy. *J. Ophthalmic Vis. Res.* **2020**. [CrossRef] [PubMed]
25. Ashinne, B.; Rajalakshmi, R.; Anjana, R.M.; Narayan, K.M.V.; Jayashri, R.; Mohan, V.; Hendrick, A.M. Association of serum vitamin D levels and diabetic retinopathy in Asian Indians with type 2 diabetes. *Diabetes Res. Clin. Pract.* **2018**, *139*, 308–313. [CrossRef]
26. Wu, W.; Weng, Y.; Guo, X.; Feng, L.; Xia, H.; Jiang, Z.; Lou, J. The Association between Serum Vitamin D Levels and Age-Related Macular Degeneration: A Systematic Meta-Analytic Review. *Investig. Opthalmol. Vis. Sci.* **2016**, *57*, 2168. [CrossRef]
27. Tohari, A.M.; Alhasani, R.H.; Biswas, L.; Patnaik, S.R.; Reilly, J.; Zeng, Z.; Shu, X. Vitamin D Attenuates Oxidative Damage and Inflammation in Retinal Pigment Epithelial Cells. *Antioxidants* **2019**, *8*, 341. [CrossRef]

28. Layana, A.; Minnella, A.; Garhöfer, G.; Aslam, T.; Holz, F.; Leys, A.; Silva, R.; Delcourt, C.; Souied, E.; Seddon, J. Vitamin D and Age-Related Macular Degeneration. *Nutrients* **2017**, *9*, 1120. [CrossRef]
29. Sun, J.K.; Keenan, H.A.; Cavallerano, J.D.; Asztalos, B.F.; Schaefer, E.J.; Sell, D.R.; Strauch, C.M.; Monnier, V.M.; Doria, A.; Aiello, L.P.; et al. Protection From Retinopathy and Other Complications in Patients With Type 1 Diabetes of Extreme Duration: The Joslin 50-Year Medalist Study. *Diabetes Care* **2011**, *34*, 968–974. [CrossRef]
30. Keenan, H.A.; Costacou, T.; Sun, J.K.; Doria, A.; Cavellerano, J.; Coney, J.; Orchard, T.J.; Aiello, L.P.; King, G.L. Clinical Factors Associated With Resistance to Microvascular Complications in Diabetic Patients of Extreme Disease Duration: The 50-year Medalist Study. *Diabetes Care* **2007**, *30*, 1995–1997. [CrossRef]
31. Barrett, E.J.; Liu, Z.; Khamaisi, M.; King, G.L.; Klein, R.; Klein, B.E.K.; Hughes, T.M.; Craft, S.; Freedman, B.I.; Bowden, D.W.; et al. Diabetic Microvascular Disease: An Endocrine Society Scientific Statement. *J. Clin. Endocrinol. Metab.* **2017**, *102*, 4343–4410. [CrossRef] [PubMed]
32. Testa, R.; Bonfigli, A.R.; Prattichizzo, F.; La Sala, L.; De Nigris, V.; Ceriello, A. The "Metabolic Memory" Theory and the Early Treatment of Hyperglycemia in Prevention of Diabetic Complications. *Nutrients* **2017**, *9*, 437. [CrossRef] [PubMed]
33. Voronova, V.; Zhudenkov, K.; Helmlinger, G.; Peskov, K. Interpretation of metabolic memory phenomenon using a physiological systems model: What drives oxidative stress following glucose normalization? *PLoS ONE* **2017**, *12*, e0171781. [CrossRef] [PubMed]
34. Jha, J.C.; Ho, F.; Dan, C.; Jandeleit-Dahm, K. A causal link between oxidative stress and inflammation in cardiovascular and renal complications of diabetes. *Clin. Sci.* **2018**, *132*, 1811–1836. [CrossRef]
35. Aghadavod, E.; Khodadadi, S.; Baradaran, A.; Nasri, P.; Bahmani, M.; Rafieian-Kopaei, M. Role of Oxidative Stress and Inflammatory Factors in Diabetic Kidney Disease. *Iran. J. Kidney Dis.* **2016**, *10*, 337–343. [PubMed]
36. Jha, J.C.; Banal, C.; Chow, B.S.M.; Cooper, M.E.; Jandeleit-Dahm, K. Diabetes and Kidney Disease: Role of Oxidative Stress. *Antioxid. Redox Signal.* **2016**, *25*, 657–684. [CrossRef] [PubMed]
37. Sifuentes-Franco, S.; Pacheco-Moisés, F.P.; Rodríguez-Carrizalez, A.D.; Miranda-Díaz, A.G. The Role of Oxidative Stress, Mitochondrial Function, and Autophagy in Diabetic Polyneuropathy. *J. Diabetes Res.* **2017**, *2017*, 1–15. [CrossRef]
38. Liyanagamage, D.S.N.K.; Martinus, R.D. Role of Mitochondrial Stress Protein HSP60 in Diabetes-Induced Neuroinflammation. *Mediators Inflamm.* **2020**, *2020*, 8073516. [CrossRef]
39. Ahmed, L.H.M.; Butler, A.E.; Dargham, S.R.; Latif, A.; Robay, A.; Chidiac, O.M.; Jayyousi, A.; Al Suwaidi, J.; Crystal, R.G.; Atkin, S.L.; et al. Association of vitamin D2 and D3 with type 2 diabetes complications. *BMC Endocr. Disord.* **2020**, *20*, 65. [CrossRef]
40. Tagliaferri, S.; Porri, D.; De Giuseppe, R.; Manuelli, M.; Alessio, F.; Cena, H. The controversial role of vitamin D as an antioxidant: Results from randomised controlled trials. *Nutr. Res. Rev.* **2019**, *32*, 99–105. [CrossRef]
41. Veldman, C.M.; Cantorna, M.T.; DeLuca, H.F. Expression of 1,25-dihydroxyvitamin D(3) receptor in the immune system. *Arch. Biochem. Biophys.* **2000**, *374*, 334–338. [CrossRef] [PubMed]
42. Christakos, S.; Ajibade, D.V.; Dhawan, P.; Fechner, A.J.; Mady, L.J. Vitamin D: Metabolism. *Endocrinol. Metab. Clin. N. Am.* **2010**, *39*, 243–253. [CrossRef]
43. Christensen, E.I.; Birn, H. Megalin and cubilin: Multifunctional endocytic receptors. *Nat. Rev. Mol. Cell Biol.* **2002**, *3*, 258–267. [CrossRef] [PubMed]
44. Labudzynskyi, D.O.; Zaitseva, O.V.; Latyshko, N.V.; Gudkova, O.O.; Veliky, M.M. Vitamin D3 contribution to the regulation of oxidative metabolism in the liver of diabetic mice. *Ukr. Biochem. J.* **2015**, *87*, 75–90. [CrossRef] [PubMed]
45. Kono, K.; Fujii, H.; Nakai, K.; Goto, S.; Kitazawa, R.; Kitazawa, S.; Shinohara, M.; Hirata, M.; Fukagawa, M.; Nishi, S. Anti-oxidative effect of vitamin D analog on incipient vascular lesion in non-obese type 2 diabetic rats. *Am. J. Nephrol.* **2013**, *37*, 167–174. [CrossRef]
46. Farhangi, M.A.; Nameni, G.; Hajiluian, G.; Mesgari-Abbasi, M. Cardiac tissue oxidative stress and inflammation after vitamin D administrations in high fat-diet induced obese rats. *BMC Cardiovasc. Disord.* **2017**, *17*, 161. [CrossRef]
47. Hajiluian, G.; Abbasalizad Farhangi, M.; Nameni, G.; Shahabi, P.; Megari-Abbasi, M. Oxidative stress-induced cognitive impairment in obesity can be reversed by vitamin D administration in rats. *Nutr. Neurosci.* **2018**, *21*, 744–752. [CrossRef]
48. Farhangi, M.A.; Mesgari-Abbasi, M.; Hajiluian, G.; Nameni, G.; Shahabi, P. Adipose Tissue Inflammation and Oxidative Stress: The Ameliorative Effects of Vitamin D. *Inflammation* **2017**, *40*, 1688–1697. [CrossRef]

49. Lin, Y.; Ubels, J.L.; Schotanus, M.P.; Yin, Z.; Pintea, V.; Hammock, B.D.; Watsky, M.A. Enhancement of Vitamin D Metabolites in the Eye Following Vitamin D3 Supplementation and UV-B Irradiation. *Curr. Eye Res.* **2012**, *37*, 871–878. [CrossRef]
50. Toda, R.; Kawazu, K.; Oyabu, M.; Miyazaki, T.; Kiuchi, Y. Comparison of drug permeabilities across the blood-retinal barrier, blood-aqueous humor barrier, and blood-brain barrier. *J. Pharm. Sci.* **2011**, *100*, 3904–3911. [CrossRef]
51. Packer, L.; Cadenas, E. Oxidants and antioxidants revisited. New concepts of oxidative stress. *Free Radic. Res.* **2007**, *41*, 951–952. [CrossRef] [PubMed]
52. Polidoro, L.; Properzi, G.; Marampon, F.; Gravina, G.L.; Festuccia, C.; Di Cesare, E.; Scarsella, L.; Ciccarelli, C.; Zani, B.M.; Ferri, C. Vitamin D Protects Human Endothelial Cells from H2O2 Oxidant Injury Through the Mek/Erk-Sirt1 Axis Activation. *J Cardiovasc. Transl. Res.* **2013**, *6*, 221–231. [CrossRef] [PubMed]
53. Bao, B.-Y.; Ting, H.-J.; Hsu, J.-W.; Lee, Y.-F. Protective role of 1α, 25-dihydroxyvitamin D3 against oxidative stress in nonmalignant human prostate epithelial cells. *Int. J. Cancer* **2008**, *122*, 2699–2706. [CrossRef] [PubMed]
54. Peng, X.; Vaishnav, A.; Murillo, G.; Alimirah, F.; Torres, K.E.O.; Mehta, R.G. Protection against cellular stress by 25-hydroxyvitamin D3 in breast epithelial cells. *J. Cell. Biochem.* **2010**, *110*, 1324–1333. [CrossRef] [PubMed]
55. Lee, H.-S.; Namkoong, K.; Kim, D.-H.; Kim, K.-J.; Cheong, Y.-H.; Kim, S.-S.; Lee, W.-B.; Kim, K.-Y. Hydrogen peroxide-induced alterations of tight junction proteins in bovine brain microvascular endothelial cells. *Microvasc. Res.* **2004**, *68*, 231–238. [CrossRef] [PubMed]
56. Maier, R.; Weger, M.; Haller-Schober, E.-M.; El-Shabrawi, Y.; Wedrich, A.; Theisl, A.; Aigner, R.; Barth, A.; Haas, A. Multiplex bead analysis of vitreous and serum concentrations of inflammatory and proangiogenic factors in diabetic patients. *Mol. Vis.* **2008**, *14*, 637–643.
57. Koleva-Georgieva, D.N.; Sivkova, N.P.; Terzieva, D. Serum inflammatory cytokines IL-1beta, IL-6, TNF-alpha and VEGF have influence on the development of diabetic retinopathy. *Folia Med.* **2011**, *53*, 44–50. [CrossRef]
58. Yoshimura, T.; Sonoda, K.; Sugahara, M.; Mochizuki, Y.; Enaida, H.; Oshima, Y.; Ueno, A.; Hata, Y.; Yoshida, H.; Ishibashi, T. Comprehensive analysis of inflammatory immune mediators in vitreoretinal diseases. *PLoS ONE* **2009**, *4*, e8158. [CrossRef]
59. Rangasamy, S.; McGuire, P.G.; Das, A. Diabetic retinopathy and inflammation: Novel therapeutic targets. *Middle East Afr. J. Ophthalmol.* **2012**, *19*, 52–59. [CrossRef]
60. Joussen, A.M.; Poulaki, V.; Le, M.L.; Koizumi, K.; Esser, C.; Janicki, H.; Schraermeyer, U.; Kociok, N.; Fauser, S.; Kirchhof, B.; et al. A central role for inflammation in the pathogenesis of diabetic retinopathy. *FASEB J.* **2004**, *18*, 1450–1452. [CrossRef]
61. Wang, J.; Xu, X.; Elliott, M.H.; Zhu, M.; Le, Y.-Z. Müller cell-derived VEGF is essential for diabetes-induced retinal inflammation and vascular leakage. *Diabetes* **2010**, *59*, 2297–2305. [CrossRef] [PubMed]
62. Murakami, T.; Felinski, E.A.; Antonetti, D.A. Occludin phosphorylation and ubiquitination regulate tight junction trafficking and vascular endothelial growth factor-induced permeability. *J. Biol. Chem.* **2009**, *284*, 21036–21046. [CrossRef] [PubMed]
63. Holick, M.F. Vitamin D Deficiency. *N. Engl. J. Med.* **2007**, *357*, 266–281. [CrossRef] [PubMed]
64. Hyppönen, E.; Läärä, E.; Reunanen, A.; Järvelin, M.-R.; Virtanen, S.M. Intake of vitamin D and risk of type 1 diabetes: A birth-cohort study. *Lancet* **2001**, *358*, 1500–1503. [CrossRef]
65. Shab-Bidar, S.; Neyestani, T.R.; Djazayery, A.; Eshraghian, M.-R.; Houshiarrad, A.; Kalayi, A.; Shariatzadeh, N.; Khalaji, N.; Gharavi, A. Improvement of vitamin D status resulted in amelioration of biomarkers of systemic inflammation in the subjects with type 2 diabetes: Vitamin D and Systemic Inflammation. *Diabetes Metab. Res. Rev.* **2012**, *28*, 424–430. [CrossRef]
66. Guillot, X.; Semerano, L.; Saidenberg-Kermanac'h, N.; Falgarone, G.; Boissier, M.-C. Vitamin D and inflammation. *Jt. Bone Spine* **2010**, *77*, 552–557. [CrossRef]
67. Hewison, M. Vitamin D and the immune system: New perspectives on an old theme. *Endocrinol. Metab. Clin. N. Am.* **2010**, *39*, 365–379. [CrossRef]
68. Hao, J.; Zhang, H.; Yu, J.; Chen, X.; Yang, L. Methylene Blue Attenuates Diabetic Retinopathy by Inhibiting NLRP3 Inflammasome Activation in STZ-Induced Diabetic Rats. *Ocul. Immunol. Inflamm.* **2019**, *27*, 836–843. [CrossRef]

69. Wooff, Y.; Man, S.M.; Aggio-Bruce, R.; Natoli, R.; Fernando, N. IL-1 Family Members Mediate Cell Death, Inflammation and Angiogenesis in Retinal Degenerative Diseases. *Front. Immunol.* **2019**, *10*. [CrossRef]
70. Schroder, K.; Tschopp, J. The Inflammasomes. *Cell* **2010**, *140*, 821–832. [CrossRef]
71. Zhou, J.; Wang, S.; Xia, X. Role of intravitreal inflammatory cytokines and angiogenic factors in proliferative diabetic retinopathy. *Curr. Eye Res.* **2012**, *37*, 416–420. [CrossRef]
72. Loukovaara, S.; Piippo, N.; Kinnunen, K.; Hytti, M.; Kaarniranta, K.; Kauppinen, A. NLRP3 inflammasome activation is associated with proliferative diabetic retinopathy. *Acta Ophthalmol.* **2017**, *95*, 803–808. [CrossRef] [PubMed]
73. An, E.; Gordish-Dressman, H.; Hathout, Y. Effect of TNF-alpha on human ARPE-19-secreted proteins. *Mol. Vis.* **2008**, *14*, 2292–2303. [PubMed]
74. Kutty, R.K.; Samuel, W.; Boyce, K.; Cherukuri, A.; Duncan, T.; Jaworski, C.; Nagineni, C.N.; Redmond, T.M. Proinflammatory cytokines decrease the expression of genes critical for RPE function. *Mol. Vis.* **2016**, *22*, 1156–1168. [PubMed]
75. Desjardins, D.M.; Yates, P.W.; Dahrouj, M.; Liu, Y.; Crosson, C.E.; Ablonczy, Z. Progressive Early Breakdown of Retinal Pigment Epithelium Function in Hyperglycemic Rats. *Investig. Opthalmol. Vis. Sci.* **2016**, *57*, 2706. [CrossRef]
76. Xia, Z.; Chen, H.; Zheng, S. Alterations of Retinal Pigment Epithelium–Photoreceptor Complex in Patients with Type 2 Diabetes Mellitus without Diabetic Retinopathy: A Cross-Sectional Study. *J. Diabetes Res.* **2020**, *2020*, 1–6. [CrossRef]
77. Yan, H.; Mao, C. Roles of elevated intravitreal IL-1β and IL-10 levels in proliferative diabetic retinopathy. *Indian J. Ophthalmol.* **2014**, *62*, 699. [CrossRef]
78. Gee, K.; Guzzo, C.; Che Mat, N.; Ma, W.; Kumar, A. The IL-12 Family of Cytokines in Infection, Inflammation and Autoimmune Disorders. *Inflamm. Allergy-Drug Targets* **2009**, *8*, 40–52. [CrossRef]
79. Santos, J.M.; Mohammad, G.; Zhong, Q.; Kowluru, R.A. Diabetic Retinopathy, Superoxide Damage and Antioxidants. *Curr. Pharm. Biotechnol.* **2011**, *12*, 352–361. [CrossRef]

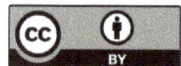

© 2020 by the authors. Licensee MDPI, Basel, Switzerland. This article is an open access article distributed under the terms and conditions of the Creative Commons Attribution (CC BY) license (http://creativecommons.org/licenses/by/4.0/).

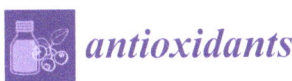

Article

Antioxidative Effects of Ascorbic Acid and Astaxanthin on ARPE-19 Cells in an Oxidative Stress Model

Sanghyeon Oh [1,†], Young Joo Kim [2,†], Eun Kyoung Lee [3,†], Sung Wook Park [3] and Hyeong Gon Yu [3,*]

1. Interdisciplinary Program in Stem Cell Biology, Graduate School of Medicine, Seoul National University, Seoul 03080, Korea; OhSaHy@hotmail.com
2. Department of Ophthalmology, Seoul National University Hospital Biomedical Research Institute, Seoul 03080, Korea; yjkim612@daum.net
3. Department of Ophthalmology, Seoul National University College of Medicine, Seoul National University Hospital, Seoul 03080, Korea; righthanded8282@gmail.com (E.K.L.); academypark@gmail.com (S.W.P.)
* Correspondence: hgonyu@snu.ac.kr; Tel.: +822-2072-3083
† These authors contributed equally to this work.

Received: 31 July 2020; Accepted: 3 September 2020; Published: 6 September 2020

Abstract: Oxidative stress has been implicated as critical pathogenic factors contributing to the etiology of diabetic retinopathy and other retinal diseases. This study investigated antioxidative effect of ascorbic acid and astaxanthin on ARPE-19 cells within an oxidative stress model induced by common biological sources of reactive oxygen species (ROS). Hydrogen peroxide (H_2O_2) at concentrations of 0.1–0.8 mM and 20–100 mJ/cm^2 of ultraviolet B (UVB) were treated to ARPE-19 cells. Cell viability and intracellular ROS level changes were measured. With the sublethal and lethal dose of each inducers, 0–750 μM of ascorbic acid and 0–40 μM of astaxanthin were treated to examine antioxidative effect on the model. Ascorbic acid at concentrations of 500 and 750 μM increased the cell viability not only in the UVB model but also in the H_2O_2 model, but 20 and 40 μM of astaxanthin only did so in the UVB model. The combination of ascorbic acid and astaxanthin showed better antioxidative effect compared to each drug alone, suggesting a synergistic effect.

Keywords: antioxidant; ascorbic acid; astaxanthin; oxidative stress; diabetic retinopathy; retinal pigment epithelium; retinal disease

1. Introduction

Diabetic retinopathy (DR) is a microvascular consequence of diabetes mellitus and remains the leading cause of blindness among the working-age population [1]. DR is defined as the progressive, irreversible deterioration of retinal microvasculature as a result of chronic hyperglycemia [2]. Studies have found the relationship between oxidative stress and DR that oxidative stress plays a role in pathogenesis of DR and DR can increase the reactive oxygen species (ROS) level. Hyperglycemia is thought to be one of the main causes of the disease and higher level of oxidative stress can accelerate the process by blocking the downstream flow of glycolysis [3,4]. DR also increases oxidative stress because high glucose level and retinal vascularization by diabetic induction elevate arginase activity which later increases oxidative stress [5].

As the relationship between ROS and various retinal pathogenesis have been studied, defense mechanisms against ROS have been also studied [6–11]. Organisms have defense mechanisms against oxygen metabolites and the mechanism includes removal of free radicals by enzymes, proteins, and pro-oxidant metal reactions, and reduction of free radicals by antioxidants (vitamin C, vitamin E, glutathione) [6]. The cellular antioxidant response element is essentially important for the amelioration of oxidative stress. It responds to hyperglycemia and can be used to evaluate the complications of diabetes. In a previous study, Busik et al. [12] suggested that diabetes-related endothelial injury in the retina may be due to glucose-induced cytokine release by other retinal cells, such as retinal pigment epithelium (RPE) and Müller cells, and not a direct effect of high glucose. Therefore, it is important to investigate the oxidative stress as well as effects of antioxidants on RPE cells in order to determine the pathogenesis regarding oxidative stress in DR.

Studies have found that with aging, endogenous antioxidants level [13] and antioxidant enzyme activity along with its gene expression and protein level decrease [14]. This alteration in the antioxidative defense system worsens the imbalance between ROS production and its removal. As a consequence, oxidatively damaged macromolecules including lipids, deoxyribonucleic acid (DNA), and proteins accumulate accelerating the aging process with oxidative-stress-induced aging [15].

For this reason, it becomes more important to maintain the antioxidant defense system and one way is to supplement antioxidants from an outer source. Supplements actively studied for their antioxidative effect are ascorbic acid (vitamin C), glutathione, alpha-tocopherol (vitamin E), and other carotenoids (i.e., astaxanthin, lutein, β-carotene) [16–18]. One frequently used way to evaluate their antioxidant activity is by studying their reactivity with free radicals and metal ions (DPPH, ABTS, FRAP, CUPRAC, ORAC, HORAC, TRAP) [19–22]. However, giving them enough credence for their antioxidant capacity assumption is often controversial since one same antioxidant can have a different relative capacity to other antioxidants when measured with different methods [23–28].

For this reason, it is necessary to study potential antioxidants' capacities and properties based on a solid oxidative stress model. A solid oxidative stress model portrays the biological environment well so that a more accurate assumption is possible, and the result is reproducible. Hydrogen peroxide (H_2O_2) [29–31] and ultraviolet B (UVB) irradiation [32–34] have been studied to establish an oxidative stress model within cells. H_2O_2 represents endogenous ROS production and UVB represents an outer source of oxidative stress to retinal cells. In this study, both a H_2O_2-induced oxidative stress model and UVB-induced oxidative stress model will be used to evaluate the antioxidative potential of ascorbic acid and astaxanthin on ARPE-19 cells.

2. Materials and Methods

2.1. ARPE-19 Cell Culture

ARPE-19 cells (american type culture collection, Manassas, VA, USA) were cultured and maintained as a monolayer in 1:1 mixture of Dulbecco's modified eagle's medium and nutrient mixture F-12 (DMEM/F-12) (Invitrogen, Gibco, Carlsbad, CA, USA) supplemented with 10% fetal bovine serum (FBS) (Invitrogen) and 1% penicillin-streptomycin (Invitrogen). Cells were incubated at 37 °C in a humidified 5% CO_2 incubator in the complete medium with a 2–3-times-a-week change until they reached 80% confluency. Cells used for this study were in a passage between 25 and 30.

2.2. Hydrogen Peroxide Exposure Procedure

Cells were seeded in a 96-well plate with a density of 2.5×10^4 cells/well and allowed to attach to the bottom of the well and to become confluent overnight. The next day, the medium was changed to a serum-free medium and cells were maintained in it up to 7 days until the day of the procedure. 30% (w/w) H_2O_2 in H_2O-containing stabilizer (Sigma Aldrich, St. Louis, MO, USA) was used to make medium with intended H_2O_2 concentration. H_2O_2 solution was diluted fresh each time. For the exposure, the used medium of the cells was changed to serum-free DMEM/F-12 without phenol red (Invitrogen) with the desired concentration of H_2O_2. The viability was checked by MTT assay after 24 h of exposure to H_2O_2.

2.3. Ultraviolet B Irradiation Procedure

Cells were seeded in a 96-well plate with a density of 2.5×10^4 cells/well and allowed to attach to the bottom of the well and to become confluent overnight. The next day, the medium was changed to serum-free medium and cells were maintained in it up to 7 days until the day of the procedure. At UVB irradiation, the medium was changed to DMEM/F-12 without phenol red without serum. As a UVB source, Sankyo Denki lamps (G15T8E, Tokyo, Japan) was used. Its irradiation intensity was $0.2\ mW/cm^2$ when measured 20 cm below the lamp where the plates were put. The intensity was measured with a UVB meter (UVX Digital Radiometer, UVP, Upland, CA, USA). Cells were irradiated with intended doses of UVB and for the control group and differential dose of UVB irradiation, remaining wells in the same plate were thoroughly masked.

2.4. DPPH Scavenging Assay

Total antioxidative capacities of ascorbic acid and astaxanthin were estimated using DPPH (2,2-diphenyl-1-picrylhydrazyl) ROS scavenging assay. DPPH solution was made by dissolving DPPH in methanol to 0.16 mM. Ascorbic acid and astaxanthin were dissolved to various concentrations in dimethyl sulfoxide (DMSO) (Sigma Aldrich). Ascorbic acid (20 µL) or astaxanthin (20 µL) solution was mixed with 100 µL DPPH solution for 30 min with vigorous shaking at room temperature. After the reaction absorbance at 517 nm was measured and the relative amount of scavenged DPPH was calculated using the following equation.

$$Scavenged\ DPPH\ fraction\ (\%) = \frac{Ab_{Control} - Ab_{AO}}{Ab_{Control}} \times 100 \tag{1}$$

$Ab_{Control}$ is the absorbance of the groups with only DPPH and Ab_{AO} is the absorbance of the groups of the mixture of DPPH and various concentrations of antioxidants.

2.5. Antioxidant Treatment

Cells were treated with either ascorbic acid (Sigma Aldrich) or astaxanthin (Sigma Aldrich) in DMEM/F-12 without phenol red to study their antioxidative effect on ARPE-19 cells. Ascorbic-acid-containing medium was made from ascorbic acid stock (0.5 M in PBS) and astaxanthin-containing medium was made from astaxanthin stock (1 mg/mL in DMSO). Cells were pretreated with ascorbic acid or astaxanthin for 6 h and then they were irradiated by UVB or exposed to H_2O_2. For UVB irradiation group, after pretreatment, used medium was changed to the fresh medium containing the same concentrations of compounds and followed the UVB irradiation ($20\ mJ/cm^2$ or $100\ mJ/cm^2$) procedure. For the H_2O_2 exposure group, after pretreatment, the used medium was changed to the fresh medium containing the same concentrations of the compounds with a sublethal or lethal dose of H_2O_2 (0.2 mM or 0.4 mM).

2.6. MTT Assay

3-(4,5-Dimethyl-2-thiazolyl)-2,5-diphenyl-2H-tetrazolium bromide (MTT) (Sigma Aldrich) was used to determine cell viability. MTT is enzymatically turned into purple formazan crystals by mitochondrial respiration activity. The procedure was done following the manufacturer's instructions. Briefly, after antioxidants, UVB, or H_2O_2 treatment to the cells, the medium was removed and MTT (0.5 mg/mL) was added diluted in serum-free medium. After 3 h of incubation at 37 °C in a humidified 5% CO_2 incubator, MTT-containing medium was carefully aspirated from the well and DMSO was added to each well to solubilize formazan crystals. Absorbance at 570 nm was measured using a microplate reader (EPOCH 2, BioTek Instruments Inc. Winoosky, VT, USA) with a reference wavelength of 630 nm. Cells untreated or treated with the only vehicle were set to be 100% cell viability for the normalization of the absorbance and experiments had more than three replicates for each condition.

2.7. Crystal Violet Assay

The relative number of cells attached to the bottom of the well was measured by crystal violet uptake assay. The procedure was done as previously described [35]. Briefly, after UVB, or H_2O_2 treatment to the cells, the medium was removed, and cells were fixed with 4% paraformaldehyde in 4 °C. After they were washed 3 times and 0.1% crystal violet (Sigma Aldrich) in 10% ethanol was added to each well for 5 min. After washing 3 times, the remaining stain was dissolved in 10% acetic acid and absorbance at 540 nm was measured.

2.8. DCFH-DA Intracellular ROS Level Assay

Intracellular ROS level was measured by 2′,7′-dichlorodihydrofluorescein diacetate (DCFH-DA) assay. DCFH-DA is cell-permeable and is not fluorescent which enters cells to be de-esterified to 2′,7′-dichlorodihydrofluorescein (DCFH), and become impermeable to the cell membrane. It then reacts with ROS to be highly fluorescent 2′,7′-dichlorofluorescein (DCF). Before UVB irradiation or H_2O_2 exposure, cells were cultured with 10 µM DCFH-DA (Sigma Aldrich) in DMEM/F-12 without phenol red for 30 min at 37 °C in a humidified 5% CO_2 incubator. After incubation, they were washed 2 times in phosphate-buffered saline (PBS) and antioxidant treatment, UVB irradiation or H_2O_2 exposure was done following measurement of fluorescence of DCF at excitation and emission wavelength of 495 nm and 529 nm, respectively, with a microplate reader (Synergy Mix, BioTek Instruments Inc. Winoosky, VT, USA). Cells untreated or treated with the only vehicle were set to be 100% intracellular ROS level for the normalization of the fluorescence intensity and experiments had more than three replicates for each condition.

2.9. Statistical Analysis

The results were expressed as mean values and standard deviation (SD). Statistical analyses were performed using the Kruskal-Wallis test for comparison between several groups and the Mann-Whitney U test for comparison between 2 subgroups to assess the effects of drug treatment, with $p < 0.05$. The analyses were done using IBM SPSS Statistics for Windows, Version 26.0 (IBM Corp., Armonk, New York, NY, USA).

3. Results

3.1. Effect of H_2O_2 on the Viability of ARPE-19 Cells and Intracellular ROS Level

To establish the H_2O_2-induced oxidative stress model in ARPE-19 cells, different concentrations of H_2O_2 were treated to the cells and their viability and intracellular ROS level were measured. Viability measured with MTT assay decreased as the concentration of treated H_2O_2 increased. When cells were treated with 0.4 mM H_2O_2, they showed the viability of 66% and the viability change was the greatest between 0.2 mM and 0.6 mM (Figure 1A). Crystal violet assay resulted in a similar aspect of viability change as MTT assay with 69% of viability at 0.4 mM (Figure 1B). Intracellular ROS level increased dependently to the concentration of H_2O_2 (Figure 1C). The mean value of the ROS level measured in 0.8 mM H_2O_2 increased to 176% compared to the control group. This trend of decreased cell viability after the H_2O_2 exposure was confirmed in bright field imaging (Figure 1D,E). As cell viability changed rapidly at 0.4 mM H_2O_2, 0.4 mM was set to be a lethal dose of H_2O_2 and 0.2 mM was set to be sublethal dose.

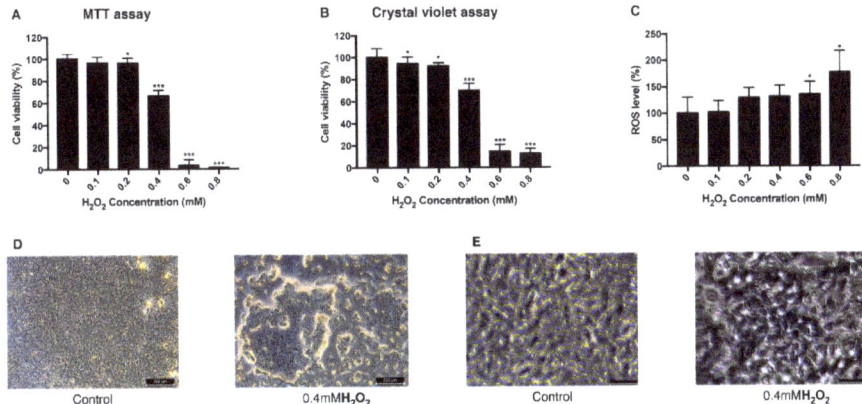

Figure 1. Change of viability and intracellular ROS level in ARPE-19 cells after exposure to H_2O_2. The response of ARPE-19 cells to 0–0.8 mM H_2O_2 exposure for MTT assay (**A**), and crystal violet assay (**B**) to determine cell viability. For intracellular ROS level, DCFH-DA was treated for 30 min after the H_2O_2 exposure. Exposure to H_2O_2 reduced the cell viability (**A**,**B**) and increased the intracellular ROS level (**C**). The cell morphology was observed with bright field microscopy (Scale bar 500 μm) (**D**) and with higher magnification (scale bar 100 μm) (**E**). Asterisks indicate a significant reduction in cell viability or increment in ROS level compared with untreated cells (* $p < 0.05$, ** $p < 0.01$, *** $p < 0.001$). MTT, 3-(4,5-dimethylthiazol-2-yl)-2,5-diphenyltetrazolium bromide; ROS, reactive oxygen species; DCFH-DA, 2′,7′-dichlorodihydrofluorescein diacetate.

3.2. Effect of UVB Irradiation on the Viability of ARPE-19 Cells and Intracellular ROS

To establish the UVB-induced oxidative stress model in ARPE-19 cells, different doses of UVB were exposed to the cells and their viability and intracellular ROS level were measured. Viability measured with MTT assay decreased as the dose of UVB irradiation increased. When cells were exposed to 20 mJ/cm² UVB, they showed the viability of 80% and with 100 mJ/cm² UVB, the viability was 60% (Figure 2A). In a crystal violet assay with the same range of UVB dose, the viability dropped to 78% at 20 mJ/cm² UVB and to 72% at 100 mJ/cm² UVB (Figure 2B). Intracellular ROS level increased dependently to the UVB dose (Figure 2C). The mean value of ROS level measured at 20 mJ/cm² UVB increased to 140% and 270% at 100 mJ/cm² UVB compared to the control group. Morphological change of the cells was observed in bright field imaging. Cells became rounder and holes in the monolayer were observed as UVB dose increased (Figure 2D,E). The sublethal dose of UVB was set to be 20 mJ/cm², where the cells show 80% of viability without significant morphological change and 100 mJ/cm² where the cells show 60% of viability with morphological change was set to be the lethal dose of UVB.

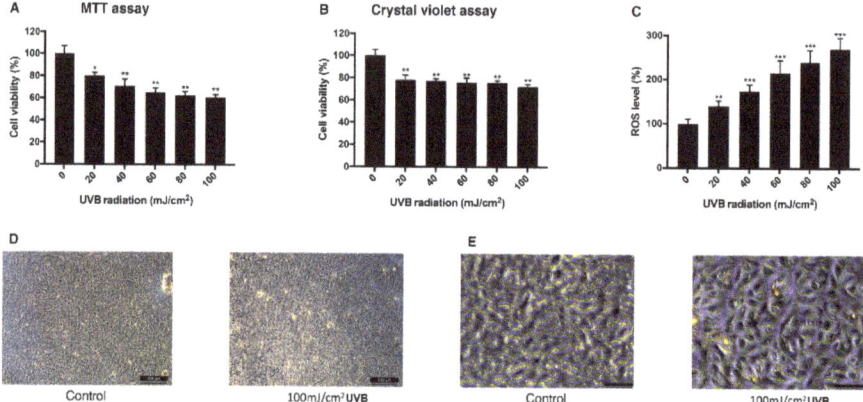

Figure 2. Change of viability and intracellular ROS level in ARPE-19 cells after UVB irradiation. The response of ARPE-19 cells 24 h after 0–100 mJ/cm^2 UVB irradiation with MTT assay (**A**), and crystal violet assay (**B**) to determine cell viability. For intracellular ROS level, DCFH-DA was treated for 30 min after the UVB irradiation. Irradiation by UVB reduced the cell viability (**A**,**B**) and increased the intracellular ROS level (**C**). The cell morphology was observed with bright field microscopy (scale bar 500 μm) (**D**) and with higher magnification (scale bar 100 μm) (**E**). Asterisks indicate a significant reduction in cell viability or increment in ROS level compared with untreated cells (* $p < 0.05$, ** $p < 0.01$, *** $p < 0.001$). UVB, ultraviolet B; MTT, 3-(4,5-dimethylthiazol-2-yl)-2,5-diphenyltetrazolium bromide; ROS, reactive oxygen species; DCFH-DA, 2′,7′-dichlorodihydrofluorescein diacetate.

3.3. Antioxidative Effect of Ascorbic Acid and Astaxanthin by Scavenging DPPH

DPPH scavenging assay was performed with ascorbic acid and astaxanthin. Ascorbic acid, at concentrations of 0.025 mM, 0.1 mM, 0.4 mM, and 1.6 mM, dissolved in DMSO was mixed with DPPH solution and each concentration scavenged 33%, 52%, 57%, 73% of DPPH, respectively, after 30 min of reaction (Figure 3A). When 75 μM, 85 μM, 95 μM, and 105 μM astaxanthin dissolved in DMSO were reacted with DPPH solution for 30 min, 44%, 50%, 64%, and 69% of DPPH were scavenged, respectively (Figure 3B). Both ascorbic acid and astaxanthin showed antioxidative effect.

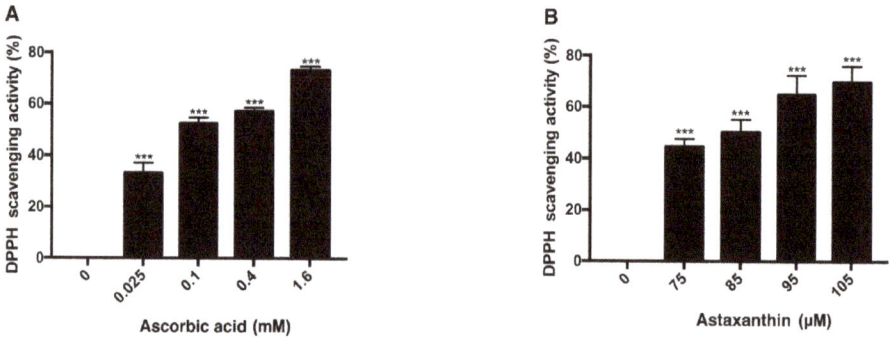

Figure 3. DPPH scavenging activity of ascorbic acid and astaxanthin. The antioxidative capacities of ascorbic acid and astaxanthin were determined by their capabilities to scavenge DPPH. Ascorbic acid (0.025–1.6 mM) was reacted with DPPH (**A**), and astaxanthin (75–105 μM) was reacted with DPPH (**B**). The compounds were diluted in DMSO. Both compounds scavenged DPPH in dose-dependent way in 30 min of reaction time. Asterisks indicate a significant increment in DPPH scavenging activity compared with controls (*** $p < 0.001$). DPPH, 2,2-diphenyl-1-picrylhydrazyl; DMSO, dimethyl sulfoxide.

3.4. Antioxidative Effect of Ascorbic Acid on ARPE-19 Cells Under H_2O_2-Induced Oxidative Stress

ARPE-19 cells were pretreated with various concentrations of ascorbic acid or astaxanthin for 6 h and then they were treated together with H_2O_2 and the same concentrations of antioxidants for another 24 h. Viability was assessed after 3 h of MTT treatment. When groups treated together with ascorbic acid and H_2O_2 they showed increased viability compared to controls. Cells treated only with 0.2 mM H_2O_2 showed the viability of 80% and groups treated together with ascorbic acid showed 81%, 107%, and 126% of viability, respectively, for 250 µM, 500 µM, and 750 µM of the drug concentration. On the other hand, astaxanthin did not show any significant effect on the viability of ARPE-19 with H_2O_2-induced oxidative stress (Figure 4A). For 0.4 mM H_2O_2 treatment, cells treated only with H_2O_2 showed 58% of viability, while 250 µM, 500 µM, and 750µM of ascorbic acid increased the viability to 64%, 72%, and 95%, respectively. On the other hand, astaxanthin did not show any significant effect on the viability of ARPE-19 with H_2O_2-induced oxidative stress (Figure 4B).

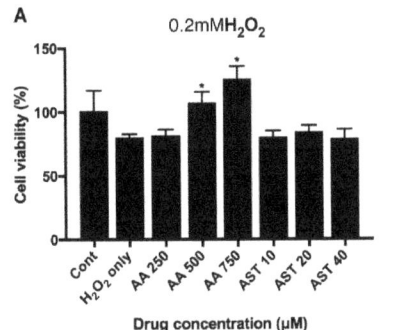
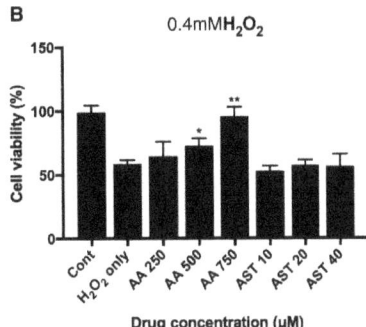

Figure 4. Effect of ascorbic acid and astaxanthin on H_2O_2-induced oxidative stress model of ARPE-19. The effect of various concentration of ascorbic acid or astaxanthin (pretreated for 6 h and co-treated with H_2O_2 for 24 h) on the response of ARPE-19 cells to sublethal dose of 0.2 mM (**A**) or lethal dose of 0.4 mM H_2O_2 (**B**). The cell viability was determined by MTT assay. Treatment of ascorbic acid (500–750 µM) significantly increased ARPE-19 cell viability following 0.2 mM H_2O_2 exposure. However, astaxanthin (10–40 µM) did not significantly affect the cell viability (**A**). Ascorbic acid (500–750 µM) also significantly increased the cell viability under 0.4 mM H_2O_2 but astaxanthin (10–40 µM) did not have significant effect on the viability (**B**). Asterisks indicate a significant increment in cell viability compared with cells treated with H_2O_2 only (* $p < 0.05$, ** $p < 0.01$). AA, ascorbic acid; AST, astaxanthin; MTT, 3-(4,5-dimethylthiazol-2-yl)-2,5-diphenyltetrazolium bromide.

3.5. Antioxidative Effect of Ascorbic Acid and Astaxanthin on ARPE-19 Cells Under UVB-induced Oxidative Stress

ARPE-19 cells were pretreated with various concentrations of ascorbic acid or astaxanthin for 6 h and then they were irradiated with UVB. Viability 24 h after the irradiation was assessed with MTT assay. When cells were pretreated with ascorbic acid and then UVB irradiated with it, the cell viability increased compared to the UVB irradiation-only group. Cells irradiated only with 20 mJ/cm^2 UVB showed the viability of 85% and groups treated together with ascorbic acid showed 92%, 102%, and 130% of viability, respectively, for 250 µM, 500 µM, and 750 µM of the drug concentration. Astaxanthin treated cells also showed increased viability compared to the cells irradiated only with UVB. The 10 µM, 20 µM, and 40 µM astaxanthin groups showed 95%, 101%, and 102%, respectively, after 20 mJ/cm^2 UVB irradiation (Figure 5A). For 100 mJ/cm^2 UVB irradiation, the cells irradiated only with UVB showed 66% of viability while 250 µM, 500 µM, and 750 µM of ascorbic acid increased the viability to 68%, 78%, and 109%, respectively. Astaxanthin-treated cells also showed increased viability compared to the cells irradiated only with UVB. The 10 µM, 20 µM, and 40 µM astaxanthin groups showed 67%, 74%, and 83% after 100 mJ/cm² UVB irradiation (Figure 5B).

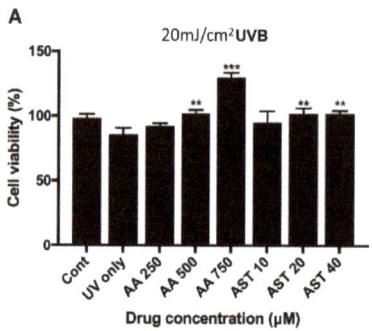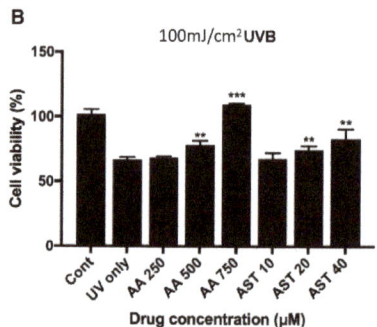

Figure 5. Effect of ascorbic acid and astaxanthin on UVB-induced oxidative stress model of ARPE-19. The effect of various concentration of ascorbic acid and astaxanthin (pretreated for 6 h and additional 24 h after UVB irradiation) on the response of ARPE-19 cells to sublethal dose of 20 mJ/cm² (**A**) or lethal dose of 100 mJ/cm² UVB (**B**). The cell viability was determined by MTT assay 24 h after the irradiation. Treatment of ascorbic acid (500–750 µM) and astaxanthin (20–40 µM) significantly increased ARPE-19 cell viability following 20 mJ/cm² UVB irradiation (**A**). Ascorbic acid (500–750 µM) and astaxanthin (20–40 µM) also significantly increased the cell viability after 100 mJ/cm² UVB irradiation (**B**). Asterisks indicate a significant increment in cell viability compared with cells treated with UVB only (* $p < 0.05$, ** $p < 0.01$, *** $p < 0.001$). UVB, ultraviolet B; AA, ascorbic acid; AST, astaxanthin; MTT, 3-(4,5-dimethylthiazol-2-yl)-2,5-diphenyltetrazolium bromide.

3.6. Effect of Ascorbic Acid on the Intracellular ROS Level of ARPE-19

The effect of ascorbic acid on the intracellular ROS level of ARPE-19 cells was studied with DCFH-DA assay. The intracellular ROS level was measured after cells were treated with UVB with or without 500 µM ascorbic acid. UVB of 20 mJ/cm² and 100 mJ/cm² increased the intracellular ROS level to 123% and 234%, respectively, and 500 µM ascorbic acid treatment reduced the ROS level to 105% and 115% (Figure 6A). This trend between groups were confirmed with fluorescence microscopy (Figure 6B).

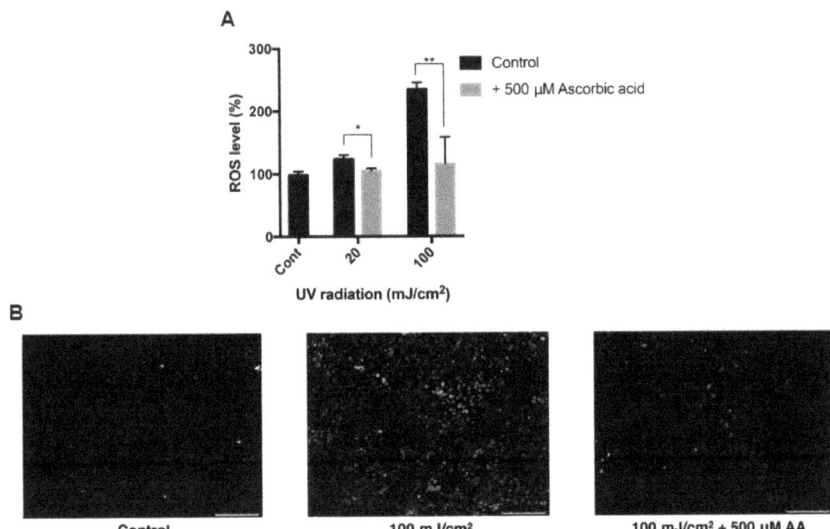

Figure 6. Intracellular ROS level of ARPE-19 after UVB treatment with ascorbic acid. The effects of ascorbic acid on the intracellular ROS level of ARPE-19 under UVB-induced oxidative stress were examined by DCFH-DA assay. Ascorbic acid at 500 µM significantly reduced the ROS level after UVB irradiation (20–100 mJ/cm^2) compared to groups with UVB irradiation only (**A**). The green fluorescence of the reacted DCFH-DA which indicates the ROS level, was observed with fluorescence microscopy (scale bar 250 µm) (**B**). Asterisks indicate a significant reduction in ROS level compared with control cells only with UVB exposure without ascorbic acid treatment (* $p < 0.05$, ** $p < 0.01$). ROS, reactive oxygen species; UVB, ultraviolet B; DCFH-DA, 2′,7′-dichlorodihydrofluorescein diacetate; AA, ascorbic acid.

3.7. Antioxidative Effect of Astaxanthin and Ascorbic Acid by Reducing Intracellular ROS in ARPE-19 Cells

H_2O_2 of 0.2 mM and 0.4 mM increased the intracellular ROS level to 123% and 135% compared to the nontreated group, while ascorbic-acid-treated group showed reduced ROS level of 33% and 34%, respectively (Figure 7A).

ARPE-19 cells were pretreated with either 20 µM astaxanthin, 90 µM ascorbic acid, or a mixture of 20 µM astaxanthin and 90 µM ascorbic acid. When cells were exposed to 0.2 mM H_2O_2 for 24 h, the viability decreased to 75%. The 20-µM-astaxanthin- and 90-µM-ascorbic-acid-treatment could increase the viability to 97% and 93%, respectively. The mixture of 20 µM astaxanthin and 90 µM ascorbic acid increased the viability to 129% (Figure 7B). Each drug could also decrease the intracellular ROS level. When cells were treated with 0.2 mM H_2O_2 for 24 h, the intracellular ROS level increased to 200%. The 20-µM-astaxanthin- and 90-µM-ascorbic-acid-treatment reduced the ROS level to 169%, and 135%, respectively. The mixture of 20 µM astaxanthin and 90 µM ascorbic acid decreased the ROS level to 104% (Figure 7C).

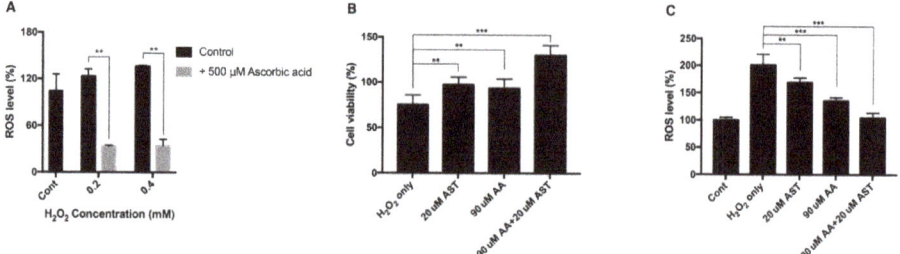

Figure 7. Intracellular ROS level and cell viability of ARPE-19 after H_2O_2 exposure with ascorbic acid and the mixture of ascorbic acid and astaxanthin. Ascorbic acid at 500 μM significantly reduced the intracellular ROS level under sublethal and lethal dose of H_2O_2 (0.2–0.4 mM) compared to the control group without ascorbic acid treatment (**A**). The effect of 20 μM astaxanthin, 90 μM ascorbic acid, and the mixture of the two compounds on the cell viability of ARPE-19 under H_2O_2-induced oxidative stress was examined by MTT assay. Cell viability was significantly increased when the cells were pretreated with 20 μM astaxanthin, 90 μM ascorbic acid, and the mixture of the two compounds for 6 h and with 0.2 mM H_2O_2 for 24 h, compared to H_2O_2 only (**B**). ROS level was significantly decreased when the cells were pretreated with 20 μM astaxanthin, 90 μM ascorbic acid, and the mixture of the two compounds for 6 h and with 0.2 mM H_2O_2 for 24 h, compared to H_2O_2 only. Asterisks indicate a significant difference between increment in cell viability and reduction in intracellular ROS level compared to control cells only with H_2O_2 exposure without antioxidant treatment (**C**). (** $p < 0.01$, *** $p < 0.001$). AST, astaxanthin; AA, ascorbic acid; ROS, reactive oxygen species; MTT, 3-(4,5-dimethylthiazol-2-yl)-2,5-diphenyltetrazolium bromide.

4. Discussion

In this study, antioxidative properties of ascorbic acid and astaxanthin were evaluated based on H_2O_2-induced and UVB-induced oxidative stress models within ARPE-19 cells. Studies have found that H_2O_2 and UVB have different effects on cells regarding oxidative stress. First, even directly adding H_2O_2 in the cell culture medium results in a short-term exposure because its concentration decreases rapidly in the presence of the cells. H_2O_2 can penetrate the cell easily, but it is also reduced rapidly by the antioxidative mechanism [29]. On the other hand, UVB has a lingering effect on the cells by directly damaging DNA, causing gene mutation, and modifying gene expression, and enzyme activity along with increasing ROS level [36]. UVB-induced damage is mediated by two different pathways. sne is by ROS generated immediately after the irradiation and the other is by reactive nitrogen species in the later time point [37]. As a result, even with a single and momentary exposure to UVB, the viability of the exposed cells decreases in the course of time [36].

Based on the precedent research, viability change of ARPE-19 cells was evaluated after 24 h for a H_2O_2 model and a UVB model [38]. H_2O_2 (0–0.8 mM) was exposed to ARPE-19 cells and their viability was dose-dependently reduced and intracellular ROS level was increased. UVB also reduced the cell viability and increased the intracellular ROS level but the H_2O_2 seemed to decrease the viability exponentially. One explanation can be that because H_2O_2 not only produces ROS, but it also affects junctional integrity of the RPE cell [39], weakening the cell adhesion to the bottom of the well—the cell viability assay result may have been affected. This can also explain the lower cell viability at 0.4 mM of H_2O_2 than 40 mJ/cm^2 UVB even though cells with H_2O_2-induced oxidative stress have a lower ROS level.

Within the condition of sublethal and lethal doses of H_2O_2 and UVB, antioxidative potencies of ascorbic acid and astaxanthin were evaluated. Although their antioxidative properties had been studied and have moved on to clinical level with patients with retinal diseases (Age-Related Eye Disease Study [AREDS] and Carotenoids in Age-Related Maculopathy Italian Study [CARMIS]) [40,41], there are controversies about whether they have a protective effect on cellular oxidative stress model.

In one study, ascorbic acid did not have a protective effect on Fenton-reaction-mediated oxidative stress model of ARPE-19 but it rather decreased the cell survival ratio at a low concentration (0.1–1 mM) compared to the group without ascorbic acid [42]. This was also the case for a *tert*-butyl hydroperoxide (t-BOOH)-induced oxidative stress model. In a study by Kagan et al., ascorbic acid (0.02–0.2 mM) also decreased the cell viability of ARPE-19 with oxidative stress induced by t-BOOH [43]. The effect of t-BOOH in porcine RPE also could not be diminished by ascorbic acid [44]. In our study, however, ascorbic acid increased the viability of the cells even at a low concentration where studies mentioned above suggest it decreases the viability and this was confirmed within two different oxidative stress models mediated by H_2O_2 and UVB. Although the central mechanism of t-BOOH to induce oxidative stress is by generating alkyl radicals [45], H_2O_2 is the central redox signaling molecule in general [30] forming hydroxy radicals [46], which can react intracellularly to generate various radicals including alkyl radical [47]. Considering H_2O_2 model reproduces more general situation of oxidative stress, and UVB model mediates H_2O_2 as the central signaling molecule [48], our result based on both models is more convincing.

Ascorbic acid neutralized the effect of the oxidative stress inducer in both H_2O_2 and UVB model but astaxanthin only did so in UVB-induced stress model. Li et al. [38] investigated the effect of astaxanthin on ARPE-19 cells against oxidative stress with H_2O_2. They incubated ARPE-19 cells with 20 µM astaxanthin for different lengths of time (6, 12, and 24 h) and then exposed to 200 µM H_2O_2 for 24 h. The cell viability increase was time-dependent, and they suggested that 24 h was the optimal time for astaxanthin treatment. In the current study, we incubated ARPE-19 cells with ascorbic acid or astaxanthin for 6 h and then exposed to H_2O_2 with antioxidants for 24 h. Our findings that astaxanthin did not show significant effect on the cell viability with H_2O_2 exposure while it did show increased viability with UVB irradiation may be due to different lengths of time from those of Li et al. [38] for astaxanthin treatment. There is also another possibility that even if astaxanthin, an extremely lipophilic compound, was dissolved in DMSO, it may be possible that the efficiency was lower than the actual concentration in an aqueous environment such as cell culture medium.

The synergistic effect of ascorbic acid and astaxanthin was also evaluated in this study. The combination of ascorbic acid and astaxanthin showed better antioxidative effect compared to each drug alone. There are few reports that investigate the effective antioxidant action of ascorbic acid and astaxanthin in combination. In a study by Guerra et al. [49], the association of astaxanthin with ascorbic acid greatly improved neutrophil phagocytic capacity and decreased ROS with pro-inflammatory cytokines. They suggested that the astaxanthin/ascorbic acid system mimics the recycling system of vitamin E/vitamin C. Astaxanthin provides cell membranes with potent protection against free radicals or other oxidative attack. Moreover, previous studies confirm that astaxanthin has a large capacity to neutralize free radicals or other oxidant activity in the nonpolar zones of phospholipid aggregates, as well as along their polar boundary zones [50]. Ascorbic acid, in turn, promotes antioxidant effects mainly in a water-phase microenvironment. The exact mechanism other than reducing the intracellular ROS production is unknown through this study, but it is assumed that the two antioxidants exhibited synergistic effects through the mechanism identified in previous experimental studies.

An elevated level of ROS is always observed in the diabetic retina. Given that the administration of antioxidants in animal models preserves retinal capillaries from hyperglycemia-induced degeneration, ROS are considered a major causative factor involved in DR development [51,52]. Meanwhile, diabetes induces mitochondrial damage in the retina and its capillary cells and mitochondrial dysfunction is also considered to play a significant role in the development of DR [53,54]. The results of this study showed that antioxidants treatment resulted in significantly improved cell viability which is perhaps due to the improved mitochondrial function, improved cellular attachment performance, and increased growth rate of the cells. However, further investigation will be required to determine more precise mechanisms and effects of antioxidants on ARPE-19 cells.

Although the role of retinal endothelial cells comprising inner blood-retinal barriers (BRB) is important in DR development, the role of RPE cells comprising outer BRB is also crucial. The flow of nutrients materials, metabolites, ions, proteins, and water flux to and from the retina is regulated by these two BRBs and disruption of inner and outer BRB causes retinal hyperpermeability and development of diabetic macular edema, which is a leading cause of vision loss in DR [55]. Therefore, current study using ARPE-19 cells is thought be closely related to BRB breakdown and the pathogenesis of DR. Oxidative damage to cells is commonly modeled using treatment with H_2O_2 for a long time [56,57], however, very little is known about the role of UV irradiation on ARPE-19 cells and especially on the development of DR. A recent population-based study investigated the association between daily sunlight exposure duration and DR [58]. The authors suggested that the risk of DR was 2.66 times higher in the group with ≥ 5 h of daily sunlight exposure than in the group with less exposure after adjusting for risk factors such as duration of diabetes, serum hemoglobin A1c level, hypertension, and dyslipidemia. Although a lot of evidence is still lacking, the results of the current study can be used as evidence that the effects of oxidative stress induced by H_2O_2 or UVB irradiation on the development of DR as well as the antioxidants can reduce disruption of outer BRB, which is represented by the viability of ARPE-19 cells.

This study successfully established an oxidative stress model of RPE which can be used to test potential antioxidative compounds. Since it has been known that oxidative stress is closely linked to diabetic retinopathy, identifying antioxidants like ascorbic acid and astaxanthin used in this study can also be beneficial to patients with diabetic retinopathy.

5. Conclusions

In summary, the antioxidative effect of ascorbic acid and astaxanthin was evaluated in this study using two different oxidative stress models achieved by H_2O_2 and UVB. Despite controversies questioning the antioxidative property of ascorbic acid, it was shown in this study that ascorbic acid diminishes the oxidative damage within human RPE oxidative stress models of H_2O_2 and UVB which reflect general circumstance of oxidatively stressed environment. This study also showed the ROS scavenging capacity of astaxanthin in a UVB-induced stress model. Synergistic effect of ascorbic acid and astaxanthin was also shown resulting in increment in cell viability and reduction in intracellular ROS level.

Author Contributions: S.O. performed the experiment and wrote the manuscript; Y.J.K. performed the experiment; E.K.L. reviewed, wrote, and edited the manuscript; S.W.P. designed the experiment; H.G.Y. designed all experiments and reviewed the manuscript. All authors have read and agreed to the published version of the manuscript.

Funding: This research was supported by a grant of the Korea Health Technology R&D Project through the Korea Health Industry Development Institute (KHIDI), funded by the Ministry of Health & Welfare, Republic of Korea (grant number: HI14C1277).

Conflicts of Interest: The authors declare no conflict of interest.

References

1. Klein, B.E. Overview of epidemiologic studies of diabetic retinopathy. *Ophthalmic Epidemiol.* **2007**, *14*, 179–183. [CrossRef] [PubMed]
2. Safi, S.Z.; Qvist, R.; Kumar, S.; Batumalaie, K.; Ismail, I.S. Molecular mechanisms of diabetic retinopathy, general preventive strategies, and novel therapeutic targets. *Biomed. Res. Int.* **2014**, *2014*, 801269. [CrossRef] [PubMed]
3. Chiu, C.J.; Taylor, A. Dietary hyperglycemia, glycemic index and metabolic retinal diseases. *Prog. Retin. Eye Res.* **2011**, *30*, 18–53. [CrossRef] [PubMed]
4. Nishikawa, M.; Inoue, M. Oxidative stress and tissue injury. *Masui* **2008**, *57*, 321–326.
5. Naruse, R.; Suetsugu, M.; Terasawa, T.; Ito, K.; Hara, K.; Takebayashi, K.; Morita, K.; Aso, Y.; Inukai, T. Oxidative stress and antioxidative potency are closely associated with diabetic retinopathy and nephropathy in patients with type 2 diabetes. *Saudi Med. J.* **2013**, *34*, 135–141.

6. Limón-Pacheco, J.; Gonsebatt, M.E. The role of antioxidants and antioxidant-related enzymes in protective responses to environmentally induced oxidative stress. *Mutat. Res. Genet. Toxicol. Environ. Mutagen.* **2009**, *674*, 137–147. [CrossRef] [PubMed]
7. Valle, I.; Álvarez-Barrientos, A.; Arza, E.; Lamas, S.; Monsalve, M. PGC-1α regulates the mitochondrial antioxidant defense system in vascular endothelial cells. *Cardiovasc. Res.* **2005**, *66*, 562–573. [CrossRef]
8. De Vries, H.E.; Witte, M.; Hondius, D.; Rozemuller, A.J.; Drukarch, B.; Hoozemans, J.; van Horssen, J. Nrf2-induced antioxidant protection: A promising target to counteract ROS-mediated damage in neurodegenerative disease? *Free Radic. Biol. Med.* **2008**, *45*, 1375–1383. [CrossRef]
9. Slemmer, J.E.; Shacka, J.J.; Sweeney, M.; Weber, J.T. Antioxidants and free radical scavengers for the treatment of stroke, traumatic brain injury and aging. *Curr. Med. Chem.* **2008**, *15*, 404–414.
10. Moradas-Ferreira, P.; Costa, V.; Piper, P.; Mager, W. The molecular defences against reactive oxygen species in yeast. *Mol. Microbiol.* **1996**, *19*, 651–658. [CrossRef]
11. Gultekin, F.; Delibas, N.; Yasar, S.; Kilinc, I. In vivo changes in antioxidant systems and protective role of melatonin and a combination of vitamin C and vitamin E on oxidative damage in erythrocytes induced by chlorpyrifos-ethyl in rats. *Arch. Toxicol.* **2001**, *75*, 88–96. [CrossRef] [PubMed]
12. Busik, J.V.; Mohr, S.; Grant, M.B. Hyperglycemia-induced reactive oxygen species toxicity to endothelial cells is dependent on paracrine mediators. *Diabetes* **2008**, *57*, 1952–1965. [CrossRef] [PubMed]
13. Okoduwa, S.I.; Umar, I.A.; Ibrahim, S.; Bello, F.; Habila, N. Age-dependent alteration of antioxidant defense system in hypertensive and type-2 diabetes patients. *J. Diabetes Metab. Disord.* **2015**, *14*, 32. [CrossRef]
14. Luo, L.; Chen, H.; Trush, M.A.; Show, M.D.; Anway, M.D.; Zirkin, B.R. Aging and the brown Norway rat leydig cell antioxidant defense system. *J. Androl.* **2006**, *27*, 240–247. [CrossRef]
15. Liguori, I.; Russo, G.; Curcio, F.; Bulli, G.; Aran, L.; Della-Morte, D.; Gargiulo, G.; Testa, G.; Cacciatore, F.; Bonaduce, D.; et al. Oxidative stress, aging, and diseases. *Clin. Interv. Aging* **2018**, *13*, 757. [CrossRef] [PubMed]
16. Halliwell, B. Antioxidants in human health and disease. *Ann. Rev. Nutr.* **1996**, *16*, 33–50. [CrossRef]
17. Noctor, G.; Foyer, C.H. Ascorbate and glutathione: Keeping active oxygen under control. *Ann. Rev. Plant Biol.* **1998**, *49*, 249–279. [CrossRef] [PubMed]
18. Naguib, Y.M. Antioxidant activities of astaxanthin and related carotenoids. *J. Agric. Food Chem.* **2000**, *48*, 1150–1154. [CrossRef]
19. Gil, M.I.; Tomás-Barberán, F.A.; Hess-Pierce, B.; Kader, A.A. Antioxidant capacities, phenolic compounds, carotenoids, and vitamin C contents of nectarine, peach, and plum cultivars from California. *J. Agric. Food Chem.* **2002**, *50*, 4976–4982. [CrossRef]
20. Marc, F.; Davin, A.; Deglène-Benbrahim, L.; Ferrand, C.; Baccaunaud, M.; Fritsch, P. Studies of several analytical methods for antioxidant potential evaluation in food. *Med. Sci.* **2004**, *20*, 458–463.
21. Ou, B.; Hampsch-Woodill, M.; Flanagan, J.; Deemer, E.K.; Prior, R.L.; Huang, D. Novel fluorometric assay for hydroxyl radical prevention capacity using fluorescein as the probe. *J. Agric. Food Chem.* **2002**, *50*, 2772–2777. [CrossRef] [PubMed]
22. Denev, P.; Ciz, M.; Ambrozova, G.; Lojek, A.; Yanakieva, I.; Kratchanova, M. Solid-phase extraction of berries' anthocyanins and evaluation of their antioxidative properties. *Food Chem.* **2010**, *123*, 1055–1061. [CrossRef]
23. Cao, G.; Prior, R.L. Comparison of different analytical methods for assessing total antioxidant capacity of human serum. *Clin. Chem.* **1998**, *44*, 1309–1315. [CrossRef] [PubMed]
24. Ozcan, T.; Sahin, S.; Akpinar-Bayizit, A.; Yilmaz-Ersan, L. Assessment of antioxidant capacity by method comparison and amino acid characterisation in buffalo milk kefir. *Int. J. Dairy Technol.* **2019**, *72*, 65–73. [CrossRef]
25. Rao, P.S.; Kiranmayi, V.; Swathi, P.; Jeyseelan, L.; Suchitra, M.; Bitla, A.R. Comparison of two analytical methods used for the measurement of total antioxidant status. *J. Antioxid. Act.* **2015**, *1*, 22.
26. Roy, M.K.; Koide, M.; Rao, T.P.; Okubo, T.; Ogasawara, Y.; Juneja, L.R. ORAC and DPPH assay comparison to assess antioxidant capacity of tea infusions: Relationship between total polyphenol and individual catechin content. *Int. J. Food Sci. Nutr.* **2010**, *61*, 109–124. [CrossRef]
27. Valverde Malaver, C.L.; Colmenares Dulcey, A.J.; Isaza Martínez, J.H. Comparison of DPPH free radical scavenging, ferric reducing antioxidant power (FRAP), and total phenolic content of two merania species (*Melastomataceae*). *Rev. Cienc.* **2015**, *19*, 117–124. [CrossRef]

28. Rácz, A.; Papp, N.; Balogh, E.; Fodor, M.; Héberger, K. Comparison of antioxidant capacity assays with chemometric methods. *Anal. Methods* **2015**, *7*, 4216–4224. [CrossRef]
29. Gille, J.; Joenje, H. Cell culture models for oxidative stress: Superoxide and hydrogen peroxide versus normobaric hyperoxia. *Mutat. Res. DNAging.* **1992**, *275*, 405–414. [CrossRef]
30. Sies, H. Hydrogen peroxide as a central redox signaling molecule in physiological oxidative stress: Oxidative eustress. *Red. Biol.* **2017**, *11*, 613–619. [CrossRef]
31. Wijeratne, S.S.; Cuppett, S.L.; Schlegel, V. Hydrogen peroxide induced oxidative stress damage and antioxidant enzyme response in Caco-2 human colon cells. *J. Agric. Food Chem.* **2005**, *53*, 8768–8774. [CrossRef] [PubMed]
32. Glickman, R.D. Ultraviolet phototoxicity to the retina. *Eye Contact Lens* **2011**, *37*, 196–205. [CrossRef] [PubMed]
33. Podda, M.; Traber, M.G.; Weber, C.; Yan, L.J.; Packer, L. UV-irradiation depletes antioxidants and causes oxidative damage in a model of human skin. *Free Radic. Biol. Med.* **1998**, *24*, 55–65. [CrossRef]
34. Wenk, J.; Brenneisen, P.; Meewes, C.; Wlaschek, M.; Peters, T.; Blaudschun, R.; Ma, W.; Kuhr, L.; Schneider, L.; Scharffetter-Kochanek, K.; et al. UV-induced oxidative stress and photoaging. *Curr. Probl. Dermatol.* **2001**, *29*, 83–94. [PubMed]
35. Cai, J.; Qi, X.; Kociok, N.; Skosyrski, S.; Emilio, A.; Ruan, Q.; Han, S.; Liu, L.; Chen, Z.; Rickman, C.B.; et al. β-Secretase (BACE1) inhibition causes retinal pathology by vascular dysregulation and accumulation of age pigment. *EMBO Mol. Med.* **2012**, *4*, 980–991. [CrossRef]
36. Zhao, L.; Man, Y.; Liu, S. Long non-coding RNA HULC promotes UVB-induced injury by up-regulation of BNIP3 in keratinocytes. *Biomed. Pharmacother.* **2018**, *104*, 672–678. [CrossRef]
37. Terra, V.; Souza-Neto, F.; Pereira, R.; Silva, T.; Costa, A.; Luiz, R.; Cecchini, R.; Cecchini, A. Time-dependent reactive species formation and oxidative stress damage in the skin after UVB irradiation. *J. Photochem. Photobiol. B Biol.* **2012**, *109*, 34–41. [CrossRef]
38. Li, Z.; Dong, X.; Liu, H.; Chen, X.; Shi, H.; Fan, Y.; Hou, D.; Zhang, X. Astaxanthin protects ARPE-19 cells from oxidative stress via upregulation of Nrf2-regulated phase II enzymes through activation of PI3K/Akt. *Mol. Vis.* **2013**, *19*, 1656–1666.
39. Bailey, T.A.; Kanuga, N.; Romero, I.A.; Greenwood, J.; Luthert, P.J.; Cheetham, M.E. Oxidative stress affects the junctional integrity of retinal pigment epithelial cells. *Investig. Ophthalmol. Vis. Sci.* **2004**, *45*, 675–684. [CrossRef]
40. Glaser, T.S.; Doss, L.E.; Shih, G.; Nigam, D.; Sperduto, R.D.; Ferris, F.L., 3rd; Agron, E.; Clemons, T.E.; Chew, E.Y. Age-related eye disease study research, g. the association of dietary lutein plus *Zeaxanthin* and B vitamins with cataracts in the age-related eye disease study: AREDS report no. 37. *Ophthalmology* **2015**, *122*, 1471–1479. [CrossRef]
41. Piermarocchi, S.; Saviano, S.; Parisi, V.; Tedeschi, M.; Panozzo, G.; Scarpa, G.; Boschi, G.; Lo Giudice, G.; Carmis Study, G. Carotenoids in Age-related Maculopathy Italian Study (CARMIS): Two-year results of a randomized study. *Eur. J. Ophthalmol.* **2012**, *22*, 216–225. [PubMed]
42. Zeitz, O.; Schlichting, L.; Richard, G.; Strauß, O. Lack of antioxidative properties of vitamin C and pyruvate in cultured retinal pigment epithelial cells. *Graefe Arch. Clin. Exp. Ophthalmol.* **2007**, *245*, 276–281. [CrossRef] [PubMed]
43. Kagan, D.B.; Liu, H.; Hutnik, C.M. Efficacy of various antioxidants in the protection of the retinal pigment epithelium from oxidative stress. *Clin. Ophthalmol.* **2012**, *6*, 1471. [PubMed]
44. Woo, K.I.; Lee, J. The effects of ascorbic acid on free radical injury in cultured retinal pigment epithelial cells. *Korean J. Ophthalmol.* **1995**, *9*, 19–25. [CrossRef] [PubMed]
45. Korte, C.S. Tert-Butyl Hydroperoxide Stimulates Parturition-Associated Pathways in a Human Placental Cell Line. Ph.D Thesis, University of Michigan, Ann Arbor, MI, USA, 17 September 2013.
46. Wang, Y.; Branicky, R.; Noë, A.; Hekimi, S. Superoxide dismutases: Dual roles in controlling ROS damage and regulating ROS signaling. *J. Cell Biol.* **2018**, *217*, 1915–1928. [CrossRef]
47. McKetta, J., Jr. *Encyclopedia of Chemical Processing and Design: Volume 65—Waste: Nuclear Reprocessing and Treatment Technologies to Wastewater Treatment: Multilateral Approach*; Routledge: London, UK, 2017.
48. Masaki, H.; Atsumi, T.; Sakurai, H. Detection of hydrogen peroxide and hydroxyl radicals in murine skin fibroblasts under UVB irradiation. *Biochem. Biophys. Res. Commun.* **1995**, *206*, 474–479. [CrossRef]
49. Guerra, B.A.; Bolin, A.P.; Otton, R. Carbonyl stress and a combination of astaxanthin/vitamin C induce biochemical changes in human neutrophils. *Toxicol Vitro.* **2012**, *26*, 1181–1190. [CrossRef]

50. Fassett, R.G.; Coombes, J.S. Astaxanthin: A potential therapeutic agent in cardiovascular disease. *Mar. Drugs.* **2011**, *9*, 447–465. [CrossRef]
51. Kowluru, R.A.; Tang, J.; Kern, T.S. Abnormalities of retinal metabolism in diabetes and experimental galactosemia. VII. Effect of long-term administration of antioxidants on the development of retinopathy. *Diabetes* **2001**, *50*, 1938–1942. [CrossRef]
52. Kanwar, M.; Chan, P.S.; Kern, T.S.; Kowluru, R.A. Oxidative damage in the retinal mitochondria of diabetic mice: Possible protection by superoxide dismutase. *Investig. Ophthalmol. Vis. Sci.* **2007**, *48*, 3805–3811. [CrossRef]
53. Kowluru, R.A.; Abbas, S.N. Diabetes-induced mitochondrial dysfunction in the retina. *Investig. Ophthalmol. Vis. Sci.* **2003**, *44*, 5327–5334. [CrossRef] [PubMed]
54. Kowluru, R.A. Diabetic retinopathy: Mitochondrial dysfunction and retinal capillary cell death. *Antioxid Redox. Signal* **2005**, *7*, 1581–1587. [CrossRef] [PubMed]
55. Wang, M.H.; Hsiao, G.; Al-Shabrawey, M. Eicosanoids and oxidative stress in diabetic retinopathy. *Antioxidants* **2020**, *9*, 520. [CrossRef] [PubMed]
56. Kaczara, P.; Sarna, T.; Burke, J.M. Dynamics of H2O2 availability to ARPE-19 cultures in models of oxidative stress. *Free Radic. Biol. Med.* **2010**, *48*, 1064–1070. [CrossRef]
57. Zheng, Y.; Liu, Y.; Ge, J.; Wang, X.; Liu, L.; Bu, Z.; Liu, P. Resveratrol protects human lens epithelial cells against H$_2$O$_2$-induced oxidative stress by increasing catalase, SOD-1, and HO-1 expression. *Mol. Vis.* **2010**, *16*, 1467–1474. [PubMed]
58. Lee, H.J.; Kim, C.O.; Lee, D.C. Association between daily sunlight exposure duration and diabetic retinopathy in Korean adults with diabetes: A nationwide population-based cross-sectional study. *PLoS ONE* **2020**, *15*, e0237149. [CrossRef]

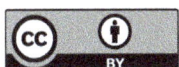

© 2020 by the authors. Licensee MDPI, Basel, Switzerland. This article is an open access article distributed under the terms and conditions of the Creative Commons Attribution (CC BY) license (http://creativecommons.org/licenses/by/4.0/).

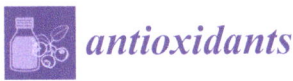

Article

Astaxanthin Protects Retinal Photoreceptor Cells against High Glucose-Induced Oxidative Stress by Induction of Antioxidant Enzymes via the PI3K/Akt/Nrf2 Pathway

Tso-Ting Lai [1,2], Chung-May Yang [1,3] and Chang-Hao Yang [1,3,*]

1. Department of Ophthalmology, National Taiwan University Hospital, Taipei 100, Taiwan; b91401005@ntu.edu.tw (T.-T.L.); chungmay@ntu.edu.tw (C.-M.Y.)
2. Graduate Institute of Clinical Medicine, College of Medicine, National Taiwan University, Taipei 100, Taiwan
3. Department of Ophthalmology, College of Medicine, National Taiwan University, Taipei 100, Taiwan
* Correspondence: chyangoph@ntu.edu.tw; Tel.: +886-2-2312-3456 (ext. 62131); Fax: +886-2-2393-4420

Received: 22 July 2020; Accepted: 7 August 2020; Published: 10 August 2020

Abstract: Diabetic retinopathy (DR) is a major microvascular complication that can lead to severe visual impairment in patients with diabetes. The elevated oxidative stress and increased reactive oxygen species (ROS) production induced by hyperglycemia have been reported to play an important role in the complex pathogenesis of DR. Astaxanthin (AST), a natural carotenoid derivative, has been recently recognized as a strong free radical scavenger and might, therefore, be beneficial in different diseases, including DR. In this study, we evaluated the potential role of AST as an antioxidative and antiapoptotic agent in protecting retinal cells and also investigated the involvement of the PI3K/Akt/Nrf2 pathway in AST-mediated effects. We treated high glucose-cultured mouse photoreceptor cells (661W) with different concentrations of AST and analyzed ROS production and cell apoptosis in the different regimens. Moreover, we also analyzed the expression of PI3K, Akt, Nrf2, and Phase II enzymes after AST treatment. Our results showed that AST dose-dependently reduced ROS production and attenuated 661W cell apoptosis in a high glucose environment. Importantly, its protective effect was abolished by treatment with PI3K or Nrf2 inhibitors, indicating the involvement of the PI3K/Akt/Nrf2 pathway. These results suggest AST as a nutritional supplement that could benefit patients with DR.

Keywords: diabetic retinopathy; hyperglycemia; oxidative stress; astaxanthin; carotenoid; reactive oxygen species; apoptosis; photoreceptor cells; PI3K; Nrf2

1. Introduction

Diabetes is a major metabolic disease that can affect different organs through microvascular and macrovascular damages [?]. Diabetic retinopathy (DR), a leading microvascular complication of diabetes, is characterized by a progressive increase in vascular permeability, retinal ischemia and edema, and neovascularization, which can result in visual impairment and even legal blindness [?]. Despite the improved understanding of its pathogenesis and the advances in available treatments, the long-term outcome of DR remains poor owing to its complex pathogenesis [? ?]. Therefore, the continuous search for new modalities to prevent and treat this debilitating complication is essential.

Hyperglycemia induces oxidative stress and generates reactive oxygen species (ROS) within the retina [? ?]; however, the activity of cellular antioxidant enzymes responding to ROS is insufficient to prevent the consequent damages. Yeh et al. reported a positive correlation between ROS levels in vitreous fluid and the severity of DR [?]. In addition, several studies have indicated chronic oxidative stress as one of the primary causes of DR [? ? ? ? ?]. Normally, the retina already presents substantial lipid oxidation and ROS production due to the high content of unsaturated fatty acids and high oxygen uptake, which render it more vulnerable to oxidative stress damage than other tissues [? ?]. Furthermore, ROS accumulation alters the homeostasis of retinal cells, triggers cellular apoptosis, and leads to increased vascular permeability and basement membrane leakage in the retina. These pathological changes may lead to a breakdown of the blood–retinal barrier and the development of DR [? ?]. Thus, reducing oxidative stress could inhibit apoptosis in retinal cells and reduce the risk of DR progression.

Astaxanthin (AST) is a member of the xanthophyll family of oxygenated carotenoid derivatives. AST has been recently recognized as a strong free radical scavenger and an excellent anti-inflammatory agent that suppresses the expression of proinflammatory chemokines and cytokines [? ?]. The unique molecular structure of AST, which contains hydroxyl and keto moieties on each ionone ring, explains its high antioxidant activity [?]. Mechanistically, AST terminates the free radical chain reaction by donating electrons and reacting with free radicals to convert them to more stable products [? ?]. AST can, therefore, act as a powerful antioxidant in numerous organisms. In fact, AST has been attributed as having the potential to defend organisms against a broad range of diseases, including cardiovascular disease [?], ischemic brain damage [?], cataracts [?], diabetes [?], and diabetic nephropathy [? ?]. AST has also shown protective effects in ocular diseases, including neuroprotection in retinal ganglion cells [?], suppression of choroid neovascularization development [?], and reduction of endotoxin-induced uveitis [?].

Recent studies have shown that AST can activate the Nrf2–antioxidant responsive element (ARE) pathway in different cell types and organs [? ? ? ? ?]. The Nrf2–ARE pathway is an important endogenous mechanism that can attenuate oxidative stress within the cell [? ?]. Nrf2 induces the expression of Phase II enzymes, including NAD(P)H dehydrogenase (NQO1) and heme oxygenase-1(HO-1), thereby limiting the subsequent generation of ROS and promoting the formation of antioxidant bilirubin [? ? ? ?]. An earlier study indicated that retinal pigment epithelial (RPE) cells could be protected against oxidative damage by activating the Nrf2–ARE pathway and increasing expression of Phase II enzymes [?]. A later study further showed the crucial role of the PI3K/Akt pathway in modulating Nrf2–ARE-dependent protection against oxidative stress in RPE cells [?].

Therefore, in this study, we hypothesized that AST could counteract high glucose-induced oxidative stress and attenuate oxidative stress-induced apoptosis by modulating Nrf2 expression in retinal photoreceptor cells. To test our hypotheses, we first investigated the role of high glucose-induced oxidative stress in initiating retinal photoreceptor cell (661W) apoptosis and evaluated the antioxidative and antiapoptotic effects of AST. Moreover, we analyzed the modulatory effect of AST on Nrf2 expression and analyzed the related signaling pathway. Our results showed that AST reduced high glucose-induced oxidative stress and attenuated apoptosis of photoreceptor cells by induction of antioxidant enzymes via the PI3K/Akt/Nrf2 pathway.

2. Materials and Methods

2.1. Cell Culture and Experimental Design

In this study, we used the 661W cell line, obtained from Dr. M. Al-Ubaidi (University of Houston), to evaluate the response of photoreceptor cells to AST treatment. The 661W cells, exhibiting biochemical features characteristic of cone photoreceptor cells, constitute an immortalized mouse photoreceptor cell line (by the expression of simian virus 40 T antigen) [?]. We cultured the 661W cells in Dulbecco's modified Eagle's media (DMEM) containing 10% phosphate buffer solution (PBS) and 1% penicillin–streptomycin (100 U/mL penicillin and 100 µg/mL streptomycin) at 37 °C and 5% CO_2. Cells were passaged by trypsinization every 3–4 days and used for experiments at the second to fifth passage. For the experiment, the cells were exposed to either normal (5 mM/mL) or high glucose (35 mM/mL) concentration. In addition, the cells were pretreated with 10, 20, or 50 µM AST (Sigma, St. Louis, MO, USA) for 2 h prior to high glucose treatment. After 24 h treatment, the cells were collected and further analyzed. Two different inhibitors, PI3K inhibitor (LY294002, 20 µM, (Sigma, St. Louis, MO, USA)) and Nrf2 inhibitor (ML385, 10 µM, (Selleck Chemicals, Houston, TX, USA)) were used to determine the causal relationship between AST and the changes in other antioxidative molecules. The cultured cells were pretreated with either of the inhibitors and 50 µM AST simultaneously for 2 h, followed by high glucose treatment for 24 h.

2.2. Cell Viability Assay

Cell viability assay was performed with CyQUANT MTT Cell Viability Assay Kit (Invitrogen-Life Technologies Inc., Gaithersburg, MD, USA). The cells were seeded in 96-well plates (1×10^4 cells per well) and incubated at 37 °C. Different concentrations of AST were added to the cells exposed to high glucose. After 24 h incubation, 5 mg/mL 3-(4,5-dimethylthiazol-2-yl)-2,5-diphenyltetrazolium bromide (MTT) was added to each well and incubated at 37 °C for 4 h. The culture medium supernatant was removed, and the formazan was dissolved with dimethyl sulfoxide (DMSO) for 30 min at 25 °C. The absorbance was measured at 570 nm with a microplate reader (Bio-Rad Laboratories, Inc., Hercules, CA, USA).

2.3. Analysis of Apoptosis by Terminal Deoxynucleotidyl Transferase dUTP Nick End Labeling (TUNEL)

We used TUNEL to detect 661W cell apoptosis. TUNEL was performed using a commercial kit (Millipore Corp., Billerica, MA, USA) according to the manufacturer's instructions. Positive controls were cultured cells incubated with DNase I prior to the labeling procedure, and sham controls were cells stained with label solution containing no terminal transferase.

2.4. Detection of Intracellular ROS

We used Image-IT Green Reactive Oxygen Species Detection Kit (Invitrogen-Life Technologies Inc., Gaithersburg, MD, USA) to determine the level of ROS under different conditions. Intracellular ROS levels were measured using 2',7'-dichlorodihydrofluorescein diacetate (2',7'-DCFDA) oxidation. For the detection of ROS, 661W cells were exposed to 10 µM 2',7'-DCFDA; in the presence of ROS, bright green fluorescence could be detected by a fluorescence microscope (Thermo Fisher Scientific Inc., Waltham, MA, USA).

2.5. Quantitative Detection of Nrf2 and ROS-Induced Cellular Oxidation Using Immunocytochemistry (ICC)

DNA oxidation, lipid peroxidation, and protein oxidation levels were determined by detecting the expression of 8-hydroxydeoxyguanosine (8-OHdG), acrolein, and nitrotyrosine, respectively, using ICC according to a previously published protocol [?]. In brief, the cultured cells were simultaneously blocked and permeabilized with 0.2% Triton in PBS containing 5% goat serum for 1 h at room temperature. Then, cells were incubated with primary antibodies diluted in blocking solution overnight at 4 °C, followed by incubation with the appropriate fluorescent secondary antibodies (all diluted 1:200) in blocking solution for 3 h at room temperature. Primary antibodies included anti-Nrf2, antiacrolein, antinitrotyrosine, and anti-8-OHdG (all from Abcam, Cambridge, MA, USA). Nuclei were counterstained with DAPI.

The quantitative protein expression measurements were done by densitometric methods as previously described [?]. The relative density of immunostaining was analyzed by an immunostaining index comparing 661W cells treated with different AST concentrations and high glucose condition versus low glucose condition (as normal reference).

2.6. Determination of Changes in Mitochondrial Membrane Potential

The mitochondrial membrane potential was measured using a fluorescence reader with JC-1 stain (Sigma, St. Louis, MO, USA) and a lipophilic cationic probe to detect the extent of mitochondrial dysfunction. The 661W cells were seeded in 96-well plates (1×10^4 cells per well) and incubated at 37 °C. Then, different concentrations of AST were added to the cells exposed to high glucose. After 24 h incubation, 5 µL of JC-1 staining solution was added to each well, and the plate was incubated at 37 °C for 15 min. The fluorescence intensity for both J-aggregates with Texas Red (healthy cells, excitation/emission = 560/595 nm) and JC-1 monomers with FITC (apoptotic or unhealthy cells, excitation/emission = 485/535 nm) were measured with a microplate reader (Bio-Rad Laboratories, Inc., Hercules, CA, USA). For microscopy, the cells were incubated in 24-well plates. Then, 50 µL of JC-1 staining buffer was added to 1 mL of culture medium. After incubation at 37 °C for 30 min, the cells were observed using fluorescence microscopy. J-aggregates and JC-1 monomers were detected with settings designed to detect Texas Red and FITC, respectively.

2.7. Preparation of RNA and cDNA

Total RNA was extracted from the retinas using TRIzol reagent (Invitrogen-Life Technologies Inc., Gaithersburg, MD, USA). For each sample, 1 µg of total RNA was incubated with 300 ng of Oligo dT for 5 min at 65 °C and reverse-transcribed into cDNA using 80 U of Moloney murine leukemia virus reverse transcriptase per 50 µg reaction sample for 1 h at 37 °C. The reaction was stopped by heating the samples for 5 min at 90 °C.

2.8. Quantitative Analysis of mRNA Levels

We performed polymerase chain reaction (PCR) on the resultant cDNA from each sample using specific primers. The amplification was performed using a thermocycler (Applied Biosystems, Waltham, MA, USA). The 25 µL reaction mixture contained 5 µL of cDNA, 1 µL of sense and antisense primers, 200 µM of each deoxynucleotide (DTT), 5 µL of 10× Taq polymerase buffer, and 1.25 U of GoTaq polymerase (Applied Biosystems, Waltham, MA, USA). The PCR reactions were performed using an annealing temperature of 56 °C with GoTaq polymerase, cDNA, and the following primers: sense 5′-ATGACACCAAGGACCAGAGC and antisense 5′-GTAAGGACCCATCGGAGAAGC for HO-1; sense 5′-TATCCTGCCGAGTCTGTTCTG and antisense 5′-AACTGGAATATCACAAGGTCTGC for NQO1; and sense 5′-CGACTTCAACAGCAACTCCCACTC and antisense 5′-TGGGTGGTCCAGGGTTTCTTACTC for glyceraldehyde 3-phosphate dehydrogenase (GAPDH). The DNA fragments were amplified for 25–30 cycles (30 s at 94 °C; 1 min at 50–52 °C; 1 min at 72 °C), followed by a final 7 min extension step at 72 °C. The amplified products were further analyzed. Levels of each mRNA were normalized to those of GAPDH mRNA.

2.9. Protein Extractions and Western Blot Analysis

We extracted total proteins from the 661W cells using radioimmunoprecipitation assay (RIPA) lysis buffer (0.5 M Tris-HCl (pH 7.4), 1.5 M NaCl, 2.5% deoxycholic acid, 10% NP-40, 10 mM EDTA, and 10% protease inhibitors). Before analysis, the protein samples were separated on a 10% sodium dodecyl sulfate (SDS)–polyacrylamide gel and transferred to a polyvinylidene difluoride membrane. The membranes were probed using the following antibodies: anti-HO-1; anti-NQO1 (from Abcam, Cambridge, MA, USA); anti-PI3K; anti-Akt; anti-phospho-Akt(p-Akt); anti-caspase-3; anti-poly(ADP-ribose) polymerase (PARP) (from Cell Signaling Technology, Danvers, MA, USA); and anti-GAPDH (Millipore Corp., Billerica, MA, USA). Immunodetections were done using enhanced chemiluminescence (Pierce Biotechnology, Rockford, IL, USA) according to the manufacturer's instructions. Protein levels were determined using densitometry analysis of the protein bands.

2.10. Nuclear Protein Extraction and Electrophoretic Mobility Shift Assay (EMSA)

The 661W cells treated with low glucose, high glucose, and different concentrations of AST were harvested separately. Nuclear proteins were prepared as described before [?]. In brief, the cells were trypsinized, resuspended, and homogenized in ice-cold buffer A (10 mM 4-(2-hydroxyethyl)-1-piperazineethanesulfonic acid (HEPES) (pH 7.9), 1.5 mM KCl, 10 mM MgCl2, 1.0 mM dithiothreitol (DTT), and 1.0 mM phenylmethylsulfonyl fluoride (PMSF)). The cell suspensions were homogenized and centrifuged for 10 min at 5000× g at 4 °C. The sediment was resuspended in 200 µL of buffer B (20 mM HEPES (pH 7.9), 25% glycerol, 1.5 mM MgCl2, 420 mM NaCl, 0.5 mM DTT, 0.2 mM EDTA, 0.5 mM PMSF, and 4 µM leupeptin). Then, the samples were incubated for 30 min on ice and centrifuged for another 30 min at 12,000× g at 4 °C. The supernatants containing the nuclear proteins were collected for further analysis. A bicinchoninic acid assay kit, with bovine serum albumin as the standard, was used to determine the protein concentration. EMSA was performed with a Nrf2 DNA-binding protein detection system (Abcam, Cambridge, MA, USA) according to the manufacturer's instructions. Ten micrograms of nuclear protein was incubated with a biotin-labeled Nrf2 consensus oligonucleotide probe (5′-GCACAAAGCGCTGAGTCACGGGGAGG-3′) for 30 min in binding buffer. The specificity of the DNA/protein binding was then determined by adding a 100-fold molar excess of unlabeled Nrf2 oligonucleotide for competitive binding, 10 min before adding the biotin-labeled probe.

2.11. Statistical Analyses

The results are expressed as the mean ± standard deviation where applicable. The data were analyzed using SPSS software (SPSS 22.0; SPSS Inc., Chicago, IL, USA). The Mann–Whitney U test was used to calculate the differences between the means of different experimental groups. p values of less than 0.05 were considered significant.

3. Results

3.1. Astaxanthin Protects 661W Cells from Apoptosis under High Glucose Conditions

To evaluate the potential role of AST as a therapeutic agent, we first tested the safety of different concentrations (1, 5, 10, 20, and 50 µM) of AST on 661W cells. The cell viability was not affected by treatment with up to 50 µM AST, as shown by MTT assay (Figure ??A). Therefore, 10, 20, and 50 µM AST were used for the following experiments. To evaluate the protective effect of AST in 661W cells under high glucose conditions, we used the TUNEL assay to detect apoptosis. The results demonstrated a dose-dependent protective effect of AST against 661W cell apoptosis in a high glucose environment (Figure ??B), with a significantly decreased number of apoptotic cells upon treatment with 20 and 50 µM AST. The antiapoptotic effect of AST was further confirmed by decreased caspase-3 cleavage and decreased PARP in AST-treated 661W cells (Figure ??C).

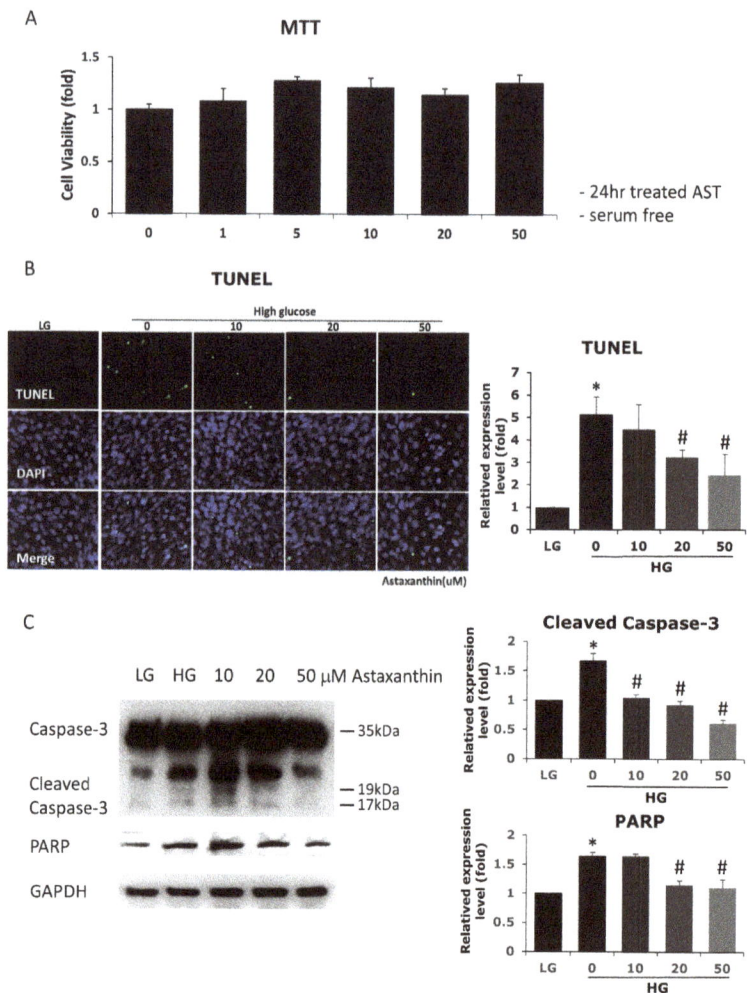

Figure 1. Effects of AST on cell viability and high glucose-induced apoptosis in 661W cells. (**A**) Cell viability was evaluated using MTT assay upon treatment with different concentrations of AST for 24 h. AST-treated and control cells showed similar cell viability. (**B**) Increased cell apoptosis was noted under high glucose environment, demonstrated by TUNEL assay and protein expression (western blots, **C**). AST reduced apoptosis at 20 and 50 μM concentration. (**C**) Decreased cleaved caspase-3 and PARP protein expression seen in western blots indicated that apoptosis was attenuated by AST. AST = astaxanthin; HG = high glucose; LG = low glucose; MTT = 3-(4,5-dimethylthiazol-2-yl)-2,5-diphenyltetrazolium bromide; TUNEL = terminal deoxynucleotidyl transferase dUTP nick end labeling; PARP = poly(ADP-ribose) polymerase; GAPDH = glyceraldehyde 3-phosphate dehydrogenase. * Significantly different from control group ($p < 0.05$); # significantly different from high glucose-treated group without AST ($p < 0.05$). The Mann–Whitney U test was used to calculate the differences between the means of different experimental groups (three repeats per experiment, three wells per repeat, five images per well analyzed).

3.2. Astaxanthin Reduces ROS and ROS-Related Mitochondrial Damage

To understand if the observed attenuation in apoptosis resulted from the antioxidative effect of AST, we measured the intracellular ROS levels in cells treated with different concentrations of this compound. AST reduced the levels of ROS increased by high glucose treatment in 661W cells at 20 µM and 50 µM concentration (Figure ??A). The ROS-related mitochondrial damages, detected by JC-1 staining, were also reduced by AST treatment (Figure ??B).

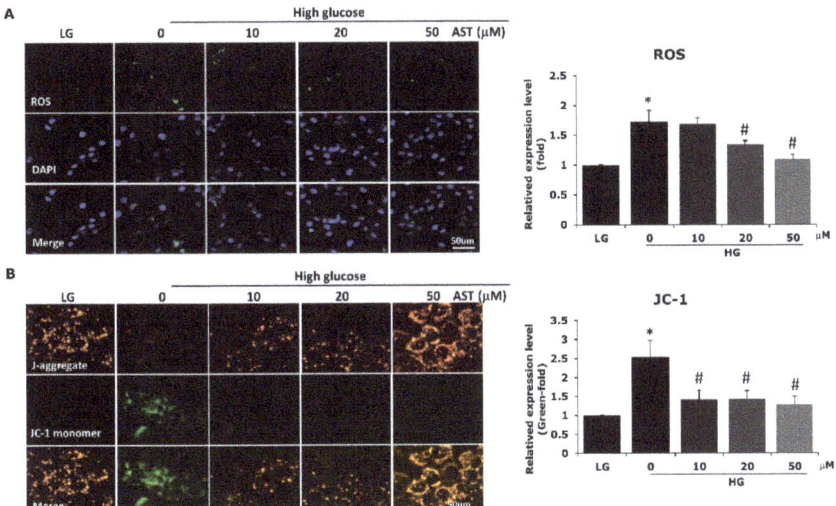

Figure 2. AST reduced ROS and ROS-related mitochondrial damage. (**A**) 661W cells pretreated with different concentrations of AST for 2 h were cultured under high glucose environment. Intracellular ROS levels were detected by measuring the green fluorescence of 2′,7′-dichlorodihydrofluorescein diacetate oxidation. ROS levels were significantly reduced in cells pretreated with 20 and 50 µM of AST. (**B**) Mitochondrial membrane potential was evaluated by JC-1 staining. The results showed decreased mitochondrial damage after AST treatment. AST = astaxanthin; HG = high glucose; LG = low glucose; ROS = reactive oxygen species. * Significantly different from control group ($p < 0.05$); # significantly different from high glucose-treated group without AST ($p < 0.05$). The Mann–Whitney U test was used to calculate the differences between the means of different experimental groups (three repeats per experiment, three wells per repeat, five images per well analyzed).

3.3. Astaxanthin Reduces ROS-Related Lipid, Protein, and DNA Damage

Increased intracellular ROS levels can cause further damage to lipids, proteins, and DNA, which may eventually lead to apoptosis. We therefore evaluated the expression of acrolein, nitrotyrosine, and 8-OHdG using different concentrations of AST. The levels of all three surrogate markers decreased with increasing concentrations of AST, indicating the antioxidative capacity of AST treatment (Figure ??). Significantly reduced damage to lipids and DNA (indicated by acrolein and 8-OHdG, respectively) and to proteins (indicated by nitrotyrosine) was observed with at least 10 or 20 µM AST, respectively.

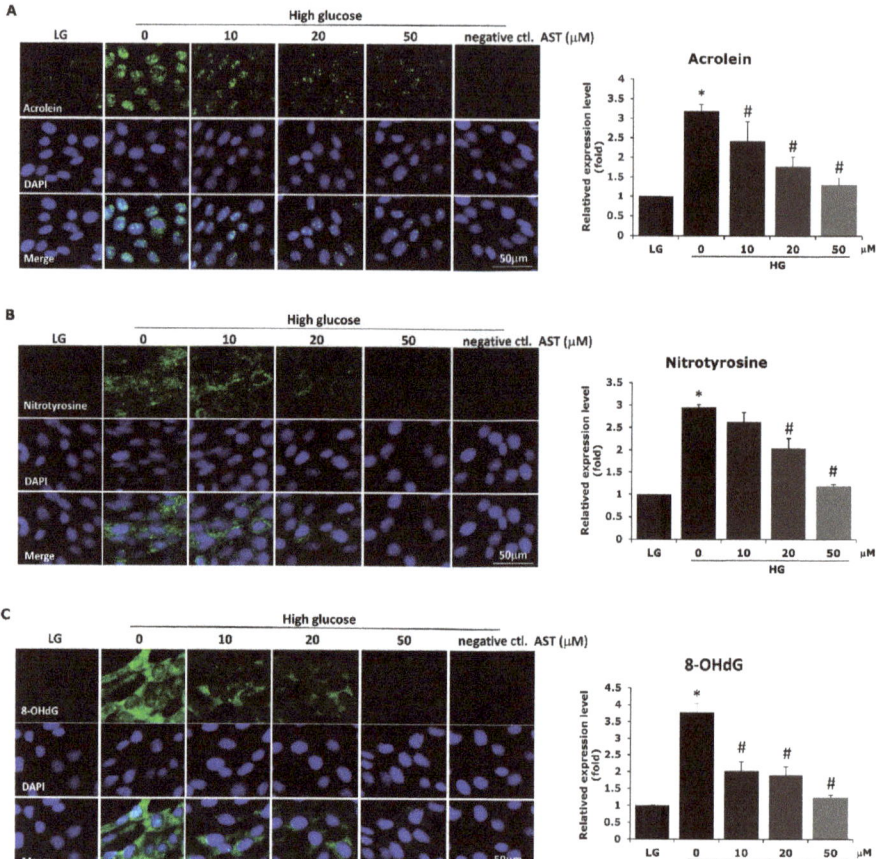

Figure 3. AST reduces ROS-related lipid, protein, and DNA damage in high glucose-treated 661W cells. To confirm that high glucose-induced ROS-related damage was also attenuated by AST treatment, we measured the expression of acrolein (**A**), nitrotyrosine (**B**), and 8-OHdG (**C**) by immunocytochemistry to indicate the oxidative damages to lipids, proteins, and DNA, respectively. Significantly decreased oxidative damage was noted under AST treatment. AST = astaxanthin; HG = high glucose; LG = low glucose; ROS = reactive oxygen species. * Significantly different from control group ($p < 0.05$); # significantly different from high glucose-treated group without AST ($p < 0.05$). The Mann–Whitney U test was used to calculate the differences between the means of different experimental groups (three repeats per experiment, three wells per repeat, five images per well analyzed).

3.4. Astaxanthin Reduces ROS through Upregulation of Phase II Enzymes

The Phase II enzymes HO-1 and NQO1, which exhibit antioxidative properties and are known to reduce intracellular ROS, have been reported to be upregulated by AST [? ? ?]. To confirm if the reduction in ROS induced by AST in our study was associated with a change in Phase II enzyme expression, we evaluated both the mRNA and protein levels of HO-1 and NQO1. We found that Phase II enzymes were upregulated both at the mRNA and protein levels after AST treatment in a dose-dependent fashion (Figure ??).

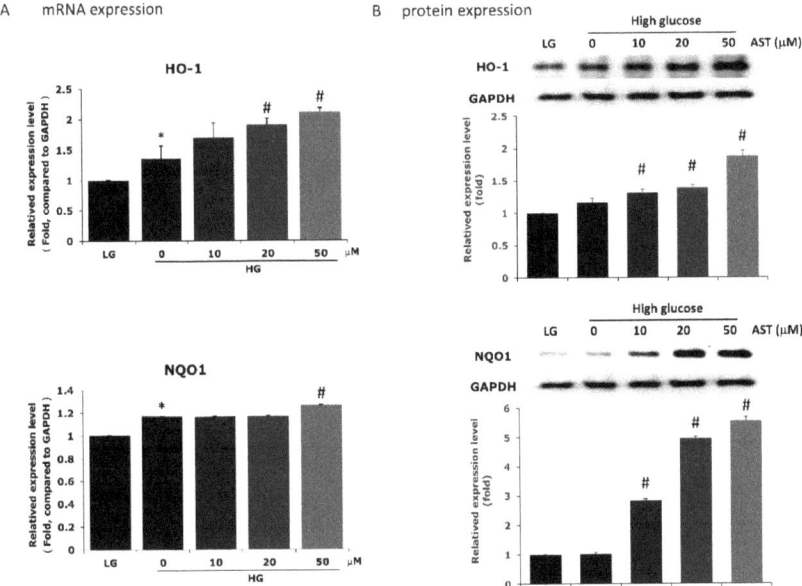

Figure 4. AST promotes the expression of Phase II enzymes HO-1 and NQO1 in 661W cells. The expression of HO-1 and NQO1 was determined in AST-treated 661W cells by measuring the mRNA levels with qPCR (**A**) and the corresponding protein levels by western blot (**B**). The measurements were normalized to GAPDH. AST = astaxanthin; HO-1 = Heme oxygenase-1; HG = high glucose; LG = low glucose; NQO1 = NAD(P)H dehydrogenase. * Significantly different from control group ($p < 0.05$); # significantly different from high glucose-treated group without AST ($p < 0.05$). The Mann–Whitney U test was used to calculate the differences between the means of different experimental groups.

3.5. Astaxanthin Activates PI3K/Akt Pathway and Upregulates the Expression of Nrf2

We further evaluated the activation of the PI3K/Akt pathway and the expression of Nrf2 under AST treatment to better understand how AST protects 661W cells from high glucose-induced damage. Treatment of 661W cells cultured in high glucose with 20 and 50 μM AST increased PI3K protein levels, which further increased the downstream p-Akt/Akt ratio (Figure ??A,B). In the same culture conditions, we found increased nuclear expression of Nrf2 upon treatment with AST (Figure ??C). Moreover, activation of Nrf2 was observed 30 min after treatment with 50 μM AST (Figure ??D). These results indicate that AST activates the PI3K/Akt/Nrf2 pathway, which further contributes to decreasing the ROS generated in a high glucose environment.

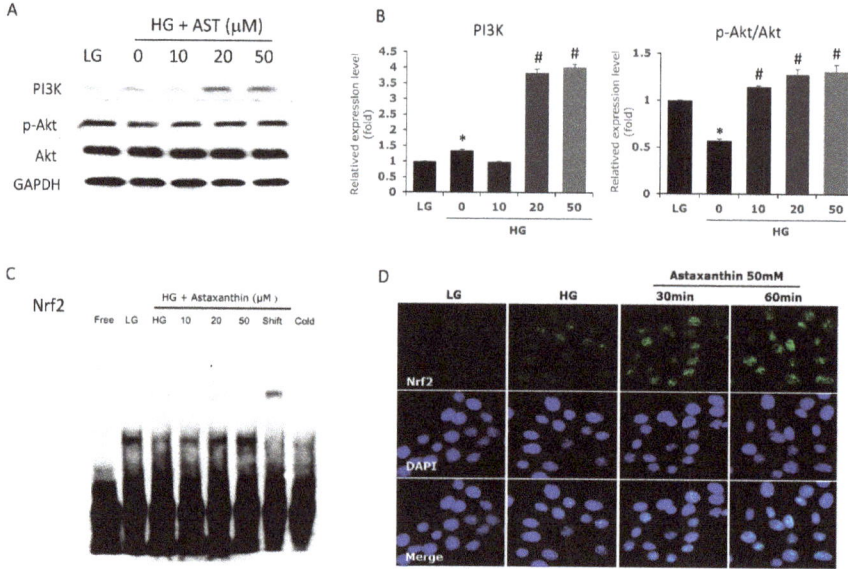

Figure 5. AST upregulates the expression of the PI3K/Akt/Nrf2 pathway in 661W cells. (**A,B**) The expression of PI3K and phosphorylated Akt proteins were detected by western blot. 661W cells were pretreated with different concentrations of AST for 2 h and grown in high glucose for 24 h. (**C**) Nrf2 levels in nuclear protein extracts were determined by electrophoretic mobility shift assay. (**D**) Immunocytochemistry confirmed the increased expression of Nrf2 after AST treatment. AST = astaxanthin; HG = high glucose; LG = low glucose. * Significantly different from control group ($p < 0.05$); # significantly different from high glucose-treated group without AST ($p < 0.05$). The Mann–Whitney U test was used to calculate the differences between the means of different experimental groups.

3.6. Inhibition of Both PI3K and Nrf2 Attenuate the Antioxidative Effect of AST

To confirm whether the protective effects of AST act through the PI3K/Akt/Nrf2 pathway, we added the PI3K inhibitor LY294002 (20 µM) and Nrf2 inhibitor ML385 (10 µM) and observed the corresponding changes in Phase II enzyme production and ROS levels. In the presence of PI3K inhibitor, downstream p-Akt decreased accordingly. Moreover, the levels of both HO-1 and NQO1 were lower upon treatment with the PI3K inhibitor than with AST alone (Figure ??A). The Nrf2 inhibitor also downregulated the AST-enhanced expression of HO-1 and NQO1 while not affecting p-Akt. Both PI3K and Nrf2 inhibitors attenuated the reduction in ROS induced by AST (Figure ??B). These results confirmed the sequential changes and causal relationship between PI3K/Akt pathway, Nrf2 and Phase II enzyme expression, and apoptosis with the protective effects of AST in photoreceptor cells.

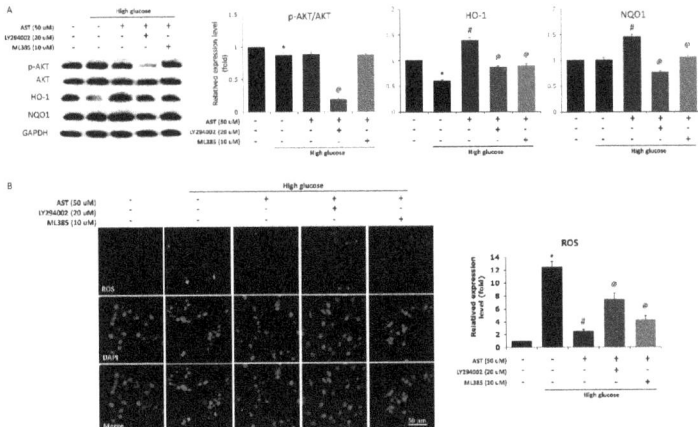

Figure 6. Blocking the PI3K/Akt/Nrf2 pathway abolishes the antioxidative effect of AST in 661W cells. Cells were administered PI3K inhibitor (LY294002, 20 µM) and Nrf2 inhibitor (ML385, 10 µM) along with AST. (**A**) The protein expression of Akt, p-Akt, HO-1, and NQO1 was detected by western blot. The PI3K inhibitor resulted in lower p-Akt/Akt ratio, HO-1, and NQO1 expression compared with AST treatment alone. Meanwhile, Nrf2 inhibition resulted in decreased expression of HO-1 and NQO1 but not the p-Akt/Akt ratio. (**B**) Both inhibitors counteracted the protective effect of AST and significantly increased the ROS levels, AST = astaxanthin; ROS = reactive oxygen species. * Significantly different from control group ($p < 0.05$); # significantly different from high glucose-treated group without AST ($p < 0.05$); @ significantly different from high glucose-treated group with 50 µM AST. The Mann–Whitney U test was used to calculate the differences between the means of different experimental groups (three repeats per experiment, three wells per repeat, five images per well analyzed).

4. Discussion

Astaxanthin possesses unique chemical properties derived from its distinctive molecular structure, including two hydroxyl groups, two carbonyl groups, and 11 conjugated ethylenic double bonds. In contrast to other carotenoids, AST can be esterified, has a more polar nature, and displays greater antioxidant capacity, which could be explained by the presence of the hydroxyl and keto moieties on each ionone ring [?]. AST was recently reported to significantly suppress oxidative stress and protect various cells from apoptosis [? ? ? ? ?]. In this study, we demonstrated that AST could protect photoreceptor cells from oxidative stress through activation of the PI3K/Akt/Nrf2 signaling pathway in high glucose environments, which further reduced apoptosis and could potentially prevent the progression of DR.

The correlation between oxidative stress and the development of DR has been previously demonstrated [? ? ? ? ? ?]. Increased oxidative stress and production of ROS cause tissue injury through peroxidation of lipids, carbohydrates, proteins, and DNA [?], with the concomitant production of oxidative biomarkers, such as acrolein, carbonylated proteins, nitrotyrosine, and 8-OHdG [? ?]. In this study, we confirmed the harmful effects of high glucose by showing an increase in ROS, oxidative biomarkers 8-OHdG, nitrotyrosine, and acrolein, as well as apoptosis. In addition, our results also demonstrated that the oxidative stress and consequent ROS-induced damage to DNA, lipids, and proteins could be ameliorated by the antioxidative effect of AST. The overall reduction in oxidative stress mediated by AST further led to decreased apoptosis of photoreceptor cells. Baccouche et al. [?] found that short-term use of AST could reduce retinal damage in fat sand rats. In their study, while the serum glucose levels were similar in the AST-treated animals and the control group, the cellular damage in Muller cells and retinal ganglion cells was reduced by AST treatment through increased HO-1 production. Dong et al. [?] also reported a protective effect of AST against the oxidative stress induced by diabetes in retinal ganglion cells. Another study using streptozotocin-induced diabetic rats demonstrated the antioxidative effect of AST in the retina in a high glucose environment [?]. In this study, after AST treatment, the retinal thickness was preserved not only in the inner but also in the outer retinal layers. The cellular damage in DR is not limited to retinal ganglion cells. Photoreceptor loss in DR due to increased apoptosis has also been reported [?]. Our results confirm that the antiapoptotic effect of AST is not limited to ganglion cells and Muller cells but also extends to photoreceptors, indicating the potential universal benefits of AST treatment in DR.

The Nrf2–ARE pathway plays an important role in cellular resistance to oxidative stress [? ? ?]. Nrf2 is a transcription factor that binds to the ARE and promotes the expression of Phase II enzymes [?]. In the absence of oxidative damage, Nrf2 interacts with the chaperone Keap1; conversely, in an oxidant environment, Nrf2 dissociates from Keap1 and translocates to the nucleus in its activated form, where it binds to the ARE and induces the expression of Phase II enzymes, such as HO-1 and NQO1 [?]. Several studies have demonstrated the beneficial effects of Nrf2 activation in DR. Fenofibrate was reported to activate Nrf2, increase HO-1 and NQO1 expression, and reduce oxidative damage in diabetic mice [?]. Sulforaphane also exhibited similar antioxidative effects in streptozotocin-induced diabetic rats and high glucose-treated Muller cells through the activation of the Nrf2 pathway [?]. Furthermore, activation of Nrf2, either through DJ-1 overexpression [?] or through Nrf2 activators [?], could provide additional benefits to improve retinal pericyte survival and reduce vascular endothelial growth factor-induced cell migration in human retinal microvascular endothelial cells, both involved in the development of DR. In the current study, we have further demonstrated that the Nrf2–ARE pathway can be activated by AST, thereby increasing the expression of HO-1 and NQO1, which in turn attenuates ROS-mediated and intracellular oxidative damage and further protects photoreceptor cells from high glucose-induced apoptosis.

AST can ameliorate cell apoptosis via more than one pathway, including ERK, NF-κB, and PI3K/Akt [? ? ?]. Among these, the PI3K/Akt pathway is a prominent regulator of numerous proteins involved in cell survival through profound antioxidative and antiapoptotic actions [?]. Studying apoptosis after burn in an animal model, Guo et al. demonstrated a dose-dependent effect of AST in increasing p-Akt and decreasing cleaved caspase-3 levels [?]. In diabetic rats, the cognitive functions could also be preserved by AST through activation of the PI3K/Akt pathway and downregulation of caspase-3 expression [?]. In RPE cells, Li et al. [?] reported that oxidative stress was attenuated by AST. They further demonstrated that AST upregulates Nrf2 and Nrf2-related Phase II enzymes through activation of the PI3K/Akt pathway. Collectively, these pieces of evidence support the involvement of the PI3K/Akt pathway in the antiapoptotic effect of AST. Nevertheless, the cellular response to AST may differ among distinct cell types and with diverse environmental stimuli. In a hamster model of oral cancer, Kavitha et al. [?] found downregulated PI3K and p-Akt in AST-treated animals, which further led to caspase-induced apoptosis. Therefore, we specifically focused here on the response of photoreceptor cells. Our study clearly demonstrated that the PI3K/Akt pathway was upregulated in the presence of AST and that downstream Nrf2 expression was enhanced along with an increased expression of HO-1 and NQO1, which eventually reduced caspase activity and ameliorated apoptosis in high glucose-treated photoreceptor cells. Both PI3K inhibitor (LY294002) and Nrf2 inhibitor (ML385) counteracted the protective effects of AST and attenuated the expression of HO-1 and NQO1, indicating the importance of PI3K/Akt/Nrf2 signaling in AST-mediated cellular protection.

Systemic AST supplementation could function in the eye and potentially protect the retina from various diseases by reducing oxidative stress. Oral AST supplementation has been used in previous randomized controlled trials and was found to suppress the aqueous vascular endothelial growth factor levels and peroxide production in humans [? ?]. An earlier trial using AST in combination with lutein and other antioxidants also reported improved central visual function in patients with age-related macular degeneration [?]. The results from our study, along with those from previous studies, imply the potential benefits of AST in DR. Taken together with the benefits of AST in increasing serum insulin and glucose metabolism [? ? ?], the role of oral AST supplementation in the prevention and treatment of DR warrants further evaluation in clinical trials.

There were a few limitations to our study. First, we treated the photoreceptor cells with AST before the high glucose administration; therefore, we evaluated only the effects of AST on the acute response of cells to high glucose but not on the cells that had already developed a certain degree of damage under the high glucose environment. Previous in vivo studies have demonstrated that AST administered after the induction of diabetes in different animal models may reduce the levels of oxidative stress mediators and preserve retinal function [? ? ?]. These results indicate that AST may potentially be used for the treatment of high glucose-induced damage, but further studies are needed to confirm the cellular responses of AST administered after the occurrence of cellular damage. Second, we only used a fluorescent probe to detect ROS. Other methods, including spectrophotometry, chromatography, and electron spin resonance, have also been proposed to increase the sensitivity and specificity of ROS detection [?]. Nevertheless, we used other ancillary tests to confirm our detection of ROS, and the results of JC-1 staining and the detection of oxidative stress mediators support our conclusions.

5. Conclusions

The data presented in this study indicate that AST could protect photoreceptor cells from apoptosis secondary to high glucose-induced oxidative stress. In addition, we have demonstrated that the protective effects of AST are mediated by upregulated Nrf2 and that increased expression of downstream Phase II enzymes results from activation of the PI3K/Akt pathway. Thus, AST should be considered as a nutritional supplement that could benefit patients with diabetes, especially in view of preventing the visual loss in DR.

Author Contributions: Conceptualization, C.-M.Y. and C.-H.Y.; methodology, T.-T.L. and C.-H.Y.; software, T.-T.L. and C.-H.Y.; validation, C.-M.Y. and C.-H.Y.; formal analysis, T.-T.L. and C.-H.Y.; investigation, T.-T.L., C.-M.Y., and C.-H.Y.; resources, C.-H.Y.; data curation, T.-T.L., C.-M.Y., and C.-H.Y.; writing—original draft preparation, T.-T.L.; writing—review and editing, C.-M.Y. and C.-H.Y.; visualization, T.-T.L.; supervision, C.-M.Y. and C.-H.Y.; funding acquisition, C.-M.Y. and C.-H.Y. All authors have read and agreed to the published version of the manuscript.

Funding: This research received no external funding.

Acknowledgments: We thank Zi-Yun Weng for the technical support.

Conflicts of Interest: The authors declare no conflict of interest.

References

1. Chen, H.Y.; Kuo, S.; Su, P.-F.; Wu, J.-S.; Ou, H.-T. Health care costs associated with macrovascular, microvascular, and metabolic complications of type 2 diabetes across time: Estimates from a population-based cohort of more than 0.8 million individuals with up to 15 years of follow-up. *Diabetes Care* **2020**, *43*, dc200072. [CrossRef] [PubMed]
2. Martinez-Zapata, M.J.; Martí-Carvajal, A.J.; Solà, I.; Pijoán, J.I.; Buil-Calvo, J.A.; Cordero, J.A.; Evans, J.R. Anti-vascular endothelial growth factor for proliferative diabetic retinopathy. *Cochrane Database Syst. Rev.* **2014**, *11*, CD008721. [CrossRef] [PubMed]
3. Stitt, A.W.; Curtis, T.M.; Chen, M.; Medina, R.J.; McKay, G.J.; Jenkins, A.; Gardiner, T.A.; Lyons, T.J.; Hammes, H.-P.; Simó, R.; et al. The progress in understanding and treatment of diabetic retinopathy. *Prog. Retin Eye Res.* **2016**, *51*, 156–186. [CrossRef] [PubMed]
4. Wang, W.; Lo, A.C.Y. Diabetic retinopathy: Pathophysiology and treatments. *Int. J. Mol. Sci.* **2018**, *19*, 1816. [CrossRef]
5. Feldman, E.L. Oxidative stress and diabetic neuropathy: A new understanding of an old problem. *J. Clin. Investig.* **2003**, *111*, 431–433. [CrossRef]
6. Brownlee, M. The pathobiology of diabetic complications: A unifying mechanism. *Diabetes* **2005**, *54*, 1615–1625. [CrossRef]
7. Yeh, P.-T.; Yang, C.-M.; Huang, J.-S.; Chien, C.-T.; Yang, C.-H.; Chiang, Y.-H.; Shih, Y.-F. Vitreous levels of reactive oxygen species in proliferative diabetic retinopathy. *Ophthalmology* **2008**, *115*, 734–737. [CrossRef]

8. Giacco, F.; Brownlee, M. Oxidative stress and diabetic complications. *Circ. Res.* **2010**, *107*, 1058–1070. [CrossRef]
9. Pan, H.-Z.; Zhang, H.; Chang, D.; Li, H.; Sui, H. The change of oxidative stress products in diabetes mellitus and diabetic retinopathy. *Br. J. Ophthalmol.* **2008**, *92*, 548–551. [CrossRef]
10. Kaneto, H.; Katakami, N.; Kawamori, D.; Miyatsuka, T.; Sakamoto, K.; Matsuoka, T.-A.; Matsuhisa, M.; Yamasaki, Y. Involvement of oxidative stress in the pathogenesis of diabetes. *Antioxid. Redox Signal.* **2007**, *9*, 355–366. [CrossRef]
11. Baynes, J.W.; Thorpe, S.R. Role of oxidative stress in diabetic complications: A new perspective on an old paradigm. *Diabetes* **1999**, *48*, 1–9. [CrossRef] [PubMed]
12. Kowluru, R.A.; Kowluru, A.; Mishra, M.; Kumar, B. Oxidative stress and epigenetic modifications in the pathogenesis of diabetic retinopathy. *Prog. Retin Eye Res.* **2015**, *48*, 40–61. [CrossRef] [PubMed]
13. Van Reyk, D.M.; Gillies, M.C.; Davies, M.J. The retina: Oxidative stress and diabetes. *Redox Rep.* **2003**, *8*, 187–192. [CrossRef]
14. Anderson, R.E.; Rapp, L.M.; Wiegand, R.D. Lipid peroxidation and retinal degeneration. *Curr. Eye Res.* **1984**, *3*, 223–227. [CrossRef] [PubMed]
15. Park, S.W.; Cho, C.S.; Jun, H.O.; Ryu, N.H.; Kim, J.H.; Yu, Y.S.; Kim, J.S.; Kim, J.H. Anti-angiogenic effect of luteolin on retinal neovascularization via blockade of reactive oxygen species production. *Investig. Ophthalmol. Vis. Sci.* **2012**, *53*, 7718–7726. [CrossRef] [PubMed]
16. Feenstra, D.J.; Yego, E.C.; Mohr, S. Modes of retinal cell death in diabetic retinopathy. *J. Clin. Exp. Ophthalmol.* **2013**, *4*, 298.
17. Jackson, H.; Braun, C.L.; Ernst, H. The chemistry of novel xanthophyll carotenoids. *Am. J. Cardiol.* **2008**, *101*, 50–57. [CrossRef]
18. Nakajima, Y.; Inokuchi, Y.; Shimazawa, M.; Otsubo, K.; Ishibashi, T.; Hara, H. Astaxanthin, a dietary carotenoid, protects retinal cells against oxidative stress in-vitro and in mice in-vivo. *J. Pharm. Pharmacol.* **2008**, *60*, 1365–1374. [CrossRef]
19. Hussein, G.; Sankawa, U.; Goto, H.; Matsumoto, K.; Watanabe, H. Astaxanthin, a carotenoid with potential in human health and nutrition. *J. Nat. Prod.* **2006**, *69*, 443–449. [CrossRef]
20. Yuan, J.P.; Peng, J.; Yin, K.; Wang, J.H. Potential health-promoting effects of astaxanthin: A high-value carotenoid mostly from microalgae. *Mol. Nutr. Food Res.* **2011**, *55*, 150–165. [CrossRef]
21. Pashkow, F.J.; Watumull, D.G.; Campbell, C.L. Astaxanthin: A novel potential treatment for oxidative stress and inflammation in cardiovascular disease. *Am. J. Cardiol.* **2008**, *101*, 58–68. [CrossRef]
22. Shen, H.; Kuo, C.-C.; Chou, J.; Delvolve, A.; Jackson, S.N.; Post, J.; Woods, A.S.; Hoffer, B.J.; Wang, Y.; Harvey, B.K. Astaxanthin reduces ischemic brain injury in adult rats. *FASEB J.* **2009**, *23*, 1958–1968. [CrossRef]
23. Wu, T.H.; Liao, J.-H.; Hou, W.-C.; Huang, F.-Y.; Maher, T.J.; Hu, C.-C. Astaxanthin protects against oxidative stress and calcium-induced porcine lens protein degradation. *J. Agric. Food Chem.* **2006**, *54*, 2418–2423. [CrossRef]
24. Uchiyama, K.; Naito, Y.; Hasegawa, G.; Nakamura, N.; Takahashi, J.; Yoshikawa, T. Astaxanthin protects beta-cells against glucose toxicity in diabetic db/db mice. *Redox Rep.* **2002**, *7*, 290–293. [CrossRef]
25. Naito, Y.; Uchiyama, K.; Aoi, W.; Hasegawa, G.; Nakamura, N.; Yoshida, N.; Maoka, T.; Takahashi, J.; Yoshikawa, T. Prevention of diabetic nephropathy by treatment with astaxanthin in diabetic db/db mice. *Biofactors* **2004**, *20*, 49–59. [CrossRef]
26. Manabe, E.; Handa, O.; Naito, Y.; Mizushima, K.; Akagiri, S.; Adachi, S.; Takagi, T.; Kokura, S.; Maoka, T.; Yoshikawa, T. Astaxanthin protects mesangial cells from hyperglycemia-induced oxidative signaling. *J. Cell Biochem.* **2008**, *103*, 1925–1937. [CrossRef]
27. Izumi-Nagai, K.; Nagai, N.; Ohgami, K.; Satofuka, S.; Ozawa, Y.; Tsubota, K.; Ohno, S.; Oike, Y.; Ishida, S. Inhibition of choroidal neovascularization with an anti-inflammatory carotenoid astaxanthin. *Investig. Ophthalmol. Vis. Sci.* **2008**, *49*, 1679–1685. [CrossRef]
28. Suzuki, Y.; Ohgami, K.; Shiratori, K.; Jin, X.-H.; Ilieva, I.; Koyama, Y.; Yazawa, K.; Yoshida, K.; Kase, S.; Ohno, S. Suppressive effects of astaxanthin against rat endotoxin-induced uveitis by inhibiting the NF-kappaB signaling pathway. *Exp. Eye Res.* **2006**, *82*, 275–281. [CrossRef]
29. Ben-Dor, A.; Steiner, M.; Gheber, L.; Danilenko, M.; Dubi, N.; Linnewiel, K.; Zick, A.; Sharoni, Y.; Levy, J. Carotenoids activate the antioxidant response element transcription system. *Mol. Cancer Ther.* **2005**, *4*, 177–186.

30. Tripathi, D.N.; Jena, G.B. Astaxanthin intervention ameliorates cyclophosphamide-induced oxidative stress, DNA damage and early hepatocarcinogenesis in rat: Role of Nrf2, p53, p38 and phase-II enzymes. *Mutat. Res.* **2010**, *696*, 69–80. [CrossRef]
31. Zhu, X.; Chen, Y.; Chen, Q.; Yang, H.; Xie, X. Astaxanthin promotes Nrf2/ARE signaling to alleviate renal fibronectin and collagen IV accumulation in diabetic rats. *J. Diabetes Res.* **2018**, *2018*, 6730315. [CrossRef]
32. Xie, X.; Chen, Q.; Tao, J. Astaxanthin promotes Nrf2/ARE signaling to inhibit HG-induced renal fibrosis in GMCs. *Mar. Drugs* **2018**, *16*, 117.
33. Niu, T.; Xuan, R.; Jiang, L.; Wu, W.; Zhen, Z.; Song, Y.; Hong, L.; Zheng, K.; Zhang, J.; Xu, Q.; et al. Astaxanthin induces the Nrf2/HO-1 antioxidant pathway in human umbilical vein endothelial cells by generating trace amounts of ROS. *J. Agric. Food Chem.* **2018**, *66*, 1551–1559. [CrossRef]
34. Park, E.J.; Lim, J.H.; Nam, S.I.; Park, J.W.; Kwon, T.K. Rottlerin induces heme oxygenase-1 (HO-1) up-regulation through reactive oxygen species (ROS) dependent and PKC delta-independent pathway in human colon cancer HT29 cells. *Biochimie* **2010**, *92*, 110–115. [CrossRef]
35. Xiao, H.; Lv, F.; Xu, W.; Zhang, L.; Jing, P.; Cao, X. Deprenyl prevents MPP(+)-induced oxidative damage in PC12 cells by the upregulation of Nrf2-mediated NQO1 expression through the activation of PI3K/Akt and Erk. *Toxicology* **2011**, *290*, 286–294. [CrossRef]
36. Feng, Z.; Liu, Z.; Li, X.; Jia, H.; Sun, L.; Tian, C.; Jia, L.; Liu, J. α-Tocopherol is an effective Phase II enzyme inducer: Protective effects on acrolein-induced oxidative stress and mitochondrial dysfunction in human retinal pigment epithelial cells. *J. Nutr. Biochem.* **2010**, *21*, 1222–1231. [CrossRef]
37. Rojo, A.I.; Sagarra, M.R.; Cuadrado, A. GSK-3β down-regulates the transcription factor Nrf2 after oxidant damage: Relevance to exposure of neuronal cells to oxidative stress. *J. Neurochem.* **2008**, *105*, 192–202. [CrossRef]
38. Li, Y.; Cao, Z.; Zhu, H. Upregulation of endogenous antioxidants and phase 2 enzymes by the red wine polyphenol, resveratrol in cultured aortic smooth muscle cells leads to cytoprotection against oxidative and electrophilic stress. *Pharmacol. Res.* **2006**, *53*, 6–15. [CrossRef]
39. Kim, J.H.; Nam, S.-W.; Kim, B.-W.; Choi, W.; Lee, J.-H.; Kim, W.-J.; Choi, Y.-H. Astaxanthin improves stem cell potency via an increase in the proliferation of neural progenitor cells. *Int. J. Mol. Sci.* **2010**, *11*, 5109–5119. [CrossRef] [PubMed]
40. Ha, K.N.; Chen, Y.; Cai, J.; Sternberg, P., Jr. Increased glutathione synthesis through an ARE-Nrf2-dependent pathway by zinc in the RPE: Implication for protection against oxidative stress. *Investig. Ophthalmol. Vis. Sci.* **2006**, *47*, 2709–2715. [CrossRef] [PubMed]
41. Li, Z.; Dong, X.; Liu, H.; Chen, X.; Shi, H.; Fan, Y.; Hou, D.; Zhang, X. Astaxanthin protects ARPE-19 cells from oxidative stress via upregulation of Nrf2-regulated phase II enzymes through activation of PI3K/Akt. *Mol. Vis.* **2013**, *19*, 1656–1666. [PubMed]
42. Tan, E.; Ding, X.Q.; Saadi, A.; Agarwal, N.; Naash, M.I.; Al-Ubaidi, M.R. Expression of cone-photoreceptor-specific antigens in a cell line derived from retinal tumors in transgenic mice. *Invest. Ophthalmol. Vis. Sci.* **2004**, *45*, 764–768. [CrossRef] [PubMed]
43. Fang, I.M.; Yang, C.-H.; Yang, C.-M.; Chen, M.-S. Chitosan oligosaccharides attenuates oxidative-stress related retinal degeneration in rats. *PLoS ONE* **2013**, *8*, e77323. [CrossRef] [PubMed]
44. Ma, Q. Role of nrf2 in oxidative stress and toxicity. *Annu. Rev. Pharmacol. Toxicol.* **2013**, *53*, 401–426. [CrossRef]
45. Fang, Q.; Guo, S.; Zhou, H.; Han, R.; Wu, P.; Han, C. Astaxanthin protects against early burn-wound progression in rats by attenuating oxidative stress-induced inflammation and mitochondria-related apoptosis. *Sci. Rep.* **2017**, *7*, 41440. [CrossRef]
46. Cutler, R.G. Oxidative stress profiling: Part I. Its potential importance in the optimization of human health. *Ann. N. Y. Acad. Sci.* **2005**, *1055*, 93–135. [CrossRef]
47. Kowluru, R.A.; Odenbach, S. Effect of long-term administration of alpha-lipoic acid on retinal capillary cell death and the development of retinopathy in diabetic rats. *Diabetes* **2004**, *53*, 3233–3238. [CrossRef]
48. Levine, R.L.; Garland, D.; Oliver, C.N.; Amici, A.; Climent, I.; Lenz, A.G.; Ahn, B.W.; Shaltiel, S.; Stadtman, E.R. Determination of carbonyl content in oxidatively modified proteins. *Methods Enzymol.* **1990**, *186*, 464–478.
49. Baccouche, B.; Benlarbi, M.; Barber, A.J.; Ben Chaouacha-Chekir, R. Short-term administration of Astaxanthin attenuates retinal changes in diet-induced diabetic *Psammomys obesus*. *Curr. Eye Res.* **2018**, *43*, 1177–1189. [CrossRef]

50. Dong, L.Y.; Jin, J.; Lu, G.; Kang, X.-L. Astaxanthin attenuates the apoptosis of retinal ganglion cells in db/db mice by inhibition of oxidative stress. *Mar. Drugs* **2013**, *11*, 960–974. [CrossRef]
51. Yeh, P.-T.; Huang, H.-W.; Yang, C.-M.; Yang, W.-S.; Yang, C.-H. Astaxanthin inhibits expression of retinal oxidative stress and inflammatory mediators in streptozotocin-induced diabetic rats. *PLoS ONE* **2016**, *11*, e0146438. [CrossRef]
52. Barber, A.J.; Baccouche, B. Neurodegeneration in diabetic retinopathy: Potential for novel therapies. *Vis. Res.* **2017**, *139*, 82–92. [CrossRef]
53. Liu, Q.; Zhang, F.; Zhang, X.; Cheng, R.; Ma, J.-X.; Yi, J.; Li, J. Fenofibrate ameliorates diabetic retinopathy by modulating Nrf2 signaling and NLRP3 inflammasome activation. *Mol. Cell Biochem.* **2018**, *445*, 105–115. [CrossRef]
54. Li, S.; Yang, H.; Chen, X. Protective effects of sulforaphane on diabetic retinopathy: Activation of the Nrf2 pathway and inhibition of NLRP3 inflammasome formation. *Exp. Anim.* **2019**, *68*, 221–231. [CrossRef]
55. Wang, W.; Zhao, H.; Chen, B. DJ-1 protects retinal pericytes against high glucose-induced oxidative stress through the Nrf2 signaling pathway. *Sci. Rep.* **2020**, *10*, 2477. [CrossRef]
56. Nakamura, S.; Noguchi, T.; Inoue, Y.; Sakurai, S.; Nishinaka, A.; Hida, Y.; Masuda, T.; Nakagami, Y.; Horai, N.; Tsusaki, H.; et al. Nrf2 activator RS9 suppresses pathological ocular angiogenesis and hyperpermeability. *Invest. Ophthalmol. Vis. Sci.* **2019**, *60*, 1943–1952. [CrossRef]
57. Kim, Y.H.; Koh, H.K.; Kim, D.S. Down-regulation of IL-6 production by astaxanthin via ERK-, MSK-, and NF-kappaB-mediated signals in activated microglia. *Int. Immunopharmacol.* **2010**, *10*, 1560–1572. [CrossRef]
58. Kim, S.H.; Kim, H. Astaxanthin modulation of signaling pathways that regulate autophagy. *Mar. Drugs* **2019**, *17*, 546. [CrossRef]
59. Yan, T.; Zhao, Y.; Zhang, X.; Lin, X. Astaxanthin inhibits acetaldehyde-induced cytotoxicity in SH-SY5Y cells by modulating Akt/CREB and p38MAPK/ERK signaling pathways. *Mar. Drugs* **2016**, *14*, 56. [CrossRef]
60. Wang, Z.-Y.; Shen, L.-J.; Hu, D.-N.; Liu, G.-Y.; Zhou, Z.-L.; Lin, Y.; Chen, L.-H.; Qu, J. Erythropoietin protects retinal pigment epithelial cells from oxidative damage. *Free Radic. Biol. Med.* **2009**, *46*, 1032–1041. [CrossRef]
61. Guo, S.-X.; Zhou, H.-L.; Huang, C.-L.; You, C.-G.; Fang, Q.; Wu, P.; Wang, X.-G.; Han, C.-H. Astaxanthin attenuates early acute kidney injury following severe burns in rats by ameliorating oxidative stress and mitochondrial-related apoptosis. *Mar. Drugs* **2015**, *13*, 2105–2123. [CrossRef] [PubMed]
62. Xu, L.; Zhu, J.; Yin, W.; Ding, X. Astaxanthin improves cognitive deficits from oxidative stress, nitric oxide synthase and inflammation through upregulation of PI3K/Akt in diabetes rat. *Int. J. Clin. Exp. Pathol.* **2015**, *8*, 6083–6094. [PubMed]
63. Kavitha, K.; Kowshik, J.; Kishore, T.K.K.; Baba, A.B.; Nagini, S. Astaxanthin inhibits NF-kappaB and Wnt/beta-catenin signaling pathways via inactivation of Erk/MAPK and PI3K/Akt to induce intrinsic apoptosis in a hamster model of oral cancer. *Biochim. Biophys. Acta* **2013**, *1830*, 4433–4444. [CrossRef]
64. Hashimoto, H.; Arai, K.; Hayashi, S.; Okamoto, H.; Takahashi, J.; Chikuda, M.; Obara, Y. Effects of astaxanthin on antioxidation in human aqueous humor. *J. Clin. Biochem. Nutr.* **2013**, *53*, 1–7. [CrossRef]
65. Hashimoto, H.; Arai, K.; Hayashi, S.; Okamoto, H.; Takahashi, J.; Chikuda, M. The effect of astaxanthin on vascular endothelial growth factor (VEGF) levels and peroxidation reactions in the aqueous humor. *J. Clin. Biochem. Nutr.* **2016**, *59*, 10–15. [CrossRef] [PubMed]
66. Parisi, V.; Tedeschi, M.; Gallinaro, G.; Varano, M.; Saviano, S.; Piermarocchi, S.; CARMIS Study Group. Carotenoids and antioxidants in age-related maculopathy italian study: Multifocal electroretinogram modifications after 1 year. *Ophthalmology* **2008**, *115*, 324–333. [CrossRef]
67. Bhuvaneswari, S.; Anuradha, C.V. Astaxanthin prevents loss of insulin signaling and improves glucose metabolism in liver of insulin resistant mice. *Can. J. Physiol. Pharmacol.* **2012**, *90*, 1544–1552. [CrossRef]
68. Mashhadi, N.S.; Zakerkish, M.; Mohammadiasl, J.; Zarei, M.; Mohammadshahi, M.; Haghighizadeh, M.H. Astaxanthin improves glucose metabolism and reduces blood pressure in patients with type 2 diabetes mellitus. *Asia Pac. J. Clin. Nutr.* **2018**, *27*, 341–346.
69. Zhang, Y.; Dai, M.; Yuan, Z. Methods for the detection of reactive oxygen species. *Anal. Methods* **2018**, *10*, 4625–4638. [CrossRef]

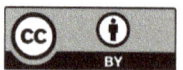

© 2020 by the authors. Licensee MDPI, Basel, Switzerland. This article is an open access article distributed under the terms and conditions of the Creative Commons Attribution (CC BY) license (http://creativecommons.org/licenses/by/4.0/).

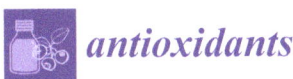

Article

Protective Effect of Fenofibrate on Oxidative Stress-Induced Apoptosis in Retinal–Choroidal Vascular Endothelial Cells: Implication for Diabetic Retinopathy Treatment

Ying-Jung Hsu [1], Chao-Wen Lin [1,2], Sheng-Li Cho [3], Wei-Shiung Yang [1,3], Chung-May Yang [2] and Chang-Hao Yang [2,*]

[1] Graduate Institute of Clinical Medicine, College of Medicine, National Taiwan University, No. 1, Jen Ai Road Section 1, Taipei 100, Taiwan; d98421005@ntu.edu.tw (Y.-J.H.); b91401108@ntu.edu.tw (C.-W.L.); wsyang@ntu.edu.tw (W.-S.Y.)
[2] Department of Ophthalmology, National Taiwan University Hospital, No. 7, Zhongshan South Road, Taipei 100, Taiwan; chungmay@ntu.edu.tw
[3] Department of Internal Medicine, National Taiwan University Hospital, No. 7, Zhongshan South Road, Taipei 100, Taiwan; leechoecho@gmail.com
* Correspondence: chyangoph@ntu.edu.tw; Tel.: +886-2-23123456 (ext. 63193)

Received: 9 July 2020; Accepted: 4 August 2020; Published: 5 August 2020

Abstract: Diabetic retinopathy (DR) is an important microvascular complication of diabetes and one of the leading causes of blindness in developed countries. Two large clinical studies showed that fenofibrate, a peroxisome proliferator-activated receptor type α (PPAR-α) agonist, reduces DR progression. We evaluated the protective effects of fenofibrate on retinal/choroidal vascular endothelial cells under oxidative stress and investigated the underlying mechanisms using RF/6A cells as the model system and paraquat (PQ) to induce oxidative stress. Pretreatment with fenofibrate suppressed reactive oxygen species (ROS) production, decreased cellular apoptosis, diminished the changes in the mitochondrial membrane potential, increased the mRNA levels of peroxiredoxin (Prx), thioredoxins (Trxs), B-cell lymphoma 2 (Bcl-2), and Bcl-xl, and reduced the level of B-cell lymphoma 2-associated X protein (Bax) in PQ-stimulated RF/6A cells. Western blot analysis revealed that fenofibrate repressed apoptosis through cytosolic and mitochondrial apoptosis signal-regulated kinase-1 (Ask)-Trx-related signaling pathways, including c-Jun amino-terminal kinase (JNK) phosphorylation, cytochrome c release, caspase 3 activation, and poly (ADP-ribose) polymerase-1 (PARP-1) cleavage. These protective effects of fenofibrate on RF/6A cells may be attributable to its anti-oxidative ability. Our research suggests that fenofibrate could serve as an effective adjunct therapy for ocular oxidative stress-related disorders, such as DR.

Keywords: apoptosis; diabetic retinopathy; fenofibrate; oxidative stress; thioredoxin

1. Introduction

Diabetic retinopathy (DR) is a very important microvascular complication of diabetes [1]. It is characterized by a progressive increase in vascular permeability, retinal ischemia and edema, and neovascularization, which results in visual impairment and legal blindness [2]. Retinal vascular endothelial cells play an important role in maintaining the blood-retinal barrier (BRB), which provides a physiological border for retinal homeostasis [3]. Previous studies demonstrated that hyperglycemia induces the activation of oxidative stress and generates reactive oxygen species (ROS) within retinal vascular endothelial cells [4,5]. The accumulation of ROS alters the homeostasis and enhances the migration of retinal vascular endothelial cells, triggers cellular apoptosis, and increases vascular permeability and basement membrane leakage in the retina. These pathological changes may lead to the breakdown of the BRB and DR development [6,7]. Therefore, suppressing oxidative stress could inhibit apoptosis in retinal vascular endothelial cells and reduce the risk of DR progression.

Fenofibrate, a peroxisome proliferator-activated receptor type α (PPAR-α) agonist [8], is used clinically to treat hypertriglyceridemia and hyperlipidemia. However, evidence from two large randomized clinical trials, the Fenofibrate Intervention and Event Lowering in Diabetes (FIELD) and Action to Control Cardiovascular Risk in Diabetes (ACCORD), has shown that fenofibrate significantly prevents DR progression and reduces the use of laser treatment in DR [9,10]. In experimental diabetic models, the expression of PPARα is significantly downregulated in retina [11]. In addition, high glucose medium downregulates PPARα expression in retinal cells [11]. Moreover, over-expression of inflammatory factors, retinal vascular leakage, and more severe DR are found in diabetic PPARα knockout mice [11]. Fenofibrate exerts anti-inflammatory and anti-oxidative effects. Treatment of retinal pigment epithelial cells with fenofibrate reduces high-glucose-induced ROS generation [12]. Fenofibrate downregulated NF-κB, significantly inhibited the expressions of inflammatory mediators and reduced the concentrations of oxidative products in a diabetic rat model [13]. Fenofibrate can significantly reduce lipopolysaccharide (LPS)-induced ROS and increase endothelial nitric oxide (eNOS) levels in human umbilical vein endothelial cells (HUVECs) [14]. Fenofibrate also decreases apoptosis in human retinal endothelial cells and pericytes by activating the AMP-activated protein kinase (AMPK) pathway and downregulating the NF-κB pathway, respectively [15,16]. PPAR-α over-expression or fenofibrate treatment has also been shown to attenuate retinal vascular permeability in diabetic animals [11,17] and may protect against BRB leakage through the down-regulation of basement membrane components [18]. Despite the persuasive results from these clinical and experimental studies, the mechanisms through which fenofibrate protects the eye from DR remain elusive, and further studies are still required to clarify the protective mechanisms of fenofibrate.

Thioredoxins (Trxs) are small proteins that are essential for embryonic development and could protect cells against oxidative stress [19]. There are two main forms of Trx. Trx-1 exists in cytosol, acts as a cofactor of peroxiredoxins (Prx), and plays a direct role in reducing oxidative stress [20,21]. Trx-2 exists in mitochondria and plays an important role in the mitochondrial cellular apoptosis pathway [22,23]. Trxs are essential for life, and Trx gene deficiency is embryonic lethal [24,25]. Trxs are involved in multiple redox-regulated signaling pathways. Trxs bind to apoptosis signal-regulated kinase-1 (Ask-1) in the cytosol and mitochondria, thereby blocking the initiation of the cellular apoptotic process and inhibiting c-Jun amino-terminal kinase (JNK/p38 mitogen-activated protein kinase [MAPK]) [26]. Furthermore, previous studies have shown that Trx is a PPAR-α target gene and that PPAR-α activation induces the translocation of Trx to the nucleus and modulates Trx expression [27]. PPAR-α activator significantly enhances the activation of the Trx promoter and increases Trx-1 expression in human macrophages [28]. However, the role of Trxs against oxidative stress in retinal vascular endothelial cells, as well as the mechanism through which fenofibrate modulates Trxs expression in DR have not been reported.

In this study, we hypothesized that fenofibrate can counteract oxidative stress and attenuate oxidative stress-induced cell apoptosis and death by modulating Trx expression in retinal vascular endothelial cells. Paraquat (PQ) is a common stimulator to induce oxidative stress in in vitro and in vivo studies about retinal degeneration [29–31]. Oxidative stress induced by PQ is thought to play an important role in type 2 diabetes through the impairment of insulin action [32–34]. Therefore, we used PQ as the inducer of oxidative stress to simulate the condition in DR. We used retinal/choroidal vascular endothelial cell (RF/6A) cells as the cell model system. RF/6A cell line is a monkey choroidal–retinal vascular endothelial cell line and has been widely used to study retinal vascular diseases and DR previously [35–44]. The study was performed in two parts. First, we investigated the role of oxidative stress in initiating apoptosis and evaluated the protective effects of fenofibrate. Second, we investigated the modulatory effect of fenofibrate on Trx expression and analyzed the related apoptosis and stress signaling pathways.

2. Materials and Methods

2.1. Cell Culture and Fenofibrate Pretreatment

The RF/6A cell line is a monkey choroidal–retinal vascular endothelial cell line. RF/6A cells were purchased from the American Type Culture Collection (Rockville, MD, USA). RF/6A cells were maintained in Dulbecco's modified Eagle's medium (DMEM) with 10% fetal bovine serum, 4.5 mg/mL glucose, 100 units/mL penicillin, and 100 μg/mL streptomycin (all from Thermo Fisher Scientific, Waltham, MA, USA) in a 5% CO_2 atmosphere at 37 °C. The cells were pretreated with different concentrations of fenofibrate (CAS Number 49562-28-9, Sigma-Aldrich, St. Louis, MO, USA) before exposure to PQ (Sigma-Aldrich, St. Louis, MO, USA).

2.2. Cell Viability Assay

The RF/6A cells were seeded at a density of 1×10^4 cells per well onto 96-well plates and incubated at 37 °C. The cells were exposed to 0, 0.2, 0.4, 0.6, 0.8 and 1.0 mM PQ for 24 h. The cells in the fenofibrate treated group were pretreated with 25, 50, 75 or 100 μM fenofibrate for 1 h prior to 24-h exposure of 1.0 mM PQ. 5 mg/mL 3-(4,5-dimethylthiazol-2-yl)-2,5-diphenyltetrazolium bromide (MTT, Chemicon, Millipore, Burlington, MA, USA) was added to each well for 4 h. Then we removed the culture medium supernatant, and formazan was dissolved with dimethyl sulfoxide (DMSO, Sigma-Aldrich, St. Louis, MO, USA) for 30 min at room temperature. The absorbance (570 nm) was measured with a microplate reader (Bio-Rad Laboratories, Hercules, CA, USA).

2.3. Analysis of Apoptosis by Flow Cytometry

The RF/6A cells were pretreated with 25, 50, 75 or 100 μM fenofibrate for 1 h prior to 1.0 mM PQ exposure. The proportion of apoptotic RF/6A cells was determined at 24 h by flow cytometry using a staining solution containing 5 μL of annexin-V-FITC and 5 μL of propidium iodide (PI) (Strong Biotech, Taipei, Taiwan) in 250 μL of binding buffer. Cells were washed with PBS and centrifuged at 200 g for 5 min. Then we resuspended the cell pellet in 100 μL of staining solution and incubated for 10 min at 20 °C. Finally, 900 μL of binding buffer was added to the samples, and the samples were analyzed on a FACScan cytometer (BD Bioscience, Franklin Lakes, NJ, USA).

2.4. Detection of Intracellular ROS

We measured intracellular ROS levels by 2′,7′-dichlorodihydrofluorescein diacetate (2′,7′-DCFDA, Sigma-Aldrich, St. Louis, MO, USA) oxidation. The RF/6A cells were pretreated with 25, 50, 75 or 100 μM fenofibrate for 1 h prior to 24-h exposure of 1.0 mM PQ. RF/6A cells were then exposed to 10 μM 2′,7′-DCFDA for 10 min. The cells were analyzed by FACScan cytometer (BD Biosciences, Franklin Lakes, NJ, USA) using the FL-1 channel (515–545 nm).

2.5. Quantitative Detection of ROS-Induced Cellular Oxidation

The RF/6A cells were pretreated with 25, 50, 75 or 100 μM fenofibrate for 1 h prior to 1.0 mM PQ treatment. After 24-h PQ exposure, DNA oxidation, lipid peroxidation, and protein oxidation levels were determined using an 8-hydroxydeoxyguanosine (8-OHdG) Check Kit (JaICA, Shizuoka, Japan), a thiobarbituric acid reactive substances (TBARS) Assay Kit (Cayman Chemical, Ann Arbor, MN, USA), and a Protein Carbonyl Colorimetric Assay Kit (Cayman Chemical, Ann Arbor, MN, USA), respectively. Cellular DNA was extracted for 8-OHdG detection using a cellular genomic DNA Extraction Kit (T-Pro Biotechenology, New Taipei County, Taiwan). Cellular homogenates were prepared for TBARS or carbonyl colorimetric assays according to the manufacturer's instructions.

2.6. Determination of Mitochondrial Dysfunction

To detect the extent of mitochondrial dysfunction, we measured the mitochondrial membrane potential of cells with JC-1 stain (Cayman Chemical, Ann Arbor, MN, USA). The RF/6A cells were seeded at a density of 1×10^4 cells per well onto 96-well plates and incubated at 37 °C. We added different concentrations of fenofibrate (25, 50, 75, 100 µM) to the cells exposed to 1.0 mM PQ. After a 24-h incubation, 50 µL of JC-1 staining solution buffer was added to 1 mL of culture medium, and the plate was incubated at 37 °C for 15 min. The fluorescence signals for J-aggregates with Texas Red (healthy cells, excitation/emission = 560/595 nm) and JC-1 monomers with FITC (apoptotic or unhealthy cells, excitation/emission = 485/535 nm) were measured with a microplate reader (Bio-Rad Laboratories, Hercules, CA, USA).

2.7. Preparation of RNA and cDNA

The RF/6A cells were incubated with 10 µM GW6471 (a PPAR-α antagonist, R&D systems, Minneapolis, MN, USA) for 1 h. After removing GW6471, the cells were then pretreated with 50 or 100 µM fenofibrate for 1 h prior to 1.0 mM PQ treatment. After 24-h PQ exposure, we extracted RNA from RF/6A cells with TRIzol reagent (Thermo Fisher Scientific, Waltham, MA, USA). 1 µg of total RNA was incubated with 300 ng of Oligo dT (Promega, Madison, WI, USA) for 5 min at 65 °C. Samples were then reverse transcribed into cDNA using Moloney murine leukemia virus reverse transcriptase (MMLV-RT; Thermo Fisher Scientific, Waltham, MA, USA) for 1 h at 37 °C. The reaction was terminated by heating the samples for 5 min at 90 °C.

2.8. Analysis of mRNA Expression Levels

The resultant cDNA product was subjected to PCR using Prx, Trx-1, Trx-2, B-cell lymphoma 2 (Bcl-2), Bcl-xl, B-cell lymphoma 2-associated X protein (Bax), and β-actin primers. The amplification was performed by thermocycler (MJ Research, Waltham, MA, USA). The 25 µL reaction mixture was composed of 5 µL of cDNA, 200 µM of each deoxynucleotide (DTT), 1 µL of sense and antisense primers, 1.25 U of GoTaq polymerase (Promega, Madison, WI, USA), and 5 µL of 10× Taq polymerase buffer. PCR was performed at an annealing temperature of 56 °C with GoTaq polymerase, cDNA, and the following primers: Prx: 5′-CTTCAGGAAATGCAAAAATTGGGCAT-3′ (forward), 5′-GAGTTTCTTAAATTC TTCTGCTCTA-3′ (reverse); Trx-1: 5′-CCCTTCTTTCA TTCCCTCTGTG-3′ (forward), 5′-GAACTCCCCAACCTTTTGACC-3′ (reverse); Trx-2: 5′-CGTACAAT GCTGGTGGTCTAAC-3′ (forward), 5′-GTCTTGAAAGTCAGGTCCATCC-3′ (reverse); Bcl-2: 5′-CTGGTGGACAACATCGCTCTG-3′ (forward), 5′-GGTCTGCTGACCTCACTTGTG-3′ (reverse); Bcl-xl: 5′-CCCCAGAAGAAACTGAACCA-3′ (forward), 5′-AGTTTACCCCAT CCCGAAAG-3′ (reverse); Bax: 5′-TGGTTGCCCTTTTCTACTTTG-3′ (forward), 5′-GAAGTAGGAAAGGAGGCCA TC-3′ (reverse); β-actin: 5′- CTGGAGAAGAGCTATGAGCTG-3′ (forward), 5′- AATCTCCTTCTGCAT CCTGTC-3′ (reverse). The DNA fragments were amplified for 25–30 cycles (30 s at 94 °C; 1 min at 50–52 °C; and 1 min at 72 °C), followed by a 7 min extension step at 72 °C. The products were then subjected to electrophoresis on a 1.5% agarose gel and analyzed by gel analyzer system. β-actin was used as the internal control.

2.9. Protein Extractions and Western Blot Analysis

The RF/6A cells were incubated with 10 µM GW6471 for 1 h. After removing GW6471, the cells were then pretreated with 50 or 100 µM fenofibrate for 1 h prior to 1.0 mM PQ exposure. After 24-h or 1-h (for phospho-Ask1 and phospho-JNK) PQ exposure, we extracted proteins from RF/6A cells with radioimmunoprecipitation assay (RIPA) lysis buffer, which contained 0.5 M Tris-HCl (pH 7.4), 2.5% deoxycholic acid, 10% NP-40, 1.5 M NaCl, 10 mM EDTA, and 10% protease inhibitors (Complete Mini; Roche Diagnostics, Indianapolis, IN, USA). Mitochondrial proteins and cytosolic proteins were isolated using a mitochondria isolation kit (Thermo Fisher Scientific, Waltham, MA, USA), following the protocol description. For the western blot analysis, the protein samples were separated by a 10% sodium dodecyl sulfate (SDS)-polyacrylamide gel and then transferred to a polyvinylidene difluoride (PVDF) membrane (Immobilon-P; Millipore, Burlington, MA, USA). The primary antibodies used in the experiment were as follows: anti-PPAR-α (at a 1:500 dilution, Santa Cruz Biotechnology, Dallas, TX, USA); anti-Prx-1 (at a 1:1000 dilution, Cell Signaling Technology, Danvers, MA, USA); anti-Trx-1 (at a 1:500 dilution, Cell Signaling Technology, Danvers, MA, USA); anti-Ask-1 (at a 1:1000 dilution, Cell Signaling Technology, Danvers, MA, USA); anti-phospho-Ask1 (at a 1:2000 dilution, Bioss, Woburn, MA, USA); anti-JNK (at a 1:3000 dilution, Cell Signaling Technology, Danvers, MA, USA); anti-phospho-JNK (at a 1:3000 dilution, Cell Signaling Technology, Danvers, MA, USA); anti-Bcl-2 (at a 1:1000 dilution, Cell Signaling Technology, Danvers, MA, USA); anti-Bcl-xl (at a 1:500 dilution, Cell Signaling Technology, Danvers, MA, USA); anti-Bax (at a 1:5000 dilution, Cell Signaling Technology, Danvers, MA, USA); anti-cytochrome c (at a 1:1000 dilution, Abcam, Hong Kong, China); anti-VDAC1 (at a 1:5000 dilution, Abcam, Hong Kong, China); anti-Trx-2 (at a 1:2000 dilution, R&D System, Minneapolis, MN, USA,); anti-apoptotic protease activating factor-1 (Apaf-1) (at a 1:1000 dilution, Cell Signaling Technology, Danvers, MA, USA); anti-caspase-9 (at a 1:1000 dilution, Cell Signaling Technology, Danvers, MA, USA); anti-caspase-7 (at a 1:1000 dilution, Cell Signaling Technology, Danvers, MA, USA); anti- poly (ADP-ribose) polymerase-1 (PARP-1) (at a 1:1000 dilution, Abcam, Hong Kong, China); and anti-β-actin (at a 1:5000 dilution, Bioss, Woburn, MA, USA). Immunodetections were performed using enhanced chemiluminescence (Pierce Biotechnology, Waltham, MA, USA). Protein levels were determined using densitometry analysis of the protein bands. Protein levels were normalized to β-actin.

2.10. Caspase-3 Activity Assay

The RF/6A cells were incubated with 10 μM GW6471 for 1 h. After removing GW6471, the cells were then pretreated with 50 or 100 μM fenofibrate for 1 h prior to 1.0 mM PQ exposure. After 24 h PQ exposure, the caspase-3 activity of RF/6A cells was analyzed by the Caspase-3/CPP32 Colorimetric Assay Kit (BioVision, Milpitas, CA, USA). Assay procedures were performed following the manufacturer's instructions.

2.11. Statistical Analyses

The results are expressed as mean ± standard deviation. We used Mann–Whitney U-test to compare the data between two groups. We used Kruskal–Wallis test with post hoc Dunn's test to compare the data among multiple different groups. P values of less than 0.05 were considered statistically significant. Statistical analysis was performed using SPSS (version 17.0, SPSS, Chicago, IL, USA).

3. Results

3.1. Fenofibrate Treatment Decreased PQ-Induced RF/6A Cell Death

MTT assay was used to evaluate cell viability. After exposure to several concentrations of PQ for 24 h, the viability of RF/6A cells reduced to 88%, 77%, and 60% at PQ concentrations of 0.6 mM, 0.8 mM, and 1.0 mM, respectively (Figure 1a). Viability decreased substantially after exposure to 1.0 mM PQ. Therefore, we chose 1.0 mM as the concentration of PQ in the following experiments. When the cells were pretreated with fenofibrate and then exposed to 1.0 mM PQ, the survival rate increased in a dose-dependent manner (from 65% in only PQ-stimulated group to 83% at 100 μM fenofibrate) (Figure 1b).

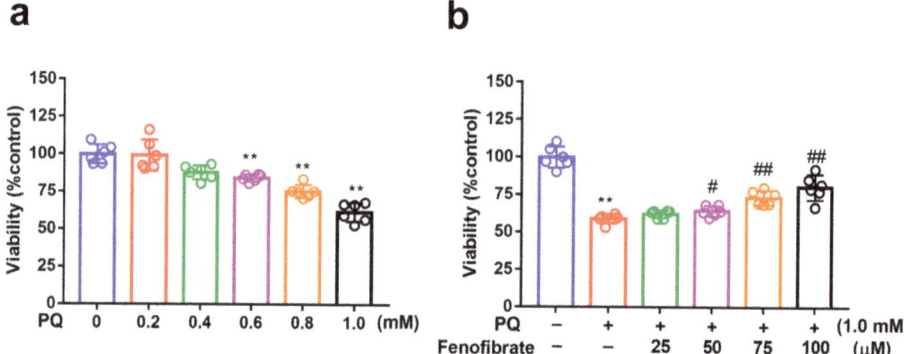

Figure 1. Effects of fenofibrate on cell viability in paraquat (PQ)-stimulated RF/6A cells assessed using MTT assay. (**a**) Cell viability after exposure to different concentrations of PQ for 24 h. (** $p < 0.01$ among the control group and 0.6, 0.8, and 1.0 mM PQ-stimulated groups using Kruskal–Wallis test with post hoc Dunn's test; $n = 6$ in each group) (**b**) Cell viability in PQ-stimulated RF/6A cells with fenofibrate pre-treatment. RF/6A cells were pretreated with different concentration of fenofibrate for 1 h, then exposed to 1.0 mM PQ for 24 h. (** $p < 0.01$ between the control group and 1.0 mM PQ-stimulated group using Mann–Whitney U-test; # $p < 0.05$, ## $p < 0.01$ compared to only 1.0 mM PQ-stimulated group using Kruskal–Wallis test with post hoc Dunn's test; $n = 6$ in each group).

3.2. Fenofibrate Treatment Suppressed PQ-Induced Apoptosis in RF/6A Cells

We investigated the effects of fenofibrate on PQ-stimulated cell apoptosis by flow cytometry. After exposure to 1.0 mM PQ, the level of cell apoptosis was significantly increased compared to that in the control group. Prior treatment with fenofibrate before PQ stimulation protected RF/6A cells and dose-dependently decreased the levels of cell apoptosis (Figure 2).

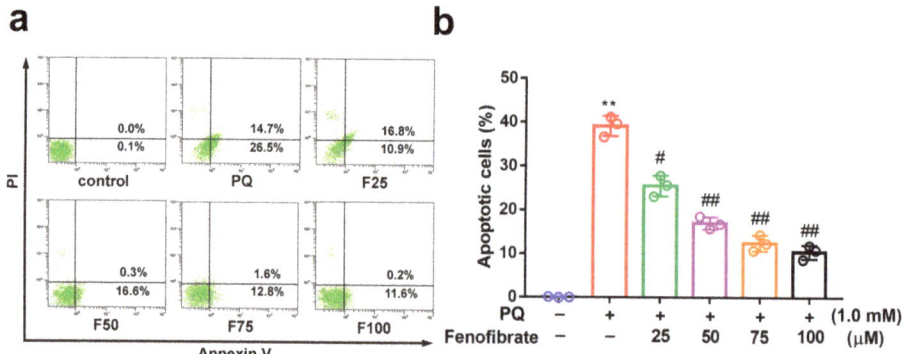

Figure 2. Effects of fenofibrate on apoptosis in paraquat (PQ)-stimulated RF/6A cells assessed by flow cytometry. (**a**) RF/6A cells were pretreated with different concentrations of fenofibrate for 1 h and then exposed to 1.0 mM PQ for 24 h. The x-axis and y-axis represent annexin V-FITC and propidium iodide (PI) staining, respectively. PQ: 1.0 mM PQ; F25: 1.0 mM PQ with 25 µM fenofibrate; F50: 1.0 mM PQ with 50 µM fenofibrate; F75: 1.0 mM PQ with 75 µM fenofibrate; F100: 1.0 mM PQ with 100 µM fenofibrate. (**b**) Percentage of apoptotic cells treated with different concentrations of fenofibrate. (** $p < 0.01$ between the control group and 1.0 mM PQ-stimulated group using Mann–Whitney U-test; # $p < 0.05$, ## $p < 0.01$ compared to only 1.0 mM PQ-stimulated group using Kruskal–Wallis test with post hoc Dunn's test; $n = 3$ in each group).

3.3. Fenofibrate Treatment Suppressed PQ-Induced ROS, 8-OHdG, Malondialdehyde, and Protein Carbonyl Content Production in RF/6A Cells

PQ stimulation can induce oxidative stress by overproducing ROS in RF/6A cells. PQ stimulation led to an increased ROS production, which was reduced by pretreatment with fenofibrate (Figure 3a,b). To further investigate the effects of fenofibrate on oxidative stress, the levels of 8-OHdG (oxidative DNA adduct), malondialdehyde (MDA, lipid peroxidation product), and protein carbonyl content (protein oxidative marker) were evaluated. The levels of 8-OHdG, MDA and protein carbonyl content were significantly increased after exposure to PQ. The levels of 8-OHdG and MDA decreased with fenofibrate pretreatment in a dose-dependent manner (Figure 3c,d). The levels of protein carbonyl content were reduced with higher concentration of fenofibrate (75 and 100 µM) (Figure 3e).

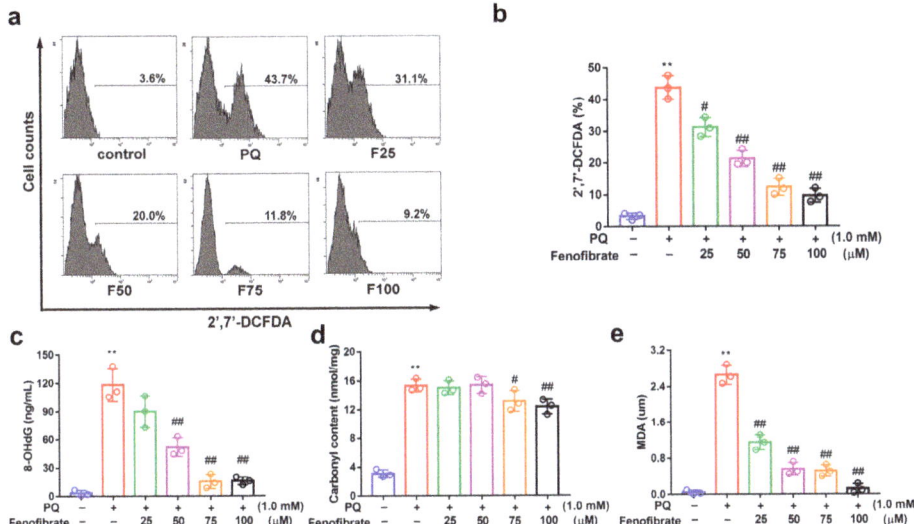

Figure 3. Effects of fenofibrate on reactive oxygen species (ROS) production and oxidative stress indicators in paraquat (PQ)-stimulated RF/6A cells assessed by flow cytometry. RF/6A cells were pretreated with different concentration of fenofibrate for 1 h, then exposed to 1 mM PQ for 24 h. (**a**) PQ-induced ROS production under fenofibrate treatment. The x-axis represents 2′,7′-dichlorodihydrofluorescein diacetate (2′,7′-DCFDA) staining, and the Y-axis represents cell numbers. PQ: 1 mM PQ; F25: 1 mM PQ with 25 µM fenofibrate; F50: 1 mM PQ with 50 µM fenofibrate; F75: 1 mM PQ with 75 µM fenofibrate; F100: 1 mM PQ with 100 µM fenofibrate. Dose-dependent effect of fenofibrate treatment on (**b**) ROS production; (**c**) the expression of 8-hydroxydeoxyguanosine (8-OHdG), a DNA oxidation indicator; (**d**) the expression of malondialdehyde (MDA), a lipid peroxidation indicator; (**e**) the expression of protein carbonyl content, a protein oxidation indicator. (** $p < 0.01$ between the control group and 1 mM PQ-stimulated group using Mann–Whitney U-test; # $p < 0.05$, ## $p < 0.01$ compared to only 1 mM PQ-stimulated group using Kruskal–Wallis test with post hoc Dunn's test; $n = 3$ in each group).

3.4. Fenofibrate Treatment Diminished Mitochondrial Damage in PQ-Induced RF/6A Cell

To determine whether fenofibrate can protect mitochondrial function, the extent of mitochondrial damage was analyzed using a JC-1 assay. JC-1 spontaneously formed J-aggregates in healthy cells. Our results showed that PQ stimulation significantly decreased the ratio of J-aggregates compared to that in control group. Fenofibrate treatment dose-dependently increased the expression of J-aggregates in RF/6A cells (Figure 4a). JC-1 remained in the monomeric form in apoptotic or unhealthy cells. After PQ exposure, the expression of JC-1 monomers had a 1.58-fold increase compared to that in control group. Fenofibrate treatment decreased the expression of JC-1 monomers in a dose-dependent manner (Figure 4b). The fluorescence signal revealed a high level of JC-1 monomers (FITC) in PQ-stimulated cells; conversely, a high level of J-aggregates (Texas Red) was detected in the control group. Fenofibrate pretreatment decreased the level of JC-1 monomers and increased the level of J-aggregates in a dose-dependent manner (Figure 4c).

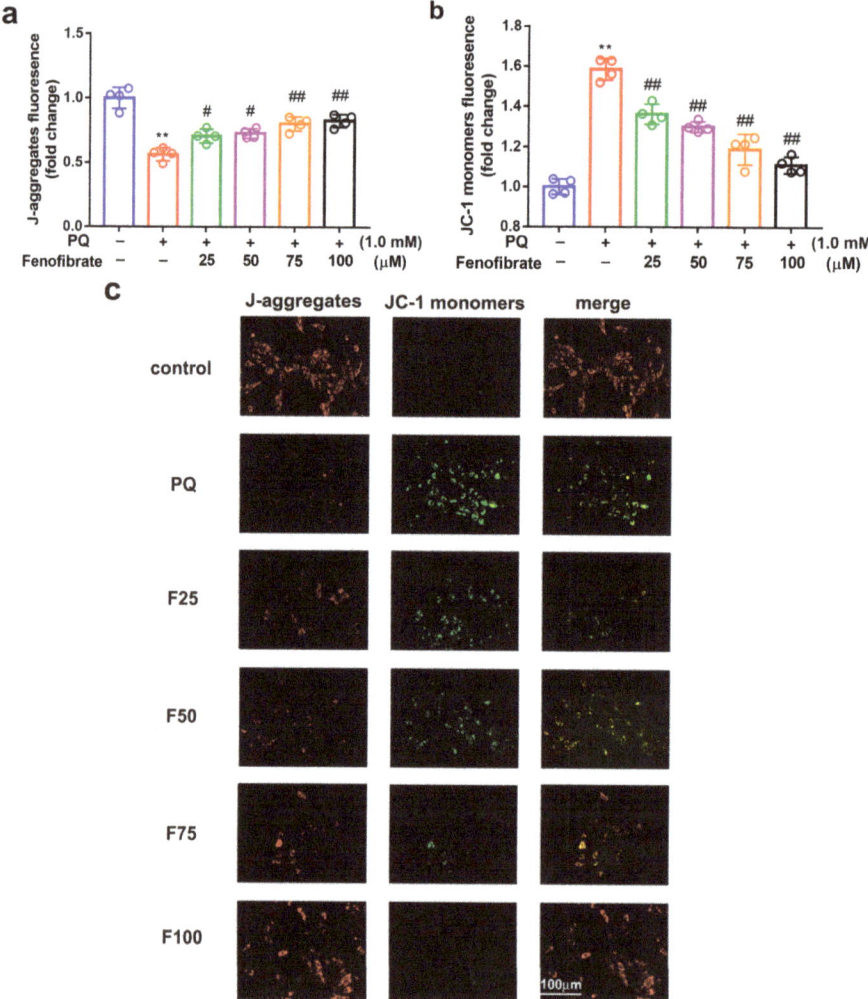

Figure 4. Effects of fenofibrate on mitochondrial damage in RF/6A cells assessed by JC-1 staining. RF/6A cells were pretreated with different concentrations of fenofibrate for 1 h, then exposed to 1 mM paraquat (PQ) for 24 h. Dose-dependent effect of fenofibrate treatment on (a) the expression of J-aggregates in PQ-stimulated RF/6A cells, and (b) JC-1 monomers in PQ-stimulated RF/6A cells. (** $p < 0.01$ between the control group and 1 mM PQ-stimulated group using Mann–Whitney U-test; # $p < 0.05$, ## $p < 0.01$ compared to only 1 mM PQ-stimulated group using Kruskal–Wallis test with post hoc Dunn's test; $n = 4$ in each group) PQ: 1 mM PQ; F25: 1 mM PQ with 25 µM fenofibrate; F50: 1 mM PQ with 50 µM fenofibrate; F75: 1 mM PQ with 75 µM fenofibrate; F100: 1 mM PQ with 100 µM fenofibrate. (c) Fluorescence microscopy images showing the expression of JC-1 monomers (FITC) and J-aggregates (Texas Red).

3.5. Effects of Fenofibrate on PQ-Induced Oxidative Stress-Related mRNA Levels in RF/6A Cells

The mRNA levels of Prx, Trx-1, Trx-2, Bcl-2, Bcl-xl, and Bax were determined using semi-quantitative PCR analysis (Figure 5). Compared to those of the control group, the expression levels of Prx, Trx-1, Trx-2, Bcl-2, and Bcl-xl mRNA were significantly lower in the PQ-stimulated group. Fenofibrate treatment significantly enhanced the expression of Prx, Trx-1, Bcl-2, and Bcl-xl mRNA levels in a dose-dependent manner (Figure 5a–e). However, the increase of Trx-1 expression was not concentration-dependent (Figure 5c). The mRNA level of Bax was significantly higher in the PQ-stimulated group than that in control group. Only high-dose fenofibrate reduced Bax mRNA level (Figure 5f). To further confirm the effects of fenofibrate, a PPAR-α antagonist, GW6471, was added to the medium before fenofibrate treatment. The results revealed that 10 μM GW6471 could attenuate the effect of fenofibrate on Prx, Trx-1, Trx-2, Bcl-2, Bcl-xl, and Bax mRNA expression (Figure 5a–f).

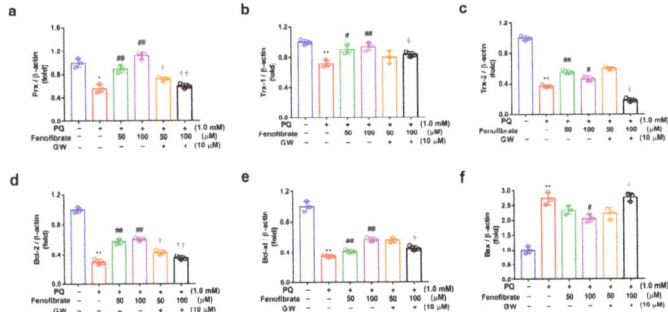

Figure 5. mRNA expression of peroxiredoxin (Prx), thioredoxin-1 (Trx-1), Trx-2, B-cell lymphoma 2 (Bcl-2), Bcl-xl, and B-cell lymphoma 2-associated X protein (Bax) in RF/6A cells detected using semi-quantitative PCR. RF/6A cells were pretreated with a high or low dose of fenofibrate or 1 h, then stimulated with 1 mM paraquat (PQ) for 24 h. In GW6471 (GW) treated groups, the cells were incubated with 10 μM GW6471 for 1 h before fenofibrate treatment. (a) Relative expression of Prx. (b) Relative expression of Trx-1. (c) Relative expression of Trx-2. (d) Relative expression of Bcl-2. (e) Relative expression of Bcl-xl. (f) Relative expression of Bax. (* $p < 0.05$, ** $p < 0.01$ between the control group and 1 mM PQ-stimulated group using Mann–Whitney U-test; # $p < 0.05$, ## $p < 0.01$ compared to only 1 mM PQ-stimulated group using Kruskal–Wallis test with post hoc Dunn's test; † $p < 0.05$, †† $p < 0.01$ between GW6471 treated group and fenofibrate treated group (the same concentration of fenofibrate) using Mann–Whitney U-test; $n = 3$ in each group; β-actin was used as an internal control.).

3.6. Effects of Fenofibrate on PQ-Induced Apoptosis and Stress-Signaling Pathway-Related Proteins in RF/6A Cells

We evaluated the effects of fenofibrate on PQ-induced apoptosis and stress-signaling pathway-related proteins in RF/6A cells. PQ stimulation decreased the expression of PPAR-α, Prx, Bcl-2, and Bcl-xl compared to that of the control group. The expression of PPAR-α, Prx, Bcl-2, and Bcl-xl increased with fenofibrate pretreatment. The expression of p-JNK and Bax increased after PQ exposure and was suppressed by fenofibrate pretreatment. The effects of fenofibrate were partially counteracted by 10 μM of GW6471 (Figure 6).

We then assessed protein expression in mitochondria and cytosol. In mitochondria, PQ stimulation enhanced p-Ask-1 expression but reduced cytochrome c and Trx-2 expression compared to that of the control group. Fenofibrate treatment enhanced cytochrome c and Trx-2 expression and suppressed p-Ask-1 expression. Stimulation of PQ facilitated cytochrome c release from the mitochondria into cytosol, and fenofibrate treatment inhibited the release of cytochrome c. In addition, PQ stimulation enhanced p-Ask-1 expression but reduced Trx-1 expression in cytosol. Fenofibrate treatment enhanced Trx-1 expression and suppressed p-Ask-1 expression in cytosol. The effects of fenofibrate were also partially counteracted by 10 μM of GW6471 (Figure 7).

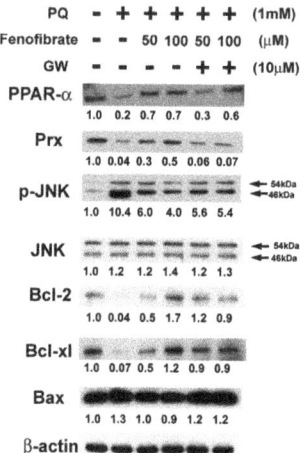

Figure 6. Effects of fenofibrate on the expression of paraquat (PQ)-induced apoptosis and stress-signaling pathway-related proteins assessed by western blot analysis. RF/6A cells were pretreated with a high or low dose of fenofibrate for 1 h, then exposed to 1 mM PQ for 1 h (for phospho-c-Jun amino-terminal kinase (p-JNK)) or 24 h. In GW6471 (GW) treated groups, the cells were incubated with 10 μM GW6471 for 1 h before fenofibrate treatment. The expression levels of peroxisome proliferator-activated receptor type α (PPAR-α), peroxiredoxin (Prx), p-JNK, JNK, B-cell lymphoma 2 (Bcl-2), Bcl-xl, and B-cell lymphoma 2-associated X protein (Bax) are shown and the fold changes compared to those in control group are presented under the protein bands. β-actin was used as an internal control.

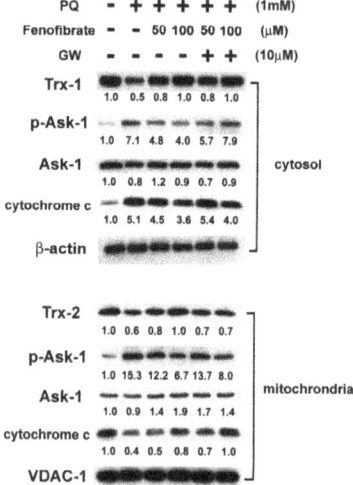

Figure 7. Effects of fenofibrate on the expression of paraquat (PQ)-induced thioredoxins (Trxs), apoptosis signal-regulated kinase-1 (Ask-1), and cytochrome c assessed by western blot analysis. RF/6A cells were pretreated with a high or low dose of fenofibrate for 1 h, then exposed to 1 mM PQ for 1 h (for phospho-Ask-1 (p-Ask-1)) or 24 h. In GW6471 (GW) treated groups, the cells were incubated with 10 μM GW6471 for 1 h before fenofibrate treatment. Mitochondrial proteins and cytosolic proteins were isolated and analyzed separately. The expression levels of mitochondrial Trx-2, Ask-1, p-Ask-1, and cytochrome c and cytosolic Trx-1, Ask-1, p-Ask-1, and cytochrome c are shown, and the fold changes compared to those in control group are presented under the protein bands. In cytosol, β-actin was used as an internal control. In mitochondria, VDAC-1 was used as an internal control.

PQ stimulation enhanced the expression of Apaf-1, cleaved caspase-9, and caspase-7 compared to that in control group, and the expression levels of these proteins were suppressed by fenofibrate treatment. The effects of fenofibrate were partially counteracted by 10 µM of GW6471. PARP-1 was cleaved in PQ-stimulated cells, and the level of cleavage form of PARP-1 was diminished by fenofibrate treatment (Figure 8a). We also assessed the activity of caspase-3 and the results demonstrated that PQ stimulation significantly increased caspase-3 activity. The activity of caspase-3 was inhibited by fenofibrate treatment in a dose-dependent manner. The effects of fenofibrate were also partially counteracted by the addition of 10 µM GW6471 (Figure 8b).

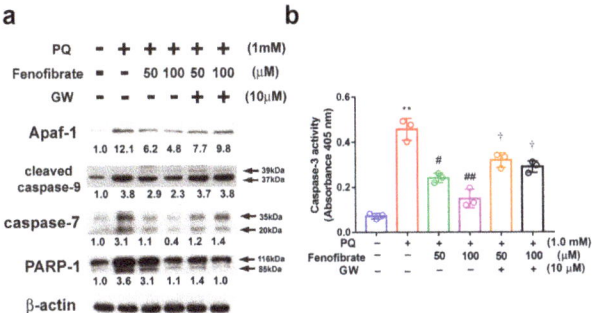

Figure 8. Effects of fenofibrate on the expression of paraquat (PQ)-induced apoptosis-related proteins assessed by western blot analysis. RF/6A cells were pretreated with a high or low dose of fenofibrate for 1 h, then exposed to 1 mM PQ for 24 h. In GW6471 (GW) treated groups, the cells were incubated with 10 µM GW6471 for 1 h before fenofibrate treatment. (**a**) The expression levels of anti-apoptotic protease activating factor-1 (Apaf-1), cleaved caspase-9, caspase-7, and poly (ADP-ribose) polymerase-1 (PARP-1) are shown. The fold changes compared to those in control group are presented under the protein bands. β-actin was used as an internal control. (**b**) Caspase-3 activity. (** $p < 0.01$ between the control group and 1 mM PQ-stimulated group using Mann–Whitney U-test; # $p < 0.05$, ## $p < 0.01$ compared to only 1 mM PQ-stimulated group using Kruskal–Wallis test with post hoc Dunn's test; † $p < 0.05$ between GW6471 treated group and fenofibrate treated group (the same concentration of fenofibrate) using Mann–Whitney U-test; $n = 3$ in each group.).

4. Discussion

In the present study, we demonstrated the protective effects of fenofibrate on RF/6A cells under oxidative stress. Fenofibrate inhibited ROS accumulation, mitochondrial dysfunction, and modulated the apoptosis and stress signaling pathway in oxidative stress-induced RF/6A cells.

Increasing evidence supports the idea that oxidative stress plays an important role in the pathogenesis of DR. PPAR-α is a regulator of inflammation and oxidative stress that induces the activation of antioxidant enzymes [45–47]. Evidence suggests that fenofibrate may modulate anti-oxidant pathways. For example, fenofibrate inhibits the production of ROS in streptozotocin-induced diabetic rats and reduces nephropathy development [48]. In the present study, the mRNA expression of anti-oxidant enzymes Prx, Trx1, and Trx-2 decreased in PQ-stimulated RF/6A cells, whereas the mRNA levels of these enzymes increased after fenofibrate treatment. This finding indicated that fenofibrate may induce the expression of anti-oxidant proteins and protect cells from oxidative stress. Endothelial cell apoptosis has been linked to oxidative damage through the production of 8-OHdG, nitrotyrosine, and MDA [49,50]. In the present study, the results showed that fenofibrate suppressed MDA production and protected vascular endothelial cells from lipid peroxidation. We also observed that fenofibrate suppressed 8-OHdG adduct formation but only inhibited protein oxidation at higher concentrations. Previous studies have also revealed that fenofibrate could suppress MDA production in rat models for low-density lipoprotein-induced endothelial dysfunction and Parkinson's disease [51,52]. Taken together, the results from the present study suggested that fenofibrate could induce the expression of anti-oxidant enzymes, reduce the production of ROS and decrease the generation of oxidant products, thus protecting endothelial cells from oxidative stress-induced damage.

Mitochondria are a major source of oxidative stress in DR because oxidative stress in the inner membrane leads to imbalance in the electron transport chain and generates superoxide and hydrogen peroxide, thereby damaging the membrane proteins. Furthermore, mitochondrial dysfunction activates the apoptosis-related signaling pathway [53]. Fenofibrate has been reported to decrease apoptosis in high-glucose-stimulated microvascular endothelial cells [54] and decrease the apoptotic rate of the ganglion cells in the mouse model for type 2 diabetes [55]. In the present study, we observed that fenofibrate reduced the apoptotic rate and could preserve mitochondrial function in PQ-stimulated RF/6A cells. Our findings suggested that fenofibrate could inhibit cell death and DR progression by preventing mitochondrial dysfunction.

Trxs belong to a group of small redox proteins that can be found in most cells. The anti-oxidative activity of Trxs is indispensable for cells [56]. Trxs exert most anti-oxidant properties in cells through thioredoxin peroxidase [18]. Niso-Santano et al. observed that PQ induces the phosphorylation of Ask-1 and suppress Trx expression in SH-SY5Y cells (human neuroblastoma cells) [57]. Trx-1 levels are also reduced in mycophenolic acid-induced apoptosis in pancreatic β-cells [58]. Fiuza et al. demonstrated that the protective effects of diphenyl diselenide on endothelial cells against oxidative stress are through the expression of different isoforms of Prx [59]. In our study, we found that the mRNA and protein expression of Prx, Trx-1, and Trx-2 decreased, and phosphorylated Ask-1 increased in PQ-stimulated RF/6A cells. In addition, thioredoxin-interacting protein (TRXIP) was reported to be significantly up-regulated in DR. TRXIP may interact with Trx, block its anti-oxidant activity, and then cause mitochondrial dysfunction and inflammation in DR [60,61]. The expression of Trx increased after fenofibrate treatment in our experiments. Our results were consistent with that of the study conducted by Billiet et al., in which PPAR-α activation induced Trx-1 expression [28]. The addition of PPAR-α antagonist could attenuate but not completely abolish the effects of fenofibrate, indicating that the effects of fenofibrate were not all PPAR-α dependent. In summary, our study suggested that the anti-oxidative activity and anti-apoptotic effects of fenofibrate could be attributed to the increase of Trx expression and the inhibition of Ask-1 phosphorylation.

We then investigated the effects of fenofibrate on the regulation of Trx-related signaling pathways. Trx binds to Ask-1 in the mitochondria and cytosol, thereby blocking the initiation of the cellular apoptotic process and inhibiting the activation of JNK/p38 MAP kinase [26]. In the cytosol, Ask-1 is required for the activation of JNK/p38 MAP kinases. Bcl-2 and Bcl-xl are known to regulate mitochondrial dynamics and play essential roles in anti-apoptosis; however, Bax promotes apoptosis [62,63]. JNK/p38 MAP kinase also regulates mitochondrial-mediated apoptosis [64] and facilitates the release of mitochondrial cytochrome c to the cytosol. Our study revealed that p-JNK and Bax expression were elevated in PQ-stimulated RF/6A cells and fenofibrate treatment suppressed their expression. Conversely, the expression of Bcl-2 and Bcl-xl increased after fenofibrate treatment. In mitochondria, Trx-2 inhibits Ask-1-mediated apoptosis, which in turn causes the inhibition of cytochrome c release to the cytosol [65]. Our findings showed that pretreatment of fenofibrate in PQ-stimulated cells increased Trx-2 expression, decreased the formation of p-Ask-1 and inhibited cytochrome c release. Cytochrome c release is an initiator of the main apoptotic pathway [66]. When cytochrome c is released from the mitochondria to cytosol, it binds to Apaf-1 and activates an apoptosis-related caspase cascade, consequently inducing PARP-1 cleavage leading to apoptosis [67]. We observed that fenofibrate treatment reduced the levels of cytosolic cytochrome c and the related caspase cascade in PQ-stimulated cells. In summary, our results indicated that fenofibrate could protect against oxidative stress-induced retinal/choroidal endothelial cell apoptosis by enhancing Trx-1 and Trx-2 expression, thereby suppressing Ask-1 activity, which in turn inhibits the activation of the subsequent apoptotic signaling pathways.

Our study has some limitations. It is an in vitro analysis, and the protective effects of fenofibrate and the underlying mechanisms need to be demonstrated with animal models. However, two large randomized controlled trials (FIELD and ACCORD study) have shown significant benefits of fenofibrate in patients with DR. Our results supported the assertion that fenofibrate can slow the progression of DR by modulating apoptosis- and stress-related signaling pathways.

5. Conclusions

Our study demonstrated that fenofibrate inhibited ROS accumulation, diminished mitochondrial dysfunction, as well as modulating several apoptotic and survival signal pathways in oxidative stress-induced RF/6A cells. The mechanism of action could be through enhancing Trxs expression and suppressing Ask-1 activity, which in turn inhibited the subsequent apoptotic signaling pathways. The anti-oxidative and anti-apoptotic beneficial effects of fenofibrate identified in this study may provide new insights into the design of therapeutic strategies concerning the imbalance between pro-apoptotic and survival pathways induced by oxidative stress in DR.

Author Contributions: Conceptualization, Y.-J.H., C.-W.L., S.-L.C., W.-S.Y. and C.-H.Y.; Data curation, Y.-J.H. and S.-L.C.; Formal analysis, Y.-J.H., C.-W.L. and C.-H.Y.; Funding acquisition, C.-M.Y. and C.-H.Y.; Investigation, Y.-J.H., C.-W.L., S.-L.C. and C.-H.Y.; Methodology, Y.-J.H., C.-W.L., S.-L.C., W.-S.Y. and C.-H.Y.; Project administration, W.-S.Y., C.-M.Y. and C.-H.Y.; Resources, C.-W.L., W.-S.Y., C.-M.Y. and C.-H.Y.; Software, C.-M.Y.; Supervision, W.-S.Y., C.-M.Y. and C.-H.Y.; Validation, Y.-J.H. and C.-W.L.; Visualization, Y.-J.H., C.-W.L. and S.-L.C.; Writing—original draft, Y.-J.H., C.-W.L. and S.-L.C.; Writing—review & editing, C.-M.Y. and C.-H.Y. All authors have read and agreed to the published version of the manuscript.

Funding: This research received no external funding.

Conflicts of Interest: The authors declare no conflict of interest.

References

1. Stitt, A.W.; Curtis, T.M.; Chen, M.; Medina, R.J.; McKay, G.J.; Jenkins, A.; Gardiner, T.A.; Lyons, T.J.; Hammes, H.P.; Simó, R.; et al. The progress in understanding and treatment of diabetic retinopathy. *Prog. Retin. Eye Res.* **2016**, *51*, 156–186. [CrossRef]
2. Martinez-Zapata, M.J.; Marti-Carvajal, A.J.; Sola, I.; Pijoan, J.I.; Buil-Calvo, J.A.; Cordero, J.A.; Evans, J.R. Anti-vascular endothelial growth factor for proliferative diabetic retinopathy. *Cochrane Database Syst. Rev.* **2014**, *11*, Cd008721. [CrossRef] [PubMed]
3. Zhang, X.; Fu, Y.; Xu, X.; Li, M.; Du, L.; Han, Y.; Ge, Y. PERK pathway are involved in NO-induced apoptosis in endothelial cells cocultured with RPE under high glucose conditions. *Nitric Oxide* **2014**, *40*, 10–16. [CrossRef] [PubMed]
4. Feldman, E.L. Oxidative stress and diabetic neuropathy: A new understanding of an old problem. *J. Clin. Investig.* **2003**, *111*, 431–433. [CrossRef] [PubMed]
5. Brownlee, M. The pathobiology of diabetic complications: A unifying mechanism. *Diabetes* **2005**, *54*, 1615–1625. [CrossRef]
6. Park, S.W.; Cho, C.S.; Jun, H.O.; Ryu, N.H.; Kim, J.H.; Yu, Y.S.; Kim, J.S.; Kim, J.H. Anti-angiogenic effect of luteolin on retinal neovascularization via blockade of reactive oxygen species production. *Investig. Ophthalmol. Vis. Sci.* **2012**, *53*, 7718–7726. [CrossRef]
7. Feenstra, D.J.; Yego, E.C.; Mohr, S. Modes of Retinal Cell Death in Diabetic Retinopathy. *J. Clin. Exp. Ophthalmol.* **2013**, *4*, 298. [CrossRef]
8. Schoonjans, K.; Martin, G.; Staels, B.; Auwerx, J. Peroxisome proliferator-activated receptors, orphans with ligands and functions. *Curr. Opin. Lipidol.* **1997**, *8*, 159–166. [CrossRef]
9. Keech, A.C.; Mitchell, P.; Summanen, P.A.; O'Day, J.; Davis, T.M.; Moffitt, M.S.; Taskinen, M.R.; Simes, R.J.; Tse, D.; Williamson, E.; et al. Effect of fenofibrate on the need for laser treatment for diabetic retinopathy (FIELD study): A randomised controlled trial. *Lancet* **2007**, *370*, 1687–1697. [CrossRef]
10. Chew, E.Y.; Ambrosius, W.T.; Davis, M.D.; Danis, R.P.; Gangaputra, S.; Greven, C.M.; Hubbard, L.; Esser, B.A.; Lovato, J.F.; Perdue, L.H.; et al. Effects of medical therapies on retinopathy progression in type 2 diabetes. *N. Engl. J. Med.* **2010**, *363*, 233–244. [CrossRef]
11. Hu, Y.; Chen, Y.; Ding, L.; He, X.; Takahashi, Y.; Gao, Y.; Shen, W.; Cheng, R.; Chen, Q.; Qi, X.; et al. Pathogenic role of diabetes-induced PPAR-alpha down-regulation in microvascular dysfunction. *Proc. Natl. Acad. Sci. USA* **2013**, *110*, 15401–15406. [CrossRef] [PubMed]

12. Miranda, S.; Gonzalez-Rodriguez, A.; Garcia-Ramirez, M.; Revuelta-Cervantes, J.; Hernandez, C.; Simo, R.; Valverde, A.M. Beneficial effects of fenofibrate in retinal pigment epithelium by the modulation of stress and survival signaling under diabetic conditions. *J. Cell. Physiol.* **2012**, *227*, 2352–2362. [CrossRef] [PubMed]
13. Yeh, P.T.; Wang, L.C.; Chang, S.W.; Yang, W.S.; Yang, C.M.; Yang, C.H. Effect of Fenofibrate on the Expression of Inflammatory Mediators in a Diabetic Rat Model. *Curr. Eye Res.* **2019**, *44*, 1121–1132. [CrossRef] [PubMed]
14. Liu, J.; Lu, C.; Li, F.; Wang, H.; He, L.; Hao, Y.; Chen, A.F.; An, H.; Wang, X.; Hong, T.; et al. PPAR-alpha Agonist Fenofibrate Upregulates Tetrahydrobiopterin Level through Increasing the Expression of Guanosine 5′-Triphosphate Cyclohydrolase-I in Human Umbilical Vein Endothelial Cells. *PPAR Res.* **2011**, *2011*, 523520. [CrossRef]
15. Kim, J.; Ahn, J.H.; Kim, J.H.; Yu, Y.S.; Kim, H.S.; Ha, J.; Shinn, S.H.; Oh, Y.S. Fenofibrate regulates retinal endothelial cell survival through the AMPK signal transduction pathway. *Exp. Eye Res.* **2007**, *84*, 886–893. [CrossRef]
16. Ding, L.; Cheng, R.; Hu, Y.; Takahashi, Y.; Jenkins, A.J.; Keech, A.C.; Humphries, K.M.; Gu, X.; Elliott, M.H.; Xia, X.; et al. Peroxisome proliferator-activated receptor α protects capillary pericytes in the retina. *Am. J. Pathol.* **2014**, *184*, 2709–2720. [CrossRef]
17. Chen, Y.; Hu, Y.; Lin, M.; Jenkins, A.J.; Keech, A.C.; Mott, R.; Lyons, T.J.; Ma, J.X. Therapeutic effects of PPARalpha agonists on diabetic retinopathy in type 1 diabetes models. *Diabetes* **2013**, *62*, 261–272. [CrossRef]
18. Trudeau, K.; Roy, S.; Guo, W.; Hernandez, C.; Villarroel, M.; Simo, R.; Roy, S. Fenofibric acid reduces fibronectin and collagen type IV overexpression in human retinal pigment epithelial cells grown in conditions mimicking the diabetic milieu: Functional implications in retinal permeability. *Investig. Ophthalmol. Vis. Sci.* **2011**, *52*, 6348–6354. [CrossRef]
19. Watson, W.H.; Yang, X.; Choi, Y.E.; Jones, D.P.; Kehrer, J.P. Thioredoxin and its role in toxicology. *Toxicol. Sci.* **2004**, *78*, 3–14. [CrossRef]
20. Powis, G.; Montfort, W.R. Properties and biological activities of thioredoxins. *Annu. Rev. Pharmacol. Toxicol.* **2001**, *41*, 261–295. [CrossRef] [PubMed]
21. Rhee, S.G.; Kang, S.W.; Chang, T.S.; Jeong, W.; Kim, K. Peroxiredoxin, a novel family of peroxidases. *IUBMB Life* **2001**, *52*, 35–41. [CrossRef]
22. Tanaka, T.; Hosoi, F.; Yamaguchi-Iwai, Y.; Nakamura, H.; Masutani, H.; Ueda, S.; Nishiyama, A.; Takeda, S.; Wada, H.; Spyrou, G.; et al. Thioredoxin-2 (TRX-2) is an essential gene regulating mitochondria-dependent apoptosis. *EMBO J.* **2002**, *21*, 1695–1703. [CrossRef] [PubMed]
23. Saxena, G.; Chen, J.; Shalev, A. Intracellular shuttling and mitochondrial function of thioredoxin-interacting protein. *J. Biol. Chem.* **2010**, *285*, 3997–4005. [CrossRef] [PubMed]
24. Matsui, M.; Oshima, M.; Oshima, H.; Takaku, K.; Maruyama, T.; Yodoi, J.; Taketo, M.M. Early embryonic lethality caused by targeted disruption of the mouse thioredoxin gene. *Dev. Biol.* **1996**, *178*, 179–185. [CrossRef] [PubMed]
25. Nonn, L.; Williams, R.R.; Erickson, R.P.; Powis, G. The absence of mitochondrial thioredoxin 2 causes massive apoptosis, exencephaly, and early embryonic lethality in homozygous mice. *Mol. Cell. Biol.* **2003**, *23*, 916–922. [CrossRef]
26. Tobiume, K.; Matsuzawa, A.; Takahashi, T.; Nishitoh, H.; Morita, K.; Takeda, K.; Minowa, O.; Miyazono, K.; Noda, T.; Ichijo, H. ASK1 is required for sustained activations of JNK/p38 MAP kinases and apoptosis. *EMBO Rep.* **2001**, *2*, 222–228. [CrossRef]
27. Liu, G.H.; Qu, J.; Shen, X. Thioredoxin-mediated negative autoregulation of peroxisome proliferator-activated receptor alpha transcriptional activity. *Mol. Biol. Cell.* **2006**, *17*, 1822–1833. [CrossRef]
28. Billiet, L.; Furman, C.; Cuaz-Perolin, C.; Paumelle, R.; Raymondjean, M.; Simmet, T.; Rouis, M. Thioredoxin-1 and its natural inhibitor, vitamin D3 up-regulated protein 1, are differentially regulated by PPARalpha in human macrophages. *J. Mol. Biol.* **2008**, *384*, 564–576. [CrossRef]
29. Fang, I.M.; Yang, C.H.; Yang, C.M.; Chen, M.S. Chitosan oligosaccharides attenuates oxidative-stress related retinal degeneration in rats. *PLoS ONE* **2013**, *8*, e77323. [CrossRef]
30. Chen, M.; Luo, C.; Penalva, R.; Xu, H. Paraquat-induced retinal degeneration is exaggerated in CX3CR1-deficient mice and is associated with increased retinal inflammation. *Investig. Ophthalmol. Vis. Sci.* **2013**, *54*, 682–690. [CrossRef]

31. Lederman, M.; Hagbi-Levi, S.; Grunin, M.; Obolensky, A.; Berenshtein, E.; Banin, E.; Chevion, M.; Chowers, I. Degeneration modulates retinal response to transient exogenous oxidative injury. *PLoS ONE* **2014**, *9*, e87751. [CrossRef] [PubMed]
32. Kimura, K.; Tawara, S.; Igarashi, K.; Takenaka, A. Effect of various radical generators on insulin-dependent regulation of hepatic gene expression. *Biosci. Biotechnol. Biochem.* **2007**, *71*, 16–22. [CrossRef] [PubMed]
33. Kimura, K.; Katsumata, Y.; Ozawa, T.; Tawara, S.; Igarashi, K.; Cho, Y.; Shibata, N.; Hakuno, F.; Takahashi, S.; Takenaka, A. Effect of paraquat-induced oxidative stress on insulin regulation of insulin-like growth factor-binding protein-1 gene expression. *J. Clin. Biochem. Nutr.* **2010**, *46*, 157–167. [CrossRef] [PubMed]
34. Shibata, M.; Hakuno, F.; Yamanaka, D.; Okajima, H.; Fukushima, T.; Hasegawa, T.; Ogata, T.; Toyoshima, Y.; Chida, K.; Kimura, K.; et al. Paraquat-induced oxidative stress represses phosphatidylinositol 3-kinase activities leading to impaired glucose uptake in 3T3-L1 adipocytes. *J. Biol. Chem.* **2010**, *285*, 20915–20925. [CrossRef] [PubMed]
35. Gendron, R.; Good, W.; Adams, L.; Paradis, H. Suppressed expression of tubedown-1 in retinal neovascularization of proliferative diabetic retinopathy. *Investig. Ophthalmol. Vis. Sci.* **2001**, *42*, 3000–3007.
36. Lukiw, W.J.; Ottlecz, A.; Lambrou, G.; Grueninger, M.; Finley, J.; Thompson, H.W.; Bazan, N.G. Coordinate activation of HIF-1 and NF-κB DNA binding and COX-2 and VEGF expression in retinal cells by hypoxia. *Investig. Ophthalmol. Vis. Sci.* **2003**, *44*, 4163–4170. [CrossRef]
37. You, J.J.; Yang, C.M.; Chen, M.S.; Yang, C.H. Regulation of Cyr61/CCN1 expression by hypoxia through cooperation of c-Jun/AP-1 and HIF-1a in retinal vascular endothelial cells. *Exp. Eye Res.* **2010**, *91*, 825–836. [CrossRef]
38. You, J.J.; Yang, C.H.; Yang, C.M.; Chen, M.S. Cyr61 induces the expression of monocyte chemoattractant protein-1 via the integrin αvβ3, FAK, PI3K/Akt, and NF-κB pathways in retinal vascular endothelial cells. *Cell. Signal.* **2014**, *26*, 133–140. [CrossRef] [PubMed]
39. Wu, T.; Xu, W.; Wang, Y.; Tao, M.; Hu, Z.; Lv, B.; Hui, Y.; Du, H. OxLDL enhances choroidal neovascularization lesion through inducing vascular endothelium to mesenchymal transition process and angiogenic factor expression. *Cell. Signal.* **2020**, *70*, 109571. [CrossRef]
40. Warden, C.; Barnett, J.M.; Brantley, M.A., Jr. Taurocholic acid inhibits features of age-related macular degeneration in vitro. *Exp. Eye Res.* **2020**, *193*, 107974. [CrossRef]
41. Xie, W.; Zhou, P.; Qu, M.; Dai, Z.; Zhang, X.; Zhang, C.; Dong, X.; Sun, G.; Sun, X. Ginsenoside Re Attenuates High Glucose-Induced RF/6A Injury via Regulating PI3K/AKT Inhibited HIF-1α/VEGF Signaling Pathway. *Front. Pharmacol.* **2020**, *11*, 695. [CrossRef]
42. Li, J.; He, J.; Zhang, X.; Li, J.; Zhao, P.; Fei, P. TSP1 ameliorates age-related macular degeneration by regulating the STAT3-iNOS signaling pathway. *Exp. Cell Res.* **2020**, *388*, 111811. [CrossRef] [PubMed]
43. Yao, G.; Li, R.; Du, J.; Yao, Y. Angiogenic factor with G patch and FHA domains 1 protects retinal vascular endothelial cells under hyperoxia by inhibiting autophagy. *J. Biochem. Mol. Toxicol.* **2020**, e22572. [CrossRef] [PubMed]
44. Wang, C.; Lin, Y.; Fu, Y.; Zhang, D.; Xin, Y. MiR-221-3p regulates the microvascular dysfunction in diabetic retinopathy by targeting TIMP3. *Pflugers Arch.* **2020**. [CrossRef]
45. Bordet, R.; Ouk, T.; Petrault, O.; Gele, P.; Gautier, S.; Laprais, M.; Deplanque, D.; Duriez, P.; Staels, B.; Fruchart, J.C.; et al. PPAR: A new pharmacological target for neuroprotection in stroke and neurodegenerative diseases. *Biochem. Soc. Trans.* **2006**, *34*, 1341–1346. [CrossRef] [PubMed]
46. Wong, T.Y.; Simo, R.; Mitchell, P. Fenofibrate—A potential systemic treatment for diabetic retinopathy? *Am. J. Ophthalmol.* **2012**, *154*, 6–12. [CrossRef]
47. Pearsall, E.A.; Cheng, R.; Matsuzaki, S.; Zhou, K.; Ding, L.; Ahn, B.; Kinter, M.; Humphries, K.M.; Quiambao, A.B.; Farjo, R.A.; et al. Neuroprotective effects of PPARα in retinopathy of type 1 diabetes. *PLoS ONE* **2019**, *14*, e0208399. [CrossRef]
48. Kadian, S.; Mahadevan, N.; Balakumar, P. Differential effects of low-dose fenofibrate treatment in diabetic rats with early onset nephropathy and established nephropathy. *Eur. J. Pharmacol.* **2013**, *698*, 388–396. [CrossRef]
49. Quagliaro, L.; Piconi, L.; Assaloni, R.; Martinelli, L.; Motz, E.; Ceriello, A. Intermittent high glucose enhances apoptosis related to oxidative stress in human umbilical vein endothelial cells: The role of protein kinase C and NAD(P)H-oxidase activation. *Diabetes* **2003**, *52*, 2795–2804. [CrossRef]

50. Chang, Y.; Chang, T.C.; Lee, J.J.; Chang, N.C.; Huang, Y.K. Sanguis draconis, a dragon's blood resin, attenuates high glucose-induced oxidative stress and endothelial dysfunction in human umbilical vein endothelial cells. *Sci. World J.* **2014**, *2014*, 423259. [CrossRef]
51. Yang, T.L.; Chen, M.F.; Luo, B.L.; Yu, J.; Jiang, J.L.; Li, Y.J. Effect of fenofibrate on LDL-induced endothelial dysfunction in rats. *Naunyn Schmiedebergs Arch. Pharmacol.* **2004**, *370*, 79–83. [CrossRef] [PubMed]
52. Uppalapati, D.; Das, N.R.; Gangwal, R.P.; Damre, M.V.; Sangamwar, A.T.; Sharma, S.S. Neuroprotective Potential of Peroxisome Proliferator Activated Receptor- alpha Agonist in Cognitive Impairment in Parkinson's Disease: Behavioral, Biochemical, and PBPK Profile. *PPAR Res.* **2014**, *2014*, 753587. [CrossRef]
53. Madsen-Bouterse, S.A.; Kowluru, R.A. Oxidative stress and diabetic retinopathy: Pathophysiological mechanisms and treatment perspectives. *Rev. Endocr. Metab. Disord.* **2008**, *9*, 315–327. [CrossRef] [PubMed]
54. Tomizawa, A.; Hattori, Y.; Inoue, T.; Hattori, S.; Kasai, K. Fenofibrate suppresses microvascular inflammation and apoptosis through adenosine monophosphate-activated protein kinase activation. *Metabolism* **2011**, *60*, 513–522. [CrossRef] [PubMed]
55. Bogdanov, P.; Hernandez, C.; Corraliza, L.; Carvalho, A.R.; Simo, R. Effect of fenofibrate on retinal neurodegeneration in an experimental model of type 2 diabetes. *Acta Diabetol.* **2015**, *52*, 113–122. [CrossRef] [PubMed]
56. Garrido, E.O.; Grant, C.M. Role of thioredoxins in the response of Saccharomyces cerevisiae to oxidative stress induced by hydroperoxides. *Mol. Microbiol.* **2002**, *43*, 993–1003. [CrossRef]
57. Niso-Santano, M.; Gonzalez-Polo, R.A.; Bravo-San Pedro, J.M.; Gomez-Sanchez, R.; Lastres-Becker, I.; Ortiz-Ortiz, M.A.; Soler, G.; Moran, J.M.; Cuadrado, A.; Fuentes, J.M. Activation of apoptosis signal-regulating kinase 1 is a key factor in paraquat-induced cell death: Modulation by the Nrf2/Trx axis. *Free Radic. Biol. Med.* **2010**, *48*, 1370–1381. [CrossRef]
58. Huh, K.H.; Cho, Y.; Kim, B.S.; Do, J.H.; Park, Y.J.; Joo, D.J.; Kim, M.S.; Kim, Y.S. The role of thioredoxin 1 in the mycophenolic acid-induced apoptosis of insulin-producing cells. *Cell Death Dis.* **2013**, *4*, e721. [CrossRef]
59. Fiuza, B.; Subelzu, N.; Calcerrada, P.; Straliotto, M.R.; Piacenza, L.; Cassina, A.; Rocha, J.B.; Radi, R.; de Bem, A.F.; Peluffo, G. Impact of SIN-1-derived peroxynitrite flux on endothelial cell redox homeostasis and bioenergetics: Protective role of diphenyl diselenide via induction of peroxiredoxins. *Free Radic. Res.* **2015**, *49*, 122–132. [CrossRef]
60. Devi, T.S.; Hosoya, K.; Terasaki, T.; Singh, L.P. Critical role of TXNIP in oxidative stress, DNA damage and retinal pericyte apoptosis under high glucose: Implications for diabetic retinopathy. *Exp. Cell Res.* **2013**, *319*, 1001–1012. [CrossRef]
61. Singh, L.P. Thioredoxin Interacting Protein (TXNIP) and Pathogenesis of Diabetic Retinopathy. *J. Clin. Exp. Ophthalmol.* **2013**, *4*. [CrossRef] [PubMed]
62. Adams, J.M.; Cory, S. The Bcl-2 protein family: Arbiters of cell survival. *Science* **1998**, *281*, 1322–1326. [CrossRef] [PubMed]
63. Jeong, H.S.; Choi, H.Y.; Choi, T.W.; Kim, B.W.; Kim, J.H.; Lee, E.R.; Cho, S.G. Differential regulation of the antiapoptotic action of B-cell lymphoma 2 (Bcl-2) and B-cell lymphoma extra long (Bcl-xL) by c-Jun N-terminal protein kinase (JNK) 1-involved pathway in neuroglioma cells. *Biol. Pharm. Bull.* **2008**, *31*, 1686–1690. [CrossRef] [PubMed]
64. Yuan, L.; Wang, J.; Xiao, H.; Wu, W.; Wang, Y.; Liu, X. MAPK signaling pathways regulate mitochondrial-mediated apoptosis induced by isoorientin in human hepatoblastoma cancer cells. *Food Chem. Toxicol.* **2013**, *53*, 62–68. [CrossRef] [PubMed]
65. Zhang, R.; Al-Lamki, R.; Bai, L.; Streb, J.W.; Miano, J.M.; Bradley, J.; Min, W. Thioredoxin-2 inhibits mitochondria-located ASK1-mediated apoptosis in a JNK-independent manner. *Circ. Res.* **2004**, *94*, 1483–1491. [CrossRef] [PubMed]
66. Friedlander, R.M. Apoptosis and caspases in neurodegenerative diseases. *N. Engl. J. Med.* **2003**, *348*, 1365–1375. [CrossRef]
67. Giacco, F.; Brownlee, M. Oxidative stress and diabetic complications. *Circ. Res.* **2010**, *107*, 1058–1070. [CrossRef]

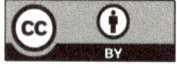

© 2020 by the authors. Licensee MDPI, Basel, Switzerland. This article is an open access article distributed under the terms and conditions of the Creative Commons Attribution (CC BY) license (http://creativecommons.org/licenses/by/4.0/).

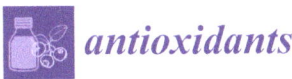

Article

A Higher Proportion of Eicosapentaenoic Acid (EPA) When Combined with Docosahexaenoic Acid (DHA) in Omega-3 Dietary Supplements Provides Higher Antioxidant Effects in Human Retinal Cells

Manuel Saenz de Viteri [1,2,3,4,†], María Hernandez [2,3,†], Valentina Bilbao-Malavé [1,2,3,†], Patricia Fernandez-Robredo [2,3,4,*], Jorge González-Zamora [1,2,3], Laura Garcia-Garcia [2], Nahia Ispizua [2], Sergio Recalde [2,3,4,‡] and Alfredo Garcia-Layana [1,2,3,4,‡]

1. Department of Ophthalmology, Clinica Universidad de Navarra, 31008 Pamplona, Spain; msaenzdevit@unav.es (M.S.d.V.); vbilbao@unav.es (V.B.-M.); jgzamora@unav.es (J.G.-Z.); aglayana@unav.es (A.G.-L.)
2. Retinal Pathologies and New Therapies Group, Experimental Ophthalmology Laboratory, Department of Ophthalmology, Clinica Universidad de Navarra, 31008 Pamplona, Spain; mahersan@unav.es (M.H.); mgarcia.6@alumni.unav.es (L.G.-G.); nispizua@alumni.unav.es (N.I.); srecalde@unav.es (S.R.)
3. Navarra Institute for Health Research, IdiSNA, 31008 Pamplona, Spain
4. Red Temática de Investigación Cooperativa Sanitaria en Enfermedades Oculares (Oftared), 31008 Pamplona, Spain
* Correspondence: pfrobredo@unav.es; Tel.: +34-9484-256-00 (ext. 806499)
† These authors contributed equally to this work.
‡ These authors also contributed equally to this work.

Received: 31 July 2020; Accepted: 1 September 2020; Published: 4 September 2020

Abstract: Retinal pigment epithelium (RPE) is a key regulator of retinal function and is directly related to the transport, delivery, and metabolism of long-chain n-3 polyunsaturated fatty acids (n3-PUFA), in the retina. Due to their functions and location, RPE cells are constantly exposed to oxidative stress. Eicosapentaenoic acid (EPA) and docosahexaenoic acid (DHA) have shown to have antioxidant effects by different mechanisms. For this reason, we designed an in vitro study to compare 10 formulations of DHA and EPA supplements from different origins and combined in different proportions, evaluating their effect on cell viability, cell proliferation, reactive oxygen species production, and cell migration using ARPE-19 cells. Furthermore, we assessed their ability to rescue RPE cells from the oxidative conditions seen in diabetic retinopathy. Our results showed that the different formulations of n3-PUFAs have a beneficial effect on cell viability and proliferation and are able to restore oxidative induced RPE damage. We observed that the n3-PUFA provided different results alone or combined in the same supplement. When combined, the best results were obtained in formulations that included a higher proportion of EPA than DHA. Moreover, n3-PUFA in the form of ethyl-esters had a worse performance when compared with triglycerides or phospholipid based formulations.

Keywords: eicosapentaenoic acid (EPA); docosahexaenoic acid (DHA); oxidative stress; diabetic retinopathy; retinal pigment epithelium

1. Introduction

Diabetes mellitus (DM) epidemic is a global public health problem and the leading cause of preventable blindness in the working-age population [1]. The International Diabetes Federation, in 2019, stated that DM affected an estimated 425 million adults worldwide and this number is likely to increase over the next few years due to urbanization, increased obesity prevalence, and sedentary lifestyles. According to epidemiologic predictions 1 in 10 adults across the globe, will live with diabetes by 2045 [2]. The physiopathology of DR is complex and several interconnecting biochemical pathways have been proposed as contributors in its development. These include the polyol pathway [3], non-enzymatic glycation [4], activation of protein kinase C (PKC) [5], oxidative stress [6–10], and inflammation through proinflammatory cytokines, chemokines, and other inflammatory mediators [11,12]. Among these, oxidative stress and inflammation are major causal factors involved in the endothelial dysfunction of the retina microvasculature that occurs in DR [6–10]. In addition, this chronic low-grade inflammation could finally lead to neovascularization [13]. While improvements in treatment have reduced the macro and microvascular complications of the disease, the increasing number of diabetic patients combined with the extended life expectancy means that more patients will live long enough to develop DR. In fact, it is expected that the number of people with DR will grow from 126.6 million in 2010 to 191.0 million by 2030 [14].

Metabolic abnormalities of diabetes cause mitochondrial superoxide overproduction [15]. This is the central and major mediator of diabetes endothelial dysfunction and tissue damage, with several pathways involved in the pathogenesis: Polyol pathway, increased formation of advanced glycation end-products (AGEs), increased expression of the receptor for AGEs and its activating ligands, activation of protein kinase C (PKC) isoforms, and overactivity of the hexosamine pathway [15].

According to the above, long-chain n-3 polyunsaturated fatty acids (n3-PUFA), including eicosapentaenoic acid (EPA), and docosahexaenoic acid (DHA) have been studied as an alternative therapy for retinal diseases due to their pleiotropic effects including anti-inflammatory, antioxidant, antiproliferative, and antiangiogenic properties. They are essential fatty acids in the human diet that exert anti-inflammatory and antioxidant effects by binding cell membrane receptors to affect downstream mediators and alter gene expression [16]. DHA is a major structural lipid in the sensory and vascular retina. In fact, the highest body concentrations of DHA per unit weight are found in phospholipids of retinal photoreceptor outer segments. Retinal pigmented epithelium (RPE) is a polarized epithelial monolayer known to synthesize DHA [17]. Moreover, the RPE plays an important role in regulation and delivery of DHA from the plasma to the photoreceptors [18]. EPA is converted intracellularly to DHA at low basal levels, yet exogenous EPA supplementation does not increase DHA levels in human plasma [19]. Rather than rapidly converting to DHA, EPA seems to have a clinically relevant biological activity itself, distinct from that of DHA [20–22].

Several clinical trials have demonstrated the beneficial effects of the administration of n3-PUFA in the development of DR. J. Howard-Williams et al. found that poorly controlled patients with low levels of n3-PUFA intake had a significantly greater frequency of retinopathy [23]. Similarly, a reduced severity of DR in well-controlled diabetes patients was observed with increasing n3-PUFA intake [24]. The primary prevention of cardiovascular disease with a Mediterranean diet (PREDIMED) demonstrated that participants taking at least 500 mg/day of long-chain v-3 PUFAs, showed a 48% relatively reduced risk of incident sight-threatening DR compared with those not fulfilling this recommendation [25]. Moreover, the addition of DHA supplement to intravitreal ranibizumab was effective to achieve better sustained improvement of central subfield macular thickness compared with ranibizumab alone [26].

In diabetic animal models, the ability of n3-PUFAs, especially EPA and DHA, to suppress IL-6, TNF-a, ICAM-1, MCP-1, and VEGF production has been demonstrated, as well as the reduction of free radical generation and the restoration of antioxidant homeostasis [27–30]. According to the conclusions of a study conducted by Mahmoudabadi and Rahbar [31], the administration of EPA increases several endogenous antioxidant enzymes, namely superoxide dismutase and glutathione peroxidase, while simultaneously decreasing the levels of malondialdehyde, a classical biomarker of oxidative stress, in type II diabetic patients.

Despite their similarities in their nutritional sources and most of their biological actions, the type of n3-PUFA formulation seems to matter in treating different diseases. DHA is associated with decreased Alzheimer disease risk in humans [32]. Conversely, EPA has a more therapeutic effect in treating depression [19–21] while cardiovascular outcomes have been shown to improve after the intake of combined EPA and DHA supplements [33]. Nevertheless, it should be noted that many of the observational studies published in DR only supplement one type of n3-PUFA (EPA or DHA), while some of them did not measure the type of omega 3 consumed, but rather frequency of fish oil consumption. In addition, the efficacy of the use of different formulations of DHA and EPA have not been studied to date. Currently, the primary dietary source of these fatty acids is fish oil; however, since the global consumption cannot be satisfied due to the increasing demand, alternative sources such as microalgae have emerged [34,35].

Given this lack of evidence, we designed an in vitro study to compare 10 formulations of DHA and EPA supplements from different origins, and assess their safety profile and their ability to rescue retinal pigment epithelium (RPE) cells from the oxidative and inflammatory conditions seen in the DR.

2. Materials and Methods

2.1. Cell Culture

ARPE-19, obtained from the American Type Culture Collection (CRL-2302, ATCC®, Manassas, VA, USA), were grown to confluence in a standard incubator at 37 °C in humidified 5% CO_2 condition in a DMEM/F12 medium (1:1) (Sigma-Aldrich, St. Louis, MO, USA) containing 10% fetal bovine serum (FBS; Sigma-Aldrich, St. Louis, MO, USA), 1% fungizone, and L-glutamine penicillin-streptomycin (Sigma-Aldrich, St. Louis, MO, USA). Cells were passaged every 3–4 days with 0.25% Trypsin-EDTA (Invitrogen, Carlsbad, CA, USA). For all assays, cells were grown to 100% confluence with the exception of BrdU, which requires non-confluent cells grown for 1–2 days.

2.2. Omega-3 Supplementation

Fatty acids (FA) were conjugated to albumin to solubilize them and to replicate the in vivo environment. Cells were seeded with a lipid-free bovine serum albumin (BSA) media in a 2:1 FA/BSA ratio.

Ten different omega-3 supplements were tested grouped in three parts as shown in Table 1: I: EPA and DHA, separately; II: EPA and DHA combined in different proportions and in the form of ethyl esters (EE) or triglycerides (TG); III: DHA-TG combined with DHA phospholipids (PL) from different origins (marine or vegetable). All the supplements were provided by Théa Laboratories (Clermont-Ferrand, France). Details of the composition of each formulation and identification of groups are displayed in Table 1.

2.3. Immunofluorescence Detection of Zonula Occludens

The effect of all FA groups on the integrity of the epithelial tight junctions was determined by ZO-1 immunofluorescence to determine if any formulations compromised these intercellular unions. One hundred thousand ARPE-19 cells were seeded onto polycarbonate inserts (Corning® Transwell®, Phoenix, AR, USA,) and kept in a culture with 1% DMEM for four weeks to allow epithelial polarization. Supplements were then added to ARPE-19 cells, which were fixed in cold methanol after 24 h. After three washes with 1% PBS, cells were submerged in 1% PBS-BSA for 20 min to block non-specific bonds before incubation with the polyclonal ZO-1 anti-rabbit antibody (1:100; Life Technologies, Gaithersburg, MD, USA) in 1% PBS-BSA at 4 °C for 24 h. The cells were washed with 1% PBS (three times of 5 min) and incubated with the secondary antibody goat anti-rabbit Alexa Fluor® 488 (1:250; A11008 Invitrogen, Thermo Fisher, Madrid, Spain) in 1% PBS-BSA for 1 h in the dark at room temperature. TOPRO-3 was used for nuclear staining. Membranes were cut from the transwell insert with a scalpel and placed on a microscope slide and mounted with PBS-Glycerol

1:1. Images were captured in the Z-stack mode with a laser scanning confocal imaging system (Zeiss LSM-510 Meta, Oberkochen, Germany) using a 40× objective.

Table 1. Composition of the different groups of n3-PUFA (long-chain n-3 polyunsaturated fatty acids) supplements. All fatty acids (FA) are presented as a percentage of n3-PUFA, the remaining percentage in each group consisted of a non n3-PUFA diluent. EPA: Eicosapentaenoic acid; DHA: Docosahexaenoic acid; TG: Triglycerides; EE: Ethylesters; PL: Phospholipids.

	n3-PUFA Supplement ID	Composition
I	DHA	80% DHA (TG)
	EPA	80% EPA (TG)
II	EPA/DHA 40/20 TG	40% EPA: 20% DHA (TG)
	EPA/DHA 20/40 TG	20% EPA: 40% DHA (TG)
	EPA/DHA 40/20 EE	40% EPA: 20% DHA (EE)
III	DHA 97/3V	97% DHA (TG): 3% DHA (PL, vegetable)
	DHA 95/5V	95% DHA (TG): 5% DHA (PL, vegetable)
	DHA 97/3M	97% DHA (TG): 3% DHA (PL, marine)
	DHA 97/3 VM 1.5	97% DHA (TG): 3% DHA (PL, 1.5% vegetable + 1.5% marine)
	DHA 95/5 VM 2.5	95% DHA (TG): 5% DHA (PL, 2.5% vegetable + 1.5% marine)

2.4. Cellular Viability and Proliferation Assays

The 3-(4,5-dimethylthiazol-2-yl)-2,5-diphenyltetrazolium bromide (MTT) reduction assay was used to determine cellular viability. Experiments were carried out on 96-well plates seeded with 10,000 ARPE-19 cells per well. Once cells were confluent, a culture medium was changed to 1% FBS and maintained for two days. At this point, cells were exposed to 100 µM of each supplement. After 96 h, cell viability was analyzed using the CellTiter 96® AQueous One Solution Cell Proliferation Assay (Promega, Madison, WI, USA), following the manufacturer's instructions. At 77 h MTT absorbance was determined at 450 and 540 nm with a Sunrise-basic Microplate reader (Tecan, Austria).

To assess the effect of the different formulations under oxidative stress conditions, at 72 h some cells were additionally exposed to 800 uM H_2O_2.

Cell proliferation was quantified by BrdU incorporation into the ARPE-19 genome using the Calbiochem® BrdU Cell Proliferation Assay (Calbiochem, La Jolla, CA, USA). Between 10,000 to 20,000 cells were seeded onto 96-well plates. After 24 h, 50 µM of the 10 supplements were added to the cells. BrdU was performed 48 h later, according to the manufacturer's protocol. Some cells were also challenged with H_2O_2 (as described above).

2.5. Reactive Oxygen Species (ROS) Detection

To measure the production of reactive oxygen species (ROS) generated by the n3-PUFA, the DCF (2′,7′-dichlorofluorescein) (H2DCFDA) test was used. Upon being oxidized, DCF emits fluorescent light at a wavelength of 540 nm when excited at 480 nm. The emitted fluorescence is captured and quantified by fluorometry. Once ARPE-19 cells reached confluence, a 10% FBS culture medium was replaced by 1% FBS medium for 24 h. Next, cells were exposed to the different supplements during 24 h. Apigenine was used as a positive control. Following this incubation, H2DCFDA was added to the medium for 30 min; cells were then harvested from the wells and transferred into a black 96-well plate to measure the emitted fluorescence.

2.6. Caspase-3 Immunofluorescence (IF)

The protein caspase-3 is an essential mediator of the activation of the apoptotic signaling cascade. To detect if the omega-3 formulations activated cell death by apoptosis, this early apoptotic mediator was visualized by confocal immunofluorescence microscopy. For these experiments, 50,000 ARPE-19 cells were cultured on 1 cm diameter cover slips (CB 100RA1, Menzel-Gläser, Braunschweig, Germany) until confluence. Then, cells were treated with a supplement for 24 h and subjected to 800 µM H_2O_2 for 3 h to activate the caspase-mediated apoptotic cascade (positive control). At the end of the experiment, glass coverslips were fixed and permeabilized in cold methanol. Afterwards, coverslips were washed with 1% PBS and submerged in 1% PBS-BSA for 20 min to block nonspecific bonds. The polyclonal rabbit anti-caspase-3 (G7481, Promega, WI, USA) was used at a 1:100 dilution in 1% PBS-BSA at 4 °C for 24 h. The coverslips were then washed with 1% PBS and incubated with an Alexa Fluor® 488 goat anti-rabbit IgG antibody (A11008, Invitrogen, Carlsbad, CA, USA) diluted in 1% PBS-BSA in the darkness for 1 h. TOPRO-3 was used as a nuclear marker. Next, the coverslips were mounted on microscope slides with PBS-glycerol and gelatin at 1:1 and observed under the confocal fluorescent microscope (LSM 750, Carl Zeiss, Oberkochen, German).

For caspase-3 quantification, each coverslip was divided into eight sectors and one image at 40× was acquired from alternate sectors. A total of four images were acquired from each cover slip and were analyzed using the LSM Zeiss software to compile them into one merged image, and caspase-3 granules per nucleus were quantified using a home-made plugin tool developed for Fiji/ImageJ, an open-source Java-based image analysis software. The plugin has been developed by the Imaging Platform of the CIMA Universidad de Navarra.

2.7. Wound Healing Cell Migration Assay

A wound healing assay was used to quantify ARPE-19 migration in the presence of n3-PUFA under standard conditions. For these experiments, 150,000 cells were seeded onto 24-well culture plates until confluence. A linear wound was then created in the middle of each well using a 20 µL sterile micropipette tip. Culture media was replaced to eliminate floating cells and debri and the different n3-PUFA formulations were added. Five points on each well were captured every hour for a total of 72 h using an automatic phase contrast inverted microscope equipped with a digital camera (Carl Zeiss, Oberkochen, Germany). Every set of images was analyzed using the Fiji software (a distribution of ImageJ) V1.48q (Fiji Wound Healing Tool by Nathalie Cahuzac, and Virginie Georget, http://dev.mri.cnrs.fr/projects/imagej-macros/wiki/Wound_Healing_Tool) to determine the speed of closure.

2.8. Western Blotting for Vascular Endothelial Growth Factor (VEGF)/Pigment Epithelium Derived Factor (PEDF) Ratio

Following 24 h of treatment with the different omega-3 formulations, 5 µg of ARPE cells homogenates were mixed with a Laemmli buffer (62.5 mM Tris-HCl, pH 6.8; 2% SDS; 10% glycerol; 0.1% bromophenol blue) and boiled for 5 min. Samples were separated on 12% SDS-PAGE gels and transferred to a nitrocellulose membrane. After blocking with 5% skimmed milk (*w/v*), 0.1% Tween-20 (*w/v*) in TBS for 1 h at room temperature, membranes were exposed to the primary antibodies (0.2 µg/µL, monoclonal anti-VEGF, sc7269, Santa Cruz Biotechnology Inc., Santa Cruz, CA, USA and 1:1000 monoclonal anti-PEDF; MAB1059; Millipore, Burlington, MA, USA), at room temperature for 1 h. Membranes where then incubated at room temperature for 1 h with a horseradish peroxidase-conjugated goat anti-mouse antibody (sc2005; 0.4 µg/µL, Santa Cruz Biotechnology Inc., Dallas, TX, USA). Signals were detected with an enhanced chemiluminescence (ECL) kit (ECL Western blotting detection kit, GE Healthcare, Fairfield, CT, USA) and with ImageQuant 400 (GE Healthcare). The relative intensities of the immunoreactive bands were analyzed with Quantity One software (version 4.2.2, Bio-Rad Laboratories, Hercules, CA, USA). The loading was verified by Ponceau S red, and the same blot was stripped and reblotted with an anti-β-actin monoclonal antibody (Sigma-Aldrich, St Louis, Mo, USA) to normalize the VEGF and PEDF levels. Protein levels were used to calculate the VEGF/PEDF ratio.

2.9. Statistical Analysis

For quantitative variables, and after assessing application conditions, all parameters were subjected to the one-way analysis of variance (ANOVA) followed by the Bonferroni post-hoc test. All groups were normalized by each pass and compared versus a control group. Data are expressed as mean ± SEM. A difference $p < 0.05$ was considered statistically significant. GraphPad Prism 6.0 (GraphPad Prism Software Inc., San Diego, CA, USA) was used for statistical analysis.

3. Results

3.1. Effect of Omega-3 Supplements on Epithelial Integrity

The distribution of the ZO-1 was similar after treatment with the 10 different n3-PUFA supplements. No difference was found among any group of study (Figure 1).

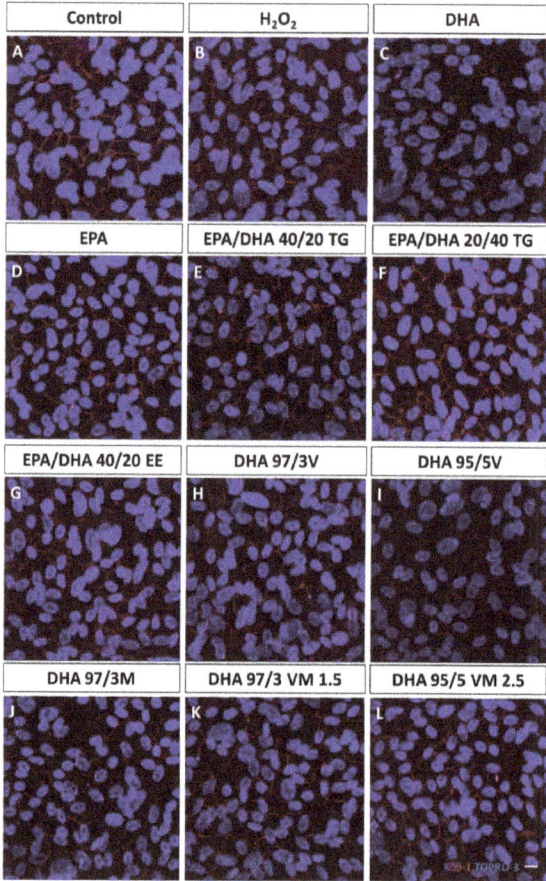

Figure 1. Effect of omega-3 supplements on epithelial tight junctions. ZO-1 (red) immunofluorescence were not affected by any of the omega-3 treatments. Nuclei are stained with TOPRO-3. Scale bar 20 μm. (**A**): Control group; (**B**): H_2O_2 treatment group; (**C**): DHA (Docosahexaenoic acid) group; (**D**): EPA (Eicosapentaenoic acid) group; (**E**): EPA/DHA 40/20; TG (Triglycerides) group; (**F**): EPA/DHA 20/40 TG group; (**G**): EPA/DHA 40/20 EE (Ethylesters) group; (**H**): DHA 97/3V (Vegetable) group; (**I**): DHA 95/5V group; (**J**): DHA 97/3M (Marine) group; (**K**): DHA 97/3 VM 1.5 group; (**L**): DHA 95/5 VM 2.5 group.

3.2. Effect of Omega-3 Supplements on Viability and Proliferation in ARPE-19

First, we wanted to evaluate the effect of Docosahexaenoic acid (DHA) and Eicosapentaenoic acid (EPA) on cell viability and proliferation. Treatment with both n3-PUFA produced a significant increase in viability (Figure 2A) of ARPE-19 cells compared to untreated controls. Proliferation also seemed to increase, but the effect was not statistically significant (Figure 2D). Secondly, we assessed the effect of different combinations of DHA and EPA on these cellular parameters. Interestingly, only the EPA/DHA 40/20 TG combination was able to significantly increase both viability (Figure 2B) and proliferation (Figure 2E), when compared to the untreated cells. Finally, we evaluated five different supplements containing a mixture of DHA in the form of TG and PL (PL from marine, vegetable, or mixed origin). In this last set of experiments, none of the formulations produced a significant change in cell viability (Figure 2C) or proliferation (Figure 2E).

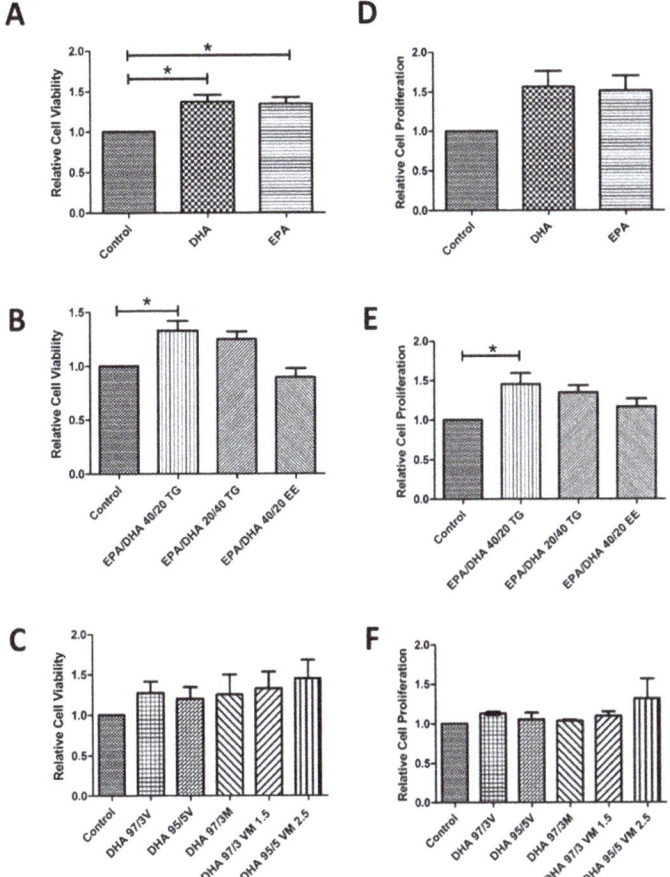

Figure 2. Graphs showing relative cell viability (**A–C**) and proliferation (**D–F**) compared to a control group under normal conditions of groups 1, 2, and 3 of eicosapentaenoic acid/docosahexaenoic acid (DHA/EPA) formulations, respectively (**D–F**). For comparisons, one-way ANOVA with the Bonferroni post-hoc test were used. Data are expressed as mean ± SEM. * $p < 0.05$. EPA: Eicosapentaenoic acid; DHA: Docosahexaenoic acid; TG: Triglycerides; EE: Ethylesters; PL: Phospholipids. V: Vegetable. M: Marine.

3.3. Effect of Omega-3 Supplements on Cell Viability and Cell Proliferation under Oxidative Stress and Inflammatory Conditions

In order to replicate the local oxidative environment of the diabetic retina, we subjected some ARPE-19 cells to H_2O_2 and measured the response after n3-PUFA treatment. As expected, exposure to 800 µM H_2O_2 produced a significant decrease in cell viability and proliferation. Treatment with EPA and DHA was able counteract the H_2O_2 induced decrease on cell viability (Figure 3A), but their effect on cell proliferation, although positive, was not statistically significant (Figure 3D). On the contrary, both n3-PUFA were able to significantly counteract the effect of H_2O_2 on cell proliferation (Figure 3D). In the combined formulations, all supplements were able to significantly reverse the oxidative effect of H_2O_2 on viability and proliferation, with the exception of the 40/20 EPA/DHA EE supplement that was not able to significantly mitigate the effect of H_2O_2 on cell viability (Figure 3B,C,E,F).

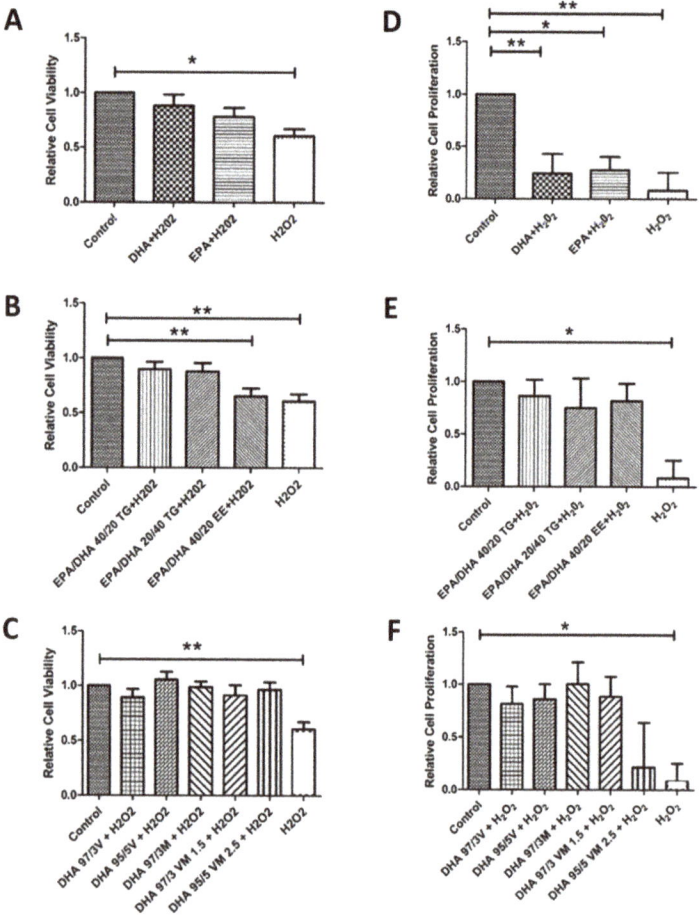

Figure 3. Graphs showing relative cell viability (**A–C**) and proliferation (**D–F**) results for ARPE-19 cells treated with different DHA and EPA treatments groups under oxidative stress conditions (H_2O_2 For comparisons, one-way ANOVA with the Bonferroni post-hoc test were used. Data are expressed as mean ± SEM. * $p < 0.05$ and ** $p < 0.01$. EPA: Eicosapentaenoic acid; DHA: Docosahexaenoic acid; TG: Triglycerides; EE: Ethylesters; PL: Phospholipids. V: Vegetable. M: Marine.

3.4. Effect of Omega-3 Supplements on ROS Production

Both DHA and EPA, alone or in combined formulations, produced a significant decrease in ROS when compared with the untreated controls. The same effect was observed in cells treated with the different DHA TG+PL formulations. The EPA/DHA 40/20 TG and DHA 95/5 VM 2.5 formulations had a stronger antioxidant effect, but this difference was not statistically significant when compared with the other combinations (Figure 4A–C).

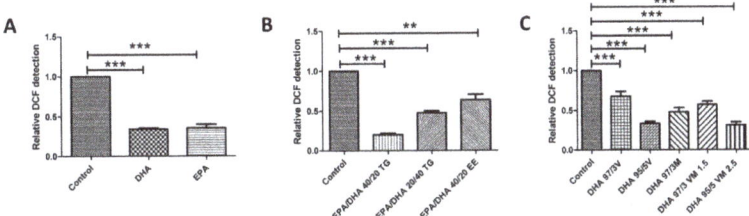

Figure 4. Graphs showing relative Dichloride fluoresceine (DCF) detection results for ARPE-19 cells in groups 1, 2, and 3 of DHA/EPA formulations, respectively (A–C). For comparisons, one-way ANOVA with the Bonferroni post-hoc test were used. Data are expressed as mean ± SEM. ** $p < 0.01$ *** $p < 0.001$. EPA: Eicosapentaenoic acid; DHA: Docosahexaenoic acid; TG: Triglycerides; EE: Ethylesters; PL: Phospholipids. V: Vegetable. M: Marine.

3.5. Effect of Omega-3 Supplements on Caspase-3 in ARPE-19

In order to test the safety of the different supplements, we evaluated their capacity to activate the early apoptotic mediator caspase-3. As expected, none of the omega-3 formulations induced a significant change in caspase-3 activation, when compared to the untreated control cells (Figure 5).

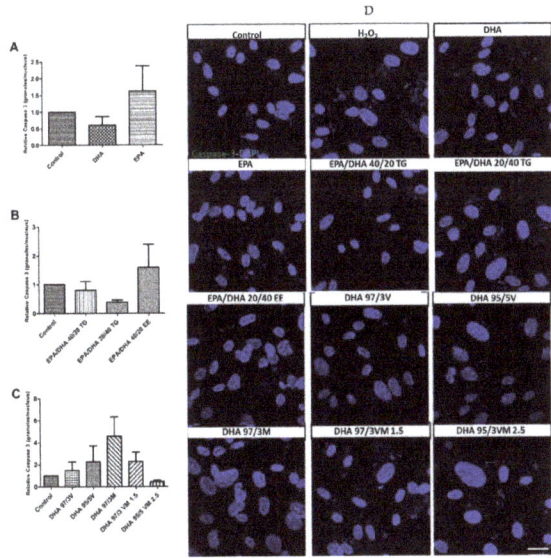

Figure 5. Graphs showing relative caspase-3 expression (positive granules per nucleus) (A–C) results for ARPE-19 cells treated with different groups 1, 2, and 3 of DHA/EPA formulations, respectively. For comparisons, one-way ANOVA with the Bonferroni post-hoc test were used. (D) Scale bar 20 µm Data are expressed as mean ± SEM. EPA: Eicosapentaenoic acid; DHA: Docosahexaenoic acid; TG: Triglycerides; EE: Ethylesters; PL: Phospholipids. V: Vegetable. M: Marine.

3.6. Effect of Omega-3 Supplements on Wound Healing Cell Migration Assay

Treatment with EPA or DHA did not produce any significant change in the migration capacity of ARPE-19 cells (Figure 5D). In the EPA/DHA formulations, the EPA/DHA 20/40 TG supplement produced a small, but significant decrease in the speed of wound closure, when compared with untreated cells. The rest of the combined EPA/DHA formulations and those combining DHA in TG and PL forms did not produce any significant changes in this cellular function (Figure 6).

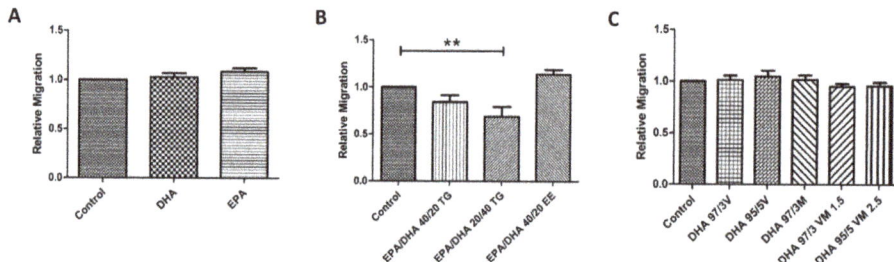

Figure 6. Graphs showing relative migration ratio (**A–C**) results for ARPE-19 cells treated with different groups 1, 2, and 3 of DHA/EPA formulations, respectively. For comparisons, one-way ANOVA with the Bonferroni post-hoc test were used. Data are expressed as mean ± SEM. ** $p < 0.01$. EPA: Eicosapentaenoic acid; DHA: Docosahexaenoic acid; TG: Triglycerides; EE: Ethylesters; PL: Phospholipids. V: Vegetable. M: Marine.

3.7. Effect of Omega-3 Supplements on the VEGF/PEDF Ratio

Treatment with the different omega-3 formulations did not produce a significant effect in the protein levels of VEGF or PEDF. However, combined formulations (especially those with EPA+DHA), showed a tendency to decrease the VEGF/PEDF ratio when compared with untreated controls, but these differences were not statistically significant (Figure 7).

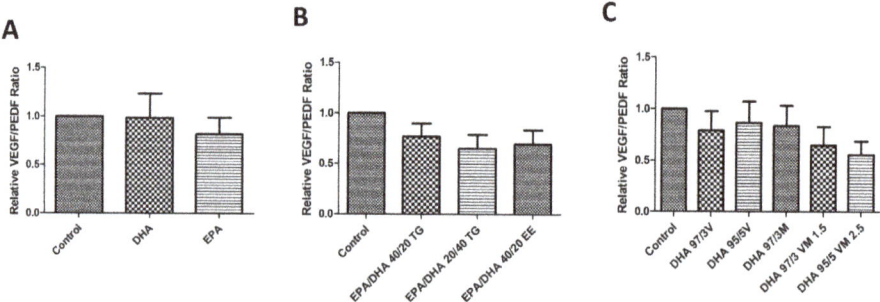

Figure 7. Graphs showing relative VEGF/PEDF ratio (**A–C**) results for ARPE-19 cells treated with different groups 1, 2, and 3 of DHA/EPA formulations, respectively. For comparisons, one-way ANOVA with the Bonferroni post-hoc test were used. Data are expressed as mean ± SEM. EPA: Eicosapentaenoic acid; DHA: Docosahexaenoic acid; TG: Triglycerides; EE: Ethylesters; PL: Phospholipids. V: Vegetable. M: Marine.

4. Discussion

RPE is a key regulator of retinal function and is directly related to the transport, delivery, and metabolism of n-3 PUFA in the retina. For this reason, we aimed to evaluate the effect of different formulations of DHA and EPA on this important cell type. Both n-3 PUFAs produced favorable effects on RPE cells by increasing cell viability and proliferation, reducing the production of ROS and decreasing oxidative damage induced by H_2O_2.

Recent research has demonstrated that the long chain n-3 PUFA, has antiangiogenic, anti-vasoproliferative, and neuroprotective actions on factors and processes implicated in the pathogenesis of degenerative/vascular retinal diseases of greatest public significance, including DR [18]. It has been demonstrated that diets with high levels of n-3 PUFA, have known anti-inflammatory properties [36] due to their ability to promote the gene expression of various inflammatory mediators via different intracellular signaling pathways [37] leading to the inhibition of the expressions of pro-inflammatory cytokines, leukocyte chemotaxis, and adhesion molecules. It is also known that they regulate the production of eicosanoids such as prostaglandins and leukotrienes and increase the synthesis of anti-inflammatory mediators such as resolvins, protectins, and maresins [38]. All these anti-inflamatory mechanisms add to their antioxidant effects by increasing the bioavailability of nitric oxide (NO) and the expression of superoxide dismutase and glutathione peroxidase, known as endogenous antioxidant enzymes, while decreasing the level of biomarkers of oxidative stress, such as malondialdehyde, in type II diabetic patients [30].

Many of the n3 supplements used in the routine clinical practice have a combination of EPA and DHA. For this reason, we explored the effect of supplements that mixed EPA and DHA in different proportions. Interestingly, EPA/DHA 40/20 TG was the only formulation that showed a significant increase in viability and proliferation of ARPE-19 cells and the most favorable antioxidant effect. This observation is in agreement with previous publications that have shown different effects of omega-3 supplements, depending on the proportion of EPA/DHA. In a study conducted on Wistar rats, it was found that the dietary intervention with 1:1 and 2:1 EPA/DHA supplements were the most effective treatments to reduce inflammation and oxidative stress when compared with a 1:2 EPA/DHA formulation [39]. Similar results were reported in a study performed in spontaneously hypertensive obese rats, where EPA/DHA supplementation at the ratios of 1:1 and 2:1 were more effective than a 1:2 formulation, lowering plasma total cholesterol and LDL concentrations, decreasing inflammation, and increasing the activity of antioxidant enzymes [40]. The reasons that underlie these differences are not completely clear, but it has been suggested that the higher unsaturation level of DHA may increase the susceptibility of the molecule to be oxidized compared to EPA, rendering a higher level of free radicals [39]. Furthermore, differences in their influence on transduction pathways, the release of inflammatory cytokines, and the expression of genes involved in lipid metabolism have also been reported [40]. In the field of ophthalmology, one article compared the effect of two different EPA/DHA formulations (1/4.5 and 1.5/1) as adjuvants to topical tacrolimus in a model of keratoconjunctivitis sicca (dry eye disease) in dogs [41]. Authors reported better clinical and biochemical outcomes after supplementation with the oral formulation containing a higher proportion of EPA.

However, the proportion of EPA/DHA is not the only factor that distinguishes one supplement from the other, and omega-3 formulations vary depending on whether they are present as TG, EE, or PL. In the body, long PUFA stores exist mainly as PL and TG and in the retina, the latter represents the predominant lipid class [18]. Although most of the large interventional studies in the field of omega-3 supplements have been conducted with EPA/DHA EE, several authors have commented on their lower bioavailability when compared to TG and PL formulations [42–44]. Possible explanations include differences in their digestion and absorption [42]. EPA and DHA may be obtained directly through the diet or can be biosynthesized from linoleic acid (an 18-carbon essential fatty acid) in the liver or the retina. However, the efficiency of tissue accretion is highest when they are ingested in the preformed state [18]. n-3 PUFA are hydrolyzed by pancreatic enzymes and are re-esterified to triglycerides and phospholipids within the intestinal epithelium. These triglycerides and phospholipids are integrated to chylomicrons and very low density lipoproteins (VLDLs) which are transported to the choriocapillaris. Further transport from the choriocapillaris to the RPE and the inner segments of photoreceptors appears to be mediated by high affinity receptors [18]. Unlike TG and PL, which are hydrolyzed mainly by a colipase dependent pancreatic lipase, EE requires additional digestion with carboxyl ester lipase, a step that can slow down their absorption by 10 to 50 times [44,45]. In our experiments, the supplement with EPA/DHA in the form of EE, did not improve cell viability or proliferation and showed a lower antioxidant effect, despite having the same proportion of EPA/DHA (40/20) than the TG supplement with the most favorable outcomes. These differences could be clinically relevant, as suggested by data from The Age-Related Eye Disease Study 2 (AREDS2), where supplementation with a 650 mg EPA/350 mg DHA EE formulation failed to show clinically significant benefits [46].

As recent evidence has suggested that dietary EPA-DHA PL are superior to TG and EE forms in exerting their functional mechanisms [43], we evaluated the effect of DHA formulations that combined TG and PL. The most relevant effect of these formulations was their antioxidant capacity. They decreased the production of ROS production, and increased viability and proliferation of cells challenged with H_2O_2. This effect is important as the oxidative stress in the human eye is also primarily due to H_2O_2, which is naturally generated in RPE cells by solar radiation and POS phagocytosis [47]. Regarding the origin of DHA PL, some authors have suggested that n3-PUFA from a marine origin might be more beneficial than those from a vegetable origin [39,43,48]. However, in our experiments we did not find an association between the origin of the DHA PL and their results. This is probably because the proportion of PL in our formulations was small (3% or 5%).

The above-mentioned beneficial effects of the n3-PUFA have been demonstrated in several clinical studies. In patients with DR and well-controlled diabetes, increasing the n3-PUFA intake was associated with a reduced likelihood of the presence and severity of DR [24]. A sub-study of the PREDIMED randomized clinical trial showed that patients with type 2 diabetes who reported an intake of at least 500 mg/d of long-chain n3-PUFA at baseline had a 46% decreased risk of sight-threatening DR compared to those not meeting this target [25]. In an early stage of DR, supplementation with a high-dose DHA plus xanthophyll carotenoid multivitamin during 90 days was associated with a progressive and significant improvement of macular function measured by microperimetry [34]. In normal ocular tissues, angiogenic homeostasis is controlled by the balance between angiogenic stimulators, mainly VEGF, and angiogenic inhibitors such as pigment epithelium derived factor (PEDF) [49]. Moreover, this balance is important in the regulation of vascular permeability. While VEGF is increased in the vitreous of patients with diabetic macular edema, the vitreous level of PEDF is significantly lower in these patients [50]. Therefore, therapeutic strategies that can lower the VEGF/PEDF ratio are clinically beneficial. In a randomized single-blind controlled trial, the addition of a DHA dietary supplement to intravitreal ranibizumab (a monoclonal antibody against VEGF) was effective to achieve better sustained improvement of central subfield macular thickness outcomes after three years of follow-up compared with intravitreal ranibizumab alone [26]. Interestingly, n3-PUFA formulations in our study produced a small decrease in the VEGF/PEDF ratio, but the results were not statistically significant. Further studies analyzing the expression of VEGF and PEDF mRNA could help clarify the effect of EPA and DHA supplementation on the VEGF/PEDF ratio and their apparent clinical benefit in the treatment of diabetic macular edema.

As with any other clinical intervention, the safety of omega-3 dietary supplements should be considered. A recent meta-analysis that specifically addressed the safety and tolerability of prescription omega-3 fatty acids did not find any definitive evidence of serious adverse events [51]. The most commonly reported treatment associated adverse reactions are digestive disturbances (mainly dysgeusia or fishy taste) and skin reactions (eruption, itching, exanthema, or eczema). Although both EPA and DHA reduce the TG levels, they can increase the concentration of low density lipoproteins (LDL) [51]. However, this mild, but negative effect in lipid profile has not been observed in patients treated with supplements that only contain EPA. Monitoring of the lipid profile may be advisable in patients undergoing omega-3 supplementation.

To our knowledge, there has not been an in vitro study or clinical trial comparing the effects of so many different formulations of EPA and DHA on ARPE-19 cells, not only under normal conditions, but also following an oxidative challenge. It was very interesting to see that DHA and EPA had different effects when applied separately than they did when used in combination. Another relevant finding of our study was that the EE formulation had worse results, which cannot be explained by a lower bioavailability due to differences in digestion and absorption. This suggests that the EE form might decrease the biological effect of EPA and DHA. However, we know that our in vitro study has certain limitations. As an in vitro study, cells were not exposed to the same physiological environment as in the functioning retina. Moreover, analyzing the effect of the supplements in other retinal cell types would have also been of interest.

5. Conclusions

In summary, the present study demonstrates that different formulations of n3-PUFAs have a beneficial effect on cell viability and proliferation, and are able to restore oxidative induced RPE damage. The protective effects of these formulations on RPE cells may translate to effective treatments to prevent or delay DR progression, which will become increasingly important with the expected rise in DM prevalence and its associated socioeconomic burden in years to come. Although differences between the formulations in our study were small, our results are in accordance with previous reports suggesting that supplements that combine both n3-PUFAs with a higher proportion of EPA might be more beneficial, especially when present in the form of triglycerides or phospholipids. Clinical trials specifically designed to confirm these observations in patients with retinal vascular pathologies are needed.

Author Contributions: Conceptualization, P.F.-R., S.R. and A.G.-L.; Data curation, M.H., P.F.-R., L.G.-G., N.I. and S.R.; Formal analysis, M.H., P.F.-R., S.R. and A.G.-L.; Funding acquisition, A.G.-L.; Investigation, M.S.d.V., M.H., J.G.-Z., L.G.-G. and N.I.; Methodology, M.S.d.V., M.H. and S.R.; Project administration, S.R.; Supervision, P.F.-R., S.R. and A.G.-L.; Validation, M.S.d.V., J.G.-Z., P.F.-R. and S.R.; Visualization, M.H., J.G.-Z., P.F.-R. and V.B.-M.; Writing—original draft, M.S.d.V., M.H., J.G.-Z. and V.B.-M.; Writing—review & editing, P.F.-R., S.R. and A.G.-L. All authors have read and agreed to the published version of the manuscript.

Funding: The present work was partially funded by Thea Laboratoires and partially supported by RETICS (RD16/0008) from ISCIII, Ministerio de Economía y Competitividad, Spain.

Acknowledgments: Authors would like to specially thank the great technician work of Maite Moreno Orduña, Edurne Albiasu Arteta and Natalia Aguado Pérez.

Conflicts of Interest: AGL is a consultant for Bayer, Novartis, Allergan, Thea, and Roche. The rest of the authors declare no conflict of interest. The funders had no role in the design of the study; in the collection, analyses, or interpretation of data; in the writing of the manuscript, or in the decision to publish the results.

References

1. Flaxman, S.R.; Bourne, R.R.A.; Resnikoff, S.; Ackland, P.; Braithwaite, T.; Cicinelli, M.V.; Das, A.; Jonas, J.B.; Keeffe, J.; Kempen, J.; et al. Global causes of blindness and distance vision impairment 1990–2020: A systematic review and meta-analysis. *Lancet Glob. Heal.* **2017**, *5*. [CrossRef]
2. Elisa D-NET—Connecting Diabetes Professionals Wordwide. Available online: https://d-net.idf.org (accessed on 29 July 2020).
3. Lorenzi, M. The polyol pathway as a mechanism for diabetic retinopathy: Attractive, elusive, and resilient. *Exp. Diabetes Res.* **2007**, *2007*, 61038. [CrossRef] [PubMed]
4. Stitt, A.W. The role of advanced glycation in the pathogenesis of diabetic retinopathy. *Exp. Mol. Pathol.* **2003**, *75*, 95–108. [CrossRef]
5. Donnelly, R. Protein kinase C inhibition and diabetic retinopathy: A shot in the dark at translational research. *Br. J. Ophthalmol.* **2004**, *88*, 145–151. [CrossRef] [PubMed]
6. Yaribeygi, H.; Sathyapalan, T.; Atkin, S.L.; Sahebkar, A. Molecular Mechanisms Linking Oxidative Stress and Diabetes Mellitus. *Oxid. Med. Cell. Longev.* **2020**, *2020*, 1–13. [CrossRef]
7. Li, C.; Miao, X.; Li, F.; Wang, S.; Liu, Q.; Wang, Y.; Sun, J. Oxidative Stress-Related Mechanisms and Antioxidant Therapy in Diabetic Retinopathy. *Oxid. Med. Cell. Longev.* **2017**, *2017*, 1–15. [CrossRef]
8. Olvera-Montaño, C.; Castellanos-González, J.A.; Navarro-Partida, J.; Cardona-Muñoz, E.G.; López-Contreras, A.K.; Roman-Pintos, L.M.; Robles-Rivera, R.R.; Rodríguez-Carrizalez, A.D. Oxidative Stress as the Main Target in Diabetic Retinopathy Pathophysiology. *J. Diabetes Res.* **2019**, *2019*, 1–21. [CrossRef]

9. Calderon, G.D.; Juarez, O.H.; Hernandez, G.E.; Punzo, S.M.; De la Cruz, Z.D. Oxidative stress and diabetic retinopathy: Development and treatment. *Eye* **2017**, *31*, 1122–1130. [CrossRef]
10. Madsen-Bouterse, S.A.; Kowluru, R.A. Oxidative stress and diabetic retinopathy: Pathophysiological mechanisms and treatment perspectives. *Rev. Endocr. Metab. Disord.* **2008**, *9*, 315–327. [CrossRef]
11. Mesquida, M.; Drawnel, F.; Fauser, S. The role of inflammation in diabetic eye disease. *Semin. Immunopathol.* **2019**, *41*, 427–445. [CrossRef]
12. Rübsam, A.; Parikh, S.; Fort, P. Role of Inflammation in Diabetic Retinopathy. *Int. J. Mol. Sci.* **2018**, *19*, 942. [CrossRef] [PubMed]
13. Abu El-Asrar, A. Role of inflammation in the pathogenesis of diabetic retinopathy. *Middle East Afr. J. Ophthalmol.* **2012**, *19*, 70. [CrossRef] [PubMed]
14. Congdon, N.; Zheng, Y.; He, M. The worldwide epidemic of diabetic retinopathy. *Indian J. Ophthalmol.* **2012**, *60*, 428. [CrossRef] [PubMed]
15. Giacco, F.; Brownlee, M. Oxidative Stress and Diabetic Complications. *Circ. Res.* **2010**, *107*, 1058–1070. [CrossRef]
16. Rajamoorthi, K.; Petrache, H.I.; McIntosh, T.J.; Brown, M.F. Packing and viscoelasticity of polyunsaturated omega-3 and omega-6 lipid bilayers as seen by (2)H NMR and X-ray diffraction. *J. Am. Chem. Soc.* **2005**, *127*, 1576–1588. [CrossRef]
17. Strauss, O. The Retinal Pigment Epithelium in Visual Function. *Physiol. Rev.* **2005**, *85*, 845–881. [CrossRef]
18. SanGiovanni, J.P.; Chew, E.Y. The role of omega-3 long-chain polyunsaturated fatty acids in health and disease of the retina. *Prog. Retin. Eye Res.* **2005**, *24*, 87–138. [CrossRef]
19. Boston, P.F.; Bennett, A.; Horrobin, D.F.; Bennett, C.N. Ethyl-EPA in Alzheimer's disease—A pilot study. *Prostaglandins Leukot. Essent. Fat. Acids* **2004**, *71*, 341–346. [CrossRef]
20. Martins, J.G. EPA but not DHA appears to be responsible for the efficacy of omega-3 long chain polyunsaturated fatty acid supplementation in depression: Evidence from a meta-analysis of randomized controlled trials. *J. Am. Coll. Nutr.* **2009**, *28*, 525–542. [CrossRef]
21. Sublette, M.E.; Ellis, S.P.; Geant, A.L.; Mann, J.J. Meta-analysis of the effects of eicosapentaenoic acid (EPA) in clinical trials in depression. *J. Clin. Psychiatry* **2011**, *72*, 1577–1584. [CrossRef]
22. Bloch, M.H.; Qawasmi, A. Omega-3 fatty acid supplementation for the treatment of children with attention-deficit/hyperactivity disorder symptomatology: Systematic review and meta-analysis. *J. Am. Acad. Child Adolesc. Psychiatry* **2011**, *50*, 991–1000. [CrossRef] [PubMed]
23. Howard-Williams, J.; Patel, P.; Jelfs, R.; Carter, R.D.; Awdry, P.; Bron, A.; Mann, J.I.; Hockaday, T.D. Polyunsaturated fatty acids and diabetic retinopathy. *Br. J. Ophthalmol.* **1985**, *69*, 15–18. [CrossRef] [PubMed]
24. Sasaki, M.; Kawasaki, R.; Rogers, S.; Man, R.E.K.; Itakura, K.; Xie, J.; Flood, V.; Tsubota, K.; Lamoureux, E.; Wang, J.J. The Associations of Dietary Intake of Polyunsaturated Fatty Acids With Diabetic Retinopathy in Well-Controlled Diabetes. *Investig. Opthalmol. Vis. Sci.* **2015**, *56*, 7473. [CrossRef]
25. Sala-Vila, A.; Díaz-López, A.; Valls-Pedret, C.; Cofán, M.; García-Layana, A.; Lamuela-Raventós, R.-M.; Castañer, O.; Zanon-Moreno, V.; Martinez-Gonzalez, M.A.; Toledo, E.; et al. Dietary Marine ω-3 Fatty Acids and Incident Sight-Threatening Retinopathy in Middle-Aged and Older Individuals With Type 2 Diabetes: Prospective Investigation From the PREDIMED Trial. *JAMA Ophthalmol.* **2016**, *134*, 1142–1149. [CrossRef] [PubMed]
26. Lafuente, M.; Ortín, L.; Argente, M.; Guindo, J.L.; López-Bernal, M.D.; López-Román, F.J.; García, M.J.; Domingo, J.C.; Lajara, J. Combined Intravitreal Ranibizumab and Oral Supplementation with Docasahexanoic and Antioxidants for Diabetic Macular Edema: Two-Year Randomized Single-Blind Controlled Trial Results. *Retina* **2017**, *37*, 1277–1286. [CrossRef] [PubMed]
27. Tikhonenko, M.; Lydic, T.A.; Wang, Y.; Chen, W.; Opreanu, M.; Sochacki, A.; McSorley, K.M.; Renis, R.L.; Kern, T.; Jump, D.B.; et al. Remodeling of retinal Fatty acids in an animal model of diabetes: A decrease in long-chain polyunsaturated fatty acids is associated with a decrease in fatty acid elongases Elovl2 and Elovl4. *Diabetes* **2010**, *59*, 219–227. [CrossRef]
28. Shen, J.; Bi, Y.-L.; Das, U.N. State of the art paper Potential role of polyunsaturated fatty acids in diabetic retinopathy. *Arch. Med. Sci.* **2014**, *6*, 1167–1174. [CrossRef]
29. Sapieha, P.; Chen, J.; Stahl, A.; Seaward, M.R.; Favazza, T.L.; Juan, A.M.; Hatton, C.J.; Joyal, J.-S.; Krah, N.M.; Dennison, R.J.; et al. Omega-3 polyunsaturated fatty acids preserve retinal function in type 2 diabetic mice. *Nutr. Diabetes* **2012**, *2*, e36. [CrossRef]

30. Behl, T.; Kotwani, A. Omega-3 fatty acids in prevention of diabetic retinopathy. *J. Pharm. Pharmacol.* **2017**, *69*, 946–954. [CrossRef]
31. Shakouri Mahmoudabadi, M.M.; Rahbar, A.R. Effect of EPA and Vitamin C on Superoxide Dismutase, Glutathione Peroxidase, Total Antioxidant Capacity and Malondialdehyde in Type 2 Diabetic Patients. *Oman Med. J.* **2014**, *29*, 39–45. [CrossRef]
32. Morris, M.C.; Evans, D.A.; Bienias, J.L.; Tangney, C.C.; Bennett, D.A.; Wilson, R.S.; Aggarwal, N.; Schneider, J. Consumption of fish and n-3 fatty acids and risk of incident Alzheimer disease. *Arch. Neurol.* **2003**, *60*, 940–946. [CrossRef] [PubMed]
33. Bradberry, J.C.; Hilleman, D.E. Overview of omega-3 Fatty Acid therapies. *Pharm. Ther.* **2013**, *38*, 681–691.
34. Rodríguez González-Herrero, M.E.; Ruiz, M.; López Román, F.J.; Marín Sánchez, J.M.; Domingo, J.C. Supplementation with a highly concentrated docosahexaenoic acid plus xanthophyll carotenoid multivitamin in nonproliferative diabetic retinopathy: Prospective controlled study of macular function by fundus microperimetry. *Clin. Ophthalmol.* **2018**, *12*, 1011–1020. [CrossRef] [PubMed]
35. Peltomaa, E.; Johnson, M.D.; Taipale, S.J. Marine Cryptophytes Are Great Sources of EPA and DHA. *Mar. Drugs* **2017**, *16*, 3. [CrossRef] [PubMed]
36. Mildenberger, J.; Johansson, I.; Sergin, I.; Kjøbli, E.; Damås, J.K.; Razani, B.; Flo, T.H.; Bjørkøy, G. N-3 PUFAs induce inflammatory tolerance by formation of KEAP1-containing SQSTM1/p62-bodies and activation of NFE2L2. *Autophagy* **2017**, *13*, 1664–1678. [CrossRef] [PubMed]
37. Yan, Y.; Jiang, W.; Spinetti, T.; Tardivel, A.; Castillo, R.; Bourquin, C.; Guarda, G.; Tian, Z.; Tschopp, J.; Zhou, R. Omega-3 fatty acids prevent inflammation and metabolic disorder through inhibition of NLRP3 inflammasome activation. *Immunity* **2013**, *38*, 1154–1163. [CrossRef]
38. Calder, P.C. Marine omega-3 fatty acids and inflammatory processes: Effects, mechanisms and clinical relevance. *Biochim. Biophys. Acta* **2015**, *1851*, 469–484. [CrossRef]
39. Dasilva, G. Healthy effect of different proportions of marineω-3 PUFAs EPA and DHA. *J. Nutr. Biochem.* **2015**, *26*, 1385–1392. [CrossRef]
40. Molinar-Toribio, E.; Pérez-Jiménez, J.; Ramos-Romero, S.; Romeu, M.; Giralt, M.; Taltavull, N.; Muñoz-Cortes, M.; Jáuregui, O.; Méndez, L.; Medina, I.; et al. Effect of n-3 PUFA supplementation at different EPA:DHA ratios on the spontaneously hypertensive obese rat model of the metabolic syndrome. *Br. J. Nutr.* **2015**, *113*, 878–887. [CrossRef]
41. Silva, D.A.; Nai, G.A.; Giuffrida, R.; Sgrignoli, M.R.; Santos, D.R.D.; Donadão, I.V.; Nascimento, F.F.; Dinallo, H.R.; Andrade, S.F. Oral omega 3 in different proportions of EPA, DHA, and antioxidants as adjuvant in treatment of keratoconjunctivitis sicca in dogs. *Arq. Bras. Oftalmol.* **2018**, *81*, 421–428. [CrossRef]
42. Neubronner, J.; Schuchardt, J.P.; Kressel, G.; Merkel, M.; Von Schacky, C.; Hahn, A. Enhanced increase of omega-3 index in response to long-term n-3 fatty acid supplementation from triacylglycerides versus ethyl esters. *Eur. J. Clin. Nutr.* **2011**, *65*, 247–254. [CrossRef] [PubMed]
43. Zhang, T.T.; Xu, J.; Wang, Y.M.; Xue, C.H. Health benefits of dietary marine DHA/EPA-enriched glycerophospholipids. *Prog. Lipid Res.* **2019**, *75*, 100997. [CrossRef] [PubMed]
44. Maki, K.C.; Dicklin, M.R. Strategies to improve bioavailability of omega-3 fatty acids from ethyl ester concentrates. *Curr. Opin. Clin. Nutr. Metab. Care* **2019**, *22*, 116–123. [CrossRef] [PubMed]
45. Dyerberg, J.; Madsen, P.; Møller, J.M.; Aardestrup, I.; Schmidt, E.B. Bioavailability of marine n-3 fatty acid formulations. *Prostaglandins Leukot. Essent. Fat. Acids* **2010**, *83*, 137–141. [CrossRef] [PubMed]
46. Chew, E.Y.; Clemons, T.E.; SanGiovanni, J.P.; Danis, R.; Ferris, F.L.; Elman, M.; Antoszyk, A.; Ruby, A.; Orth, D.; Bressler, S.; et al. Lutein + zeaxanthin and omega-3 fatty acids for age-related macular degeneration: The Age-Related Eye Disease Study 2 (AREDS2) randomized clinical trial. *J. Am. Med. Assoc.* **2013**, *309*, 2005–2015. [CrossRef]
47. Miceli, M.V.; Liles, M.R.; Newsome, D.A. Evaluation of oxidative processes in human pigment epithelial cells associated with retinal outer segment phagocytosis. *Exp. Cell Res.* **1994**, *214*, 242–249. [CrossRef]
48. Williams, C.M.; Burdge, G. Long-chain n−3 PUFA: Plant v. marine sources. *Proc. Nutr. Soc.* **2006**, *65*, 42–50. [CrossRef]
49. Funatsu, H.; Yamashita, H.; Nakamura, S.; Mimura, T.; Eguchi, S.; Noma, H.; Hori, S. Vitreous levels of pigment epithelium-derived factor and vascular endothelial growth factor are related to diabetic macular edema. *Ophthalmology* **2006**, *113*, 294–301. [CrossRef]

50. Chang, C.H.; Tseng, P.T.; Chen, N.Y.; Lin, P.C.; Lin, P.Y.; Chang, J.P.C.; Kuo, F.Y.; Lin, J.; Wu, M.C.; Su, K.P. Safety and tolerability of prescription omega-3 fatty acids: A systematic review and meta-analysis of randomized controlled trials. *Prostaglandins Leukot. Essent. Fat. Acids* **2018**, *129*, 1–12. [CrossRef]
51. Brinton, E.A.; Mason, R.P. Prescription omega-3 fatty acid products containing highly purified eicosapentaenoic acid (EPA). *Lipids Health Dis.* **2017**, *16*, 1–13. [CrossRef]

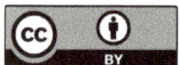

© 2020 by the authors. Licensee MDPI, Basel, Switzerland. This article is an open access article distributed under the terms and conditions of the Creative Commons Attribution (CC BY) license (http://creativecommons.org/licenses/by/4.0/).

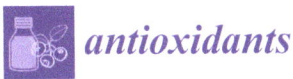

Article

The Herbal Combination CPA4-1 Inhibits Changes in Retinal Capillaries and Reduction of Retinal Occludin in db/db Mice

Young Sook Kim [1,†], Junghyun Kim [2,3,†], Chan-Sik Kim [4], Ik Soo Lee [1], Kyuhyung Jo [1], Dong Ho Jung [2], Yun Mi Lee [2] and Jin Sook Kim [2,*]

1. Research Infrastructure Team, Herbal Medicine Division, Korea Institute of Oriental Medicine, Daejeon 34054, Korea; ykim@kiom.re.kr (Y.S.K.); knifer48@kiom.re.kr (I.S.L.); jopd7414@kiom.re.kr (K.J.)
2. Herbal Medicine Research Division, Korea Institute of Oriental Medicine, Daejeon 34054, Korea; dvmhyun@jbnu.ac.kr (J.K.); jdh9636@kiom.re.kr (D.H.J.); candykomg@kiom.re.kr (Y.M.L.)
3. Department of Oral pathology, School of Dentistry, Chonbuk National University, Jeonju 54896, Korea
4. Clinical Medicine Division, Korea Institute of Oriental Medicine, Daejeon 34054, Korea; chskim@kiom.re.kr
* Correspondence: jskim@kiom.re.kr; Tel.: +82-42-868-9465
† These authors contributed equally to this work.

Received: 24 June 2020; Accepted: 14 July 2020; Published: 16 July 2020

Abstract: Increased formation of advanced glycation end products (AGEs) plays an important role in the development of diabetic retinopathy (DR) via blood-retinal barrier (BRB) dysfunction, and reduction of AGEs has been suggested as a therapeutic target for DR. In this study, we examined whether CPA4-1, a herbal combination of Cinnamomi Ramulus and Paeoniae Radix, inhibits AGE formation. CPA4-1 and fenofibrate were tested to ameliorate changes in retinal capillaries and retinal occludin expression in db/db mice, a mouse model of obesity-induced type 2 diabetes. CPA4-1 (100 mg/kg) or fenofibrate (100 mg/kg) were orally administered once a day for 12 weeks. CPA4-1 (the half maximal inhibitory concentration, IC_{50} = 6.84 ± 0.08 μg/mL) showed approximately 11.44-fold higher inhibitory effect on AGE formation than that of aminoguanidine (AG, the inhibitor of AGEs, IC_{50} = 78.28 ± 4.24 μg/mL), as well as breaking effect on AGE-bovine serum albumin crosslinking with collagen (IC_{50} = 1.30 ± 0.37 μg/mL). CPA4-1 treatment ameliorated BRB leakage and tended to increase retinal occludin expression in db/db mice. CPA4-1 or fenofibrate treatment significantly reduced retinal acellular capillary formation in db/db mice. These findings suggested the potential of CPA4-1 as a therapeutic supplement for protection against retinal vascular permeability diseases.

Keywords: diabetic retinopathy; db/db mice; Cinnamomi Ramulus; Paeoniae Radix; CPA4-1; blood-retinal barrier; occludin

1. Introduction

Hyperglycemia induces the formation and accumulation of advanced glycation end products (AGEs), and these products are present at high levels in the blood and tissue of diabetic patients [1,2]. AGEs are accumulated at high levels in the tissues of patients with age-related diseases, such as chronic obstructive pulmonary disease, cardiovascular diseases, osteoporosis, and neurodegenerative diseases [3]. AGEs are formed by oxidative and non-oxidative reactions, and they affect the biochemical and physical properties of proteins in tissues. AGE formation is triggered by high glucose-induced oxidative stress and fluorescent protein cross-linking [4].

Diabetic retinopathy (DR) is a complication of diabetes that causes damage to retinal blood vessels [5]. Elevated AGE levels increase the breakdown of the blood-retinal barrier (BRB), adhesion of leukocytes, and retinal vascular injury, leading to serious impairment of vision. The BRB consists of inner and outer nuclear layers. The inner nuclear layer of the BRB consists of tight junctions between endothelial cells and pericytes, whereas the outer nuclear layer of the BRB is formed by tight junctions between retinal pigment epithelial cells [6]. The advent of anti-vascular endothelial growth factor (VEGF) has shown a remarkable effect in DR patients; however, most of DR patients have failed to achieve significant clinical visual improvement. The treatment of DR remains challenging. Inhibition of AGE formation has been suggested as a therapeutic target for improving insulin resistance in diabetes with obesity [7]. For example, fenofibrate, a peroxisome proliferator-activated receptor alpha (PPARα) agonist, was approved for slowing down the progression of DR in patients with type 2 diabetes mellitus in October 2013 in Australia [8]. Moreover, pyridoxamine, an inhibitor of AGE formation, has been shown to ameliorate insulin resistance in obese, type 2 diabetic mice [9]. The identification of inhibitors of AGE formation from natural sources has gained much attention.

During the last 15 years, we have screened inhibitors of AGE formation from natural products [10–12]. *Aster koraiensis* extract prevents retinal pericyte apoptosis in streptozotocin (STZ)-induced diabetic rats [13]. *Osteomeles schweinae* extract inhibits methylglyoxal (an active precursor in the formation of AGEs)-induced apoptosis in human retinal pigment epithelial cells [14]. Cinnamomi Ramulus (the twig of *Cinnamomum cassia* Blume; Lauraceae) and Paeoniae Radix (the root of *Paeonia lactiflora* Pallas; Paeoniaceae) have been shown to exert efficacy in inhibiting the formation of AGEs in our previous study. Cinnamomi Ramulus has traditionally been used for its anti-inflammatory, antioxidant, and neuroinflammatory effects [15]. Its marker compounds include coumarin, cinnamyl alcohol, and cinnamic acid. In humans, the effect of cinnamon is controversial; it significantly decreases plasma glucose to the baseline levels, without causing adverse effects nor significant glycemic and inflammatory indicators in patients with type 2 diabetes [16,17]. Paeoniae Radix has been used in traditional medicine for treating inflammatory diseases owing to its anti-allergic, immunoregulatory, and analgesic effects [18]. The marker compounds of Paeoniae Radix include gallic acid, albiflorin, paeoniflorin, and benzoic acid [19]. In a preliminary study, we evaluated the efficacy of inhibition of AGE formation with different combinations of the two herbs to obtain the best formulation. It showed a different inhibitory effect according to the ratio, and it was the best at CPA 4-1 (Cinnamomi Ramulus:Paeoniae Radix = 1:8). Here, we tested a mixture of the CPA4-1 to investigate the optimum ratio for inhibiting AGE formation in the human retinal pigment epithelial cells (ARPE-19). In addition, we examined the therapeutic efficacy of CPA4-1 in preventing DR in db/db mice, a well-established model of obesity-induced type 2 diabetes with retinal neurodegeneration [20,21].

2. Materials and Methods

2.1. Preparation of the CPA4-1

Cinnamomi Ramulus and Paeoniae Radix were purchased from a traditional herbal medicine store in Daejeon, Republic of Korea, in April 2016 and identified by Prof. Ki Hwan Bae (College of Pharmacy, Chungnam National University, Republic of Korea). Voucher specimens of Cinnamomi Ramulus (KIOM-CIRA-2016) and Paeoniae Radix (KIOM-PARA-2016) have been deposited in the Herbarium of Korea Institute of Oriental Medicine (KIOM), Republic of Korea. The herbal combination was prepared at a Cinnamomi Ramulus to Paeoniae Radix ratio of 1:8 (m/m). For preparing CPA4-1 extract, 20 g of Cinnamomi Ramulus and 160 g of Paeoniae Radix were weighed accurately and mixed. Distilled water (1080 mL) was added to the mixed herbs (180 g) and extracted at 100 °C for 3 h using a reflux extractor (MS-DM607, M-TOPS, Seoul, Korea). The extract solutions were filtered and evaporated under reduced pressure using a rotary evaporator (N-1200A; Eyela, Tokyo, Japan) at 50 °C and then freeze-dried using a freeze dryer (FDU-2100; Eyela) at −80 °C for 72 h to obtain an extract powder of CPA4-1 (18.5 g; yield, 10.3%). This sample extract (100 mg) was dissolved in 50% methanol (10 mL), and the solution was filtered through a 0.45-μm syringe filter (Whatman, Clifton, NJ) prior to injection. Standard stock solutions of five reference standards (all at 1 mg/mL) were prepared in HPLC-grade MeOH, stored at <4 °C, and used for HPLC analyses after serial dilution in MeOH.

2.2. HPLC Analysis

HPLC analyses were performed using an Agilent 1200 HPLC instrument (Agilent Technologies, Santa Clara, CA, USA) equipped with a binary pump (G1312A), vacuum degasser (G1322A), auto-sampler (G1329A), column compartment (G1316A), and diode array detector (DAD, 1365B). Data were collected and analyzed using the Agilent ChemStation software. Chromatographic separation was conducted using a Luna C18(2) (250 × 4.6 mm, 5.0 µm; Phenomenex, Torrance, CA, USA), and the column temperature was maintained at 40 °C. The mobile phase consisted of 0.1% formic acid in water (A) and acetonitrile (B) with gradient elution for better separation. The gradient solvent system was optimized as follows: 95–55% A (0–40 min), 55–0% A (40–41 min), 100% B (41–45 min), and 95% A (45–55 min). The flow rate was 1 mL/min. The detection was conducted at 240 nm, and the injection volume of each sample was 10 µL. To test for linearity, standard solutions at five levels were prepared by serially diluting the stock solution. Each analysis was repeated three times, and the calibration curves were fitted by linear regression. The limit of detection (LOD) and limit of quantification (LOQ) data obtained under the optimal chromatographic conditions were determined using signal-to-noise (S/N) ratios of 3 and 10, respectively.

2.3. Determination of Preventive Effect of CPA4-1 on AGE Formation

Bovine serum albumin (BSA) (Sigma-Aldrich, St. Louis, MO, USA) was mixed with 0.2 M glucose or fructose in 50 µM phosphate buffer at 10 mg/mL. Various concentrations of CPA4-1 extract or aminoguanidine (AG) (Sigma-Aldrich) were added, and the mixture was incubated at 37 °C for 14 days. After incubation, the fluorescence products of glycated BSA was determined using a spectrofluorometer (Synergy HT; BIO-TEK, Winooski, VT, USA) at excitation/emission wavelength of 350/450 nm. The 50% inhibition concentration (IC_{50}) for AGE formation was calculated via interpolation from the concentration-inhibition curve.

2.4. Breaking Effect of CPA4-1 on Preformed AGE-Collagen Complexes

The ability of CPA4-1 to break preformed AGEs was evaluated using a previously described method [22]. Briefly, 1 µg of glycated BSA (AGEs-BSA) (MBL International, Woburn, MA, USA) was pre-incubated in collagen-coated 96-well plates for 24 h, and the collagen-AGEs-BSA complexes were then incubated with CPA4-1. Collagen-AGE-BSA crosslinking was detected using mouse anti-AGEs primary antibody (Clone No. 6D12; Trans Genic Inc., Kobe, Japan), horseradish peroxidase-linked goat anti-mouse IgG secondary antibody, and H_2O_2 substrate containing 2,2'-azino-bis (3-ethylbenzothiazoline-6-sulfonic acid) (ABTS) chromogen. Breakdown levels were measured as the percentage of decrease in optical density (OD = 410 nm). We calculated the IC_{50} (µg/mL) as 50% inhibition of collagen-AGE-BSA crosslinking, in which the crosslinking inhibition percent was calculated as follows:

$$\text{Inhibition of collagen-AGE-BSA crosslinking (\%)} = 100 - \frac{\text{abserbance of sample}}{\text{abserbance of control}} \times 100.$$

Breaking of AGE-induced crosslinking was expressed as the percentage decrease in optical density. The breaking percentage was calculated according to the above equation.

2.5. Cell Culture and Determination of Preventive Effect of CPA4-1 on AGE Formation in ARPE-19 Cells

ARPE-19 cells were purchased from the American Type Culture Collection (ATCC CRL-2302; Manassas, VA, USA) and maintained at 37 °C in a humidified 5% CO_2 incubator [23]. To examine the inhibitory effect of CPA4-1 on AGE formation, the cells were treated with CPA4-1 (10, 20, or 50 µg/mL in DMSO) for 1 h before the addition of 25 mM glucose and 500 µg/mL BSA (Roche Diagnostics, Basel, Swiss). After that, the cells were incubated for 48 h and then subjected to Western blotting analysis.

2.6. Western Blot Analysis

Sodium dodecyl sulfate-polyacrylamide gel electrophoresis (SDS-PAGE) was performed, as described previously [4]. Each sample (25 µg/mL) was fractionated on a 10% SDS-PAGE, after which the proteins were transferred to a polyvinylamide gel membrane (Millipore, Billerica, MA, USA) using traditional tank transfer system (Mini Trans-Blot cell, Bio-rad, Hercules, CA, USA). Membranes were probed with antibodies against AGEs (Clone No. 6D12; Trans Genic Inc.), occludin (Invitrogen, Carlsbad, CA, USA), and β-actin (Sigma-Aldrich), each at 1:1000 dilution. Signals were detected using a WEST-one ECL solution (Intron, Korea) and captured on a Fuji Film LAS-3000 (Tokyo, Japan).

2.7. Animals and Experimental Design

Animal experiments were conducted by Qu-Best Bio Co., Ltd. (Yongin City, Korea), according to the National Institutes of Health Guide for the Care and Use of Laboratory Animals (Approval number: QJE14015). Male C57BL/KsJ db/db mice and their age-matched lean littermates (db/+) were purchased from Japan SLC (Shizuoka, Japan). At 8 weeks of age, the db/db mice were randomly assigned into four groups (n = 10): NOR, normal control mice; DM, db/db mice; FENO, db/db mice treated with fenofibrate (100 mg/kg); CPA4-1-100, db/db mice treated with CPA4-1 (100 mg/kg). CPA4-1 was dissolved in the vehicle (0.5% w/v carboxymethyl cellulose solution) at a concentration of 5 mg/mL. The mice received daily gastric gavage of fenofibrate (100 mg/kg) or CPA4-1-100 (100 mg/kg), and db/+ mice received the same vehicle treatment for 12 weeks. Blood glucose level was measured with an automated biochemistry analyzer (HITACHI917; Hitachi, Japan), and the glycated hemoglobin (Hb1Ac) level was determined by a commercial kit (Roche Diagnostic, Mannheim, Germany).

2.8. Measurement of BRB Permeability

At autopsy, mice were anesthetized by intraperitoneal injection of 10 mg/kg zolazepam (Zoletil, Virbac, Carros, France) and 10 mg/kg xylazine hydrochloride (Rumpun, Bayer, Frankfurt, Germany). The peritoneal and thoracic cavities were opened to secure the heart, and 50 mg/mL fluorescein-dextran (10 kDa Mw, Sigma-Aldrich) and 10 mg/mL Hoechst 33342 (Sigma-Aldrich) dissolved in 1 mL sterile phosphate-buffered saline (PBS) were injected into the left ventricle. After 5 min, the eyeballs were removed, fixed in 4% paraformaldehyde for 2 h, and the retina was separated from the eyecup. The separated retina was placed on a slide, mounted with an aqueous mounting medium, and observed under a fluorescence microscope with digital capture (BX41 microscope; Olympus, Tokyo, Japan).

2.9. Preparation of Trypsin-Digested Retinal Vessel

The isolated retinas were placed in 10% formalin for 2 days. After fixation, the retina was incubated in trypsin (3% in sodium phosphate buffer containing 0.1 M sodium fluoride) for 60 min. The vessel structures were separated from retinal cells by gentle rinsing in distilled water. The vascular specimens were mounted on a slide and subjected to periodic acid-Schiff staining. The specimens were then analyzed under a microscope with digital capture (BX41 microscope; Olympus). The number of acellular capillaries per mm^2 of the capillary area was determined by counting 10 selected microscopic fields.

2.10. Immunohistochemical Staining

Each eye was enucleated and fixed with 4% paraformaldehyde for 24 h. The retina was isolated under a dissecting microscope and entirely washed with water and incubated in 3% trypsin in sodium phosphate buffer for 1 h. The trypsin digests were subjected to immunofluorescence staining, as previously described [13]. The slides were incubated with a mouse anti-occludin antibody (Invitrogen) for 1 h at room temperature. Signals were detected using a rhodamine-conjugated goat anti-mouse antibody (Santa Cruz Biotechnology, Paso Robles, CA, USA) and detected by fluorescence microscopy (BX51; Olympus).

2.11. Statistical Analysis

Data were expressed as mean ± SD or mean ± SE. ANOVA with Tukey's test was used for multiple comparisons using the Prism 7.0 software (GraphPad software, San Diego, CA, USA).

3. Results

3.1. HPLC Analysis of CPA4-1

The regression equations for the five reference standards, together with the LOD and LOQ values, are shown in Table 1. All of the calibration curves showed good linearity ($R^2 > 0.999$) within the test ranges. An established analytical HPLC method was applied to quantitatively analyze five compounds in CPA4-1. The main chromatographic peaks in CPA4-1 were identified by comparing their retention times and UV spectra with those of the corresponding commercial standards. Representative chromatograms of CPA4-1 and five standard compounds monitored at a wavelength of 240 nm are shown in Figure 1. The content of the five compounds, namely, gallic acid, albiflorin, paeoniflorin, benzoic acid, and cinnamic acid, in CPA4-1 were 1.1%, 5.3%, 8.5%, 0.4%, and 0.1%, respectively (Table 2).

Table 1. Regression equation, linearity, LOD, and LOQ for five marker compounds (n = 3).

Compound	Regression Equation [a]	Linear Range (μg/mL)	Linearity (R^2)	LOD [b] (μg/mL)	LOQ [c] (μg/mL)
Gallic acid	y = 11.507x − 8.142	6.25–200	0.9998	0.06	0.20
Albiflorin	y = 7.425x − 7.816	31.25–1000	0.9998	0.35	1.17
Paeoniflorin	y = 6.751x − 46.907	31.25–1000	0.9998	0.38	1.27
Benzoic acid	y = 29.191x − 0.899	3.15–100	0.9999	0.02	0.07
Cinnamic acid	y = 22.359x − 2.634	1.0–50	0.9997	0.01	0.03

[a] y, the peak area of the compound; x, concentration (μg/mL) of the compound. [b] LOD, limit of detection, signal-to-noise, S/N = 3. [c] LOQ, limit of quantification, S/N = 10.

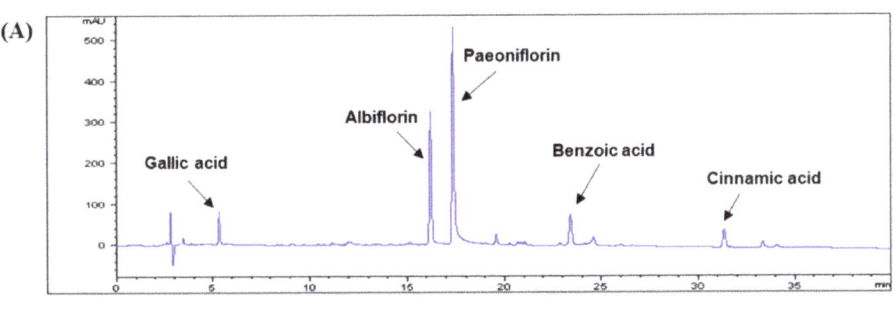

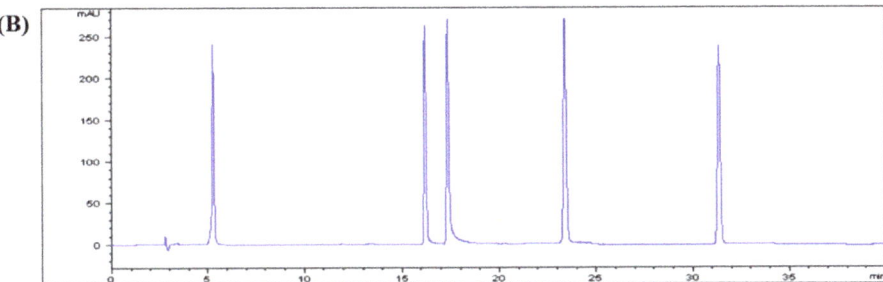

Figure 1. HPLC chromatograms of CPA4-1 (Cinnamomi Ramulus:Paeoniae Radix = 1:8) (**A**) and five standard compound mixtures (**B**). The chromatographic conditions are described in the text. Detection was conducted at 240 nm.

Table 2. Content of the five compounds in CPA4-1 as determined by HPLC analysis.

Compounds	Source	Content in CPA4-1 (%)
Gallic acid	Paeoniae Radix	1.1
Albiflorin	Paeoniae Radix	5.3
Paeoniflorin	Paeoniae Radix	8.5
Benzoic acid	Paeoniae Radix	0.4
Cinnamic acid	Cinnamomi Ramulus	0.1

CPA4-1 (Cinnamomi Ramulus:Paeoniae Radix = 1:8).

3.2. Inhibitory Effects of CPA4-1 on AGE Formation In Vitro and in ARPE-19 Cells

As shown in Table 3, CPA4-1 inhibited AGE formation compared with the positive control, AG. The IC$_{50}$ value of CPA4-1 was 6.84 ± 0.08 µg/mL, and that of AG was 78.28 ± 4.24 µg/mL. CPA4-1 was approximately 11.44-fold more potent than AG in inhibiting AGE formation.

Table 3. Inhibitory effect of CPA4-1 on the formation of advanced glycation end product (AGE).

Sample	Conc., µg/mL	Inhibition, %	IC$_{50}$, µg/mL
CPA4-1	2.5	16.64 ± 0.58	
	5	43.06 ± 0.71	6.84 ± 0.08
	10	69.68 ± 1.67	
AG	55.55 (750 µM)	44.53 ± 2.33	
	74.06 (1000 µM)	49.97 ± 0.59	78.28 ± 4.24 (1056.47 ± 57.25 µM)
	111.10 (1500 µM)	56.37 ± 0.67	

CPA4-1 was added into BSA solution and 0.2 M glucose and fructose and incubated for 14 days. AGE-specific fluorescence was analyzed using a spectrofluorometer, as described in the Methods section. IC$_{50}$ (50% inhibition concentration) value was calculated from the dose-inhibition curve (n = 3). Aminoguanidine (AG) was used as a positive control.

AGE-specific fluorescence was detected after incubation of AGEs-BSA with CPA4-1. The results showed that CPA4-1 was inhibited in a dose-dependent manner (Figure 2A). As shown in Figure 2B,C, CPA4-1 inhibited AGE formation in ARPE-19 cells in a dose-dependent manner.

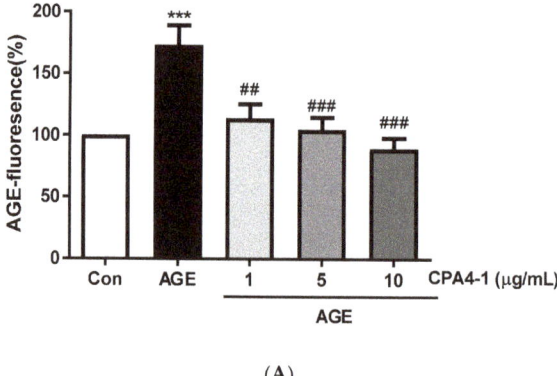

(A)

Figure 2. *Cont.*

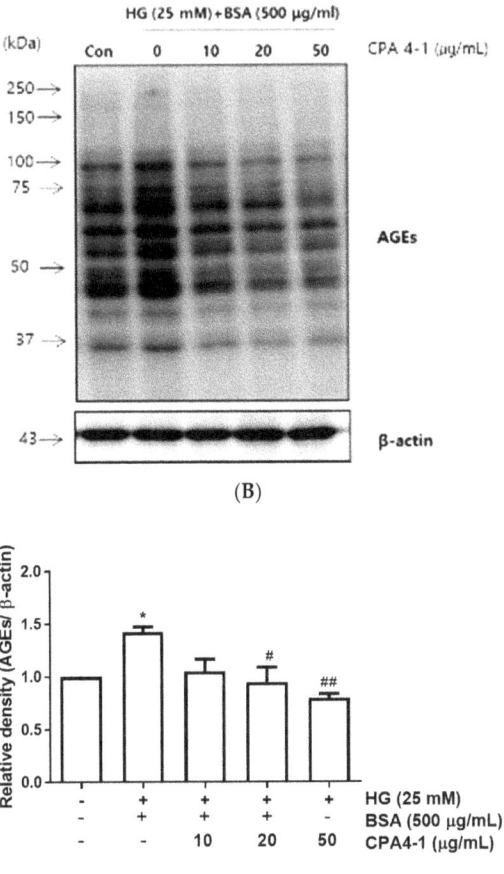

Figure 2. Inhibitory effect of CPA4-1 on the formation of advanced glycation end product (AGE). (**A**) AGE-fluorescence. *** $p < 0.001$ vs. Con; ## $p < 0.01$, ### $p < 0.001$ vs. AGE (n = 8). (**B**,**C**) Inhibitory effect of CPA4-1 on AGE formation in ARPE-19 cells. Data are expressed as mean ± SD. * $p < 0.05$ vs. Con; ## $p < 0.01$, # $p < 0.05$ vs. High glucose (HG) + BSA (n = 4).

3.3. Breaking Effect of CPA4-1 on Preformed AGE-Collagen Complexes

The ability of CPA4-1 to break the cross-links in the preformed AGE-collagen complexes was tested (Figure 3). CPA4-1 destroyed the cross-links in the complexes in a dose-dependent manner (IC$_{50}$ = 1.30 ± 0.37 µg/mL).

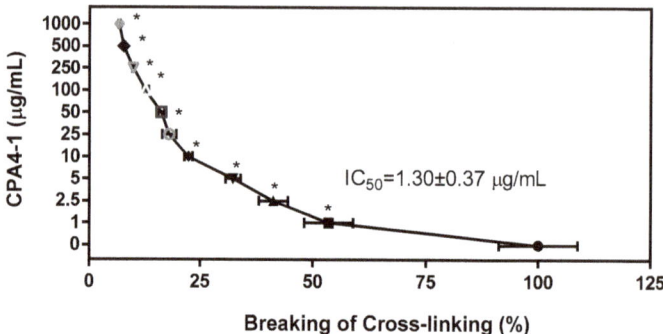

Figure 3. Breaking effect of CPA4-1 on AGE-BSA cross-linking with collagen. IC$_{50}$ (50% inhibition concentration) values were calculated from the dose-inhibition curve. Data are expressed as mean ± SD (n = 4). * $p < 0.001$ vs. Con (0 μg/mL).

3.4. Metabolic and Physical Parameters

Blood glucose and HbA1c levels are summarized in Table 4. Blood glucose and HbA1c levels significantly increased in the DM group ($p < 0.05$), but decreased in the FENO group. However, in the CPA4-1 group, glucose level was not changed, and HbA1c was slightly reduced, although not significant (Table 4).

Table 4. Blood and liver parameters in the serum of db/db mice treated with FENO and CPA4-1.

	NOR	DM	FENO	CPA4-1
Blood glucose (mg/dl)	137.6 ± 16.2	447.2 ± 113.7 *	423.5 ± 266.4 #	459.6 ± 146.9
HbA1c (%)	2.66 ± 1.74	11.29 ± 3.81 *	6.32 ± 5.14 #	10.63 ± 1.96

NOR, normal control mice; DM, db/db mice; FENO, db/db mice treated with fenofibrate (100 mg/kg); CPA4-1-100, db/db mice treated with CPA4-1 (100 mg/kg). All data are expressed as mean ± SD. * $p < 0.05$ vs. Nor group, # $p < 0.05$ vs. DM group. HbA1c, glycated hemoglobin.

As shown in Figure 4, compared with the normal mice group, the DM mice group exhibited significantly elevated body weight. However, treatment with CPA4-1 or FENO did not lead to any significant changes in body weight compared with that of DM mice.

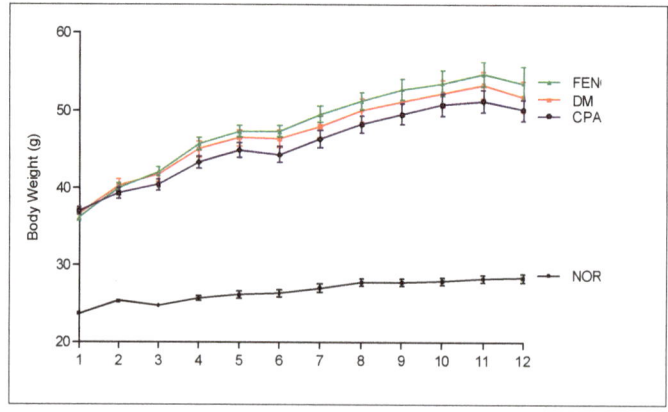

Figure 4. Body weight. NOR, normal control mice; DM, db/db mice; FENO, db/db mice treated with fenofibrate (100 mg/kg); CPA4-1, db/db mice treated with CPA4-1-100 (100 mg/kg). All data are expressed as mean ± SE.

3.5. Preventive Effects of CPA4-1 on BRB Breakage in db/db Mice

Fluorescence leakage due to BRB damage was observed and analyzed. In the normal group, no fluorescence leakage was observed. However, in the db/db mice group (DM), retinal vessels showed bright fluorescence due to the BRB breakage. As shown in Figure 5, the DM group showed a significant increase in BRB leakage compared with the normal group. FENO- or CPA4-1-treated db/db mice groups showed a significant decrease in BRB leakage compared with the db/db mice group.

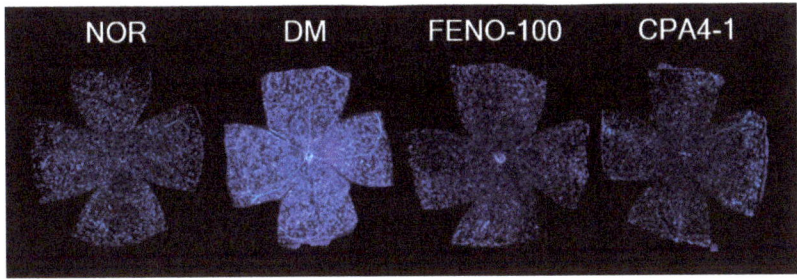

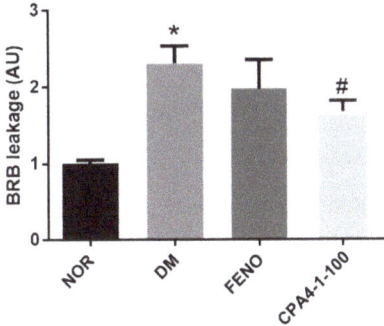

Figure 5. Effects of FENO and CPA4-1 on blood-retinal barrier (BRB) breakage in db/db mice. NOR, normal control mice; DM, db/db mice; FENO, db/db mice treated with fenofibrate (100 mg/kg); CPA4-1, db/db mice treated with CPA4-1-100 (100 mg/kg). All data are expressed as mean ± SE. * $p < 0.05$ vs. NOR group. # $p < 0.05$ vs. DM group.

3.6. Preventive Effects of CPA4-1 on Tight Junction Protein Loss in db/db Mice

To examine the therapeutic efficacy of CPA4-1 on the BRB, we detected loss of tight junction proteins in the retinal vascular endothelial cells of db/db mice. These proteins are important factors that increase the permeability of blood vessels. As shown in Figure 6A, the damage of vessels significantly increased in the retinas of db/db mice compared with that of the normal group. To elucidate whether this phenomenon was related to the expression of tight junction proteins, we assessed occludin levels in the retina of db/db mice. Figure 6B shows that the expression of occludin was downregulated in db/db mice compared with that in the normal control group. However, CPA4-1 treatment restored occludin expression in db/db mice.

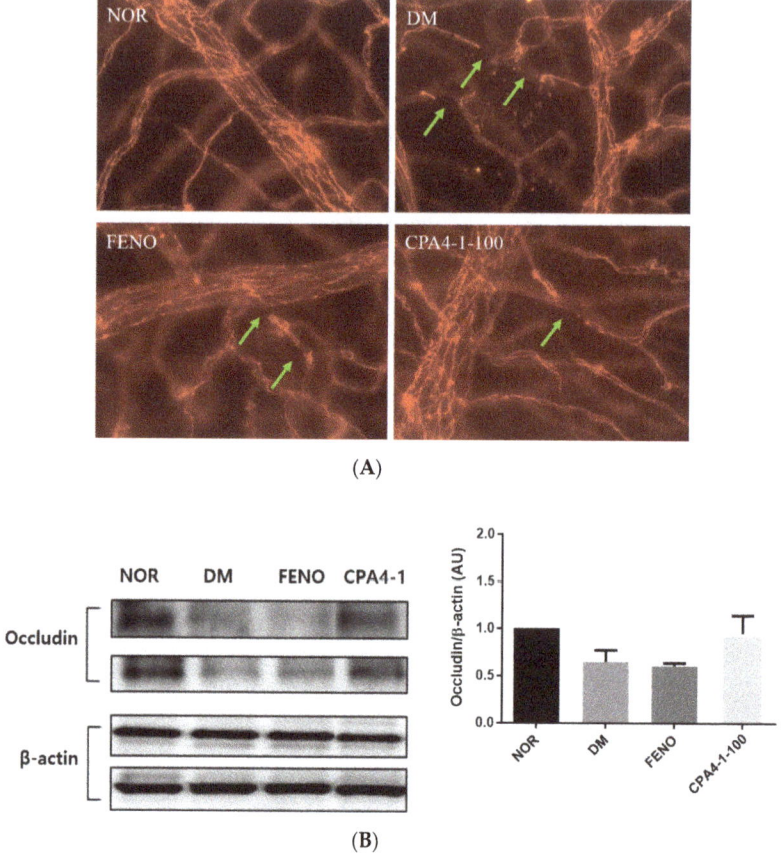

Figure 6. Effect of CPA4-1 on tight junction protein loss. (**A**) Immunofluorescence staining for occludin in trypsin-digested retinal vessels acellular capillaries (green arrow). (**B**) Expression of retinal occludin. The total protein was isolated from retinal tissues and subjected to Western blotting using occludin and beta-actin antibodies. Values in the bar graphs represent the mean (n = 2).

3.7. Effects of CPA4-1 on Acellular Capillary Formation in db/db Mice

The formation of the acellular capillary, due to the loss of vascular endothelial cells and pericytes among blood vessels, occurred in DR. As shown in Figure 7, the db/db mice group showed a significant increase in retinal acellular capillary formation (black arrow) compared with the normal group. As expected, the acellular capillary of FENO- or CPA4-1-treated db/db mice significantly decreased compared with that of vehicle-treated db/db mice.

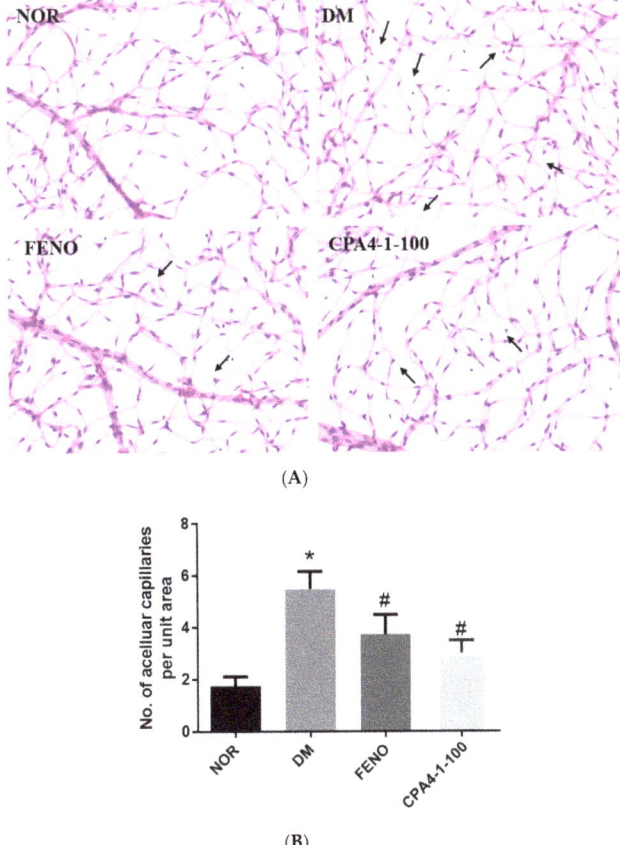

Figure 7. Effects of FENO and CPA4-1 on retinal acellular capillary formation in db/db mice. Retinal vessels were stained with H&E (**A**). Acellular capillaries (black arrow) were measured to assess the extent of retinopathy (**B**). NOR, normal control mice; DM, db/db mice; FENO, db/db mice treated with fenofibrate (100 mg/kg); CPA4-1, db/db mice treated with CPA4-1-100 (100 mg/kg). All data are expressed as mean ± SE (n = 6 ~ 7). * $p < 0.05$ vs. NOR group. # $p < 0.05$ vs. DM group.

4. Discussion

In our previous studies, we examined the effects of herbal extracts in inhibiting AGE formation (CPA1-1 (1:1) IC_{50} = 9.94 ± 0.20 μg/mL; CPA2-1 (1:2) IC_{50} = 7.54 ± 0.18 μg/mL; CPA3-1 (1:4) IC_{50} = 8.16 ± 0.23 μg/mL; CPA4-1 (1:8) IC_{50} = 6.84 ± 0.08 μg/mL) and we showed potential therapeutic targets of DR in animal and in vitro models. In this study, we investigated whether CPA4-1, a herbal combination, inhibits AGE formation and breaks the cross-linking of AGE with collagen in vitro. We tested whether CPA4-1 affects the expression of occludin in the retina and whether this effect is correlated with inhibition of BRB breakage. Our findings showed that CPA4-1 significantly prevented retinal vascular leakage and retinal acellular capillary formation. These results indicated that CPA4-1 attenuated the downregulation of tight junction protein occludin in the retinas of db/db mice. The tight junction acts as a semipermeable barrier for paracellular transports of solutes, ions, water, and cells. Occludin is the first identified component of the tight junction strand, a transmembrane protein of approximately 60 kDa [24]. In diabetic patients, retinal occludin protein expression is selectively decreased, and BRB permeability is increased [25]. Decreased expression of tight junction proteins is important in diabetic patients, as it causes increased vascular permeability, vasodilation, and edema.

As CPA4-1 was shown to increase the expression of occludin in the retina of db/db mice in this study, CPA4-1 might serve as an inhibitor of AGE formation to protect against DR.

Fasting blood glucose and HbA1c levels are important factors in diabetes. HbA1c is monitored in the long-term follow-up of patients with DR, and diabetic patients are primarily treated with insulin to lower blood glucose levels. Fenofibrate decreased blood glucose level and HbA1c level in the db/db mice group (Table 3). Fenofibrate treatment induces lowing of blood glucose levels and HbA1c by reducing adiposity, thus improving peripheral insulin action [26]. Previous studies have suggested that that fenofibrate exerts robust protective effects against DR in type 2 diabetic patients and type 1 diabetic animal models [27,28]. The potential therapeutic mechanisms of fenofibrate on retinal microvascular dysfunctions induced by diabetes include the restoration of VEGF and the reduction of oxidative stress in diabetic rats [29]. As CPA4-1 did not alter blood glucose level and HbA1c of db/db mice compared with those of the db/db mice group, CPA4-1 might act as a supplement for the prevention of BRB breakage and retinal acellular capillary formation, without altering blood glucose level or HbA1c of diabetic patients.

Herbal medicine has been used to treat diabetes and diabetic complications, including DR, for thousands of years worldwide. Many researchers have tried to provide evidence of the therapeutic effectiveness and mechanisms of herbal medicine. *Panax notoginseng* (Araliaceae) has been reported to exert antidiabetic activities, and it contains saponins, such as ginsenoside Re 14, ginsenoside Rd, ginsenoside Rg1, ginsenoside Rb1, and notoginsenoside R1. These saponins have also been reported to exert antioxidant action [30]. As free radical damage is critically involved in the pathophysiology of DR, *P. notoginseng* saponins can be used in the treatment of DR owing to their beneficial effects. *Pueraria lobata* (Fabaceae) is one of the most used herbs in traditional Korean medicine, and it contains puerarin, genistein, and daidzein. Puerarin directly inhibits the formation of AGEs in vitro [31]. CPA4-1 is formulated at the optimum conditions to inhibit AGE formation. Cinnamic acid from Cinnamomi Ramulus promotes the management of diabetes and its complications [32]. Cinnamic acid and its derivatives stimulate insulin and hepatic gluconeogenesis, enhance glucose uptake, and inhibit AGE formation [33,34]. Paeoniae Radix extract contains 5% paeoniflorin, the most important component that suppresses high glucose-induced retinal microglial matrix metalloproteinase 9 (MMP-9) expression and inflammation by reducing capillary permeability [35]. Paeoniflorin also exerts a neuroprotective effect on inflammation and apoptosis in Alzheimer's disease and regulates hepatic cholesterol synthesis and metabolism by reducing oxidative stress [36,37].

5. Conclusions

The present study showed that CPA4-1 exerted an inhibitory effect on AGE formation and breaking effect on AGE-collagen cross-linking. CPA4-1 treatment ameliorated BRB leakage and retinal acellular capillary formation in db/db mice. These results suggested the potential of CPA4-1 as a therapeutic supplement for protection against retinal vascular permeability diseases.

6. Patents

The patent related to this study has been registered in Korea (no. 10-2015-0176274).

Author Contributions: Y.S.K. designed the in vitro experiment and wrote the manuscript; J.K. designed the in vivo experiments; I.S.L. confirmed the HPLC chromatogram; C.-S.K., K.J., and Y.M.L. performed the animal experiments; D.H.J. performed the in vitro experiments; G.H.B. identified the herbs; J.S.K. designed all experiments and reviewed the manuscript. All authors have read and agreed to the published version of the manuscript.

Funding: This research was funded by the Korea Institute of Oriental Medicine (grant number K18270 and KSN20134261).

Conflicts of Interest: The authors declare no conflict of interest.

Data Availability: All data generated or analyzed during this study are included in this published article.

References

1. Brownlee, M. Advanced protein glycosylation in diabetes and aging. *Annu. Rev. Med.* **1995**, *46*, 223–234. [CrossRef] [PubMed]
2. Brownlee, M. The pathological implications of protein glycation. *Clin. Investig. Med.* **1995**, *18*, 275–281.
3. Reynaert, N.L.; Gopal, P.; Rutten, E.P.A.; Wouters, E.F.M.; Schalkwijk, C.G. Advanced glycation end products and their receptor in age-related, non-communicable chronic inflammatory diseases; Overview of clinical evidence and potential contributions to disease. *Int. J. Biochem. Cell Biol.* **2016**, *81 (Pt B)*, 403–418. [CrossRef]
4. Baynes, J.W. Role of oxidative stress in development of complications in diabetes. *Diabetes* **1991**, *40*, 405–412. [CrossRef] [PubMed]
5. Shin, E.S.; Sorenson, C.M.; Sheibani, N. Diabetes and retinal vascular dysfunction. *J. Ophthalmic. Vis. Res.* **2014**, *9*, 362–373.
6. Kaur, C.; Foulds, W.S.; Ling, E.A. Blood-retinal barrier in hypoxic ischaemic conditions: Basic concepts, clinical features and management. *Prog. Retin. Eye Res.* **2008**, *27*, 622–647. [CrossRef]
7. Song, F.; Schmidt, A.M. Glycation and insulin resistance: Novel mechanisms and unique targets? *Arterioscler. Thromb. Vasc. Biol.* **2012**, *32*, 1760–1765. [CrossRef]
8. Sharma, N.; Ooi, J.L.; Ong, J.; Newman, D. The use of fenofibrate in the management of patients with diabetic retinopathy: An evidence-based review. *Aust. Fam. Physician* **2015**, *44*, 367–370.
9. Unoki-Kubota, H.; Yamagishi, S.; Takeuchi, M.; Bujo, H.; Saito, Y. Pyridoxamine, an inhibitor of advanced glycation end product (AGE) formation ameliorates insulin resistance in obese, type 2 diabetic mice. *Protein Pept. Lett.* **2010**, *17*, 1177–1181. [CrossRef]
10. Lee, I.S.; Jung, S.H.; Kim, J.S. Polyphenols from Euphorbia pekinensis Inhibit AGEs Formation In Vitro and Vessel Dilation in Larval Zebrafish In Vivo. *Planta Med.* **2018**, *84*, 176–181. [CrossRef]
11. Lee, I.S.; Kim, Y.J.; Jung, S.H.; Kim, J.H.; Kim, J.S. Flavonoids from Litsea japonica Inhibit AGEs Formation and Rat Lense Aldose Reductase In Vitro and Vessel Dilation in Zebrafish. *Planta Med.* **2017**, *83*, 318–325. [CrossRef] [PubMed]
12. Jang, D.S.; Yoo, N.H.; Kim, N.H.; Lee, Y.M.; Kim, C.S.; Kim, J.; Kim, J.H.; Kim, J.S. 3,5-Di-O-caffeoyl-epi-quinic acid from the leaves and stems of Erigeron annuus inhibits protein glycation, aldose reductase, and cataractogenesis. *Biol. Pharm. Bull.* **2010**, *33*, 329–333. [CrossRef] [PubMed]
13. Kim, J.; Jo, K.; Lee, I.S.; Kim, C.S.; Kim, J.S. The Extract of Aster Koraiensis Prevents Retinal Pericyte Apoptosis in Diabetic Rats and Its Active Compound, Chlorogenic Acid Inhibits AGE Formation and AGE/RAGE Interaction. *Nutrients* **2016**, *8*, 585. [CrossRef] [PubMed]
14. Pyun, B.J.; Kim, Y.S.; Lee, I.S.; Jung, D.H.; Kim, J.H.; Kim, J.S. Osteomeles schwerinae Extract and Its Major Compounds Inhibit Methylglyoxal-Induced Apoptosis in Human Retinal Pigment Epithelial Cells. *Molecules* **2020**, *25*, 2605. [CrossRef]
15. Momtaz, S.; Hassani, S.; Khan, F.; Ziaee, M.; Abdollahi, M. Cinnamon, a promising prospect towards Alzheimer's disease. *Pharmacol. Res.* **2018**, *130*, 241–258. [CrossRef] [PubMed]
16. Mang, B.; Wolters, M.; Schmitt, B.; Kelb, K.; Lichtinghagen, R.; Stichtenoth, D.O.; Hahn, A. Effects of a cinnamon extract on plasma glucose, HbA, and serum lipids in diabetes mellitus type. *Eur. J. Clin. Investig.* **2006**, *36*, 340–344. [CrossRef]
17. Talaei, B.; Amouzegar, A.; Sahranavard, S.; Hedayati, M.; Mirmiran, P.; Azizi, F. Effects of Cinnamon Consumption on Glycemic Indicators, Advanced Glycation End Products, and Antioxidant Status in Type 2 Diabetic Patients. *Nutrients* **2017**, *9*, 991. [CrossRef]
18. Wu, X.; He, J.; Xu, H.; Bi, K.; Li, Q. Quality assessment of Cinnamomi Ramulus by the simultaneous analysis of multiple active components using high-performance thin-layer chromatography and high-performance liquid chromatography. *J. Sep. Sci.* **2014**, *37*, 2490–2498. [CrossRef]
19. Chuang, W.C.; Lin, W.C.; Sheu, S.J.; Chiou, S.H.; Chang, H.C.; Chen, Y.P. A comparative study on commercial samples of the roots of Paeonia vitchii and, P. lactiflora. *Planta Med.* **1996**, *62*, 347–351. [CrossRef]
20. Bogdanov, P.; Corraliza, L.; Villena, J.A.; Carvalho, A.R.; Garcia-Arumi, J.; Ramos, D.; Ruberte, J.; Simo, R.; Hernandez, C. The db/db mouse: A useful model for the study of diabetic retinal neurodegeneration. *PLoS ONE* **2014**, *9*, e97302. [CrossRef]

21. Tang, L.; Zhang, Y.; Jiang, Y.; Willard, L.; Ortiz, E.; Wark, L. Dietary wolfberry ameliorates retinal structure abnormalities in db/db mice at the early stage of diabetes. *Exp. Biol. Med. (Maywood)* **2011**, *236*, 1051–1063. [CrossRef] [PubMed]
22. Kim, J.; Kim, C.S.; Kim, Y.S.; Lee, I.S.; Kim, J.S. Jakyakgamcho-tang and Its Major Component, Paeonia Lactiflora, Exhibit Potent Anti-glycation Properties. *J. Exerc. Nutr. Biochem.* **2016**, *20*, 60–64. [CrossRef] [PubMed]
23. Kim, Y.S.; Jung, D.H.; Kim, N.H.; Lee, Y.M.; Jang, D.S.; Song, G.Y.; Kim, J.S. KIOM-79 inhibits high glucose or AGEs-induced VEGF expression in human retinal pigment epithelial cells. *J. Ethnopharmacol.* **2007**, *112*, 166–172. [CrossRef] [PubMed]
24. Furuse, M.; Hirase, T.; Itoh, M.; Nagafuchi, A.; Yonemura, S.; Tsukita, S. Occludin: A novel integral membrane protein localizing at tight junctions. *J. Cell Biol.* **1993**, *123*, 1777–1788. [CrossRef]
25. Antonetti, D.A.; Barber, A.J.; Khin, S.; Lieth, E.; Tarbell, J.M.; Gardner, T.W. Vascular permeability in experimental diabetes is associated with reduced endothelial occludin content: Vascular endothelial growth factor decreases occludin in retinal endothelial cells. Penn State Retina Research Group. *Diabetes* **1998**, *47*, 1953–1959. [CrossRef]
26. Koh, E.H.; Kim, M.S.; Park, J.Y.; Kim, H.S.; Youn, J.Y.; Park, H.S.; Youn, J.H.; Lee, K.U. Peroxisome proliferator-activated receptor (PPAR)-alpha activation prevents diabetes in OLETF rats: Comparison with PPAR-gamma activation. *Diabetes* **2003**, *52*, 2331–2337. [CrossRef]
27. Chen, Y.; Hu, Y.; Lin, M.; Jenkins, A.J.; Keech, A.C.; Mott, R.; Lyons, T.J.; Ma, J.X. Therapeutic effects of PPARalpha agonists on diabetic retinopathy in type 1 diabetes models. *Diabetes* **2013**, *62*, 261–272. [CrossRef]
28. Keech, A.C.; Mitchell, P.; Summanen, P.A.; O'Day, J.; Davis, T.M.; Moffitt, M.S.; Taskinen, M.R.; Simes, R.J.; Tse, D.; Williamson, E.; et al. Effect of fenofibrate on the need for laser treatment for diabetic retinopathy (FIELD study): A randomised controlled trial. *Lancet* **2007**, *370*, 1687–1697. [CrossRef]
29. Li, J.; Wang, P.; Chen, Z.; Yu, S.; Xu, H. Fenofibrate Ameliorates Oxidative Stress-Induced Retinal Microvascular Dysfunction in Diabetic Rats. *Curr. Eye Res.* **2018**, *43*, 1395–1403. [CrossRef]
30. Bermudez, V.; Finol, F.; Parra, N.; Parra, M.; Perez, A.; Penaranda, L.; Vílchez, D.; Rojas, J.; Arráiz, N.; Velasco, M. PPAR-gamma agonists and their role in type 2 diabetes mellitus management. *Am. J. Ther.* **2010**, *17*, 274–283. [CrossRef]
31. Kim, J.M.; Lee, Y.M.; Lee, G.Y.; Jang, D.S.; Bae, K.H.; Kim, J.S. Constituents of the roots of Pueraria lobata inhibit formation of advanced glycation end products (AGEs). *Arch. Pharm. Res.* **2006**, *29*, 821–825. [CrossRef] [PubMed]
32. Adisakwattana, S. Cinnamic Acid and Its Derivatives: Mechanisms for Prevention and Management of Diabetes and Its Complications. *Nutrients.* **2017**, *9*, 163. [CrossRef]
33. Adisakwattana, S.; Moonsan, P.; Yibchok-Anun, S. Insulin-releasing properties of a series of cinnamic acid derivatives in vitro and in vivo. *J. Agric. Food Chem.* **2008**, *56*, 7838–7844. [CrossRef] [PubMed]
34. Gugliucci, A.; Bastos, D.H.; Schulze, J.; Souza, M.F. Caffeic and chlorogenic acids in Ilex paraguariensis extracts are the main inhibitors of AGE generation by methylglyoxal in model proteins. *Fitoterapia* **2009**, *80*, 339–344. [CrossRef] [PubMed]
35. Zhu, S.H.; Liu, B.Q.; Hao, M.J.; Fan, Y.X.; Qian, C.; Teng, P.; Zhou, X.W.; Hu, L.; Liu, W.T.; Yuan, Z.L.; et al. Paeoniflorin Suppressed High Glucose-Induced Retinal Microglia MMP-9 Expression and Inflammatory Response via Inhibition of TLR4/NF-kappaB Pathway Through Upregulation of SOCS3 in Diabetic Retinopathy. *Inflammation* **2017**, *40*, 1475–1486. [CrossRef] [PubMed]
36. Gu, X.; Cai, Z.; Cai, M.; Liu, K.; Liu, D.; Zhang, Q.; Tan, J.; Ma, Q. Protective effect of paeoniflorin on inflammation and apoptosis in the cerebral cortex of a transgenic mouse model of Alzheimer's disease. *Mol. Med. Rep.* **2016**, *13*, 2247–2252. [CrossRef]
37. Hu, H.; Zhu, Q.; Su, J.; Wu, Y.; Zhu, Y.; Wang, Y.; Fang, H.; Pang, M.; Li, B.; Chen, S.; et al. Effects of an Enriched Extract of Paeoniflorin, a Monoterpene Glycoside used in Chinese Herbal Medicine, on Cholesterol Metabolism in a Hyperlipidemic Rat Model. *Med. Sci. Monit.* **2017**, *23*, 3412–3427. [CrossRef]

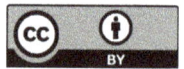

© 2020 by the authors. Licensee MDPI, Basel, Switzerland. This article is an open access article distributed under the terms and conditions of the Creative Commons Attribution (CC BY) license (http://creativecommons.org/licenses/by/4.0/).

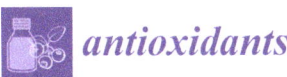

Article

Beneficial Effects of Glucagon-Like Peptide-1 (GLP-1) in Diabetes-Induced Retinal Abnormalities: Involvement of Oxidative Stress

Hugo Ramos [1,2,†], Patricia Bogdanov [1,2,†], Joel Sampedro [1], Jordi Huerta [1,2], Rafael Simó [1,2,3,*] and Cristina Hernández [1,2,3,*]

1. Diabetes and Metabolism Research Unit, Vall d'Hebron Research Institute (VHIR), 08035 Barcelona, Spain; hugo.ramos@vhir.org (H.R.); patricia.bogdanov@vhir.org (P.B.); joel.sampedro@vhir.org (J.S.); jordi.huerta@vhir.org (J.H.)
2. Centro de Investigación Biomédica en Red de Diabetes y Enfermedades Metabólicas Asociadas (CIBERDEM), Instituto de Salud Carlos III (ICSIII), 28029 Madrid, Spain
3. Department of Medicine, Universitat Autònoma de Barcelona, 08193 Barcelona, Spain
* Correspondence: rafael.simo@vhir.org (R.S.); cristina.hernandez@vhir.org (C.H.); Tel.: +34-934-894-172 (C.H.)
† These authors contributed equally to this study.

Received: 29 July 2020; Accepted: 7 September 2020; Published: 10 September 2020

Abstract: Background: Hyperglycemia-induced oxidative stress plays a key role in diabetic complications, including diabetic retinopathy. The main goal of this study was to assess whether the topical administration (eye drops) of glucagon-like peptide-1 (GLP-1) has any effect on oxidative stress in the retina. Methods: db/db mice were treated with eye drops of GLP-1 or vehicle for three weeks, with db/+ mice being used as control. Studies included the assessment by western blot of the antioxidant defense markers CuZnSOD, MnSOD, glutathione peroxidase and reductase; immunofluorescence measurements of DNA/RNA damage, nitro tyrosine and Ki67 and Babam2 proteins. Results: GLP-1 eye drops protected from oxidative stress by increasing the protein levels of glutathione reductase, glutathione peroxidase and CuZnSOD and MnSOD in diabetic retinas. This was associated with a significant reduction of DNA/RNA damage and the activation of proteins involved in DNA repair in the retina (Babam2) and Ki67 (a biomarker of cell proliferation). Conclusions: GLP-1 modulates the antioxidant defense system in the diabetic retina and has a neuroprotective action favoring DNA repair and neuron cells proliferation.

Keywords: diabetic retinopathy; GLP-1; oxidative stress; superoxide dismutase; free radicals

1. Introduction

In recent years emerging evidence has indicated that glucagon-like peptide 1 (GLP-1) exerts beneficial effects in experimental diabetic retinopathy (DR) [1–4]. The underlying mechanisms involve a downregulation of vascular endothelial growth factor (VEGF), proinflammatory cytokines and proapoptotic signaling, reduction of the excitotoxicity mediated by glutamate and a protective role for the tight junctions and cells of the blood-retinal barrier [1–4]. However, little is known regarding he effect of GLP-1 on oxidative stress.

Oxidative stress as a result of chronic hyperglycemia play a key role in diabetic complications, including DR [5]. Reactive oxygen species (ROS) and reactive nitrogen species (RNS) are physiologically produced and are needed for redox signaling, but they can also alter the normal cellular homeostasis. For this reason, a precise balance between ROS/RNS production and antioxidant activity is required [6]. The retina is more susceptible to oxidative events than other tissues due to high oxygen uptake and glucose oxidation. In fact, it has been shown that diabetic patients present lower activity of antioxidant enzymes (superoxide dismutase (SOD), glutathione reductase and glutathione peroxidase) and high ROS/RNS levels in the retina [7,8]. Recent experimental evidence suggests that oxidative stress not only contributes to the DR development, but also causes resistance to the beneficial effects of good glycemic control [9].

The aim of this study was to investigate the antioxidant and antinitrosative properties of topical GLP-1 in an experimental model of DR.

2. Experimental Section

2.1. Experimental Design

A total of 30 diabetic male db/db [BKS.Cg-Dock7m +/+ Leprdb/J] mice and 15 non-diabetic mice db/+; [BKS.Cg-Dock7m + Leprdb/+] were purchased at the age of 8 weeks (Charles River Laboratories, Calco, Italy). Db/db mice present a mutation in the leptin receptor that triggers obesity-induced type 2 diabetes. The mice had access to ad libitum food (ENVIGO Global Diet Complete Feed for Rodents, Mucedola, Milan, Italy) and filtered water. They were housed at 20 °C temperature and 60% humidity throughout all the study. With the aim of minimizing variability, the animals were randomly distributed (block randomization) in groups of 4 mice per cage. Each cage held absorbent bedding and nesting material (BioFresh Performance Bedding 1/800 pelleted cellulose, Absorption Corp, Ferndale, WA, USA).

2.2. Interventional Study

When the mice reached the age of 21 weeks, GLP-1 eye drops ($n = 15$) and vehicle (phosphate-buffered saline (PBS) eye drops ($n = 15$) were randomly dispensed directly onto the superior corneal surface of both eyes with the help of a micropipette. They received one drop in each eye (5 µL) twice daily for 21 days. On the last day of treatment, at the age of 24 weeks, a drop of GLP-1 (2 mg/mL) or vehicle was administered to each eye 1 h before euthanasia. This study obtained the approval of the Animal Care and Use Committee of VHIR (Vall d'Hebron Research Institute, Barcelona, Spain). All experiments were performed in accordance with the guidelines of the European Community (86/609/CEE) and the Association for Research in Vision and Ophthalmology (ARVO).

2.3. Retinal Tissue Processing

On the last day of the topical administrations, 8 db/db mice and 4 db/+ were transcardially perfused with paraformaldehyde 4% (Santa Cruz Biotechnology, Dallas, TX, USA), and the eyes were promptly enucleated, fixed again in paraformaldehyde 4% for 5 h and embedded in paraffin blocks. Previously, each animal had received an intraperitoneal injection of 200 µL of anesthesia (a mix containing 1 mL ketamine (GmbH, Hameln, Germany) and 0.3 mL xylazine (Laboratorios Calier S.A., Barcelona, Spain)). The remaining mice (22 db/db and 11 db/+ mice) were euthanized through cervical dislocation, their eyes were instantaneously enucleated, and retinas were separated depending on the experimental purposes. For experiments that required protein samples, retinas were introduced in sterilized PBS pH 7.4 and frozen in nitrogen liquid. For RNA assessments retinas were submerged in TRIzol reagent (Invitrogen™, Carlsbad, CA, USA) and stored at −80 °C until analysis.

2.4. Western Blotting

Retinal proteins were extracted through sonication in 80 µL of lysis buffer (phenylmethanesulfonylfluoride (PMSF), 1 mM; NaF, 100 mM; Na_3VO_4, 2 mM; all diluted in RIPA buffer (Sigma, St Louis, MO, USA)) and containing 1X protease inhibitor cocktail (Sigma, St Louis, MO, USA). Twenty-five micrograms protein of each sample were loaded in a 10% (w/v) SDS-PAGE, and electrophoresis was assessed at 90 V and 120 V for 30 and 60 min, respectively. The proteins were then transferred to a polyvinylidene difluoride (PVDF) membrane (Bio-Rad Laboratories, Madrid, Spain) at 400 mA for 90 min at 4 °C and blocked in 5% skimmed milk powder (Central Lechera

Asturiana, Siero, Spain) in 0.1% TBS-Tween. Primary antibodies (Table 1) were incubated at 4 °C overnight. Secondary antibodies goat anti-rabbit and goat anti-mouse (Dako Agilent, Santa Clara, CA, USA) were diluted 1:10,000 and the following day they were applied for 1 h at room temperature. Immunoreactive bands were detected using WesternBright ECL kit (WesternBright ECL HRP substrate, K-12045-D50, Advansta, CA, USA). Anti-vinculin (1:7000; sc-73,614; Santa Cruz, Dallas, TX, USA) and anti-cyclophilin A (1:10,000; BML-SA296; Enzo, NY, USA) were used to normalize protein levels. The densitometric analysis was carried out with Image J software (National Institutes of Health, Bethesda, MD, USA).

Table 1. Primary antibodies, targets, specific dilutions and sources used in western blot analysis.

Antibodies	Description
Babam2	Rabbit monoclonal; 1:1000; ab177960; Abcam, Cambridge, UK
Cyclophilin A	Rabbit polyclonal; 1:10,000; BML-SA296; Enzo Life Sciences, Lausen, Switzerland
CuZnSOD	Rabbit polyclonal; 1:1000; GTX100554; GeneTex, Hsinchu, Taiwan
Gadph	Mouse monoclonal; 1:10,000; sc-32233; Santa Cruz, Dallas, Texas, USA
Glutathione peroxidase	Rabbit polyclonal; 1:1000; GTX116040; GeneTex, Hsinchu, Taiwan
Glutathione reductase	Rabbit polyclonal; 1:1000; GTX114199; GeneTex, Hsinchu, Taiwan
MnSOD	Rabbit polyclonal; 1:1000; ab13533; Abcam, Cambridge, UK
Vinculin	Mouse monoclonal; 1:7000; sc-73614; Santa Cruz, Dallas, Texas, USA

2.5. Immunofluorescence Analysis

Ocular globes were paraffined, sectioned (4 μm) and mounted on poly L-lysine positive charged slides (Leica Biosystems, Nussloch, Germany). The samples were deparaffinized in xylene (VWR, Barcelona, Spain), rehydrated in grade ethanol series (100%, 96%, 70% and 50%), fixed again in ice-cold acid methanol (−20 °C) and washed 3 × 5′ with phosphate-buffered saline 0.01 M (PBS) at pH 7.4. Successively, slides were warmed in a pressure cooker for 4 min at 150 °C in 250 mL of antigen retrieval with sodium citrate 10 mM, pH 6. Then, the sections were blocked with blocking solution (protein block serum-free, X0909 Agilent, Santa Clara, CA, USA) for 1 h at room temperature and they were subsequently incubated overnight at 4 °C with specific primary antibodies (Table 2). Next day, after 3 × 10′ washes in PBS, the samples were incubated for 1 h in darkness with secondary antibodies (Alexa 488 and Alexa 594; 1/600, Molecular Probes, Eugene, OR, USA). The sections were washed again 3 × 5′ with PBS, counterstained with Hoechst 33,342 (bisbenzimide) (Thermo Fisher Scientific, Eugene, OR, USA) and mounted with mounting medium fluorescence (Prolong, Invitrogen, Thermo Fisher Scientific, Eugene, OR, USA) and coverslips. Images were acquired using laser confocal microscopy (Fluoview FV 1000 laser scanning confocal microscope Olympus, Hamburg, Germany) at a resolution of 1024 × 1024 pixels. Immunofluorescence was quantified with Image J software.

Table 2. Targets, dilutions and sources of applied antibodies used in the immunofluorescence analysis.

Primary Antibodies	Description
DNA/RNA damage (8-hydroxy-guanosine)	Mouse monoclonal; 1:100; ab62623; Abcam, Cambridge, UK
Babam2	Rabbit monoclonal; 1:100; ab177960; Abcam, Cambridge, UK
CuZnSOD	Rabbit polyclonal; 1:100; GTX100554; GeneTex, Hsinchu, Taiwan
Ki67	Rabbit polyclonal; 1:500; ab15580 (Abcam, Cambridge, UK)
MnSOD	Rabbit polyclonal; 1:100; ab13533; Abcam, Cambridge, UK
NeuN	Mouse monoclonal; 1:200; ab104224; Abcam, Cambridge, UK
Nitro tyrosine	Mouse monoclonal; 1:100; ab7048; Abcam, Cambridge, UK

Table 2. *Cont.*

Secondary Antibodies	Description
Alexa Fluor 488 Goat anti-mouse	Goat polyclonal; 1:600; #A-11032; Abcam, Cambridge, UK
Alexa Fluor 488 Goat anti-rabbit	Goat polyclonal; 1:600; ab150081; Abcam, Cambridge, UK
Alexa Fluor 594 Goat anti-mouse	Goat polyclonal; 1:600; ab150113; Life Technologies (Thermo Fisher Scientific) Waltham, MA, USA
Alexa Fluor 594 Goat anti-rabbit	Goat polyclonal; 1:600; A-110012; Life Technologies (Thermo Fisher Scientific) Waltham, MA, USA

2.6. Statistical Analysis

Data are presented as mean ± SEM. Quantitative comparisons were analyzed by using Student's *t*-test and one-way ANOVA followed by Bonferroni's multiple comparison post hoc test. Statistical significance was set at $p < 0.05$ (*).

3. Results

3.1. Topical Administration of GLP-1 has no Effect on Body Weight and Systemic Blood Glucose Levels

No significant difference was observed in body weight and blood glucose concentrations during the experiment between db/db mice treated with GLP-1 eye drops and db/db mice treated with vehicle (Figure 1A,B).

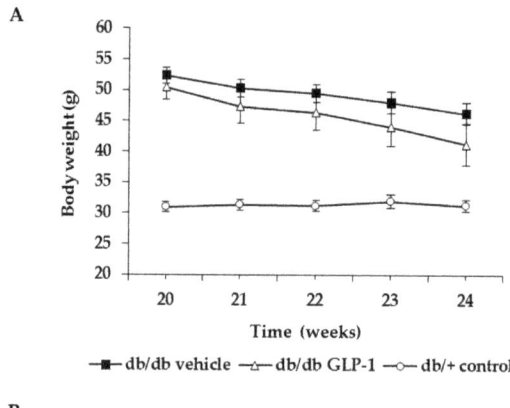

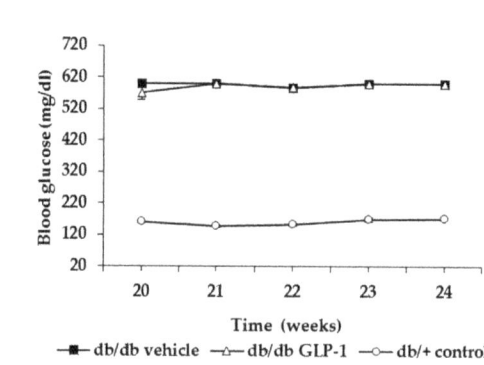

Figure 1. Evolution of (**A**) body weight and (**B**) blood glucose levels in the experimental groups.

3.2. Topical Administration of GLP-1 Reduces DNA/RNA Damage through the Decrease of Reactive Oxygen Species (ROS) and Reactive Nitrogen Species (RNS) Induced by Diabetes in the Retina

The impaired equilibrium between ROS and the antioxidant defenses promotes oxidative stress that affects the structure of several molecules, including nucleic acids. The hydroxyl radicals can damage DNA by converting deoxyguanosine into 8-hydroxyguanosine. Here we provide evidence that this phenomenon occurred in an experimental model of DR (db/db mice) and that the topical administration of GLP-1 could prevented this process (Figure 2A,B).

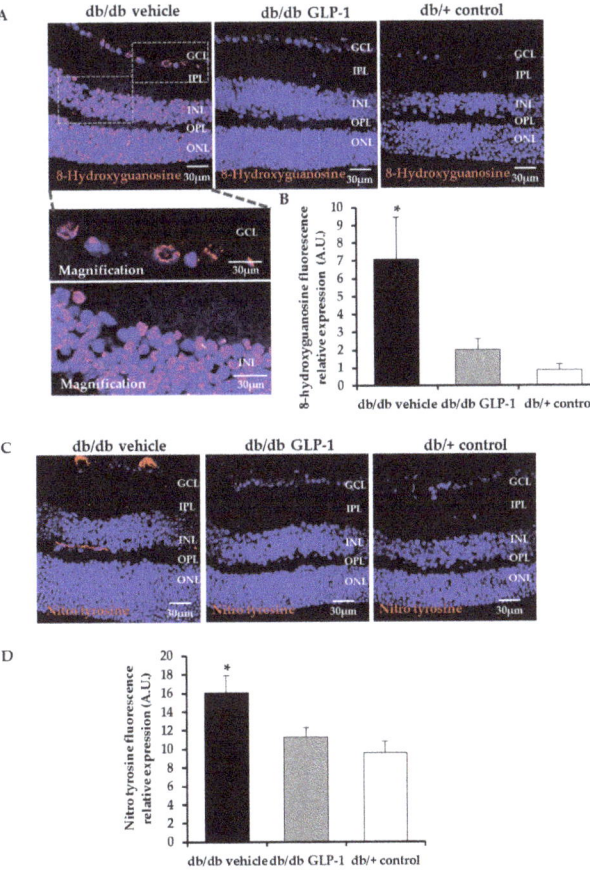

Figure 2. Immunofluorescence analysis of DNA/RNA damage (8-hydroxiguanosine) and nitro tyrosine. (**A,B**) Comparison and quantification of 8-hydroxiguanosine (red) protein levels through immunofluorescence among representative samples of diabetic retinas treated with vehicle eye drops (black bars) or GLP-1 eye drops (gray bars) and non-diabetic retinas (white bars). Hoechst staining (blue) was used for nuclei labeling. Optical magnifications of the ganglion cell layer (GCL) and the inner nuclear layer (INL) are also displayed. Scale bars, 30 µm. $n = 4$; (**C,D**) comparison and quantification of nitro tyrosine (red) protein levels through immunofluorescence among representative samples of diabetic retinas treated with vehicle eye drops (black bars) or GLP-1 eye drops (gray bars) and non-diabetic retinas (white bars). Hoechst staining (blue) used for nuclei labeling. Scale bars, 30 µm. $n = 4$; * $p < 0.05$. GCL—ganglion cell layer; INL—inner nuclear layer; IPL—inner plexiform layer; ONL—outer nuclear layer; OPL—outer plexiform layer.

RNS act similar to ROS in terms of cell damage. In fact, nitro tyrosine protein levels were also increased in the retinas of diabetic mice in comparison with non-diabetic mice. GLP-1 significantly reduced them too (Figure 2C,D).

3.3. GLP-1 Eyedrops Protect from Oxidative Stress by Increasing the Protein Levels of Glutathione Reductase, Glutathione Peroxidase and Copper–Zinc and Manganese Superoxide Dismutases (CuZnSOD and MnSOD) in Diabetic Retinas

Glutathione (GSH) effectively scavenges free radicals and other ROS and RNS (e.g., hydroxyl radical, lipid peroxyl radical, superoxide anion and hydrogen peroxide) directly and indirectly through enzymatic reactions. The reduced GSH can be regenerated from oxidized GSH by glutathione redox cycle. However, in the diabetic retina, the enzymes responsible for glutathione redox cycle (glutathione peroxidase and glutathione reductase) are compromised [6,8,10]. We observed a statistically insignificant increase of protein levels of glutathione peroxidase (Figure 3A,B) and glutathione reductase (Figure 3C,D) in diabetic retinas treated with GLP-1 eye drops in comparison with those treated with vehicle.

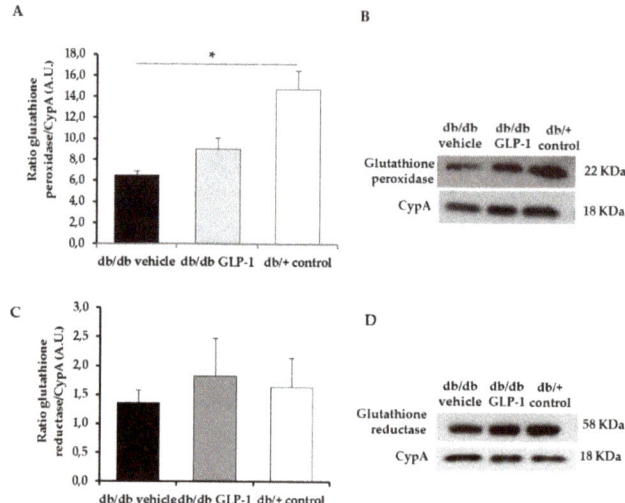

Figure 3. Protein levels of glutathione peroxidase and glutathione reductase. (**A,B**) Densitometric analysis and western blot bands of glutathione peroxidase corresponding to retinas of db/db mice treated with vehicle eye drops (black bars), GLP-1 eye drops (gray bars) and to non-diabetic mice retinas (white bars). Protein levels normalized with cyclophilin A. $n = 3$; (**C,D**) densitometric analysis and western blot bands of glutathione reductase corresponding to retinas of db/db mice treated with vehicle eye drops (black bars), GLP-1 eye drops (gray bars) and to non-diabetic mice retinas (white bars). Protein levels normalized with cyclophilin A. $n = 3$; * $p < 0.05$.

Ultimately, the radical chain reactions will be blocked by the antioxidant enzymes superoxide dismutase (SOD). The activities of both CuZnSOD, located in the cytosol, and MnSOD in the mitochondria are decreased in diabetic retina [6,8,10]. In the present study, we found that CuZnSOD and MnSOD levels were significantly increased by the topical administration of GLP-1 (Figure 4A–D and Figure 4E–H, respectively); ($p < 0.05$).

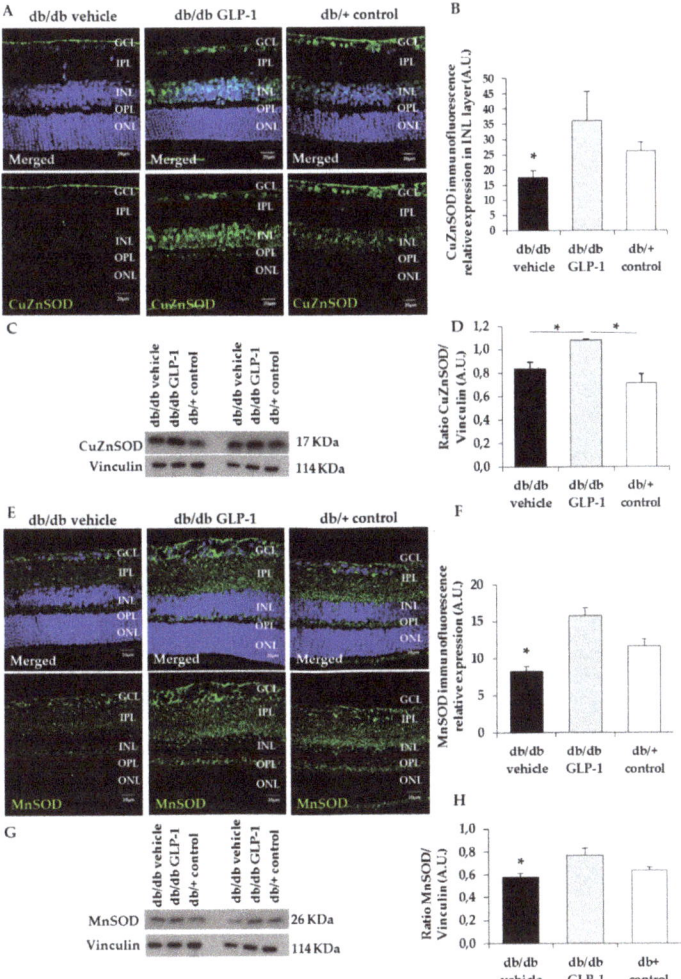

Figure 4. Protein levels of copper–zinc and manganese superoxide dismutase (CuZnSOD and MnSOD) (**A**,**B**) Comparison and quantification of CuZnSOD (green) protein levels through immunofluorescence among representative samples of diabetic retinas treated with vehicle eye drops (black bars) or GLP-1 eye drops (gray bars) and non-diabetic retinas (white bars). Hoechst staining (blue) used for nuclei labeling. GCL—ganglion cell layer; INL—inner nuclear layer; IPL—inner plexiform layer; ONL—outer nuclear layer; OPL—outer plexiform layer. Scale bars, 20 µm. $n = 4$; (**C**,**D**) densitometric analysis and western blot bands of CuZnSOD corresponding to retinas of db/db mice treated with vehicle eye drops (black bars), GLP-1 eye drops (gray bars) and to non-diabetic mice retinas (white bars). Protein levels normalized with vinculin. $n = 3$; (**E**,**F**) comparison and quantification of MnSOD (green) protein levels through immunofluorescence among representative samples of diabetic retinas treated with vehicle eye drops (black bars) or GLP-1 eye drops (gray bars) and non-diabetic retinas (white bars). Hoechst staining (blue) used for nuclei labeling. Scale bars, 20 µm. $n = 4$; (**G**,**H**) densitometric analysis and western blot bands of MnSOD corresponding to retinas of db/db mice treated with vehicle eye drops (black bars), GLP-1 eye drops (gray bars) and to non-diabetic mice retinas (white bars). Protein levels normalized with vinculin. $n = 3$; * $p < 0.05$. GCL—ganglion cell layer; INL—inner nuclear layer; IPL—inner plexiform layer; ONL—outer nuclear layer; OPL—outer plexiform layer.

3.4. Topical Administration of GLP-1 Activates the Expression in the Retina of Proteins Involved in DNA Repair (Babam2) and Cell Proliferation (Ki67)

Reactive oxygen and nitrogen species damage cellular macromolecules including DNA. Babam2 or BRE (brain and reproductive organ-expressed protein) is part of the BRCA1, a complex which is implicated in both DNA repair and maintenance of G2/M arrest in reaction to DNA damage [11,12]. For this reason, we wanted to assess Babam2 in our experiment. We found that the retina of untreated diabetic mice had considerably increased DNA/RNA damage compared with controls and that treatment with GLP-1 eye drops significantly increased the protein levels of Babam2 in retina in diabetic mice (Figure 5A–C). Moreover, GLP-1 increases Ki67 protein levels in neuroretina and favors its translocation to the nucleus, thus indicating the promotion of neurogenesis in the diabetic retina (Figure 6A,B).

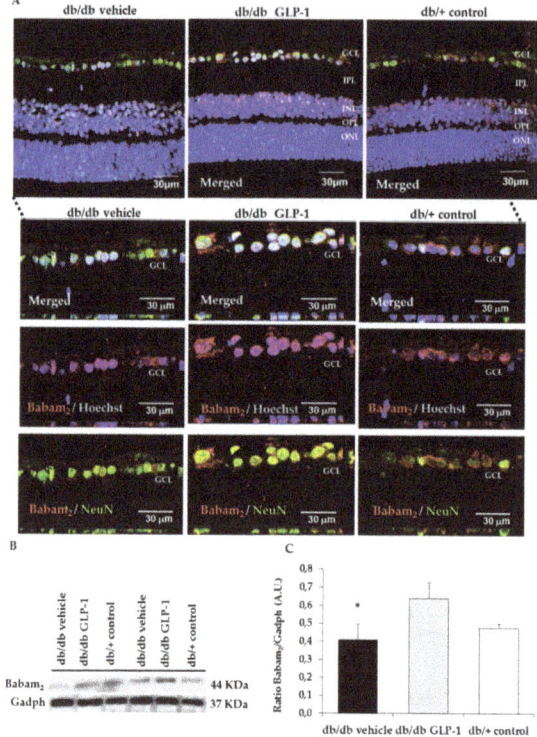

Figure 5. Babam2 protein levels. (**A**) Comparison of colabelling immunofluorescence assay for Babam2 (red) with NeuN (neuronal specific marker) (green) in db/db mice among representative samples of diabetic retinas treated with vehicle eye drops or GLP-1 eye drops and non-diabetic retinas. Nuclei labeled with Hoechst stain nuclei specific marker) (blue). GCL—ganglion cell layer; INL—inner nuclear layer; IPL—inner plexiform layer; ONL—outer nuclear layer; OPL—outer plexiform layer. An orthogonal view of Babam2 to analyze nuclear translocation in GCL of db/db mice treated with vehicle, db/bb mice treated with GLP-1 eye drops and non-diabetic mice are also displayed in this figure. Scale bars, 30 μm. $n = 4$; (**B,C**) densitometric analysis and western blot bands of babam$_2$ corresponding to retinas of db/db mice treated with vehicle eye drops (black bars), GLP-1 eye drops (gray bars) and to non-diabetic mice retinas (white bars). Protein levels normalized with Gadph. $n = 3$; * $p < 0.05$. GCL—ganglion cell layer; INL—inner nuclear layer; IPL—inner plexiform layer; ONL—outer nuclear layer; OPL—outer plexiform layer.

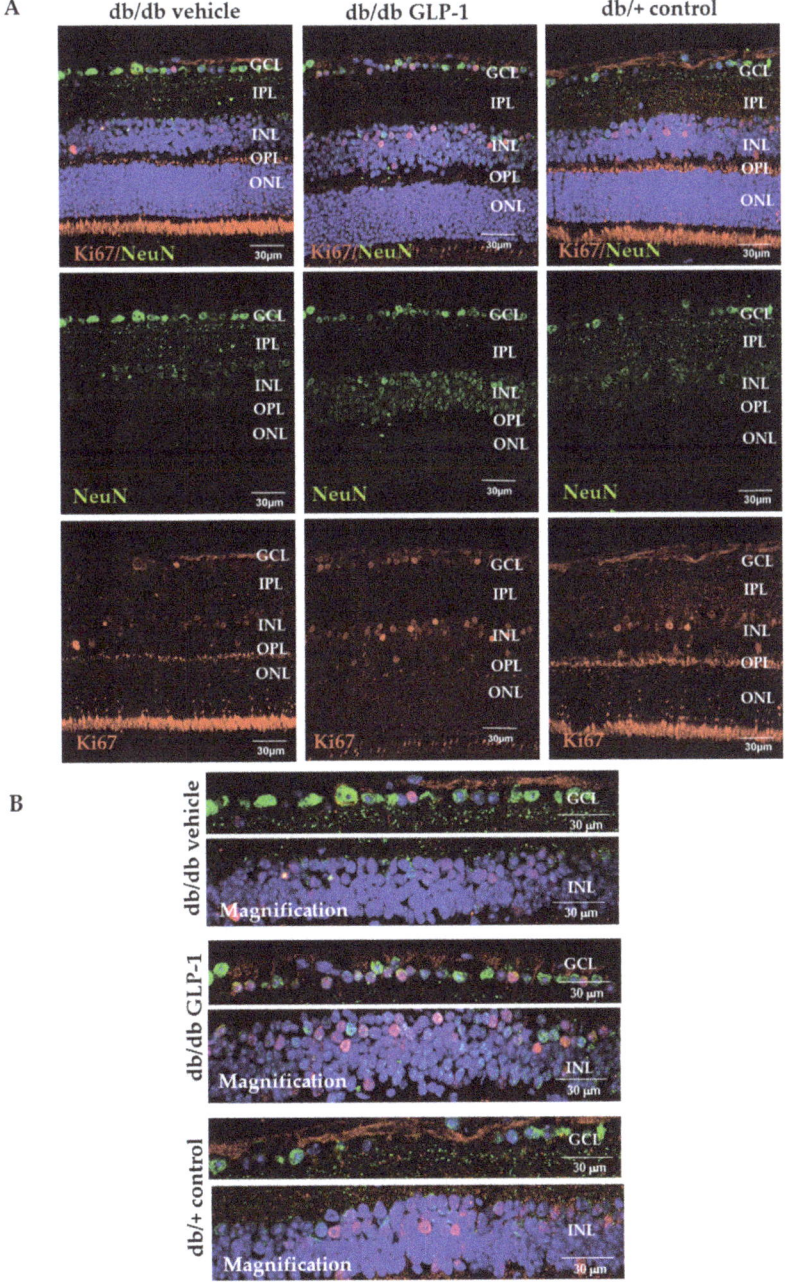

Figure 6. (**A**) Comparison of ki67 (red) protein levels through immunofluorescence among representative samples of diabetic retinas treated with vehicle eye drops or GLP-1 eye drops and non-diabetic retinas. Ki67 is colabelled with NeuN (neuronal specific marker) (green) and Hoechst staining (nuclei specific marker) (blue); (**B**) Optical magnifications of GCL and INL are also presented in this figure. Scale bars, 30 μm. $n = 4$. GCL—ganglion cell layer; INL—inner nuclear layer; IPL—inner plexiform layer; ONL—outer nuclear layer; OPL—outer plexiform layer.

4. Discussion

DR physiopathology embraces several metabolic pathways triggered by the hyperglycemic state. One of them is the overproduction of free radicals and the consequent nitro-oxidative imbalance that leads to cell damage [5]. GLP-1 and GLP-1R agonists have emerged as potential drugs against DR due to their neuroprotective properties, but their effect on DR oxidative stress has not been assessed [1,3,13]. Herein, we provide evidence that an antioxidant effect can be added to the underlying mechanism by which GLP-1R agonists exert their beneficial action on the diabetic retina.

In the present study, we found diabetes-induced oxidative stress resulting in DNA/RNA damage through guanine oxidation and protein damage by tyrosine nitration. In this regard, retinas of diabetic mice presented higher levels of both markers (8-hydroxy-2'-deoxyguanosine and nitrotyrosine, respectively) in comparison with non-diabetic mice, which implies the appearance of nitro-oxidative stress as a consequence of the DR state. Notably, these deleterious effects were prevented by the topical administration of GLP-1. Several studies have reported the relationship between GLP-1 and the decrease of cellular ROS levels [14]. Wang et al. showed that GLP-1 could reduce high-glucose-induced ROS in cardiac microvascular endothelial cells and Erdogdu et al. obtained similar results with exendin-4 (GLP-1 receptor agonist) using human coronary artery endothelial cells [15,16]. Here we demonstrate that the topical administration of GLP-1 prevents the RNA/DNA and proteins damage induced by RNS and ROS in an experimental model of DR. To the best of our knowledge this is the first study showing these beneficial effect of GLP-1 in the diabetic retina. It should be noted that systemic administration of GLP-1 analogs, by reducing blood glucose levels, may led to similar results in terms of oxidative stress, but our study provides evidence that these effects are directly mediated by GLP-1 and cannot be attributed to an improvement of blood glucose levels. In this regard, it should be emphasized that the topical (eye drops) administration of GLP-1 does not alter the blood glucose levels and that, therefore, the effects cannot be attributed to an improvement in these levels.

In the present study, we evaluated the protein levels in the retina of some antioxidant enzymes such as glutathione peroxidase, glutathione reductase, CuZnSOD and MnSOD after topical treatment with GLP-1. We found that glutathione peroxidase and glutathione reductase were higher in diabetic mice treated with GLP-1 eye drops, but without reach the statistical significance. This result agree with those obtained by Fernández-Millán et al. who found that GLP-1 was able to enhance the activity of both enzymes in beta cells (rat INS-1E cells) [17]. Regarding CuZnSOD and MnSOD, significantly higher levels in db/db mice treated with GLP-1 eye drops in comparison with vehicle were observed. Therefore, the topical administration of GLP-1 was able to prevent the diabetes-induced downregulation of CuZnSOD and MnSOD in the retina. Overall, our findings point to the enhancement of all these antioxidant enzymes as a significant mechanism of action of GLP-1.

In order to investigate the potential role of GLP-1 in the process of DNA repair we measured the Babam2 protein, which is encoded by the *Babam2* gene, also named *Bre*. The *Babam2* gene forms the Brca1-a complex in the nucleus of multiple cell types where its function consists in repairing DNA double strands breaks. Babam2 enables the Brca1-a complex to reach DNA damage sites. Shi et al. demonstrated that the deletion of Babam2 in fibroblasts leads to the accumulation of unrepaired DNA damage [11]. In the present study, we provide first evidence that GLP-1 increases the Babam2 protein, thus suggesting that DNA repair is another pleiotropic action of GLP-1. Co-labeling with the specific neuronal marker NeuN points to the ganglion cells as the main neuronal source of the Babam2 protein. In addition, we have confirmed our previous observation that GLP-1 upregulates Ki67 (an excellent marker of cellular proliferation), which also colocalized with NeuN. Taken together these findings suggest that the antioxidant properties of GLP-1 are linked to its capacity to promote neurogenesis.

5. Conclusions

Topical administration of GLP-1 in an experimental model of DR (db/db mice) confers protection against the damage caused by nitro-oxidative stress. The GLP-1-mediated increase of some antioxidant enzymes such as MnSOD and CuZnSOD is an important contributing factor. The prevention of

DNA/RNA damage, the increase in DNA repair and the enhancement of cellular proliferation observed after treating with GLP-1 all reinforce the concept that GLP-1 promotes neurogenesis in the diabetic retina. However, further studies not only to confirm this important issue, but also to unravel the underlying mechanisms linking the antioxidant effects and cellular proliferation are needed.

Author Contributions: Conceptualization, P.B., R.S. and C.H.; methodology, H.R., P.B., J.S. and C.H.; formal analysis, H.R., P.B., J.S., J.H., R.S. and C.H.; investigation, H.R., P.B., J.S., J.H., R.S. and C.H.; resources, R.S. and C.H.; data curation, H.R., P.B., R.S. and C.H.; writing—original draft preparation, H.R., P.B.; writing—review and editing, R.S. and C.H.; supervision, P.B., R.S. and C.H.; project administration, C.H.; funding acquisition, R.S. and C.H. All authors have read and agreed to the published version of the manuscript.

Funding: This research was funded by grants from the Ministerio de Economía y Competitividad (DTS15/00151, PI16/00541, SAF2016-77784) and the Fundació La Marató TV3 (201629-10). The funders had no role in the design of the study; in the collection, analyses or the interpretation of the data; in the writing of the manuscript or in the decision to publish the results.

Acknowledgments: H.R. is the recipient of a grant from the Ministerio de Economía y Competitividad (BES-2017-081690). J.S. is the recipient of a grant from the Agència de Gestió d'Ajuts Universitaris i de Recerca (AGAUR). The histological processing was performed by ICTS "NANBIOSIS", more specifically by Unit 20 of CIBER in Bioengineering, Biomaterials & Nanomedicne (CIBER-BBN) at the Vall d'Hebron Research Institute.

Conflicts of Interest: The authors declare no conflict of interest.

References

1. Hernández, C.; Bogdanov, P.; Corraliza, L.; García-Ramírez, M.; Solà-Adell, C.; Arranz, J.A.; Arroba, A.I.; Valverde, A.M.; Simó, R. Topical administration of GLP-1 receptor agonists prevents retinal neurodegeneration in experimental diabetes. *Diabetes* **2016**, *65*, 172–187. [CrossRef] [PubMed]
2. Simó, R.; Hernández, C. GLP-1R as a Target for the Treatment of Diabetic Retinopathy: Friend or Foe? *Diabetes* **2017**, *66*, 1453–1460. [CrossRef] [PubMed]
3. Sampedro, J.; Bogdanov, P.; Ramos, H.; Solà-Adell, C.; Turch, M.; Valeri, M.; Simó-Servat, O.; Lagunas, C.; Simó, R.; Hernández, C. New Insights into the Mechanisms of Action of Topical Administration of GLP-1 in an Experimental Model of Diabetic Retinopathy. *J. Clin. Med.* **2019**, *8*, 339. [CrossRef] [PubMed]
4. Pang, B.; Zhou, H.; Kuang, H. The potential benefits of glucagon-like peptide-1 receptor agonists for diabetic retinopathy. *Peptides* **2018**, *100*, 123–126. [CrossRef] [PubMed]
5. Wong, T.Y.; Cheung, C.M.; Larsen, M.; Sharma, S.; Simó, R. Diabetic retinopathy. *Nat. Rev. Dis. Primers* **2016**, *17*, 16012. [CrossRef] [PubMed]
6. Kowluru, R.A.; Mishra, M. Oxidative stress, mitochondrial damage and diabetic retinopathy. *BBA Mol. Basis Dis.* **2015**, *1582*, 2474–2483. [CrossRef] [PubMed]
7. Du, Y.; Smith, M.A.; Miller, C.M.; Kern, T.S. Diabetes-induced nitrative stress in the retina, and correction by aminoguanidine. *J. Neurochem.* **2002**, *80*, 771–779. [CrossRef] [PubMed]
8. Kowluru, R.A.; Chan, P.S. Oxidative stress and diabetic retinopathy. *Exp. Diabetes Res.* **2007**, *2007*, 43603. [CrossRef] [PubMed]
9. Kowluru, R.A. Effect of reinstitution of good glycemic control on retinal oxidative stress and nitrative stress in diabetic rats. *Diabetes* **2003**, *52*, 818–823. [CrossRef] [PubMed]
10. Kowluru, R.A.; Atasi, L.; Ho, Y.S. Role of mitochondrial superoxide dismutase in the development of diabetic retinopathy. *Investig. Ophthalmol. Vis. Sci.* **2006**, *47*, 1594–1599. [CrossRef] [PubMed]
11. Shi, W.; Tang, M.K.; Yao, Y.; Tang, C.; Chui, Y.L.; Lee, K.K.H. BRE plays an essential role in preventing replicative and DNA damage-induced premature senescence. *Sci. Rep.* **2016**, *6*, 23506. [CrossRef] [PubMed]
12. Chan, J.Y.; Li, L.; Miao, J.; Cai, D.Q.; Lee, K.K.; Chui, Y.L. Differential expression of a novel gene BRE (TNFRSF1A modulator/BRCC45) in response to stress and biological signals. *Mol. Biol. Rep.* **2010**, *37*, 363–368. [CrossRef] [PubMed]
13. Holst, J.J.; Burcelin, R.; Nathanson, E. Neuroprotective properties of GLP-1: Theoretical and practical applications. *Curr. Med. Res. Opin.* **2011**, *27*, 547–558. [CrossRef] [PubMed]
14. Petersen, K.E.; Rakipovski, G.; Raun, K.; Lykkesfeldt, J. Does Glucagon-like Peptide-1 Ameliorate Oxidative Stress in Diabetes? Evidence Based on Experimental and Clinical Studies. *Curr. Diabetes Rev.* **2016**, *12*, 331–358. [CrossRef] [PubMed]

15. Wang, D.; Luo, P.; Wang, Y.; Li, W.; Wang, C.; Sun, D.; Zhang, R.; Su, T.; Ma, X.; Zeng, C.; et al. Glucagon-like peptide-1 protects against cardiac microvascular injury in diabetes via a cAMP/PKA/Rho-dependent mechanism. *Diabetes* **2013**, *62*, 1697–1708. [CrossRef] [PubMed]
16. Erdogdu, Ö.; Eriksson, L.; Xu, H.; Sjöholm, Å.; Zhang, Q.; Nyström, T. Exendin-4 protects endothelial cells from lipoapoptosis by PKA, PI3K, eNOS, p38 MAPK, and JNK pathways. *J. Mol. Endocrinol.* **2013**, *50*, 229–241. [CrossRef] [PubMed]
17. Fernández-Millán, E.; Martín, M.A.; Goya, L.; Lizárraga-Mollinedo, E.; Escrivá, F.; Ramos, S.; Álvarez, C. Glucagon-like peptide-1 improves beta-cell antioxidant capacity via extracellular regulated kinases pathway and Nrf2 translocation. *Free Radic. Biol. Med.* **2016**, *95*, 16–26. [CrossRef] [PubMed]

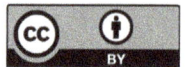

© 2020 by the authors. Licensee MDPI, Basel, Switzerland. This article is an open access article distributed under the terms and conditions of the Creative Commons Attribution (CC BY) license (http://creativecommons.org/licenses/by/4.0/).

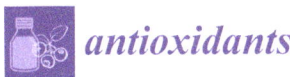

Article

Molecular Assessment of Epiretinal Membrane: Activated Microglia, Oxidative Stress and Inflammation

Sushma Vishwakarma [1,2,†], Rishikesh Kumar Gupta [1,†,‡], Saumya Jakati [3], Mudit Tyagi [4], Rajeev Reddy Pappuru [4], Keith Reddig [5], Gregory Hendricks [5], Michael R. Volkert [6], Hemant Khanna [7], Jay Chhablani [4,*,§] and Inderjeet Kaur [1,*]

1. Prof Brien Holden Eye Research Centre, LV Prasad Eye Institute, Hyderabad 500034, India; svishwakarma17@gmail.com (S.V.); rkgupta@iimcb.gov.pl (R.K.G.)
2. Manipal Academy of Higher Education, Manipal, Karnataka 576104, India
3. Ophthalmic Pathology Laboratory, L.V. Prasad Eye Institute, Hyderabad 500034, India; saumyajakati@lvpei.org
4. Smt. Kanuri Santhamma Retina Vitreous Centre, L.V. Prasad Eye Institute, Hyderabad 500034, India; drmudit@lvpei.org (M.T.); rajeev@lvpei.org (R.R.P.)
5. Department of Radiology, University of Massachusetts Medical School, Worcester, MA 01655, USA; keith.reddig@umassmed.edu (K.R.); Gregory.Hendricks@umassmed.edu (G.H.)
6. Department of Microbiology & Physiological Systems, University of Massachusetts Medical School, Worcester, MA 01655, USA; michael.volkert@umassmed.edu
7. Department of Ophthalmology & Visual Sciences, University of Massachusetts Medical School, Worcester, MA 01655, USA; hemant.khanna@umassmed.edu
* Correspondence: jay.chhablani@gmail.com (J.C.); inderjeet@lvpei.org (I.K.); Tel.: +91-40-306-12607 or +91-40-306-12345 (J.C. & I.K.); Fax: +91-40-2354-8271 (J.C. & I.K.)
† These authors contributed equally to this work.
‡ Present address: Laboratory of Neurodegeneration, International Institute of Molecular and Cell Biology in Warsaw, 02-109 Warsaw, Poland.
§ Present address: Medical Retina and Vitreoretinal Surgery, University of Pittsburgh School of Medicine, Pittsburgh, PA 15213, USA.

Received: 27 June 2020; Accepted: 21 July 2020; Published: 23 July 2020

Abstract: Fibrocellular membrane or epiretinal membrane (ERM) forms on the surface of the inner limiting membrane (ILM) in the inner retina and alters the structure and function of the retina. ERM formation is frequently observed in ocular inflammatory conditions, such as proliferative diabetic retinopathy (PDR) and retinal detachment (RD). Although peeling of the ERM is used as a surgical intervention, it can inadvertently distort the retina. Our goal is to design alternative strategies to tackle ERMs. As a first step, we sought to determine the composition of the ERMs by identifying the constituent cell-types and gene expression signature in patient samples. Using ultrastructural microscopy and immunofluorescence analyses, we found activated microglia, astrocytes, and Müller glia in the ERMs from PDR and RD patients. Moreover, oxidative stress and inflammation associated gene expression was significantly higher in the RD and PDR membranes as compared to the macular hole samples, which are not associated with inflammation. We specifically detected differential expression of hypoxia inducible factor 1-α (*HIF1-α*), proinflammatory cytokines, and Notch, Wnt, and ERK signaling pathway-associated genes in the RD and PDR samples. Taken together, our results provide new information to potentially develop methods to tackle ERM formation.

Keywords: human retina; epiretinal membrane; internal limiting membrane; vitreoretinal surgery; macular hole; proliferative diabetic retinopathy

1. Introduction

The retina is a multilayered light-sensing neural tissue located at the back of the eye [1]. The outer retina is composed of photoreceptors, which convert light into electrical signals and transmit them to the inner neurons and to the ganglion cells in the inner retina. The ganglion cell layer is also composed of Muller glia, whose foot processes are embedded into a thin transparent layer in the basal lamina of the inner retina called the inner limiting membrane (ILM). The ILM forms a boundary between the retina and the underlying vitreous [2–4].

Epiretinal membrane (ERM), a fibrocellular tissues forms on the surface of ILM, mainly on the macula. ERMs can be either: (a) idiopathic or (b) associated with ocular inflammatory diseases such as diabetic retinopathy and retinal detachment [5,6]. ERMs distort the underlying ILM and alter retinal morphology and function. Survival and proliferation of the cells present on the ERM also depends upon the oxygen level. Ischemic conditions lead to accumulation/activation of the transcription factor, hypoxia-inducible factor (HIF-1α), which causes secretion of vasoactive cytokines vascular leakage and macular edema [7]. Growth factors such as hepatocyte growth factor (HGF), heparin-binding epidermal growth factor (HB-EGF), and epidermal growth factor (EGF) others and other inflammatory molecules released due to any retinal insults also induce the migration of retinal cells like RPE to the vitreous to proliferate and induce the retinal membrane formation.

Currently, ILM removal along with ERM peeling is considered the gold standard treatment and results in minimal recurrence of the ERMs. However, the extent of successful restoration of vision varies as ERM peel can lead to retinal breaks and perturb outer retina function. Therefore, ILM peeling requires a decision on the inevitability of ERM removal only for selected needful patients.

We propose that understanding the cellular composition and gene expression signature of the ERMs will assist in designing strategies to tackle ERM formation with minimal effects on the ILM or avoid ERM peeling in patient where it may play a beneficial role, such as in preventing macular hole formation [8,9]. Previous remarkable studies have identified hyalocytes, glial cells, retinal pigment epithelial cells, fibrocytes and myofibroblast along with non-cellular component like fibronectin, and actin [10,11]. However, a comprehensive analysis of the different components and a gene expression profile related to oxidative stress and pro-inflammatory signaling associated genes have not been investigated.

In the present study, we carried out a comparative histological, ultrastructural and gene expression analysis of fibrocellular membranes associated with inflammatory conditions of the eye. Our results expand our understanding on the role of activated microglia in ERMs and suggest that immunomodulation by targeting microglia could be a potential therapy for a better clinical management of the condition.

2. Materials and Methods

2.1. Enrollment of Subjects

Initially, ILM specimens ($n = 30$) were collected during vitreo-retinal surgery from June 2016 to September 2017 at the L.V. Prasad Eye Institute by a single vitreoretinal surgeon (Jay Chhablani) and were used for Hematoxylin and Eosin (H&E), transmission electron microscopy (TEM) and immunohistochemistry (IHC)-based evaluations. Additional membranes ($n = 15$, 3 in MH, 8 in PDR and 4 in RD) were collected from the additional ORs of two other vitreo-retinal surgeons (Mudit Tyagi and Rajeev Reddy Pappuru) for the targeted gene expression profiling. This prospective study was approved (Ethic Ref No. LEC 02-14-029) by the Institutional Review Board (IRB) of L.V. Prasad Eye Institute, Hyderabad, India (LVPEI) and adhered to the tests of the Declaration of Helsinki. A prior informed consent was obtained from each study subject. All subjects underwent a comprehensive ophthalmic examination with Snellen's visual acuity, slit lamp examination, intraocular pressure measurement using applanation tonometry and dilated fundus examination. All eyes except eyes with RRD underwent preoperative spectral domain optical coherence tomography (OCT) Cirrus

High Definition-OCT (Carl Zeiss Meditec, Dublin, CA, USA). Five-line high definition raster scan was performed.

The membranes removed as part of the routine surgical management were collected from different pathological conditions. Subjects with the diagnosis of vitreoretinal interface disorders including idiopathic macular hole (MH), proliferative diabetic retinopathy (PDR) and rhegmatogenous retinal detachment (RD) who underwent pars plana vitrectomy (PPV) with Brilliant blue-G (BBG)—assisted inner limiting membrane peeling (ILM peeling) were included in the study.

2.2. Surgical Details

Surgical procedure included 23- or 25-gauge vitrectomy. After induction of posterior vitreous detachment, vitrectomy was completed. Epiretinal membranes were removed using end-gripping forceps. For ILM staining, 0.02% brilliant blue was used under air infusion. After one minute of staining, ILM at the macular area was removed using ILM forceps. In eyes undergoing macular hole repair, C3F8 gas (12–15%) was used as tamponade. Cataract surgery was performed during the follow-up in cases where it was needed with standard phacoemulsification procedure, and posterior chamber intraocular lens was implanted. In cases with rhematogenous RD, brilliant blue staining of ILM was performed under fluid with infusion canula off.

2.3. Histopathological Investigation

All surgically peeled membrane samples were embedded in the optimal cutting temperature compound (OCT)-medium (Leica Biosystems, Nussloch GmbH, Germany) and stored at −20 °C initially for slow freezing. After freezing, sections of 4 μm thickness were prepared using cryostat (Leica CM1950 Clinical Cryostat-Leica Biosystems, Nussloch GmbH, Germany) for each subject. The sections were stained with hematoxylin and eosin (H&E) dyes and images were taken at 4× and 10× with an inverted microscope (Olympus Corporation, Shinjuku, Tokyo, Japan).

2.4. Ultrastructural Evaluations of Membranes Using Transmission Electron Microscopy

The surgically excised membranes were stored in 3% glutaraldehyde at room temperature for 24 h followed by the standard procedures [11,12] for sample preparation. Ultra-thin (70 nm) sections were made with a diamond knife on ultramicrotome (Leica Ultra cut UCT-GA-D/E-1/00), mounted on gold grids and stained with saturated aqueous uranyl acetate (UA) and counter stained with Reynolds lead citrate (LC) and viewed under TEM (Model: CM10,Philips, North Worcester, MA, USA).

2.5. Cellular Characterization Using Immunohistochemistry

The tissue sections were processed for immunohistochemistry using cell type specific primary antibodies including rabbit anti-glial fibrillary acid protein antibody (GFAP) (glial marker, 1:400, Z0334, Dako, Glostrup, Denmark), rabbit anti-ALDH1L1 (astrocytes, 1:500, ab190298, Abcam, Cambridge, MA, USA), mouse anti-cellular retinaldehyde-binding protein (CRALBP) (retinal astrocytes, 1:80, ab15051, Abcam), rat anti-F4/80 (macrophages, 1:30, ab16911, Abcam,), and rabbit anti-oxidation resistance 1 (Oxidative stress, 1:100, HPA027395,Sigma, St. Louis, MO, USA), against OXR1; a protein that controls the resistance of neuronal cells to oxidative stress. After sectioning the slides were stored at −20 °C. For the experiment, slides were taken out from the −20 °C and kept at room temperature for 30 min to bring them to room temperature. Next, the slides were dipped in fixative (chilled methanol: acetone (95:5) solution) for 15 min and dired for 30 min at room temperature. The slides were then washed three times with 1× PBS. 1% BSA (Himedia, Lab Pvt. Ltd., Mumbai, Maharashtra, India) and incubated with blocking buffer containing 0.1%-Tween20 (Fisher Scientific, Guldensporenpark, Merelbeke, Belgium) for 2 h. The sections were then incubated with the primary antibody overnight. The primary antibodies were diluted in 0.1% blocking buffer. After overnight incubation, the slides were washed three times with 1X PBS, for 5 min each, followed by secondary antibody incubation at a dilution 1:300 (Alexa Fluor® 488 Goat Anti-Rabbit IgG, (A-11008, Invitrogen, Waltham, MA, USA) and Alexa Fluor® 488 Goat Anti-Mouse IgG, (ab150117, Abcam). Negative control IHC was done to test the specificity of antibody and to identify false positive results shown in Figure S1. Details of the antibodies are provided in Table S1.

2.6. Imaging and Image Analysis

The digital inverted microscope (EVOS FL Cell Imaging System, Life Technology, Paisley, UK) was used for the imaging at X200 final magnification. Further, total number of cells based on DAPI staining and the total number of positively stained cells for each marker were counted on individual sections corresponding to different pathological conditions. Average and standard deviation of the mean number of cells for each marker from specimens ($n = 3$) in different pathological conditions were calculated. Percentage of OXR1 positive cells was calculated using: (total number of OXR1 positive cells divided by total number of DAPI stained cells) × 100.

2.7. Targeted Gene Expression Profiling by qRT-PCR

Total RNA was isolated from membranes using PureLink™ RNA Mini Kit (Invitrogen™, catalog no. 12183018A) following the manuals as instructed. RNA was converted to cDNA using verso cDNA synthesis kit (Thermo Scientific™, Waltham, MA, USA, catalog no. AB1453B). A reaction mixture of volume 10µL was made using iTaq™ Universal SYBR® Green Supermix (BIO-RAD, Hercules, CA, USA, catalog no. 38220090), 200nM of primer and cDNA and further, subjected to Applied Biosystems 7900 HT system. A relative measurement of the concentration of target gene (CT) was calculated by using software SDS 2.4 (Applied Biosystems, Foster City, CA, USA). Differential gene expression was analyzed using the $2^{-\Delta\Delta C_T}$ method. Statistical analyses were performed using the $2^{-\Delta\Delta C_T} \pm$ SEM. β-actin; a housekeeping gene was used as a normalizing control. The primer sequences used for semi-quantitative real time PCRs are given in the Table S2.

2.8. Statistical Analysis

The total number of cells were counted manually in a defined fixed quadrant and equal area of each images. Average number of the cells were accounted for further the descriptive statistical analysis included mean and standard deviation (SD) described in Section 2.6. *t*-Test was used to calculate significance for qPCR data and mean fold changes ± SE were plotted in a graph. A *p*-value less than 0.05 was taken as statistically significant.

2.9. Bioinformatic Analysis

For gene expression analysis, a heat map was generated using the online tool Heatmapper (http://www.heatmapper.ca/expression/). Protein-protein interaction was predicted using STRING (v 11.0) (https://www.string-db.org/). Where network edges were defined based on evidence. The minimum required interaction score was kept at minimum confidence of 0.400, with no more than 50 interactors. The active interaction sources were text mining, experimentally proved, database, co-expression data, neighborhood joining, gene fusion, and co-occurrence.

3. Results

3.1. Demographical Data

The mean age (mean age ± standard deviation) of the subjects included in this study was 55.22 ± 7.35. The number of males and females were 33 and 12 respectively.

3.2. Histological Evaluations and Cellular Profiling

Histological analysis of the ERMs revealed spindle cells with round or oval hyperchromatic nuclei (black arrow; Figure 1 and Figure S1) and pale eosinophilic cytoplasm with or without uveal pigment.

The cellularity varied among specimens; it was lower in macular hole samples as compared to PDR and RD. We did not detect a significant difference in cellularity between PDR and RD samples.

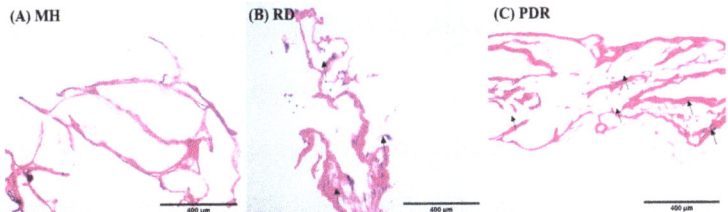

Figure 1. H&E staining of epiretinal membrane (**A**) macular hole, (**B**) retinal detachment, (**C**) proliferative diabetic retinopathy. Photomicrographs in all except macular hole show the presence of spindle shaped cells (black pointed arrows) and the adjacent fibro-collagenous tissue. (H&E; scale bar = 400 μm).

3.3. Ultrastructural Characterizations

Next, we performed ultrastructural characterization by TEM of the membranes extracted from three subjects belonging to the PDR and MH groups. The membranes from RD cases were not included due to insufficient numbers.

The retinal cell-types were characterized based on previously published morphological details [13–18]. Varying thickness of collagen fibrils, the main component of the ERMs was observed in both PDR and MH. We frequently detected astrocytes, Müller glia with long processes, microglia like cells with thick dark heterochomatic cell body and a few dark pigmented cells (Figure 2) in the PDR versus the MH specimens.

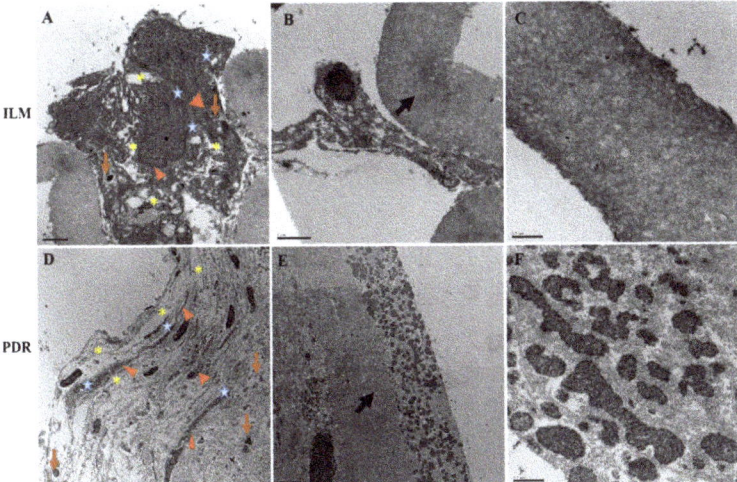

Figure 2. Transmission electron microscopy images of fibrocellular membranes from; (**A–C**); macular hole, and (**D–E**); proliferative diabetic retinopathy membrane showing the presence of astrocytes, Müller glia processes and microglia. The cell body of a Müller cell can be identified by its nucleus and dark cytoplasm (red color filled triangular shape). An astroglial cell process with flattened intermediate filaments (yellow colored asterisk) can be observed next to the Müller cell. The microglia can be seen with round shaped dark cell bodies (brown arrow) and glial cells processes with skyblue star shaped structure. (**B,E**) show collagenous fibrils of membrane indicated by black arrow and; (**C,F**) show their corresponding magnified image.

3.4. Characterization of Different Cell Types in Each Group

We next validated the presence of the specific cell types by indirect immunofluorescence using appropriate marker antibodies. We used nine samples, with three samples from each group (MH, RD and PDR). The MH samples were used as negative controls.

Our analyses confirmed the presence of both macroglial and microglial cells along with other proliferative spindle shaped cells. While GFAP and ALDH1L1, markers for astrocytes (and gliosis) were mostly detected in all specimens, the PDR samples showed greater number of GFAP positive cells present in the membrane as compared to MH and RD specimens (Figure 3 and Figure S2). CRALBP staining did not significantly differ in the Müller glia among PDR and RD samples. The number of CD11b (microglia marker) positive cells was higher in the RD membranes as compared to the others.

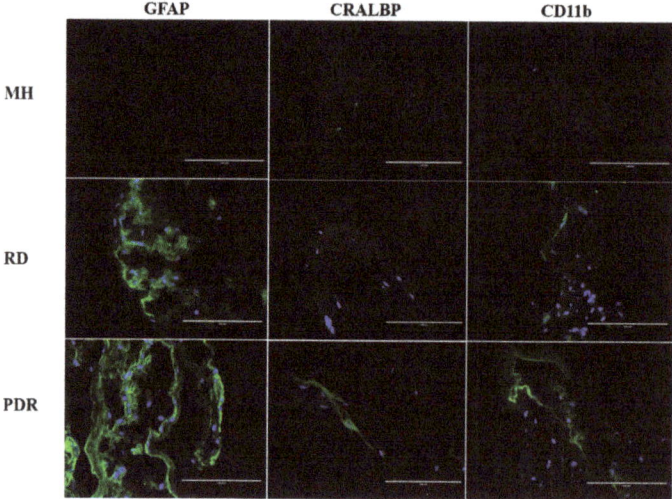

Figure 3. Representative images showing IHC of membranes from pathological conditions MH, RD and PDR with intense cytoplasmic and membranous expression of GFAP, CRALBP, and CD11b proteins. (Scale bar; 100 µm).

Quantification of the cells present on the membrane validated the higher number of CD11b positive cells in RD than MH and PDR. On the other hand, increased number of GFAP positive cells was seen in PDR as compared to all cases (Table 1).

Table 1. The number of different cell types identified by immunohistochemistry using different specific markers where GFAP; astrocytes/gliotic changes, CRALBP; Müller glia, CD11b; microglia are used.

S. No.	Pathology	H&E	Cell Specific Marker	Mean no. of Positive Cells ($n = 3$) ± SD
1.	MH	No pigmentation	GFAP	0 ± 0
			CRALBP	0 ± 0
			CD11b	0 ± 0
2.	RD	Pigmentation	GFAP	8 ± 8.4
			CRALBP	19 ± 7.0
			CD11b	2.5 ± 3.5
3.	PDR	No pigmentation	GFAP	11 ± 8.7
			CRALBP	6.3 ± 6.6
			CD11b	1.6 ± 1.5

3.5. Evaluation of Oxidative Stress among Different Pathological Condition

To further explore the involvement of oxidative stress in the ERMs, we performed immunofluorescence analysis using anti-OXR1 antibody in the same tissue specimens ($n = 3$) of MH, RD and PDR cases. OXR1 is expressed at elevated levels in cells undergoing oxidative stress [19]. We found a greater number of OXR1-positive cells in the RD sample than PDR ($p = 0.04$) shown in Figure 4; none of the cells was positive for OXR1 in the membranes from MH.

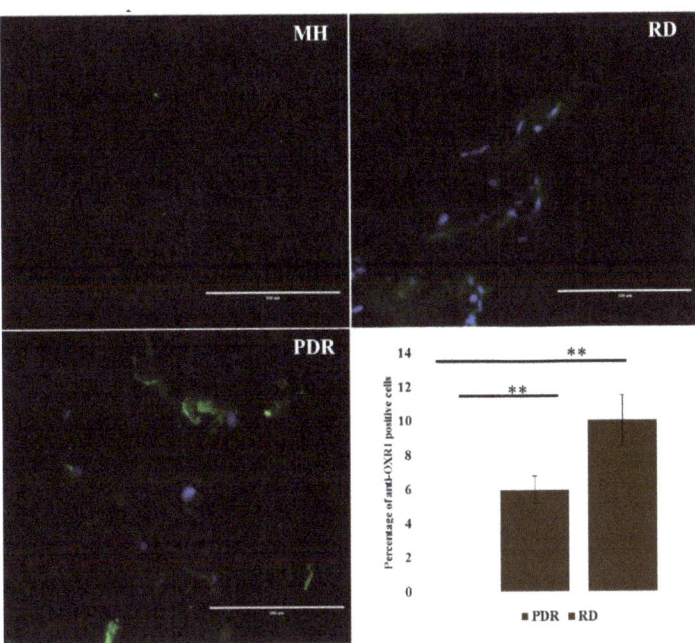

Figure 4. Representative images of IHC showing the expression of OXR1 in MH, RD, and PDR. The graph shows the mean percentage of OXR1 positive cells for each pathological condition ($n = 3$) (scale bar; 100 µm) ** p-value < 0.05.

3.6. Gene Expression Analysis of Oxidative Stress and Inflammation-Related Pathway Genes

Oxidative stress though being closely interlinked to inflammation, could also be the cumulative effect of continued insults to the eye such as ischemia and hyperglycemia [20]. To further quantitate the underlying oxidative stress and inflammation in membrane formation and DR pathogenesis, a targeted gene expression profiling was undertaken by semi-quantitative real time PCR using SYBR green chemistry. We used MH as control and the expression was measured among MH, PDR and RD. Initially, to measure the underlying oxidative stress, we used *Nrf2*, and *HIF1-α* while *MMP9*, and *IL1-β* were used as markers of inflammation. Expression of *CD11b* and *VEGF* was also measured for activated microglia and angiogenesis. In comparison to MH, the gene expression of *Nrf2*, *HIF1-α* and *MMP9* was higher in the RD (*Nrf2*: 31.81 ± 0.76, *** $p = 0.00066$; *HIF1-α*: 13.423 ± 0.63, *** $p = 0.005$; *MMP9*: 8.851 ± 0.86, * $p = 0.04$) followed by PDR (*Nrf2*: 2.76 ± 0.16, ** $p = 0.007$; *HIF1-α*: 3.88 ± 0.47, ns, $p \geq 0.05$ and; *MMP9*: 4.901 ± 0.86, * $p = 0.03$). Consistently, we noticed increased expression of *IL1-β* in RD (8.648 ± 0.43, * $p = 0.03$) and PDR (5.282 ± 0.27, ns, $p \geq 0.05$) compared to MH. *VEGF*, an angiogenic marker showed almost similar elevated level of expression in both RD (2.542 ± 0.63, * $p = 0.031$) and PDR (1.42 ± 0.13, * $p = 0.01$). Likewise, *CD11b*, also showed significantly higher expression in RD (10.333 ± 0.23, *** $p = 0.000076$), and PDR (3.092 ± 0.25, * $p = 0.011$) than MH (Figure 5a).

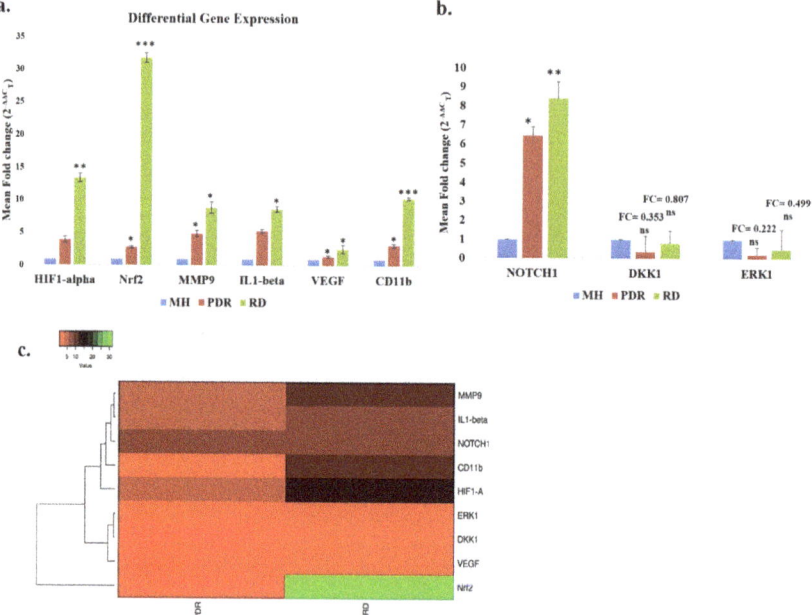

Figure 5. (**a**,**b**) Differential gene expression analysis of oxidative stress, inflammatory markers and their associated pathway involved in the pathogenesis of epiretinal membrane of RD, PDR compared to macular hole (* $p \leq 0.05$, ** $p \leq 0.01$, *** $p \leq 0.001$) (**c**) Heat map showing the expression pattern of the differentially expressed genes in PDR and RD.

We then analysed the expression of the genes associated with major signaling pathways including *NOTCH1*, *DKK1* and *ERK1* in the ERMs from RD and PDR. Besides oxidative stress and inflammation, the additional genes and pathway chosen for this analysis were selected based on the existing proposed pathogenic theories in the literature and those known to be involved in retinal cellular proliferation and maintenance. There was significant upregulation of *NOTCH1* gene expression in RD (8.427 ± 0.64, ** p-value=0.008) and PDR (6.459 ± 0.81, * p-value = 0.02) as compared to control (MH) (Figure 5b). Although *DKK1* and *ERK1* were downregulated, the effect was not statistically significant.

Further, the heatmap, a clustering based method that groups genes and/or samples together based on the similarity of their gene expression pattern, showed the differential expression profile of the genes for PDR and RD shown in Figure 5c. Except for *NRF2* all other genes that clustered together seems to be regulated by common processes.

To further validate the presence of activated microglial, we again performed immunofluorescence analyses of both resting microglia and activated microglia markers: F4/80 and Iba1 respectively. The results showed the presence of both resting as well as activated microglia in all pathologies except MH as shown in Figure 6.

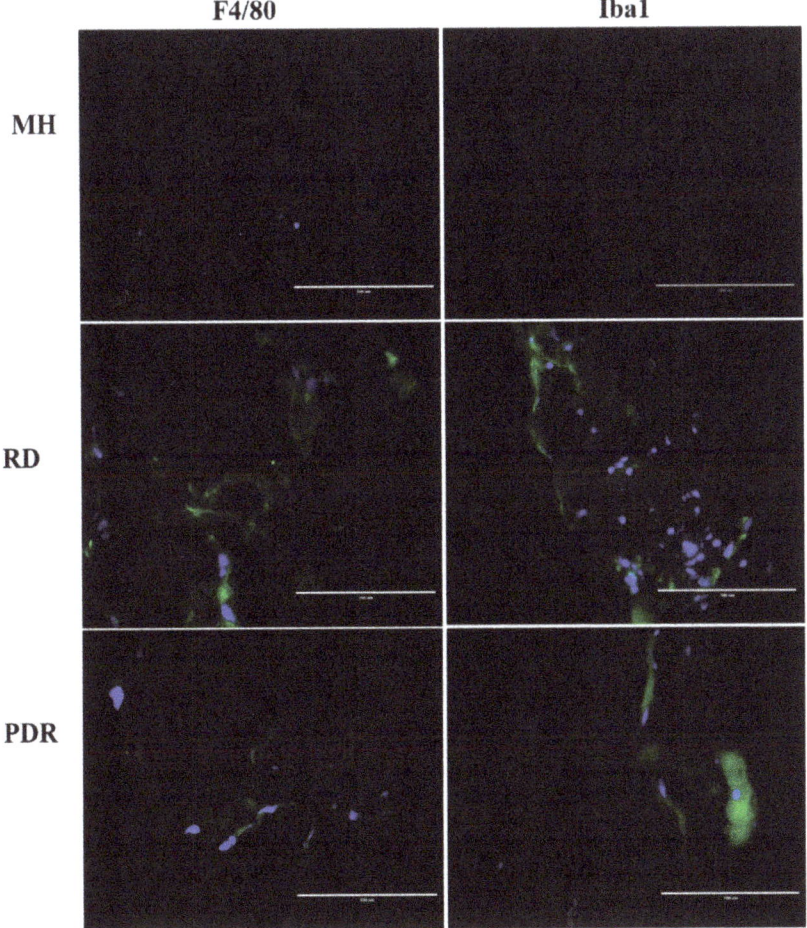

Figure 6. Validation of activation of microglia on the membrane shown by immunohistochemistry using marker for resting; F4/80 and activated stage; Iba1 in different pathological conditions MH, RD and PDR; scale bar; 100 μm.

3.7. Protein-Protein Interactions for the Differentially Expressed Genes by In-Silico Analysis

To further understand functional overlap among the significantly expressed genes in different pathways, we performed bioinformatic analysis using STRING (v 11.0). The examined genes (*HIF1-α, Nrf2, VEGF, IL1-β, CD11b, NOTCH1, MMP9, ERK1,* and *DKK1*) showed interaction among each at the protein level (Figure 7a). Several other proteins were also identified that interact with the studied proteins to modulate specific signaling pathways. Genes differentially expressed in the ERMs of PDR and RD are also shared with the genes belonging to the innate immune system, hypoxia related signaling, inflammatory pathways mediated by microglia, VEGF signaling, *TNF-α* signaling, MAP kinase signaling and extra cellular reorganization (Table 2).

Further, functionally associated proteins involved in the disease pathogenesis were also determined by studying their co-expression. We found *MMP9, IL1-β* and *ITGAM* (alias for CD11B) are functionally associated and co-expressed. Similarly, *HIF1-α,* and *Nrf2* were co-expressed together showing their strong association in disease pathogenesis (Figure 7b).

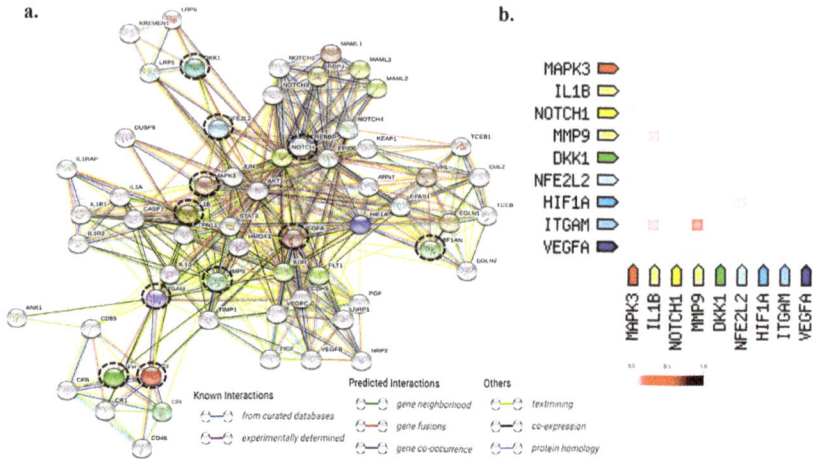

Figure 7. (a) Prediction of protein-protein interaction for the differentially expressed genes among PDR and RD in the present study. Protein 3D structure are enclosed in the circles. The colors of bond between the proteins indicate the evidences for their interaction (known interactions; skyblue-curated database, purple-experimentally determined, other predicted interactions; lime-textmining, black-co-expression). Protein of interest studied are enclosed in dotted black circle (b) triangle-matrices, where the intensity of color indicates the level of confidence of two proteins which are functionally associated.

Table 2. List of the important pathways involved in ERM pathogenesis.

S. No.	#Term ID	Term Description	Observed Gene Count	Background Gene Count	False Discovery Rate	Matching Proteins in the Network (Labels)
1	hsa04066	HIF-1 signaling pathway	17	98	7.73×10^{-23}	AKT1,ARNT,CREBBP,CUL2,EGLN1, EGLN2,EP300,FLT1,HIF1A,HMOX1, MAPK3,STAT3,TCEB1,TCEB2, TIMP1,VEGFA,VHL
2	hsa04330	Notch signaling pathway	10	48	5.83×10^{-14}	CREBBP,EP300,MAML1,MAML2, MAML3,NOTCH1,NOTCH2, NOTCH3,NOTCH4,RBPJ
3	hsa04010	MAPK signaling pathway	14	293	1.23×10^{-11}	AKT1,DUSP6,FIGF,FLT1,IL1A, IL1B,IL1R1,JUN,KDR,MAPK3, PGF,VEGFA,VEGFB,VEGFC
4	hsa04933	AGE-RAGE signaling pathway in diabetic complications	10	98	2.75×10^{-11}	AKT1,FIGF,IL1A,IL1B,JUN,MAPK3, STAT3,VEGFA,VEGFB,VEGFC
5	hsa04610	Complement and coagulation cascades	8	78	2.56×10^{-9}	C3,CD46,CD55,CFB,CFH,CFI, CR1,ITGAM
6	hsa04060	Cytokine-cytokine receptor interaction	11	263	7.33×10^{-9}	FIGF,FLT1,IL10,IL1A,IL1B,IL1R1, IL1R2,KDR,VEGFA,VEGFB,VEGFC
7	hsa04014	Ras signaling pathway	10	228	2.3×10^{-8}	AKT1,FIGF,FLT1,KDR,MAPK3,PGF, PTPN11,VEGFA,VEGFB,VEGFC
8	hsa04668	TNF signaling pathway	6	108	6.86×10^{-6}	AKT1,IL1B,JUN,MAPK3, MMP9,VEGFC
9	hsa04151	PI3K-Akt signaling pathway	9	348	6.87×10^{-6}	AKT1,FIGF,FLT1,KDR,MAPK3,PGF, VEGFA,VEGFB,VEGFC
10	hsa04310	Wnt signaling pathway	6	143	2.51×10^{-5}	CREBBP,DKK1,EP300,JUN, LRP5,LRP6
11	hsa04630	Jak-STAT signaling pathway	6	160	4.36×10^{-5}	AKT1,CREBBP,EP300,IL10, PTPN11,STAT3
12	hsa04370	VEGF signaling pathway	4	59	1.4×10^{-4}	AKT1,KDR,MAPK3,VEGFA

4. Discussion

Here, we show that activated microglia are a major component of the ERMs from RD and PDR patient samples. Microglial cells are involved in neurotrophic and neurodegenerative disease mechanisms in the retina under stress conditions. In mature retina, microglia reside in the inner and outer plexiform layers and exhibit an abundantly ramified morphology spanning the complete nuclear layers with their long protrusions [21]. Their most important role is to maintain a constant active surveillance of retinal homeostasis where they are indispensable for the immune response and synaptic pruning and transmission [22,23]. Under injury or ischemic stress, they get activated, proliferate and migrate to the site of damage, while releasing pro-inflammatory cytokines and ROS to counter the damage [24]. We recently demonstrated the role of microglial mediated aberrant complement activation in the pathogenesis of DR [25]. That study showed that a gradual increase in the expression of CFH (inhibitor of alternate complement pathway) and CD11b (activated microglial marker) in the retina (at an early stage) culminated in epiretinal membranes changes in DR patients further supporting for a major role of microglia and the alternative complement pathway in disease progression.

While there were not many differences in the cell types present in the membranes from different pathologies, higher number of GFAP positive cells in PDR and RD confirmed the presence of astrocytes and Müller glia and the glial activation (reactive gliosis). Reactive gliosis is known to cause inflammation, which leads to neurodegeneration [26]. The presence of GFAP positive cells could be due to phagocytosis and gliotic responses of Müller glia in the retina. Astrocytes are predominantly localized to the subretinal space near the ILM, where they activate and proliferate during vascular injury and neovascularization. Along with endothelial cells and pericytes, they are also involved in the formation of epiretinal vessels under ischemic condition [27,28]. Besides Müller glia and astrocytes, a large number of activated microglia was also detected in these membranes (RD and PDR). The presence of these cells indicates their role in ERM formation besides underlying gliosis. Such mechanisms may underlie the extensive gliotic changes, which pose surgical challenges.

Activated microglia secrete different types of cytokines [29]. Underlying gliosis causes the induction of inflammation, which in turn promotes oxidative stress. This is supported by our results of immunohistochemistry using anti-OXR1, an oxidative stress responsive gene. The fibrocellular membranes from RD and PDR showed significantly higher number of anti-OXR1 positive cells as compared to MH. Higher expression of CD11b along with significant increase of oxidative stress markers ($HIF1$-α and $Nrf2$), inflammatory markers ($IL1$-β and $MMP9$) and vascular endothelial growth factor (VEGF) in RD and PDR further suggested oxidative stress activates the resident microglia in the retina and adopt inflammatory phenotype. The activated ramified microglia migrate and secrete inflammatory cytokines and growth factors that promote cellular proliferation, neuronal apoptosis and phagocytosis. Inflammatory cytokines could serve as chemoattractants for invading macrophages. Higher expression of VEGF increases the endothelial cell permeability that would leads to further immune cell recruitment and disease manifestation. A study on histopathological analysis of eyes from patients with non-PDR and PDR showed increased numbers of hypertrophic microglia which correlated with disease severity [30].

Activated microglia also express activated C3a and C3b receptors on cell surface and in turn, induce astrocytes to adopt a reactive and proinflammatory phenotype. Such phenomena compromise the ability of neurons to form synapses and phagocytose dead neurons in the central nervous system. Increased deposition of dead neurons could further induce neuroinflammation and neovascularization [31]. We therefore, propose that activated microglia and astrocytes in the ERMs from RD and PDR could result from the proinflammatory phenotype of activated astrocytes in the retina. Further studies are needed to test this hypothesis.

In retinal pigment epithelium cells, Notch2 has been shown to be the major Notch receptor, and its inhibition significantly reduces the intracellular ROS production and cellular apoptosis upon ultraviolet B-induced damage. On the other hand, hypoxic stress to retinal ganglion cells induces Notch1 expression and activation. A study by Jiao et al. 2018, examined the effects of $NOX4$ mediated Notch signaling under hyperglycemic (HG) stress. The study observed that HG upregulates Nox4 expression via the activation of Notch signaling, resulting in increased ROS production and cell death in HRECs and thus the inhibition of Notch signaling or Nox4 expression was suggested to be potential therapeutic strategy for the treatment of DR [32].

Several theories have been suggested based on cellular evidences for the processes involved in the membrane formation. Some studies reported that PVR exposes the retina to blood derived fibroblast and other cytokines that causes RPE cells to undergo epithelial to mesenchymal transition and forming proliferative spindle like cells that initiate retinal remodelling and membrane formation over the ILM. Epithelial to Mesenchymal Transition (EMT) facilitates the adoption of a mesenchymal phenotype by an epithelial cell by undergoing multiple biochemical changes. The process of EMT has been well-documented in different types of cancers, leading to tumor progression and increased tumor invasiveness. Besides the other know mechanisms, release of inflammatory cytokines by immune cells has also been shown to cause EMT. Recently, a link between MMP9 and NOTCH1 signalling was also demonstrated [33]. Overexpression of MMP9 acts as a strong activator of NOTCH1 signalling. An earlier study by our group demonstrated increased expression of MMP 9 in PDR vitreous humor that is contributed by activated microglia. The present study also demonstrated an increased expression of CDllb, MMP9, IL-1β and Notch in the membranes as seen by heatmap and co expression using STRING analysis. All together these observations definitely provide a link between increased activation of microglia with RPE undergoing EMT thereby leading to membrane formation as seen in PDR and RD cases by activating Notch 1 signaling and thus inhibiting Notch 1/MMP9 signaling can be a potential therapy to prevent DR severity.

Studies have shown that ERMs impair oxygen and nutrient supply to the retina under ischemic condition [34]. It may also cause tractional retinal detachment by pulling on the neurosensory retina. Our study demonstrated higher level of oxidative stress along with inflammation in RD. Hence, the removal of ERMs may help in improving the oxygenation, nutrient supply and ion transport for retinal potassium buffering [35]. Interestingly, the surgical treatment ILM peeling is found to significantly depend on the type of ERM adherence and area where ERM attaches to the retina. ILM peeling causes mechanical trauma to the retinal nerve fiber layer (RNFL) [36], making this procedure controversial [37].

Our study shows overexpression of oxidative stress-related pathways genes in the fibrocellular membranes (Figure 8). We suggest that modulating the levels of oxidative stress and inflammation in PDR and RD could assist in predicting the need of simultaneous ERM/ILM peeling and may be helpful in improving surgical outcomes.

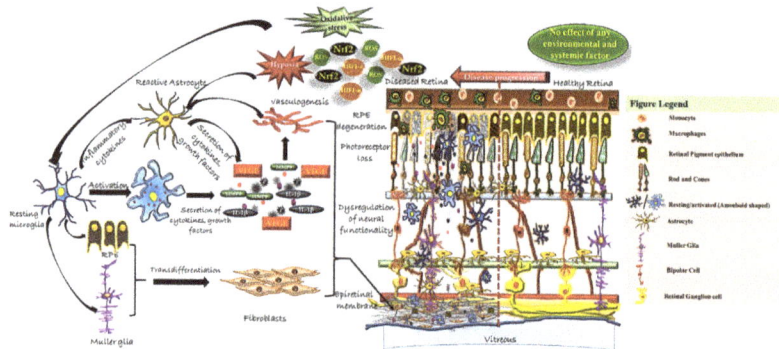

Figure 8. Schematic representation of proposed microglial activity in the epiretinal membrane of the retina. In healthy retina, resident microglia are involved in immune surveillance of all the layers of the retina and maintain retinal homeostatis by synaptic pruning, regulation of neurogenesis and axonal growth. With their phenotypic change of shape, they phagocytose cellular debris. Different kinds of stress/insults lead to abnormal functioning of retinal neurons, microglia, astrocyte, Müller glia and RPE cells. The resident/resting microglia in the retina get activated by transforming into an amoeboid shape and further interact with other neighboring retinal cells, causing abnormal functioning and trans-differentiation into proliferative cells types [10,11]. It also induces the secretion of several chemokines, proinflammatory cytokines and growth factors etc (results from the present study) that could aid in membrane formation by remodeling of the extracellular matrix proteins in retina and thereby contribute to disease pathogenesis.

5. Conclusions and Future Scope

We have shown the involvement of microglial cells, inflammation and oxidative stress in fibrocellular membranes (ERM/ILM) of different pathological conditions. Under oxidative stress microglia cells get activated and interact with other glial cells and retinal cells to cause neuroinflammation and neurodegeneration. Reducing oxidative stress and resultant inflammation may help in reducing the risk of ERM formation. Since ILM peeling also has detrimental role on the retina, these findings not only expand our knowledge about ERM pathogenesis but are helpful in identifying newer potential therapies to clinically manage blinding diseases like RD and PDR.

Further investigations on role of microglia and immunomodulation of its phenotype are underway to expand our understanding of its role in DR pathogenesis and better management of this disease and related retinopathies.

Supplementary Materials: The following are available online at http://www.mdpi.com/2076-3921/9/8/654/s1, Table S1: List of antibodies, Table S2: List of qPCR primers, Figure S1: Representative images of ERMs after H&E at 40X showing the glial cells with clear spindle shaped structure of the cells and their long thin processes. Macrophages were also seen with round darkly stained structure. Pigmentation was also observed in the membranes. Figure S2: Characterization of Müller glia cells using AldH1L1 (a specific marker for Müller glia) in MH, iERM, PDR and RD membranes.

Author Contributions: Conceptualization, I.K. and J.C.; Data curation, I.K., S.V., R.K.G., S.J., M.T., R.R.P. and J.C.; Formal analysis, I.K., S.V., R.K.G., S.J. and H.K.; Funding acquisition, I.K., H.K. and J.C.; Investigation, S.V., S.J., M.T., R.R.P., K.R. and J.C.; Methodology, I.K., S.V., R.K.G., G.H. and M.R.V.; Project administration, I.K. and J.C.; Resources, I.K., M.T., R.R.P., K.R., G.H., M.R.V. and J.C.; Software, I.K., S.V., R.K.G and H.K.; Supervision, I.K. and J.C.; Validation, I.K., S.V., R.K.G., S.J., M.T., R.R.P. and H.K.; Visualization, I.K., S.V. and M.R.V.; Writing –original draft, I.K., S.V. and J.C.; Writing–review & editing, I.K., R.K.G., S.J., K.R., G.H., M.R.V. and H.K. All authors have read and agreed to the published version of the manuscript.

Funding: This work was supported by grants from the Department of Biotechnology, Government of India (BT/01/COE/06/02/10), Hyderabad Eye Research Foundation and the Department of Biotechnology (BT/PR/16582/BID/667/2016) to IK, Department of Science and Technology, Government of India (SB/YS/LS-183/2014) to JC and from the National Institutes of Health: SI0OD021580 (to GH) and R01-EY022372 to HK.

Acknowledgments: We thank the patients and their families for their participation in this study. We also thank Subhabrata Chakrabarti and Shahna Shahulhamed at LVPEI for his help during the course of this study and Wei Zhang at UMMS for help with tissue procurement for TEM analyses. We are thankful to Sreedhar and Naidu, department of Pathology at LVPEI for their support in procuring frozen tissue sections. We sincerely thank the fellow doctors Chetan Videkar, Hitesh Agrawal, Mahima Jhingan, and Komal Agrawal for their support incollecting the membranes.

Conflicts of Interest: The authors declare no conflict of interest.

References

1. Hoon, M.; Okawa, H.; Della Santina, L.; Wong, R.O. Functional architecture of the retina: Development and disease. *Prog. Retin. Eye Res.* **2014**, *42*, 44–84. [CrossRef] [PubMed]
2. Bishop, P.N. Structural macromolecules and supramolecular organisation of the vitreous gel. *Prog. Retin. Eye Res.* **2000**, *19*, 323–344. [CrossRef]
3. Fraser-Bell, S.; Guzowski, M.; Rochtchina, E.; Wang, J.J.; Mitchell, P. Five-year cumulative incidence and progression of epiretinal membranes: The Blue Mountains Eye Study. *Ophthalmology* **2003**, *110*, 34–40. [CrossRef]
4. Hisatomi, T.; Enaida, H.; Sakamoto, T.; Kagimoto, T.; Ueno, A.; Nakamura, T.; Hata, Y.; Ishibashi, T. A new method for comprehensive bird's-eye analysis of the surgically excised internal limiting membrane. *Am. J. Ophthalmol.* **2005**, *139*, 1121–1122. [CrossRef]
5. Bu, S.C.; Kuijer, R.; Li, X.R.; Hooymans, J.M.; Los, L.I. Idiopathic epiretinal membrane. *Retina* **2014**, *34*, 2317–2335. [CrossRef]
6. Sandali, O.; El Sanharawi, M.; Basli, E.; Bonnel, S.; Lecuen, N.; Barale, P.O.; Borderie, V.; Laroche, L.; Monin, C. Epiretinal membrane recurrence: Incidence, characteristics, evolution, and preventive and risk factors. *Retina* **2013**, *33*, 2032–2038. [CrossRef]

7. Anderson, R.E.; Rapp, L.M.; Wiegand, R.D. Lipid peroxidation and retinal degeneration. *Curr. Eye Res.* **1984**, *3*, 223–227. [CrossRef]
8. Schechet, S.A.; DeVience, E.; Thompson, J.T. The Effect of Internal Limiting Membrane Peeling on Idiopathic Epiretinal Membrane Surgery, with a Review of the Literature. *Retina* **2017**, *37*, 873–880. [CrossRef]
9. Kwok, A.; Lai, T.Y.; Yuen, K.S. Epiretinal membrane surgery with or without internal limiting membrane peeling. *Clin. Exp. Ophthalmol.* **2005**, *33*, 379–385. [CrossRef]
10. Morino, I.; Hiscott, P.; McKechnie, N.; Grierson, I. Variation in epiretinal membrane components with clinical duration of the proliferative tissue. *Br. J. Ophthalmol.* **1990**, *74*, 393–399. [CrossRef]
11. Bellhorn, M.B.; Friedman, A.H.; Wise, G.N.; Henkind, P. Ultrastructure and clinicopathologic correlation of idiopathic preretinal macular fibrosis. *Am. J. Ophthalmol.* **1975**, *79*, 366–373. [CrossRef]
12. Cheville, N.F.; Stasko, J. Techniques in electron microscopy of animal tissue. *Vet. Pathol.* **2014**, *51*, 28–41. [CrossRef] [PubMed]
13. Verardo, M.R.; Lewis, G.P.; Takeda, M.; Linberg, K.A.; Byun, J.; Luna, G.; Wilhelmsson, U.; Pekny, M.; Chen, D.F.; Fisher, S.K. Abnormal reactivity of muller cells after retinal detachment in mice deficient in GFAP and vimentin. *Investig. Ophthalmol. Vis. Sci.* **2008**, *49*, 3659–3665. [CrossRef] [PubMed]
14. Uga, S.; Ikui, H.; Kono, T. Electron microscope study on astrocytes in the human retina (author's transl). *Nippon Ganka Gakkai Zasshi* **1974**, *78*, 681–685. [PubMed]
15. Castejon, O.J. Electron microscopy of astrocyte changes and subtypes in traumatic human edematous cerebral cortex: A review. *Ultrastruct. Pathol.* **2013**, *37*, 417–424. [CrossRef]
16. Mori, S.; Leblond, C.P. Identification of microglia in light and electron microscopy. *J. Comp. Neurol.* **1969**, *135*, 57–80. [CrossRef]
17. García-Cabezas, M.Á.; John, Y.J.; Barbas, H.; Zikopoulos, B. Distinction of Neurons, Glia and Endothelial Cells in the Cerebral Cortex: An Algorithm Based on Cytological Features. *Front. Neuroanat.* **2016**, *10*, 107. [CrossRef]
18. Savage, J.C.; Picard, K.; González-Ibáñez, F.; Tremblay, M.È. A Brief History of Microglial Ultrastructure: Distinctive Features, Phenotypes, and Functions Discovered Over the Past 60 Years by Electron Microscopy. *Front. Immunol.* **2018**, *9*, 803. [CrossRef]
19. Shahid, M.; Idrees, M.; Butt, A.M.; Raza, S.M.; Amin, I.; Rasul, A.; Afzal, S. Blood-based gene expression profile of oxidative stress and antioxidant genes for identifying surrogate markers of liver tissue injury in chronic hepatitis C patients. *Arch. Virol.* **2020**, *165*, 809–822. [CrossRef]
20. Wu, M.Y.; Yiang, G.T.; Lai, T.T.; Li, C.J. The Oxidative Stress and Mitochondrial Dysfunction during the Pathogenesis of Diabetic Retinopathy. *Oxid. Med. Cell. Longev.* **2018**, *18*, 3420187. [CrossRef]
21. Karlstetter, M.; Scholz, R.; Rutar, M.; Wong, W.T.; Provis, J.M.; Langmann, T. Retinal microglia: Just bystander or target for therapy? *Prog. Retin. Eye Res.* **2015**, *45*, 30–57. [CrossRef] [PubMed]
22. Akhtar-Schäfer, I.; Wang, L.; Krohne, T.U.; Xu, H.; Langmann, T. Modulation of three key innate immune pathways for the most common retinal degenerative diseases. *EMBO Mol. Med.* **2018**, *10*, e8259. [CrossRef] [PubMed]
23. Wang, Y.; Ulland, T.K.; Ulrich, J.D.; Song, W.; Tzaferis, J.A.; Hole, J.T.; Yuan, P.; Mahan, T.E.; Shi, Y.; Gilfillan, S.; et al. TREM2-mediated early microglial response limits diffusion and toxicity of amyloid plaques. *J. Exp. Med.* **2016**, *213*, 667–675. [CrossRef] [PubMed]
24. Ferrer-Martín, R.M.; Martín-Oliva, D.; Sierra-Martín, A.; Carrasco, M.C.; Martín-Estebané, M.; Calvente, R.; Martín-Guerrero, S.M.; Marín-Teva, J.L.; Navascués, J.; Cuadros, M.A. Microglial Activation Promotes Cell Survival in Organotypic Cultures of Postnatal Mouse Retinal Explants. *PLoS ONE* **2015**, *10*, e0135238. [CrossRef]
25. Shahulhameed, S.; Vishwakarma, S.; Chhablani, J.; Tyagi, M.; Pappuru, R.R.; Jakati, S.; Chakrabarti, S.; Kaur, I. A Systematic Investigation on Complement Pathway Activation in Diabetic Retinopathy. *Front. Immunol.* **2020**, *11*, 154. [CrossRef]
26. Vázquez-Chona, F.R.; Swan, A.; Ferrell, W.D.; Jiang, L.; Baehr, W.; Chien, W.M.; Fero, M.; Marc, R.E.; Levine, E.M. Proliferative reactive gliosis is compatible with glial metabolic support and neuronal function. *BMC Neurosci.* **2011**, *12*, 98. [CrossRef]
27. Méhes, E.; Czirók, A.; Hegedüs, B.; Szabó, B.; Vicsek, T.; Satz, J.; Campbell, K.; Jancsik, V. Dystroglycan is involved in laminin-1-stimulated motility of Müller glial cells: Combined velocity and directionality analysis. *Glia* **2005**, *49*, 492–500. [CrossRef]

28. Caspi, R.R.; Roberge, F.G. Glial cells as suppressor cells: Characterization of the inhibitory function. *J. Autoimmun.* **1989**, *2*, 709–722. [CrossRef]
29. Wang, W.Y.; Tan, M.S.; Yu, J.T.; Tan, L. Role of pro-inflammatory cytokines released from microglia in Alzheimer's disease. *Ann. Transl. Med.* **2015**, *3*, 136.
30. Zeng, H.Y.; Green, W.R.; Tso, M.O. Microglial activation in human diabetic retinopathy. *Arch. Ophthalmol.* **2008**, *126*, 227–232. [CrossRef]
31. Liddelow, S.A.; Guttenplan, K.A.; Clarke, L.E.; Bennett, F.C.; Bohlen, C.J.; Schirmer, L.; Bennett, M.L.; Münch, A.E.; Chung, W.S.; Peterson, T.C.; et al. Neurotoxic reactive astrocytes are induced by activated microglia. *Nature* **2017**, *541*, 481–487. [CrossRef] [PubMed]
32. Jiao, W.; Ji, J.; Li, F.; Guo, J.; Zheng, Y.; Li, S.; Xu, W. Activation of the Notch Nox4 reactive oxygen species signaling pathway induces cell death in high glucose treated human retinal endothelial cells. *Mol. Med. Rep.* **2019**, *19*, 667–677. [CrossRef] [PubMed]
33. Fazio, C.; Piazzi, G.; Vitaglione, P.; Fogliano, V.; Munarini, A.; Prossomariti, A.; Milazzo, M.; D'Angelo, L.; Napolitano, M.; Chieco, P.; et al. Inflammation increases NOTCH1 activity via MMP9 and is counteracted by Eicosapentaenoic Acid-free fatty acid in colon cancer cells. *Sci. Rep.* **2017**, *6*, 20670. [CrossRef] [PubMed]
34. Oliver, P.L.; Finelli, M.J.; Edwards, B.; Bitoun, E.; Butts, D.L.; Becker, E.B.; Cheeseman, M.T.; Davies, B.; Davies, K.E. Oxr1 is essential for protection against oxidative stress-induced neurodegeneration. *PLoS Genet.* **2011**, *7*, e1002338. [CrossRef]
35. Robaszkiewicz, J.; Chmielewska, K.; Figurska, M.; Wierzbowska, J.; Stankiewicz, A. Müller glial cells–the mediators of vascular disorders with vitreomacular interface pathology in diabetic maculopathy. *Klin. Ocz.* **2010**, *112*, 328–332.
36. Clark, A.; Balducci, N.; Pichi, F.; Veronese, C.; Morara, M.; Torrazza, C.; Ciardella, A.P. Swelling of the arcuate nerve fiber layer after internal limiting membrane peeling. *Retina* **2012**, *32*, 1608–1613. [CrossRef]
37. Bovey, E.H.; Uffer, S.; Achache, F. Surgery for epimacular membrane: Impact of retinal internal limiting membrane removal on functional outcome. *Retina* **2004**, *24*, 728–735. [CrossRef]

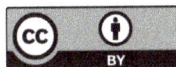

© 2020 by the authors. Licensee MDPI, Basel, Switzerland. This article is an open access article distributed under the terms and conditions of the Creative Commons Attribution (CC BY) license (http://creativecommons.org/licenses/by/4.0/).

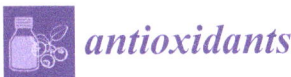 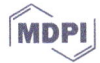

Article

Inhibition of HDAC6 Attenuates Diabetes-Induced Retinal Redox Imbalance and Microangiopathy

Hossameldin Abouhish [1,2], Menaka C. Thounaojam [1], Ravirajsinh N. Jadeja [3], Diana R. Gutsaeva [1], Folami L. Powell [3], Mohamed Khriza [2], Pamela M. Martin [3] and Manuela Bartoli [1,*]

1. Department of Ophthalmology, Medical College of Georgia, Augusta University, Augusta, GA 30912, USA; habouhish@augusta.edu (H.A.); mthounaojam@augusta.edu (M.C.T.); dgutsaeva@augusta.edu (D.R.G.)
2. Department of Clinical Pharmacology, Faculty of Medicine, Mansoura University, Mansoura 35516, Egypt; mohamedkhriza@gmail.com
3. Department of Biochemistry and Molecular Biology, Medical College of Georgia, Augusta University, Augusta, GA 30912, USA; rjadeja@augusta.edu (R.N.J.); FPOWELL@augusta.edu (F.L.P.); pmmartin@augusta.edu (P.M.M.)
* Correspondence: mbartoli@augusta.edu; Tel.: +706-721-9797 or +706-721-7910; Fax: +706-721-9799

Received: 1 July 2020; Accepted: 7 July 2020; Published: 9 July 2020

Abstract: We investigated the contributing role of the histone deacetylase 6 (HDAC6) to the early stages of diabetic retinopathy (DR). Furthermore, we examined the mechanism of action of HDAC6 in human retinal endothelial cells (HuREC) exposed to glucidic stress. Streptozotocin-induced diabetic rats (STZ-rats), a rat model of type 1 diabetes, were used as model of DR. HDAC6 expression and activity were increased in human diabetic postmortem donors and STZ-rat retinas and were augmented in HuREC exposed to glucidic stress (25 mM glucose). Administration of the HDAC6 specific inhibitor Tubastatin A (TS) (10 mg/kg) prevented retinal microvascular hyperpermeability and up-regulation of inflammatory markers. Furthermore, in STZ-rats, TS decreased the levels of senescence markers and rescued the expression and activity of the histone deacetylase sirtuin 1 (SIRT1), while downregulating the levels of free radicals and of the redox stress markers 4-hydroxynonenal (4-HNE) and nitrotyrosine (NT). The antioxidant effects of TS, consequent to HDAC6 inhibition, were associated with preservation of Nrf2-dependent gene expression and up-regulation of thioredoxin-1 activity. In vitro data, obtained from HuREC, exposed to glucidic stress, largely replicated the in vivo results further confirming the antioxidant effects of HDAC6 inhibition by TS in the diabetic rat retina. In summary, our data implicate HDAC6 activation in mediating hyperglycemia-induced retinal oxidative/nitrative stress leading to retinal microangiopathy and, potentially, DR.

Keywords: diabetic retinopathy; HDAC6; oxidative stress; tubastatin A; retinal endothelial cells; retinal endothelial cell senescence

---

1. Introduction

Diabetic retinopathy (DR) is a neurovascular complication of diabetes mellitus and the leading cause of blindness in working age adults [1]. Diabetic retinal microangiopathy significantly contributes to DR pathogenesis and strategies targeting its occurrence and progression are important for preventing vision loss in affected patients [2,3].

Hyperglycemia-induced retinal vascular pathology is a multi-step process characterized by retinal endothelial cell dysfunction and death, increased vascular permeability leading to diabetic macular edema (DME), and abnormal retinal neovascularization, as seen in proliferative diabetic retinopathy (PDR) [2,3]. Prolonged hyperglycemia affects the retinal microvasculature by altering multiple molecular pathways involving redox imbalance and induction of pro-inflammatory responses [3].

Previously, we showed that hyperglycemia-induced oxidative/nitrative stress accelerates retinal endothelial cell senescence and that this is an important early pathogenic event during the development of diabetic retinal microangiopathy [4]. Retinal oxidative/nitrative stress results from increased production of reactive oxygen and nitrogen species (ROS and RNS, respectively) from cellular and mitochondrial oxidases [5,6] as well as from loss of endogenous antioxidant activities [7,8].

Histone deacetylase 6 (HDAC6) is a class IIb histone deacetylase known to exert important biological functions due to its ability to regulate the acetylation state of nuclear and cytoplasmic proteins [9]. Most known targets of HDAC6 are cytoskeletal proteins, transcription factors [9] and endogenous antioxidants such as peroxiredoxin 1 (Prx1) [10,11]. As a consequence of its multiple biological targets, altered HDAC6 expression and activity is linked to inflammation, oxidative stress and the pathogenesis of a number of neurodegenerative [12] and cardiovascular disorders [13] as well as cancer [14].

The potential impact of HDAC6 on diabetic microvascular complications is understudied. Previous studies have shown beneficial effects of HDAC6 inhibition in diabetic kidney disease [15] and diabetic heart disease [16]. Moreover, while little is known on HDAC6 contribution to retinal diabetic disorders, studies have implicated pro-oxidative effects of HDAC6 in animal models of retinal neurodegenerative diseases [17,18], potentially suggesting a role for this histone deacetylase in retinal pathologies involving oxidative stress, such as DR.

Based on this evidence, we assessed the effects of diabetes on HDAC6 retinal expression and activity in human and experimental DR and we investigated the molecular mechanisms involved in this process in a rat model of type 1 diabetes (streptozotocin-induced diabetic rat = STZ-rat) and in cultures of human retinal microvascular endothelial cells exposed to glucidic stress.

2. Materials and Methods

2.1. Human Postmortem Samples

De-identified human postmortem retinal samples were obtained from Georgia Eye Bank, Inc. (Alanta, GA, USA). Retinas were obtained from a total of 8 diabetic and 8 non-diabetic donors that were selected based on DR history or lack of reported ocular pathologies (control). Supplementary Table S1 summarizes the demographic and clinical history information available for all donors.

2.2. Animals and Treatment

All animal experiments strictly adhered to the Statement of the Association for Research in Vision and Ophthalmology (ARVO) for the humane use of laboratory animals for ophthalmological research and to Augusta University approved protocols (#2009-0181). All animals were housed in the vivarium of Augusta University with a 12-h day/night light cycle with light intensity in the room maintained at 130 lux at cage level, and fed ad libitum. Adult male Sprague–Dawley (SD) rats (250–300 g) obtained from Envigo (Indianapolis, IN, USA) were made diabetic by a single intraperitoneal injection of streptozotocin (STZ) (55 mg/kg dissolved in 0.1 mol/L sodium citrate, pH 4.5) (Sigma-Aldrich, St. Louis, MO, USA). Control rats received injections of vehicle alone. Rats with fasting blood glucose ≥250 mg/dL were considered diabetic. A group of STZ-rats was injected intraperitoneally with 10 mg/kg Tubastatin A (TS) (MedChemExpress, Monmouth Junction, NJ, USA) starting two weeks after the STZ injections and continuing every other day for the next six weeks. Control rats received vehicle phosphate-buffered saline (PBS) injection. The diabetic rats were sacrificed by an overdose of anesthesia (ketamine 200 mg/kg and xylazine 60 mg/kg) followed by thoracotomy. Blood glucose levels were measured by ReliOn prime blood glucose monitoring system (Bentonville, AR, USA) and glycated hemoglobin A1c (HbA1c) was measured using A1c Now+ System (PTS Diagnostic, Winter Park, FL, USA). A number of other metabolites were also monitored in diabetic and control rat plasma using a biochemistry panel analyzer (Piccolo Xpress analyzer, Princeton, NJ, USA). Rats metabolic profiles in response to the different treatment protocols are reported in Supplementary Table S2.

2.3. Cells and Treatment

Human retinal endothelial cells (HuREC) were purchased from Cell Systems Corporation (Kirkland, WA, USA) and maintained using complete medium with normal glucose formulation (Cell Systems) at 37 °C and 5% CO_2 in a humidified atmosphere. All the experiments were carried out using HuREC between passages 3 to 7 and all the tissue culture flasks/plates were pre-coated with attachment factor (Cell Systems). The cells were switched to serum-free medium (Cell Systems) 10 to 12 h before the experiments. To mimic the effects of the hyperglycemia (glucidic stress), HuREC were cultured for 48 h in serum-free medium containing 25 mM D-glucose (high glucose, HG). Similarly, control cells were cultured in serum-free and normal glucose medium (5.5 mM D-glucose, NG). Cells grown in normal glucose media with the addition of L-glucose (5.5 mM D-glucose + 19.5 mM L-glucose, LG) served as an osmotic control. Some of the HuREC were treated with 5 µM TS. To determine TS toxicity towards HuREC, a dose-response curve using MTT cell viability assay (Abcam, Cambridge, MA, country) was conducted following the manufacturer's instructions. MTT dye absorbance was read using a microplate reader at 540 nm (Supplementary Figure S1).

2.4. Histology

Rat eyes from each experimental group were enucleated and embedded in optimal cutting temperature (OCT) mounting medium (Tissue-Tek, Torrance, CA, USA). Samples were then sectioned (10 µm), stained with hematoxylin and eosin (H&E), and examined centrally and on each side (temporal and nasal) of the optic nerve. Retinas were examined using a Zeiss Axioplan-2 microscope (Carl Zeiss, Göttingen, Germany) equipped with a high-resolution camera and processed using imaging Spot Software (version 4.0.2; Diagnostic Instruments, Sterling Heights, MI). Morphometric analysis was conducted to measure total retinal thickness.

2.5. Immunofluorescence

Rat eyes were embedded in OCT mounting medium (Tissue-Tek), frozen on dry ice and then cryostat sectioned. A 4% paraformaldehyde fixative was applied to the slides for 10 min. Slides were incubated overnight at 4 °C with one of the following primary antibodies: Rabbit anti-HDAC6 (Lifespan Biosciences, Seattle, WA, USA) and mouse anti-phosphorylated form of H2A histone family member X (γH2AX) (Cell Signaling Technology, Danvers, MA, USA). Slides were washed three times with 0.1% Triton X-100 in 0.1 M PBS (pH 7.4) followed by a 1-h incubation with one of the following secondary antibodies, all purchased from Molecular Probes-Life Technologies (Grand Island, NY, USA): goat anti-rabbit IgG-conjugated Alexa Fluor 488, goat anti-mouse IgG-conjugated Alexa Fluor 488. Slides were mounted using Fluoroshield mounting medium containing 4′,6-diamidino-2-phenylindole (DAPI) to visualize nuclei (Sigma-Aldrich). Sections were examined for epifluorescence using a Zeiss Axioplan-2 fluorescence microscope (Carl Zeiss) equipped with the Axiovision program (version 4.7; Carl Zeiss).

2.6. Assessment of HDAC6 Activity

HDAC6 activity was assessed in both rat and human cell samples using a commercially available fluorimetric assay kit (Biovision, Milpitas, CA, USA), employing a synthetic acetylated-peptide substrate resulting in the release of an AFC fluorophore, which can be detected and quantified with Ex/Em, 380/490 nm at 37 °C.

2.7. Assessment of Thioredoxin-1 Activity

Thioredoxin activity fluorescent assay kit (Cayman Chemical, Ann Arbor, MI, USA) was used to assess the activity of thioredoxin-1 (Trx-1) in rat retinal extracts and HuREC lysates. This assay measures the ability of endogenous Trx-1 to reduce the disulfides of fluorescently labeled insulin.

The resulting fluorescent signal, measured at Ex/Em, 520/545 nm, is a direct measurement of Trx-1 reducing activity.

2.8. Protein Analysis

Retinal tissue was homogenized in lysis buffer (ThermoFisher, Waltham, MA, USA) containing 1% phosphatase and protease inhibitor cocktail (Sigma-Aldrich). Protein concentration was measured using the Bio-Rad protein assay kit (Bio-Rad, Hercules, CA, USA) according to the manufacturer's recommendation. Proteins from whole rat retinal tissue and HuREC lysates were separated by sodium dodecyl sulfate-polyacrylamide gel electrophoresis (SDS-PAGE) and transferred onto polyvinylidene difluoride (PVDF) membrane. The membrane was blocked using 5% skim milk and incubated with the following primary antibodies: anti-HDAC6 (Abcam, Cambridge, MA, USA), anti-Trx-1, anti-sirtuin 1 (SIRT1) and anti-albumin (all from Cell Signaling Technology). After incubation with horseradish peroxidase–conjugated secondary antibody (GE Healthcare, Pittsburg, PA, USA), bands were detected using the enzymatic chemiluminescence reagent, ECL (GE Healthcare). Subsequently, the membranes were stripped using stripping buffer (Bio-Rad) and re-probed with anti-β-actin antibody (Sigma-Aldrich) to assess equal loading. Scanned images of blots were used to quantify protein expression using NIH ImageJ software (http://rsb.info.nih.gov/ij/).

2.9. Dot BlotAanalysis

Equivalent amount of proteins prepared from whole rat retinas and HuREC lysates were spotted on nitrocellulose membranes and dried for 5 min at room temperature. The membranes were blocked for 1 h by using 5 % non-fat dry milk in PBS and then probed for 1 h with either anti-3-nitrotyrosine (NT, Cayman) or anti 4-hydroxynonenal (4-HNE, Abcam) antibodies in PBS-tween buffer. The membranes were then washed three times in PBS-tween buffer and probed again with horseradish peroxidase-conjugate secondary antibody (Cell Signaling). After washing the membrane, the immuno-positive spots were visualized by using Clarity ECL- Blotting substrate (Bio-Rad). Scanned images of blots were used to quantify protein expression using NIH ImageJ software (http://rsb.info.nih.gov/ij/).

2.10. Quantitative PCR Analysis

Gene expression at mRNA level was assessed in retinal and HuREC extracts by quantitative polymerase chain reaction (qPCR). Total RNA was isolated from the HuREC and rat retinas using RNeasy Kit (Qiagen, Germantown, MD, USA). cDNA was prepared using iScript™ cDNA Synthesis Kit (Bio-Rad). Amplification of HDAC6, Trx-1, GCLC, GCLM, NQO1, and HO-1 mRNA was performed using power SYBR green PCR master mix (Applied Biosystems, Foster City, CA, USA). The conditions used for the PCR were as it follows: 95 °C for 3 min (1 cycle) and 94 °C for 20 s, 55 °C for 30 s, and 72 °C for 40 s (40 cycles). The relative mRNA abundance was determined by normalizing to mRNA for hypoxanthine phosphoribosyltransferase 1 (HPRT-1) for tissue or 18 s for cells, using the 2Ct method (Ct refers to the threshold value). A complete list of the different primers used in this study is included in Supplementary Table S3.

2.11. Reactive Oxygen Species Assays

For detection of superoxide in retinal tissue, 10 μm-thick retinal cryosections, from different experimental groups, were covered (at room temperature) with a 10 μM dihydroethidium (DHE) solution and incubated in a light-protected humidified incubator at 37 °C for 30 min. At the end of the incubation, sections were mounted with a coverslip and images were taken using Zeiss Axioplan-2 fluorescence microscope (Carl Zeiss). The fluorescence intensity was measured using NIH ImageJ software (http://rsb.info.nih.gov/ij/).

ROS detection from cellular sources was accomplished by CellROX green assay (ThermoFisher) performed according to the manufacturer's protocol. HuREC were loaded with 5 μM CellROX green in culture medium and stained in the dark for 30 min at 37 °C. Stained cells were washed in PBS twice, mounted using Fluoroshield mounting medium containing DAPI (Sigma-Aldrich) to visualize nuclei. Images were then immediately captured using a Zeiss Axioplan-2 fluorescence microscope (Carl Zeiss).

Mitochondrial superoxide production was measured using MitoSOX Red (ThermoFisher). HuREC were loaded with 5 µM MitoSOX red in Hank's balanced salt solution (HBSS) with calcium and magnesium for 30 min at 37 °C in the dark. Stained cells were then washed and suspended in HBSS, mounted using Fluoroshield mounting medium containing DAPI (Sigma-Aldrich) and immediately analyzed under a Zeiss Axioplan-2 fluorescence microscope (Carl Zeiss).

2.12. Assessment of Senescence Markers

To evidence senescent HuREC, we used senescence-associated β-Galactosidase (SA-β-Gal) reactivity-based assay using a commercially available kit (Cell Signaling) as previously shown [7]. Positive reactivity to SA-β-Gal, assessed at pH 6, is measured on images captured (10 frames per well) at 20× magnification by light microscopy using Zeiss Axioplan-2 microscope (Carl Zeiss). Percentage of SA-β-Gal positive cells/well was determined as number of cells positive for a blue color versus total number of cells counted in a blind fashion.

2.13. Statistical Analysis

Graphs were prepared using Graph Pad Prism 8.0 software for Windows (Graph Pad Software, San Diego, CA, USA). Data are shown as means ± standard error of mean (SEM). Statistical significance among experimental groups was established using one-way ANOVA, followed by the Bonferroni multiple-comparison test. Differences were considered significant when p was <0.05.

3. Results

3.1. HDAC6 Expression and Activity are Increased in the Diabetic Retina

HDAC6 expression and activity were measured in human DR using postmortem human retinas from diabetic and non-diabetic donors and STZ-rats compared to normoglycemic age-matched control. As shown in Figure 1A,B, Western blotting analysis showed a 2.5-fold increase in HDAC6 expression in retinas of postmortem diabetic donors as compared to retinas of non-diabetic donors ($p < 0.003$; $n = 8$). We then measured the expression and retinal tissue distribution of HDAC6 in STZ-rats (8 weeks of hyperglycemia) compared to normoglycemic age-matched control rats. Western blotting analysis (Figure 1C,D) showed a 2.2-fold increase of HDAC6 protein levels in retinas of STZ-rats at 8 weeks of hyperglycemia in comparison to age-matched normoglycemic control rats ($p < 0.006$; $n = 6$). Further, HDAC6 enzymatic activity, measured with a fluorimetric assay, was significantly increased in retinas of STZ-rats when compared to normoglycemic age-matched control rats ($p < 0.001$; $n = 6$) (Figure 1E). Finally, immunohistochemical analysis of normal and diabetic rat retinal sections (Figure 1F), confirmed HDAC6 increased expression in diabetic rat retinas and showed its immunolocalization in several retinal layers, particularly in the inner nuclear layer (INL), retinal pigmented epithelium (RPE), and around retinal blood vessels in the ganglion cell layer (GCL) (white arrows in Figure 1F).

3.2. Tubastatin A Decreases the Expression and Activity of HDAC6 in the Diabetic Retina

Next, we determined the effect of the HDAC6 specific inhibitor Tubastatin A (TS), on diabetes-induced increase in HDAC6 expression and activity in the retina of diabetic rats. STZ-rats were treated with 10 mg/kg of TS, administered intraperitoneally every other day starting two weeks after the onset of diabetes and prolonged for another 6 weeks (total 8 weeks of diabetes). As shown in Figure 2A, TS treatment resulted in a marked reduction of HDAC6-specific immunoreactivity in comparison to untreated STZ-rats (DB). Western blotting analysis confirmed these data by showing a significant reduction in HDAC6 protein levels in retinas of TS-treated STZ-rats (DB + TS) in comparison with untreated STZ-diabetic rats (DB) ($p < 0.05$; $n = 6$) (Figure 2B,C). As expected, we also observed a significant decrease in HDAC6 enzymatic activity (Figure 2D) in retinas of TS-treated STZ-rats (DB + TS) in comparison to untreated STZ-rats (DB) ($p < 0.01$; $n = 6$).

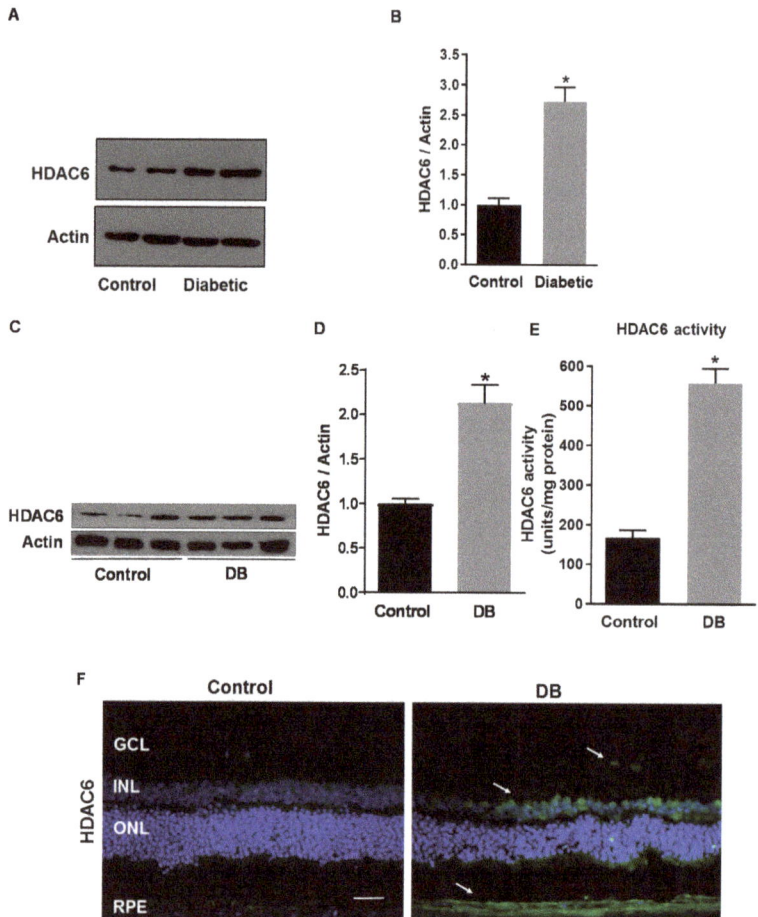

Figure 1. Histone deacetylase 6 (HDAC6) expression in the diabetic retina. (**A**) Western blotting analysis measuring HDAC6 protein levels in human postmortem retinas from diabetic and non-diabetic donors (control). (**B**) Bar histograms representing relative optical densities from the immunoblotting shown in (A) and normalized versus the loading control actin. Values are expressed as mean ± SEM for $n = 8$. * $p < 0.01$ vs. control. (**C**) Western analysis of HDAC6 protein expression in retinas of streptozotocin-induced diabetic rats (STZ-rats) (DB) at 8 weeks of hyperglycemia and age-matched normoglycemic control rats (control). (**D**) Bar histograms representing densitometric quantification of HDAC6 protein levels normalized to actin. (**E**) HDAC6 activity measured, by a fluorimetric assay, in retinas of STZ-rats and control normoglycemic rats. (**F**) Representative microimages of immunohistochemical analysis of HDAC6 (green) in retinas of STZ-rats at 8 weeks of hyperglycemia and of age-matched normoglycemic control rats. Nuclei were stained with 4′,6-diamidino-2-phenylindole (DAPI). White arrows indicate areas of increased immunoreactivity. Scale bar, 50 µm. Values are expressed as mean ± SEM for $n = 6$. * $p < 0.01$ vs. control.

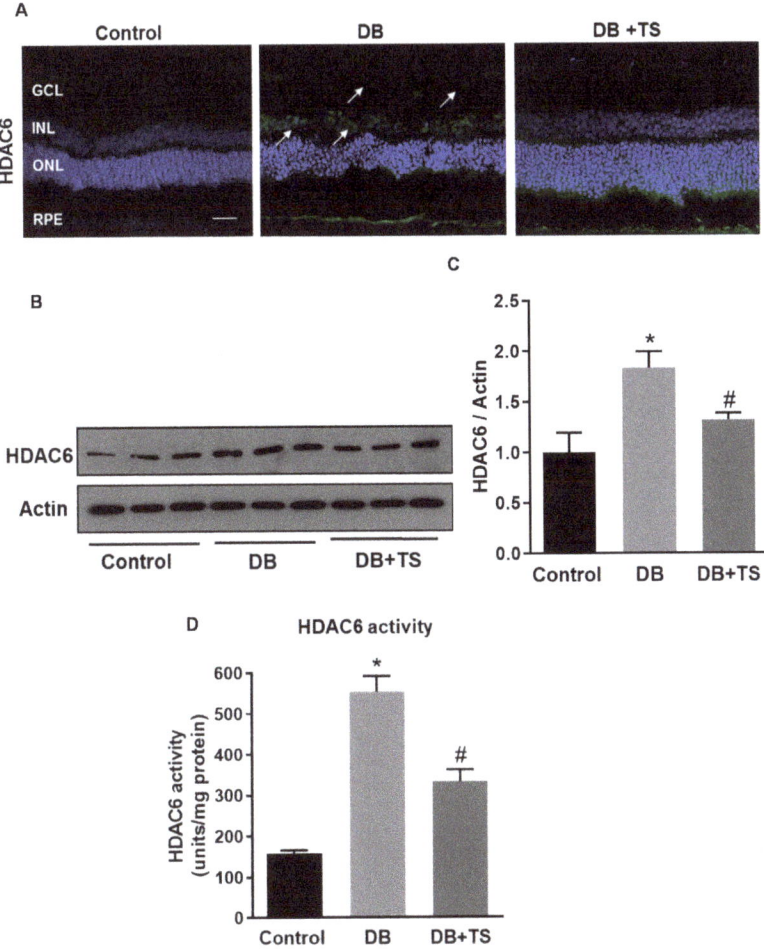

Figure 2. Effects of Tubastatin A on HDAC6 expression and activity. (**A**) Representative images of immunohistochemical analysis of HDAC6 (green) of retinal cryosections of STZ-rats (DB) (8 weeks of hyperglycemia), age-matched normoglycemic control rats, and STZ-rats receiving TS 10 mg/kg (DB + tubastatin A (TS)). Nuclei were stained with DAPI. Scale bar, 50 µm. (**B**) Western analysis assessing HDAC6 protein levels in STZ-rats after 8 weeks of hyperglycemia (DB), STZ-rats treated with 10 mg/kg TS (DB +TS) and age-matched normoglycemic rats (control). (**C**) Bar histograms representing densitometric values of HDAC6 protein expression measured in the different experimental groups and normalized to actin. (**D**) HDAC6 activity measured, by fluorimetric assay, in the three experimental groups (control, DB and DB + TS). Values are mean ± SEM for $n = 6$. * $p < 0.05$ vs. control and # $p < 0.05$ vs. DB.

3.3. Tubastatin A Preserves Retinal Structural Morphology and Reduces Vascular Leakage in Diabetic Retina

Morphological and morphometric analyses were conducted evaluating retinal cryosections stained with hematoxylin and eosin to assess the effects of TS treatment on retinal histopathology (Figure 3A,B). Figure 3B shows that total retinal thickness was significantly reduced in diabetic rats after 8 weeks of hyperglycemia (DB) in comparison to control age-matched normoglycemic rats (control) ($p < 0.03$). Treatment of diabetic rats with TS (DB + TS) normalized the morphology of the retinal layers as shown by a significant preservation of total retinal thickness (Figure 3B) ($p < 0.05$) compared to untreated diabetic rats (DB).

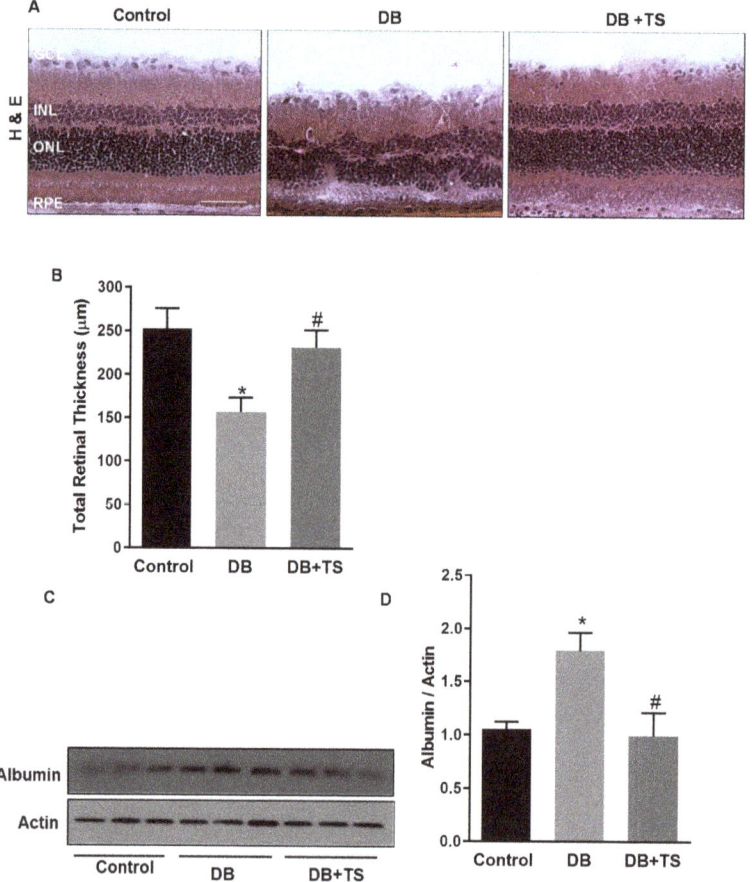

Figure 3. Effects of Tubastatin A on retinal histopathology and vascular leakage. (**A**) Hematoxylin and eosin (H&E) staining of retinal cryosections assessing retinal morphology of STZ-rats (DB), STZ-rats receiving TS (10 mg/kg) (DB + TS) and normoglycemic control rats (control). Scale bar, 50 μm. (**B**) The bars represent retinal thickness values measured in H&E retinal cryosections obtained from the different treatment groups. (**C**) Western analysis of albumin extravasation in retinas of diabetic STZ-rats (DB), STZ-rats receiving 10 mg/kg TS (DB + TS) and normoglycemic control rats (control). (**D**) Bar histograms representing optical density of albumin normalized to actin. Values are mean ± SEM for $n = 6$. * $p < 0.05$ vs. control and # $p < 0.05$ vs. DB.

Blood–retinal barrier (BRB) dysfunction, measured as an increase in vascular permeability, is an important evidence of diabetes-induced retinal vascular abnormalities [19,20]. To determine the effect of TS on hyperglycemia-induced vascular leakage in the diabetic retina, we assessed albumin extravasation after perfusion in retinas of control, DB and DB + TS rats by Western blotting. As shown in Figure 3C,D, extravascular albumin levels were significantly higher in retinas of STZ rats (DB) when compared to normoglycemic age-matched rats (control), whereas treatments with TS (DB + TS) significantly reduced albumin leakage in diabetic rats ($p < 0.02$ vs. control and $p < 0.05$ vs. DB; $n = 6$).

3.4. Tubastatin A Decreases the Levels of Senescence Markers in the Diabetic Retina

We previously showed that diabetes promotes retinal vascular senescence and this effect is associated with loss of the NAD+-dependent histone deacetylase sirtuin 1 (SIRT1) and up-regulation of senescence markers [4,7]. We, therefore, determined whether inhibition of HDAC6 by TS affected this mechanism in the diabetic retina.

Expression of SIRT1 was analyzed by Western blotting in retinas of rats from the different experimental groups (control, DB and DB + TS rats). As shown in Figure 4A,B, we found that SIRT1 expression was significantly decreased in the diabetic group (DB) compared to normoglycemic control and treatments of the diabetic rats with TS partially rescued it ($p < 0.05$ vs. control and $p < 0.01$ vs. DB; $n = 6$). Furthermore, immunohistochemical analysis of the senescence marker the phosphorylated form of H2A histone family member X (γH2AX) showed (Figure 4C) increased immunoreactivity in the diabetic rat retinas as compared to control group, particularly in the INL and in GCL (white arrows, Figure 4C). However, in TS-treated diabetic retinas, γH2AX-specific immunofluorescence was markedly decreased compared to STZ-rat retinas (Figure 4C).

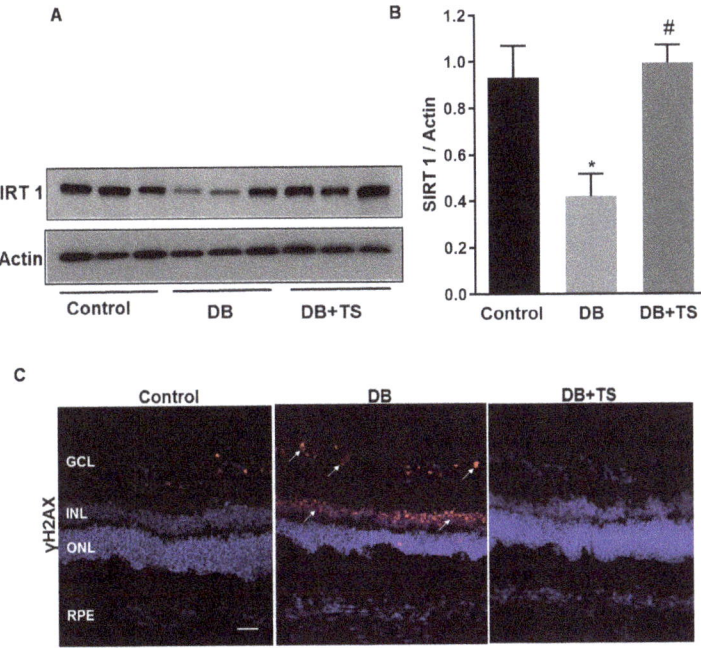

Figure 4. Effects of Tubastatin A on senescence in diabetic retina. (**A**) Immunoblot showing protein expression levels of SIRT1 measured in retinal extracts of STZ-rats (DB), STZ-rats receiving TS (10 mg/kg) (DB + TS) and age-matched normoglycemic control rats. (**B**) Bar histograms representing densitometric quantification of SIRT1 immunoblotting normalized to the loading control actin. (**C**) Representative images of immunohistochemical analysis of γH2AX (red) in retinas of STZ-rats (DB), STZ-rats treated with TS (DB + TS) and age-matched normoglycemic control rats (control). Nuclei were stained with DAPI. Scale bar, 50 µm. Values are mean ± SEM for $n = 6$. * $p < 0.05$ vs. control and # $p < 0.01$ vs. DB.

3.5. Tubastatin A Decreases Hyperglycemia-Induced Oxidative/Nitrative Stress in Retina

Increased oxidative/nitrative stress has been shown to be a key pathogenic hub for the development of DR [4,21]. To understand the potential role of HDAC6 in this process, we investigated TS effects on hyperglycemia-induced oxidative/nitrative stress by measuring retinal levels of superoxide, by dihydroethidium (DHE) staining and nitrotyrosine (NT) and 4-hydroxynonenal (4-HNE) by dot-blot analysis. Retinal cryosections probed with DHE fluorescent staining, showed increased fluorescence intensity in the diabetic rat retinas (DB) compared to normoglycemic group (control) (Figure 5A). This effect was markedly reduced by treatment of the diabetic rats with TS (Figure 5A). Quantification of fluorescence intensity confirmed our staining data ($p < 0.01$ vs. control and $p < 0.01$ vs. DB; $n = 6$) (Figure 5B). Accordingly, dot blot analysis of retinal levels of NT and 4-HNE showed that TS treatment prevented the increase of both these markers that we observed in diabetic rats ($p < 0.05$ vs. control and $p < 0.05$ vs. DB for NT and $p < 0.01$ vs. control and $p < 0.01$ vs. DB for 4-HNE; $n = 6$) (Figure 5C–E).

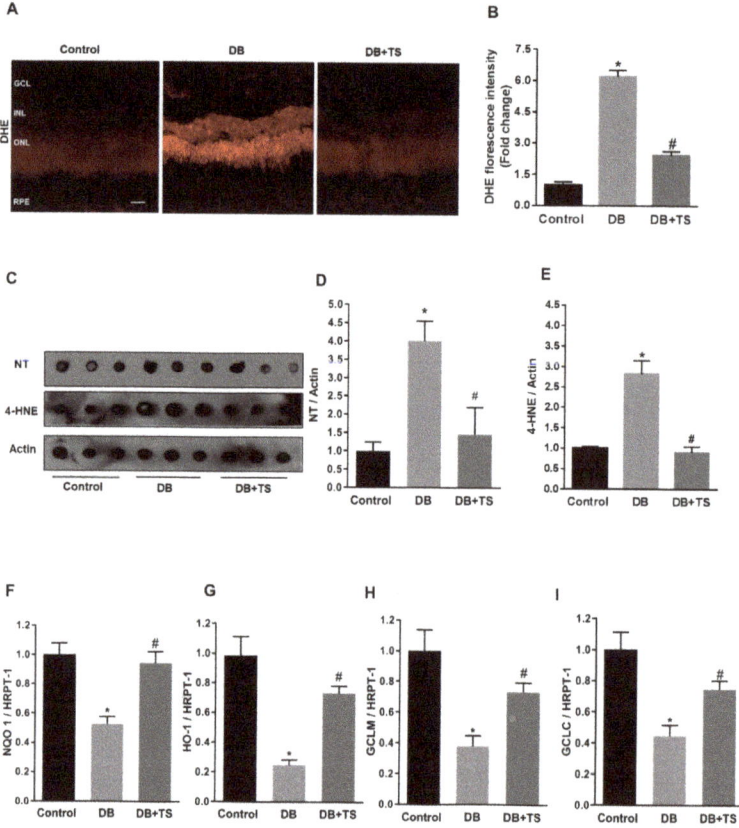

Figure 5. Effects of Tubastatin A on retinal redox homeostasis. (**A**) Representative images of retinal cryosections from the different experimental groups (control, DB and DB + TS) probed with dihydroethidium (DHE) to detect superoxide. Scale bar, 50 µm. (**B**) Quantification of relative fluorescence intensity of DHE staining. Values are mean ± SEM for $n = 6$. Results are presented as a fold change of control. * $p < 0.01$ vs. control and # $p < 0.01$ vs. DB. (**C**) Dot blot analysis assessing levels of nitrotyrosine (NT) and 4-hydroxynonenal (4-HNE) in retinas of three experimental groups (control, DB and DB + TS rats). (**D**,**E**) Quantification of optical density of NT and 4-HNE immunoblotting normalized versus actin. Values are mean ± SEM for $n = 6$. * $p < 0.05$ vs. control and # $p < 0.05$ vs. DB for NT. * $p < 0.01$ vs. control and # $p < 0.01$ vs. DB for 4-HNE. (**F**–**I**) mRNA levels of heme oxygenase-1 (HO-1), NAD(p)H dehydrogenase quinone 1 (NQO1), glutamate-cysteine ligase regulatory subunit (GCLM) and glutamate-cysteine ligase (GCLC) evaluated by qPCR and normalized to mRNA for hypoxanthine phosphoribosyltransferase 1 (HPRT-1). Values are mean ± SEM for $n = 6$. * $p < 0.05$ vs. control and # $p < 0.05$ vs. DB.

3.6. Tubastatin A Restores Antioxidant Activity in the Diabetic Retina

Redox stress in the diabetic retina could result from increased oxidase activities, but also from reduced endogenous antioxidant activities. Nuclear factor erythroid-2-related factor 2 (Nrf2) is a master regulator of endogenous antioxidants gene expression [22], therefore, we tested the effect of TS on the regulation of Nrf2-dependent antioxidant signaling, by monitoring, the expression levels of well-established Nrf2–dependent gene targets. QPCR analysis revealed that diabetes promoted a significant reduction in the expression levels of the Nrf2-dependent genes: Heme oxygenase-1 (HO-1), NAD(p)H dehydrogenase quinone 1 (NQO1), glutamate-cysteine ligase regulatory subunit (GCLM), and glutamate-cysteine ligase (GCLC) (Figure 5F–I) However, treatment of diabetic rats with TS restored the mRNA levels of all these genes ($p < 0.005$ (HO-1), $p < 0.01$ (NQO1), $p < 0.02$ (GCLM), $p < 0.02$ (GCLC) vs. control and $p < 0.002$ (HO-1), $p < 0.01$ (NQO1), $p < 0.02$ (GCLM), $p < 0.03$ (GCLC) vs. DB; $n = 6$), thus, suggesting that TS restored Nrf2-dependent signaling in the diabetic retina.

Furthermore, we assessed the expression and activity of the endogenous antioxidant Trx-1 (Figure 6A,B). As previously reported [8], Trx-1 expression was significantly increased in retinas of STZ-rats (DB) in comparison to normoglycemic control rats (Figure 6A,B). Treatment of the diabetic rats with TS, however, significantly decreased Trx-1 expression in diabetic rats ($p < 0.0051$; $n = 6$). Trx-1 activity, measured with a fluorimetric assay, was found to be significantly lower in retinas of STZ-rats (DB) than in normoglycemic age-matched rats (control) (Figure 6C). However, treatment of diabetic rats with TS rescued/normalized this antioxidant enzymatic activity ($p < 0.01$ vs. DB; $n = 6$) (Figure 6C).

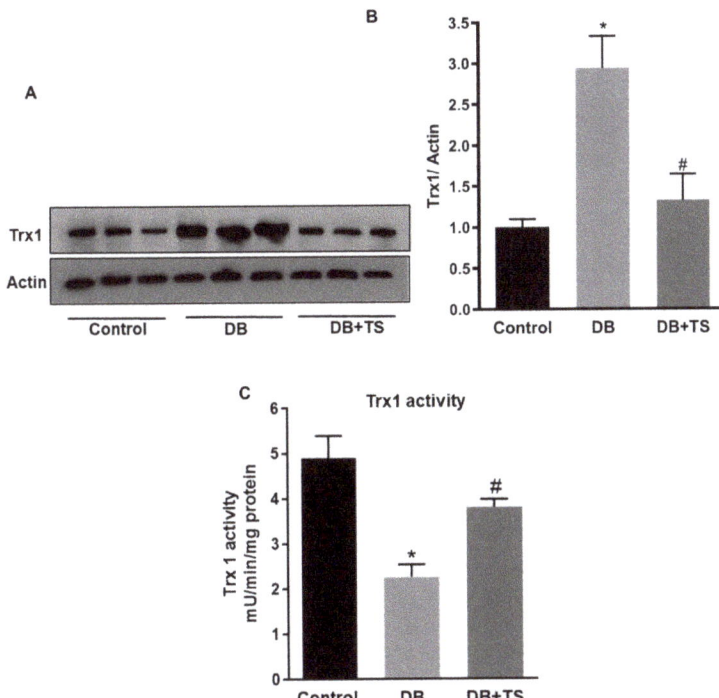

Figure 6. Effect of Tubastatin A on thioredoxin-1 expression and activity. (**A**) Western analysis of thioredoxin-1 (Trx-1) protein expression measured in retinas of STZ-rats (DB), STZ-rats receiving TS (10 mg/kg) (DB + TS) and normoglycemic control rats (control). (**B**) Quantification of optical density of Trx-1 immunoblotting normalized versus actin. (**C**) Trx-1 enzymatic activity measured in STZ-rats (DB), STZ-rats treated with TS (10 mg/kg) (DB + TS). Values are mean ± SEM for $n = 6$. * $p < 0.01$ vs. control and # $p < 0.01$ vs. DB.

3.7. Effect of High Glucose and Tubastatin A on HDAC6 Expression and Activity in Human Retinal Endothelial Cells

To determine the specific impact of HDAC6 on retinal endothelial cells and microvascular dysfunction, we performed experiments in vitro using HuREC exposed to different glucose levels. First, we confirmed that HDAC6 mRNA expression levels, measured in HuREC by qPCR analysis, were significantly increased when the cells were treated with high glucose concentrations (HG, 25 mM) as compared to cells treated with the osmotic control L-glucose (LG) or exposed to normal glucose containing media (NG, 5.5 mM) ($p < 0.01$ vs. NG; $n = 3$) (Figure 7A). Accordingly, HDAC6 protein expression (Figure 7B) was also significantly augmented in HG-treated HuREC in comparison with LG or NG ($p < 0.01$; $n = 3$). Parallel to HDAC6 protein up-regulation, we also found that HG increased HDAC6 activity 48 h post-treatment in comparison to NG and LG controls (Figure 7C) ($p < 0.005$; $n = 3$). Moreover, treatment of HuREC with TS (5 µM, 6 h pre-treatment + 48 h in combination with HG) significantly down-regulated the activity of HDAC6 in HuREC exposed to HG ($p < 0.01$; $n = 3$) and had no significant effects on cells exposed to normal glucose control (NG) (Figure 7D).

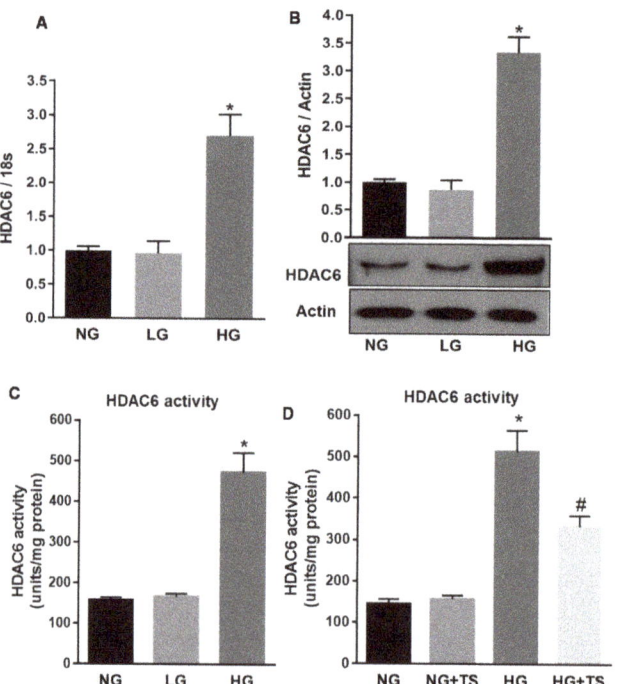

Figure 7. Effects of high glucose and Tubastatin A on HDAC6 expression and activity in HuREC. (**A**) HDAC6 mRNA expression, measured by qPCR, in HuREC exposed to different glucose levels (NG = 5.5 mM D-glucose, HG = 25 mM D-glucose) and the osmotic control L-glucose (25 mM) for 48 and 72 h. (**B**) Immunoblotting showing HDAC6 protein levels measured 48 h after exposure of HuREC to HG or the controls NG or LG. (**C**) HDAC6 activity measured in HuREC by fluorimetric assay at 48 h exposure of the cells to HG, NG or LG. (**D**) HDAC6 activity measured in HuREC by fluorimetric assay after 48 h of exposure of the cells to HG or HG plus TS (5 µM starting 6 h before HG treatment) and compared to the controls NG or LG. Values are mean ± SEM for $n = 3$. * $p < 0.01$ vs. NG and # $p < 0.01$ vs. HG.

3.8. Effects of HDAC6 Inhibition on Oxidative/Nitrative Stress and Endogenous Antioxidants in HuREC

To explore the potential contribution of HDAC6 to HG-induced redox imbalance in HuREC, we assessed the formation of ROS from cellular sources by determining CellROX deep green fluorescence intensity in HuREC exposed to NG or HG for 48 h with or without TS (5 µM) (Figure 8A). We found that HG increased superoxide-dependent fluorescence intensity in HuREC as compared to NG group, however, this effect was largely blocked by TS (Figure 8A).

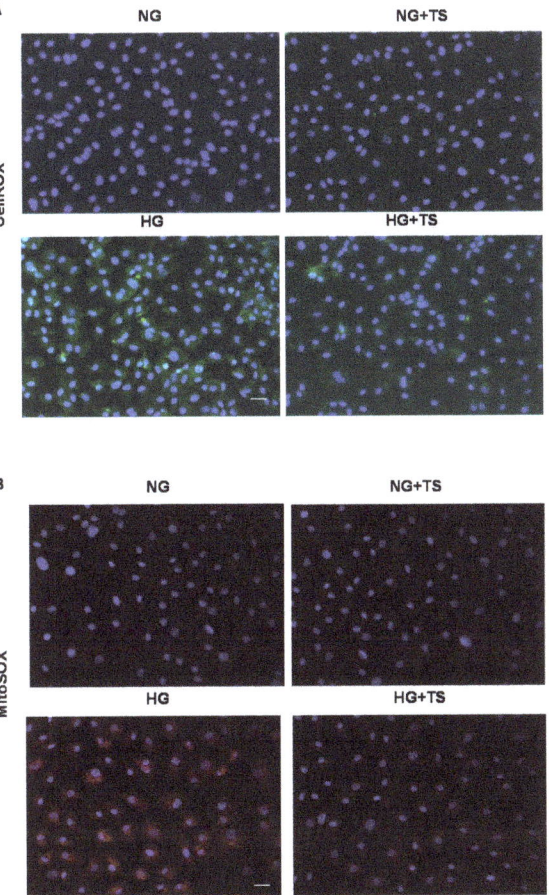

Figure 8. Effects of Tubastatin A on cellular and mitochondrial oxidases activities in HuREC. (**A**) CellROX fluorescent assay showing superoxide formation (green) in HuREC exposed to HG for 48 h or to HG in the presence of 5 µM of TS (HG + TS) and compared to HuREC cultured in NG conditions in the absence (NG) or in presence of 5 µM TS (NG + TS). (**B**) Images of MitoSOX assay showing superoxide formation from mitochondria oxidase (red) in HuREC exposed to HG for 48 h or HG in the presence of 5 µM of TS (HG + TS), also for 48 h, and compared to HuREC cultured in NG conditions in the absence (NG) or in the presence of 5 µM TS (NG + TS). In A and B blue fluorescence show cell nuclei counterstained with DAPI. Scale bar, 50 µm.

Same results were obtained while monitoring the effects of HG and TS on superoxide production from mitochondrial sources (Figure 8B). Analysis of mitochondrial oxidases activity by MitoSOX, showed that exposure of HuREC to HG for 48 h increased mitochondrial superoxide-dependent reactivity; however, TS prevented this effect (Figure 8B). In all cases, TS treatment did not affect the response of the cells to NG (NG + TS).

Furthermore, dot blot analysis showed that the levels of the oxidative/nitrative stress markers NT and 4-HNE, were increased by HG, however treatment of the cells with TS halted this effect of HG

($p < 0.0001$ vs. NG and $p < 0.0001$ vs. HG; $n = 3$) (Figure 9A–C). To ascertain whether TS was also able to normalize endogenous antioxidants, we determined the effects of HG in presence and/or absence of TS on Trx-1 activity (Figure 9D). Similarly, to what was observed in the diabetic rats, glucidic stress (HG) significantly decreased Trx-1 activity in HuREC and this was rescued by TS ($p < 0.001$ vs. NG and $p < 0.01$ vs. HG; $n = 3$) (Figure 9D).

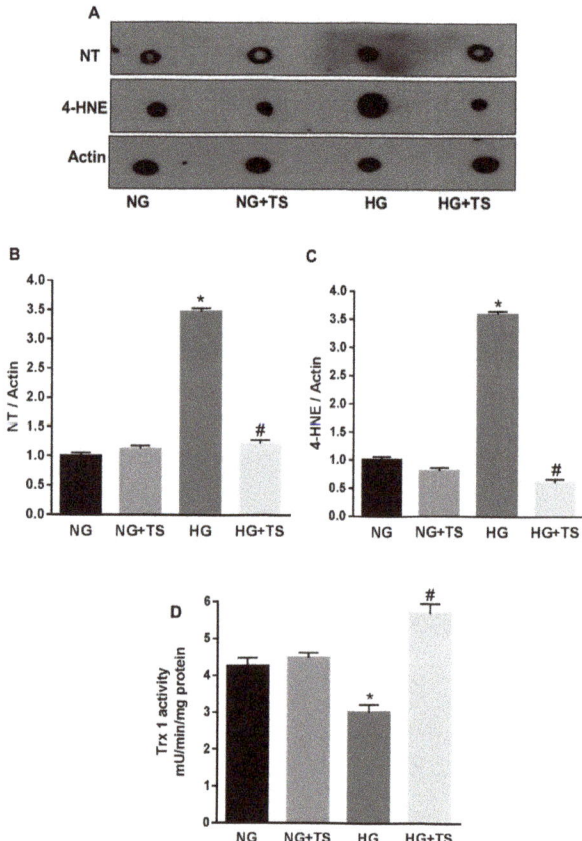

Figure 9. Effects of Tubastatin A on high glucose-induced redox imbalance in HuREC. (**A**) Representative images of dot blot analysis demonstrating nitrotyrosine (NT) and 4-hydroxynonenal (4-HNE) formation in HuREC exposed to HG for 48 h or HG in the presence of 5 µM of TS (HG + TS), also for 48 h, and compared to HuREC cultured in NG conditions in the absence (NG) or presence of 5 µM TS (NG + TS). (**B**,**C**) Quantification of optical density of NT and 4-HNE immunoblotting normalized versus actin. Values are mean ± SEM for $n = 3$. * $p < 0.0001$ vs. NG and # $p < 0.0001$ vs. HG. (**D**) Fluorimetric assay results representing Trx-1 activity in HuREC assessed after 48 h of exposure to different glucose levels (NG = 5.5 mM D-glucose, HG = 25 mM D-glucose) in the presence or absence of TS (5 µM). Values are mean ± SEM for $n = 3$. * $p < 0.01$ vs. NG and # $p < 0.01$ vs. HG.

3.9. Effects of HDAC6 Inhibition on HG-induced HuREC Senescence

Finally, we examined the effects of HDAC6 inhibition by TS on HG-induced HuREC senescence. Assessment of SA-β-Gal activity in HuREC exposed to different glucose conditions showed increased number of positive cells in the HG treatment group compared to the NG control ($p < 0.001$; $n = 3$)

(Figure 10A,B). However, treatment of HuREC with TS prevented the increase of SA-β-Gal–reactive cells in HG conditions ($p < 0.005$; $n = 3$) (Figure 10A,B).

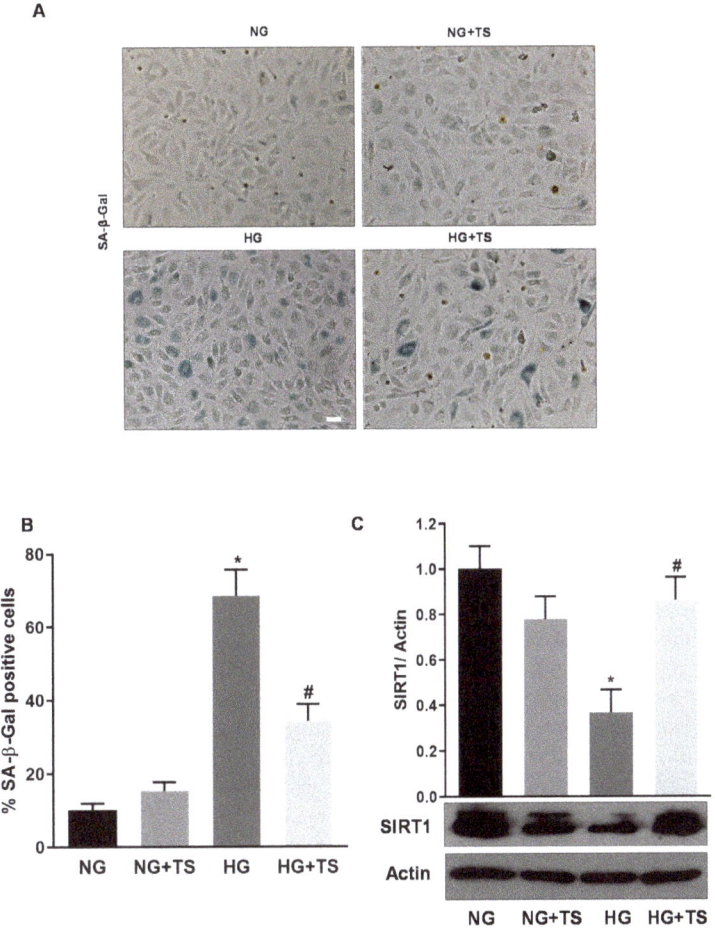

Figure 10. Tubastatin A effects on HG-induced senescence markers in HuREC. (**A**) Representative images of senescence-associated β-Galactosidase (SA-β-Gal) reactivity assay in HuREC exposed to HG for 48 h or HG plus 5 μM of TS (HG + TS), also for 48 h, and compared to HuREC cultured in NG conditions in the absence (NG) or presence of 5 μM TS (NG + TS). Positive cells develop the blue color. Scale bar, 50 μm. (**B**) Quantification of SA-β-Gal-positive cells. Values are number of positive cells per well versus total number of cells expressed as a percent. $n = 3$. * $p < 0.001$ vs. NG and # $p < 0.001$ vs. HG. (**C**) Western blotting analysis showing protein levels of the histone deacetylase SIRT1 in HuREC treated in the same experimental conditions as described in (**A**). Bar histograms represent optical density values of the blots normalized for the loading control actin. Values are mean ± SEM for $n = 3$. * $p < 0.01$ vs. NG and # $p < 0.01$ vs. HG.

Moreover, Western analysis of protein levels of the histone deacetylase SIRT1 showed that this was significantly down-regulated in HG-treated HuREC in comparison to NG. Treatment of the cells with TS significantly reduced the effects of HG by rescuing SIRT1 protein levels ($p < 0.005$ vs. HG; $n = 3$) (Figure 10C).

4. Discussion

The increased incidence of diabetes and DR, urges the realization of early interventional therapeutic strategies. In this study, we investigated the role of the histone deacetylase HDAC6 in the early events characterizing the progression of an experimental model of DR. Dysregulation of the processes of acetylation/deacetylation of nuclear and cellular proteins has been shown to be associated with different pathologic conditions including diabetes [12–18,23]. Previous findings linked the activity of several histone deacetylases to the pathogenesis of DR [23,24]. A specific contribution of HDAC1, 2, and 8 to global acetylation of retinal histones in the diabetic retina was found to be involved not only to progression of DR but also to the metabolic memory phenomenon [23]. When compared to the other members of the large family of the histone deacetylases HDAC6 presents unique structural and functional properties, including a double catalytic domain and cytosolic and nuclear intracellular localization and sites of action [9]. Among other unique functions, HDAC6 can influence the redox state of the cells through deacetylation of endogenous antioxidants and modulation of oxidase activities [16].

Our results show that HDAC6 expression and activity are upregulated in the diabetic retinas of STZ-rats and, most importantly, in postmortem retinas of diabetic donors. Using an interventional approach, we assessed the effects of pharmacological inhibition of HDAC6 by administration of the specific inhibitor TS in an experimental model of Type 1 diabetes (STZ-rats). Pharmacological inhibition of HDAC6 by TS lessened DR pathology in STZ-rats, as evidenced by maintenance of total retinal thickness and amelioration of vascular hyperpermeability, a key feature of DR microangiopathy [2,3]. The observed effects of TS on BRB stabilization in STZ-rats, are in agreement with previous studies that have underscored the role of HDAC6 activity in altering endothelial and epithelial cells permeability and the stability of intercellular junctions [25–27].

While the specific role of HDAC6 in the diabetic retina has not been studied before, HDAC6 inhibition has been shown to alleviate myocardial ischemia-reperfusion injury in diabetic rats [16] and to ameliorate diabetic kidney disease [15], predominantly through antioxidant effects. Interestingly, in the diabetic retina, downregulation of HDAC6 was linked to the effects of exogenous GLP-1 in alleviating oxidative stress-induced apoptosis and autophagy of retinal cells [24].

The results of our studies show that HDAC6 inhibition by TS decreased the appearance of the senescence marker γH2AX and significantly augmented the expression of the redox homeostatic histone deacetylase SIRT1, of which expression levels are inversely correlated with the induction of endothelial cell senescence [4,7]. A contrasting balance between HDAC6 and SIRT1 could significantly impact the redox status of a number of cells including endothelial and other retinal cells [28].

Previous studies have shown that increased HDAC6 activity results in oxidative stress due to mitochondrial dysfunction [16,29] and to altered endogenous antioxidant function [11]. Increased oxidative/nitrative stress has been shown to play a key contributing role to the pathogenesis of DR due to its effects in promoting retinal chronic inflammation, microvascular injury, and accelerated endothelial cell senescence [4]. Inhibition of HDAC6 by TS, significantly reduced superoxide formation, diminished the levels of oxidative and nitrative stress markers (4-HNE and NT, respectively) and rescued the activity of endogenous antioxidants such as Nrf2 and Trx-1. Taken together, these antioxidant properties of TS further confirm the pro-oxidative capacity of overactive HDAC6 in the diabetic retina.

The results of our experiments in vitro, specifically addressing HDCA6 role in HuREC, largely recapitulated the results obtained in the in vivo experiments as TS prevented high glucose-induced HuREC senescence (SA-β-Gal activity assay) and halted high glucose effects in downregulating SIRT1 expression. These protective effects correlated with significant reduction of superoxide production from cellular and mitochondrial sources as well as with the rescuing of the activity of the endogenous antioxidant Trx-1. Consistent with our results, blocking of HDAC6 activity was shown to be protective against high glucose-induced oxidative stress in RPE via mechanisms involving inhibition NF-κB and NLRP3 inflammasome pathway [30].

The potential role of HDAC6 in regulating cellular redox homeostasis has been previously implicated in the pathogenesis of several neurodegenerative diseases [31,32]. In addition, similar findings have been obtained in studies showing beneficial antioxidant effects of HDAC6 inhibitors in models of retinal neurodegenerative diseases [17,18]. Thus, the results here described are in agreement with these previous findings by demonstrating a role for HDAC6 in DR and retinal microangiopathy through pro-oxidant effects.

5. Conclusions

In summary, the results of the studies described herein, are the first to demonstrate the impact of HDAC6 activation in the diabetic retina and to suggest the potential therapeutic efficacy of HDAC6 specific inhibitors for the prevention of redox imbalance and injury to the retinal microvasculature in the diabetic milieu.

Supplementary Materials: The following are available online at http://www.mdpi.com/2076-3921/9/7/599/s1, Table S1: Demographics and clinical history of human postmortem retinal donors. Table S2: Biochemical parameters measured in the experimental rat groups. Table S3: Primer sequences used in the study. Figure S1: MTT Assay.

Author Contributions: Conceptualization, M.B. and F.L.P.; methodology, H.A., M.C.T., R.N.J. and D.R.G.; formal analysis, H.A. and M.C.T.; data curation, H.A., M.C.T., R.N.J.; writing—original draft preparation, H.A., M.C.T. and M.B.; writing—review and editing, D.R.G., M.C.T. and M.B.; supervision, M.K. and M.B.; funding acquisition, P.M.M. and M.B. All authors have read and agreed to the published version of the manuscript.

Funding: This research was funded by the National Eye Institute for the financial support to M.B. (EY022416, EY028714) and P.M.M. (EY022704).

Acknowledgments: The authors acknowledge the outstanding technical support of Jianghe Yuan and Shubhra Rajpurohit.

Conflicts of Interest: The authors declare no conflict of interest.

References

1. Ogurtsova, K.; da Rocha Fernandes, J.D.; Huang, Y.; Linnenkamp, U.; Guariguata, L.; Cho, N.H.; Cavan, D.; Shaw, J.E.; Makaroff, L.E. IDF Diabetes Atlas: Global estimates for the prevalence of diabetes for 2015 and 2040. *Diabetes Res.Clin. Pr.* **2017**, *128*, 40–50. [CrossRef] [PubMed]
2. Antonetti, D.A.; Klein, R.; Gardner, T.W. Diabetic retinopathy. *New Engl. J. Med.* **2012**, *366*, 1227–1239. [CrossRef] [PubMed]
3. Duh, E.J.; Sun, J.K.; Stitt, A.W. Diabetic retinopathy: Current understanding, mechanisms, and treatment strategies. *JCI Insight* **2017**, *2*. [CrossRef] [PubMed]
4. Lamoke, F.; Shaw, S.; Yuan, J.; Ananth, S.; Duncan, M.; Martin, P.; Bartoli, M. Increased oxidative and nitrative stress accelerates aging of the retinal vasculature in the diabetic retina. *PLoS ONE* **2015**, *10*, e0139664. [CrossRef] [PubMed]
5. Kowluru, R.A. Mitochondrial stability in diabetic retinopathy: Lessons learned from epigenetics. *Diabetes* **2019**, *68*, 241–247. [CrossRef]
6. Kowluru, R.A.; Mishra, M. Oxidative stress, mitochondrial damage and diabetic retinopathy. *Biochim. Biophys. Acta* **2015**, *1852*, 2474–2483. [CrossRef]
7. Thounaojam, M.C.; Jadeja, R.N.; Warren, M.; Powell, F.L.; Raju, R.; Gutsaeva, D.; Khurana, S.; Martin, P.M.; Bartoli, M. MicroRNA-34a (miR-34a) mediates retinal endothelial cell premature senescence through mitochondrial dysfunction and loss of antioxidant activities. *Antioxidants* **2019**, *8*, 328. [CrossRef]
8. Thounaojam, M.C.; Powell, F.L.; Patel, S.; Gutsaeva, D.R.; Tawfik, A.; Smith, S.B.; Nussbaum, J.; Block, N.L.; Martin, P.M.; Schally, A.V.; et al. Protective effects of agonists of growth hormone-releasing hormone (GHRH) in early experimental diabetic retinopathy. *Proc. Natl. Acad. Sci. USA* **2017**, *114*, 13248–13253. [CrossRef]
9. Liang, T.; Fang, H. Structure, functions and selective inhibitors of HDAC6. *Curr. Top. Med. Chem.* **2018**, *18*, 2429–2447. [CrossRef]

10. Choi, H.; Kim, H.J.; Kim, J.; Kim, S.; Yang, J.; Lee, W.; Park, Y.; Hyeon, S.J.; Lee, D.S.; Ryu, H.; et al. Increased acetylation of Peroxiredoxin1 by HDAC6 inhibition leads to recovery of Abeta-induced impaired axonal transport. *Mol. Neurodegener.* **2017**, *12*, 23. [CrossRef]
11. Parmigiani, R.B.; Xu, W.S.; Venta-Perez, G.; Erdjument-Bromage, H.; Yaneva, M.; Tempst, P.; Marks, P.A. HDAC6 is a specific deacetylase of peroxiredoxins and is involved in redox regulation. *Proc. Natl. Acad. Sci. USA* **2008**, *105*, 9633–9638. [CrossRef] [PubMed]
12. Simoes-Pires, C.; Zwick, V.; Nurisso, A.; Schenker, E.; Carrupt, P.A.; Cuendet, M. HDAC6 as a target for neurodegenerative diseases: What makes it different from the other HDACs? *Mol. Neurodegener.* **2013**, *8*, 7. [CrossRef] [PubMed]
13. Ferguson, B.S.; McKinsey, T.A. Non-sirtuin histone deacetylases in the control of cardiac aging. *J. Mol. Cell. Cardiol.* **2015**, *83*, 14–20. [CrossRef] [PubMed]
14. Li, T.; Zhang, C.; Hassan, S.; Liu, X.; Song, F.; Chen, K.; Zhang, W.; Yang, J. Histone deacetylase 6 in cancer. *J. Hematol. Oncol.* **2018**, *11*, 111. [CrossRef] [PubMed]
15. Brijmohan, A.S.; Batchu, S.N.; Majumder, S.; Alghamdi, T.A.; Thieme, K.; McGaugh, S.; Liu, Y.; Advani, S.L.; Bowskill, B.B.; Kabir, M.G.; et al. HDAC6 inhibition promotes transcription factor EB activation and is protective in experimental kidney disease. *Front. Pharmacol.* **2018**, *9*, 34. [CrossRef]
16. Leng, Y.; Wu, Y.; Lei, S.; Zhou, B.; Qiu, Z.; Wang, K.; Xia, Z. Inhibition of HDAC6 activity alleviates myocardial ischemia/reperfusion injury in diabetic rats: Potential role of peroxiredoxin 1 acetylation and redox regulation. *Oxidative Med. Cell. Longev.* **2018**, *2018*, 9494052. [CrossRef]
17. Leyk, J.; Daly, C.; Janssen-Bienhold, U.; Kennedy, B.N.; Richter-Landsberg, C. HDAC6 inhibition by tubastatin A is protective against oxidative stress in a photoreceptor cell line and restores visual function in a zebrafish model of inherited blindness. *Cell Death Dis.* **2017**, *8*, e3028. [CrossRef]
18. Yuan, H.; Li, H.; Yu, P.; Fan, Q.; Zhang, X.; Huang, W.; Shen, J.; Cui, Y.; Zhou, W. Involvement of HDAC6 in ischaemia and reperfusion-induced rat retinal injury. *BMC Ophthalmol.* **2018**, *18*, 300. [CrossRef]
19. Semeraro, F.; Morescalchi, F.; Cancarini, A.; Russo, A.; Rezzola, S.; Costagliola, C. Diabetic retinopathy, a vascular and inflammatory disease: Therapeutic implications. *Diabetes Metab.* **2019**, *45*, 517–527. [CrossRef]
20. Shin, E.S.; Sorenson, C.M.; Sheibani, N. Diabetes and retinal vascular dysfunction. *J. Ophthalmic Vis. Res.* **2014**, *9*, 362–373. [CrossRef]
21. Kowluru, R.A.; Chan, P.S. Oxidative stress and diabetic retinopathy. *Exp. Diabetes Res.* **2007**, *2007*, 43603. [CrossRef] [PubMed]
22. Francisqueti-Ferron, F.V.; Ferron, A.J.T.; Garcia, J.L.; Silva, C.; Costa, M.R.; Gregolin, C.S.; Moreto, F.; Ferreira, A.L.A.; Minatel, I.O.; Correa, C.R. Basic concepts on the role of nuclear factor erythroid-derived 2-like 2 (Nrf2) in age-related diseases. *Int. J. Mol. Sci.* **2019**, *20*, 3208. [CrossRef] [PubMed]
23. Zhong, Q.; Kowluru, R.A. Role of histone acetylation in the development of diabetic retinopathy and the metabolic memory phenomenon. *J. Cell. Biochem.* **2010**, *110*, 1306–1313. [CrossRef]
24. Cai, X.; Li, J.; Wang, M.; She, M.; Tang, Y.; Li, J.; Li, H.; Hui, H. GLP-1 treatment improves diabetic retinopathy by alleviating autophagy through GLP-1R-ERK1/2-HDAC6 signaling pathway. *Int. J. Med. Sci.* **2017**, *14*, 1203–1212. [CrossRef] [PubMed]
25. Friedrich, M.; Gerbeth, L.; Gerling, M.; Rosenthal, R.; Steiger, K.; Weidinger, C.; Keye, J.; Wu, H.; Schmidt, F.; Weichert, W.; et al. HDAC inhibitors promote intestinal epithelial regeneration via autocrine TGFbeta1 signalling in inflammation. *Mucosal Immunol.* **2019**, *12*, 656–667. [CrossRef]
26. Borgas, D.; Chambers, E.; Newton, J.; Ko, J.; Rivera, S.; Rounds, S.; Lu, Q. Cigarette smoke disrupted lung endothelial barrier integrity and increased susceptibility to acute lung injury via histone deacetylase 6. *Am. J. Respir. Cell Mol. Biol.* **2016**, *54*, 683–696. [CrossRef]
27. Lu, Q.; Sakhatskyy, P.; Grinnell, K.; Newton, J.; Ortiz, M.; Wang, Y.; Sanchez-Esteban, J.; Harrington, E.O.; Rounds, S. Cigarette smoke causes lung vascular barrier dysfunction via oxidative stress-mediated inhibition of RhoA and focal adhesion kinase. *Am. J. Physiol. Lung Cell. Mol. Physiol.* **2011**, *301*, L847–L857. [CrossRef]
28. Siwak, M.; Maslankiewicz, M.; Nowak-Zdunczyk, A.; Rozpedek, W.; Wojtczak, R.; Szymanek, K.; Szaflik, M.; Szaflik, J.; Szaflik, J.P.; Majsterek, I. The relationship between HDAC6, CXCR3, and SIRT1 genes expression levels with progression of primary open-angle glaucoma. *Ophthalmic Genet.* **2018**, *39*, 325–331. [CrossRef]
29. Bai, J.; Lei, Y.; An, G.L.; He, L. Down-regulation of deacetylase HDAC6 inhibits the melanoma cell line A375.S2 growth through ROS-dependent mitochondrial pathway. *PLoS ONE* **2015**, *10*, e0121247. [CrossRef]

30. Yang, Q.; Li, S.; Zhou, Z.; Fu, M.; Yang, X.; Hao, K.; Liu, Y. HDAC6 inhibitor Cay10603 inhibits high glucose-induced oxidative stress, inflammation and apoptosis in retinal pigment epithelial cells via regulating NF-kappaB and NLRP3 inflammasome pathway. *Gen. Physiol. Biophys.* **2020**, *39*, 169–177. [CrossRef]
31. Guedes-Dias, P.; Oliveira, J.M. Lysine deacetylases and mitochondrial dynamics in neurodegeneration. *Biochim. Biophys. Acta* **2013**, *1832*, 1345–1359. [CrossRef] [PubMed]
32. Yan, J. Interplay between HDAC6 and its interacting partners: Essential roles in the aggresome-autophagy pathway and neurodegenerative diseases. *DNA Cell Biol.* **2014**, *33*, 567–580. [CrossRef] [PubMed]

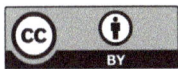

© 2020 by the authors. Licensee MDPI, Basel, Switzerland. This article is an open access article distributed under the terms and conditions of the Creative Commons Attribution (CC BY) license (http://creativecommons.org/licenses/by/4.0/).

MDPI
St. Alban-Anlage 66
4052 Basel
Switzerland
Tel. +41 61 683 77 34
Fax +41 61 302 89 18
www.mdpi.com

Antioxidants Editorial Office
E-mail: antioxidants@mdpi.com
www.mdpi.com/journal/antioxidants

www.ingramcontent.com/pod-product-compliance
Lightning Source LLC
LaVergne TN
LVHW070207100526
838202LV00015B/2014